KU-415-353

www.harcourt-international.com

Bringing you products from all Harcourt Health Sciences companies including Baillière Tindall, Churchill Livingstone, Mosby and W.B. Saunders

- ▶ **Browse** for latest information on new books, journals and electronic products

- ▶ **Search** for information on over 20 000 published titles with full product information including tables of contents and sample chapters

- ▶ **Keep up to date** with our extensive publishing programme in your field by registering with eAlert or requesting postal updates

- ▶ **Secure online ordering** with prompt delivery, as well as full contact details to order by phone, fax or post

- ▶ **News** of special features and promotions

If you are based in the following countries, please visit the country-specific site to receive full details of product availability and local ordering information

USA: www.harcourthealth.com

Canada: www.harcourtcanada.com

Australia: www.harcourt.com.au

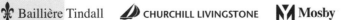

Baillière Tindall   CHURCHILL LIVINGSTONE   Mosby   W.B. SAUNDERS

Myofascial Pain and Fibromyalgia Syndromes

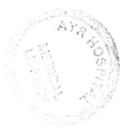

Pain is one of the most challenging problems
in medicine and biology . . . In recent years our
understanding of pain mechanisms has
increased enormously . . . we are
appalled by the needless pain that plagues
so many people. Part of the problem lies with
the health professionals who have failed to
keep up with the advances in our field . . .

Ronald Melzack & Patrick Wall, 1988

For Churchill Livingstone:

Publishing Manager: Inta Ozols
Project Manager: Gail Murray
Project Development Manager: Dinah Thom
Designer: George Ajayi

Myofascial Pain and Fibromyalgia Syndromes

A Clinical Guide to Diagnosis and Management

P E Baldry MB FRCP
Emeritus Consultant Physician and Postgraduate Clinical Tutor,
Ashford Hospital, London, UK;
Member of the British and Irish Chapter of the International
Association for the Study of Pain;
Member of the International Myopain Society

with contributions by

Muhammad B Yunus MD FACP FACR FRCPE
Professor of Medicine, Section of Rheumatology,
University of Illinois College of Medicine, Peoria, Illinois, USA

and

Fatma İnanıcı MD
Department of Physical Medicine and Rehabilitation,
Hacettepe University Medical School, Ankara, Turkey

Foreword by

Brian Hazleman MA MB FRCP
Consultant Rheumatologist and Director, Rheumatology Research Unit,
Addenbrooke's Hospital; Honorary Consultant,
Strangeways Research Laboratories; Associate Lecturer,
Department of Medicine, University of Cambridge;
Fellow, Corpus Christi College, Cambridge, UK

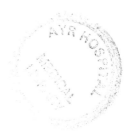

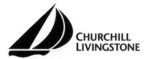

CHURCHILL
LIVINGSTONE

EDINBURGH LONDON NEW YORK PHILADELPHIA ST LOUIS SYDNEY TORONTO 2001

CHURCHILL LIVINGSTONE
An imprint of Harcourt Publishers Limited

© Harcourt Publishers Limited 2001

 is a registered trademark of Harcourt Publishers Limited

The right of Peter Baldry to be identified as author of this work has
been asserted by him in accordance with the Copyright, Designs and
Patents Act 1988

All rights reserved. No part of this publication may be reproduced,
stored in a retrieval system, or transmitted in any form or by any
means, electronic, mechanical, photocopying, recording or otherwise,
without either the prior permission of the publishers (Harcourt
Publishers Limited, Harcourt Place, 32 Jamestown Road, London
NW1 7BY), or a licence permitting restricted copying in the United
Kingdom issued by the Copyright Licensing Agency, 90 Tottenham
Court Road, London W1P 0LP.

First published 2001

ISBN 0 443 07003 2

British Library Cataloguing in Publication Data
A catalogue record for this book is available from the British Library

Library of Congress Cataloging in Publication Data
A catalog record for this book is available from the Library of
Congress

Note
Medical knowledge is constantly changing. As new information
becomes available, changes in treatment, procedures, equipment and
the use of drugs become necessary. The author, contributors and the
publishers have taken care to ensure that the information given in this
text is accurate and up to date. However, readers are strongly advised
to confirm that the information, especially with regard to drug usage,
complies with the latest legislation and standards of practice.

The
publisher's
policy is to use
**paper manufactured
from sustainable forests**

Printed in China

Contents

Contributors

Peter Baldry MB FRCP
Chapters 1–15

Address for correspondence:

Millstream House
Fladbury
Pershore
Worcestershire
WR10 2QX
UK

Fax: +44 (0)1386 861228
E-mail: p.baldry@ukonline.co.uk

Muhammad B Yunus MD FACP FACR FRCPE
Chapters 16 and 17

Address for correspondence:

Professor of Medicine
Section of Rheumatology
University of Illinois College of Medicine
Peoria IL 61656-1649
USA

Fax: +1 309 671 8513
E-mail: yunus@uic.edu

Fatma İnanıcı MD
Chapters 16 and 17

Address for correspondence:

Department of Physical Medicine and
Rehabilitation
Hacettepe University Medical School
06100 Ankara
Turkey

Fax: +90 312 3105 769
E-mail: finanici@tr.net

Foreword

Nonarticular musculoskeletal pain is common. One in ten adults in Britain will consult a general practitioner at least once in the course of a year with these symptoms. Half of them present because of low back pain, and the rest have a mixture of conditions which are considered under the rubric of soft tissue rheumatism.

The majority of these complaints are regional disorders for which there are no clear guidelines for investigation and management, nor indications for referral to secondary care. Most patients who seek treatment will be treated in primary care. Although often considered inconsequential, many cases become chronic and pose a major socioeconomic burden as a result of significant morbidity and loss of productivity.

Chronic musculoskeletal pain is not a disease, nor in most cases is it symptomatic of a single diagnosable condition. It represents a state of distress with a complex interaction of physical and emotional factors: some understood but many ill-defined.

One of the difficulties encountered with defining the nature of the burden that soft tissue lesions present has been variation in definition and diagnostic criteria for specific disorders. The diagnostic challenge that many cases present may be one explanation for the apparent lack of effect of many current conventional management approaches.

There are few studies that have evaluated the relative frequency of different disorders at different sites. In one survey by questionnaire the majority of subjects who reported pain had pain at more than one site. The use of investigations in soft tissue disorders is generally low in comparison with the other rheumatic complaints. Soft tissue lesions are often diagnosed on clinical grounds. The literature of soft tissue rheumatism contains a varied list of clinical descriptions and broad-based treatment strategies. Much of it derives from descriptive studies in specialised clinics. There are few epidemiological studies reported outside the clinic.

Fibromyalgia has taken over the mantle of what at varying times in the past has been called fibrositis or psychogenic rheumatism. The common thread that runs through accounts of these conditions is that these are always patients with generalised muscle pain, stiffness and fatiguability, which do not have a classical pathophysiological explanation. The modern concept of fibromyalgia adds a distinctive clinical characteristic to a symptomatic syndrome. This is the finding of tenderness at a minimum number of specified parts around the body. This generalised syndrome has its mirror in the idea, also developed in the post-war years, that much regional non-articular pain can be characterised by trigger points in muscles and their origins which produce patterns of referred pain. These have been labelled myofascial pain syndromes. Their relationship to fibromyalgia and to the other categories of soft tissue pain is uncertain and their epidemiology is only just being tackled.

It is easy to criticise many of the clinical studies. Out of them, however, and through the persistence of their authors, has emerged the concept of the American College of Rheumatology criteria for fibromyalgia, published in 1990. During the next few years the population patterns of generalized soft tissue pain and tender points, their associated features and predictors of their onset and persistence will emerge.

Despite the recognition of fibromyalgia by the World Health Organization in 1992, it remains a controversial condition. Its very existence is a matter of considerable debate. Doubts have been expressed about the validity of both the symptoms reported by patients and the signs observed; some deny the existence of the condition because no objective pathological findings are demonstrable.

In drawing up the criteria for the diagnosis of fibromyalgia syndrome there has been much emphasis on the presence of tender points. It might be asked, therefore, whether it is possible to distinguish between fibromyalgia and myofascial trigger point pain syndrome. Myofascial trigger point pain syndromes usually develop after trauma to the affected muscle or muscles and the pain is alleviated by deactivating the hyperactive nerve endings at trigger points by one or other of various methods. Some authors regard myofascial pain as being distinct from regional musculoskeletal pain while others regard these as synonymous. With the availability of sensitive imaging techniques and the awareness that soft tissue disorders encompass a wide spectrum of often complex pathologies, however, it is likely that imaging will become recognised as an important part of the evaluation of these disorders.

It is clear that there is considerable overlap between the myofascial pain syndromes and fibromyalgia syndrome. It is possible that they represent parts of a spectrum of muscle pain and fatiguability; however, the pathological basis for these conditions remains uncertain. Myofascial pain syndromes are clearly identified by the presence of local pain that is associated with a tense, shortened muscle which can be located by palpation, defined as a 'trigger point'. Trigger points are thought characteristically to refer pain in predictable patterns, so that digital pressure or needling of the point will reproduce symptoms. The trigger point may be distant from the pain complaint but is responsible for it.

Many patients with chronic myofascial pain syndrome fulfil the criteria for fibromyalgia syndrome. This could be because they represent a slightly different symptomatic manifestation of the same spectrum of disorders, or they could be aetiologically distinct entities that result in similar symptoms. Whatever the relationship, they certainly are among the most common of all causes of pain. These syndromes are all too common and are a neglected subject of medicine. They are barely mentioned in many textbooks of medicine, and when they are, are often passed off as trivial or untreatable. This book provides a welcome insight to an important area of musculoskeletal medicine.

Brian Hazleman

Preface

The purpose of this book is to draw to the attention of anaesthetists, orthopaedic surgeons, rheumatologists, general physicians, general practitioners, physiotherapists and other health professionals the pathophysiology, clinical manifestations and management of the myofascial trigger point pain syndromes and fibromyalgia. For although both are commonly occurring disabling disorders, they are still all too often misdiagnosed and, as a consequence, inappropriately treated.

One of the main reasons for this is that, until recently, there has been no clear-cut conception as to their fundamental nature. Recent clinical, electromyographic, biochemical and histological studies, together with concomitant advances in knowledge concerning the neurophysiology of pain in general, have changed all this by providing insight into their pathogenesis, pathophysiology, clinical manifestations and natural history. They have also assisted in the development of rational approaches to their treatment.

The outcome of all this has been the publication in a variety of different journals of numerous papers dealing with all the various aspects of these two disorders. My contributors and I hope that by bringing all this information together in one volume, we will enable those whose task it is to deal with musculoskeletal pain disorders to be better equipped to diagnose and manage these two erstwhile poorly understood syndromes.

London 2001   Peter Baldry

Acknowledgements

My sincere thanks are due to Dr Alexander Mcdonald for having, in the late 1970s when working at Charing Cross Hospital, London, aroused in me such considerable interest in myofascial trigger points as to cause me to continue to make a special study of them during the ensuing years.

I wish to express my gratitude to Dr David Simons and the late Dr Janet Travell for the very considerable contribution they have made to my knowledge of specific patterns of myofascial trigger point pain referral, for it has largely been from studying their descriptions and illustrations of these patterns that I have, during the last 20 years, learned to recognise them in my own patients.

I should also like to take this opportunity of paying tribute to Dr David Simons for having, by his pioneering work, contributed so much in the past few years to what is currently known concerning the pathophysiology of the myofascial trigger point pain syndrome.

I wish to acknowledge my indebtedness to Dr David Bowsher, Research Director of the Pain Research Foundation in Liverpool, for all he has taught me about the neurophysiology of pain, and for having provided me with much constructive criticism and guidance during the formative stages of several of the chapters in this book.

I wish to say how grateful I am to Professor John Thompson for having given me much-appreciated encouragement and advice during the preparation of this book.

I wish to thank most sincerely Mrs Bonnie Clifford not only for her secretarial skills but also for her long-suffering patience, humour and enthusiasm, which have so considerably facilitated the writing of this book.

I thank the Wellcome Library for permission to publish Figures 1.1 and 1.2; Professor Kellgren for permission to publish Figure 1.3; Professor Kellgren and Portland Press for permission to publish Figures 1.4 and 1.5; Professor Kellgren and BMJ Publishing Group for permission to publish Figure 1.6; Professor Mense and NRC Research Press for permission to publish Figure 2.3; Dr David Bowsher and British Medical Acupuncture Council for permission to publish Figure 2.5; Professor Edwards for permission to publish Figure 4.1; Dr David Simons and The Haworth Press for permission to publish Figure 4.3; Dr David Simons and Elsevier Science for permission to publish Figures 8.17 and 8.18; Dr David Simons and Lippincott Williams & Wilkins for permission to publish Figure 11.17; Professor Porter for permission to publish Figures 12.17 and 12.18.

I thank Professor Martin Berry, Chairman of the Educational Board of Gray's Anatomy and its publishers Churchill Livingstone for permission to reproduce Figures 8.13, 9.1, 9.10, 10.12, 10.18, 10.19, 10.25, 11.10, 11.15, 12.1, 13.1*, 13.9, 13.13*, 13.17*, 13.21*, 13.26, 13.30, 13.32, 13.35, 14.2, 14.6, 14.9, 15.1, 15.3, 15.5*, 15.6. The illustrations from Gray's Anatomy marked with an asterisk originally appeared in Quain's Anatomy, 11th edition.

PART 1

Myofascial trigger point pain syndromes – pathophysiology and management

1

The evolution of current concepts

INTRODUCTION

Whilst present-day views as to the aetiology, pathophysiology, diagnosis, clinical manifestations and management of the myofascial trigger point pain syndromes and fibromyalgia will be discussed in subsequent chapters, the purpose of this one is to provide a historical review of the various observations which, over the course of time, have led to the evolution of our current concepts concerning these disorders.

TERMINOLOGICAL CONFUSION

Over the years the study of these disorders has been bedevilled by terminological confusion. Originally they were grouped together under the name muscular rheumatism, a term first introduced in the latter part of the 16th century by Guillaume de Baillou (1538–1616) (Fig. 1.1) when he was dean of the medical faculty at the University of Paris. Unfortunately, as Ruhmann (1940) has pointed out in his introduction to an English translation of de Baillou's book *Liber de Rheumatismo*, the French physician used the term rheumatism in this monograph not only when describing clinical manifestations of muscular rheumatism but also when writing about what has since become known as acute rheumatic fever.

Thomas Sydenham (1624–1689), the so-called 'Father of English Medicine', then added to this nosological obfuscation by including in his *Observationes Medicae* published in 1676 a chapter

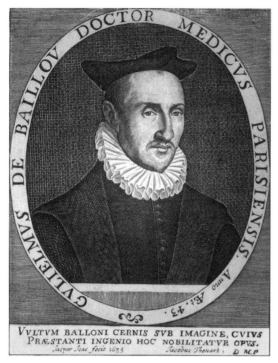

VVLTVM BALLONI CERNIS SVB IMAGINE, CVIVS
PRÆSTANTI INGENIO HOC NOBILITATVR OPVS.
Jaspar Isac fecit 1625   *Jacobus Thouart,* D M. P

Figure 1.1 Guillaume de Baillou (1538–1616).
(Reproduced by permission of The Wellcome Trust.)

entitled 'Rheumatism' which dealt only with the characteristic migratory type of arthropathy seen in acute rheumatic fever. This confusion was further compounded when, in 1810, William Wells, a physician at St Thomas' Hospital, London, called the carditis that develops in this febrile disorder, rheumatism of the heart (Baldry 1971). Fortunately, Jean Bouillaud (1796–1881), nine years after he had been appointed Professor of Medicine at the University of Paris, helped to clarify the situation when, in 1840, he made a clear distinction between rheumatic fever and muscular rheumatism (Reynolds 1983).

By that time two British physicians, Balfour (1815) and Scudamore (1827), had put forward the idea that the pain of muscular rheumatism occurs as a result of inflammation developing in the fibrous connective tissue in muscle. This concept differed from the one held by the 19th century German and Scandinavian physicians who believed that the pain develops as a result of an inflammatory process in the muscle fibres them-

selves. Nevertheless it was one that was to persist throughout England and France for the rest of that century and in 1904 caused Sir William Gowers (1845–1915) to recommend that the disorder hitherto known as muscular rheumatism should be called fibrositis.

Gowers did this during the course of a lecture on lumbago at what was then called the National Hospital for the Paralysed and Epileptic, London, (later the National Hospital for Nervous Diseases, and now the National Hospital for Neurology and Neurosurgery, London). The arguments he put forward in support of his proposition were in retrospect distinctly specious, but nevertheless they led him to conclude: 'We are thus compelled to regard lumbago in particular, and muscular rheumatism in general, as a form of inflammation of the fibrous tissues of the muscles…(and thus)…we may conveniently follow the analogy of "cellulitis" and term it "fibrositis".'

Ralph Stockman, then Professor of Medicine at Glasgow University, seemed to provide him with the pathological confirmation he required when, on examining microscopically some nodules removed from the muscles of patients affected by this disorder, he reported the presence of 'inflammatory hyperplasia…confined to white fibrous tissue' (Stockman 1904).

Although Stockman's findings have never subsequently been confirmed, their publication at that particular time helped to ensure that the term fibrositis became widely adopted. Any diagnostic specificity Gowers may have hoped to confer upon this term, however, was soon removed when in 1915 Llewellyn, a physician at the Royal Mineral Water Hospital in Bath, and Jones, a surgeon in that city, published a book entitled *Fibrositis*. In this they included a variety of disorders including gout and rheumatoid arthritis; and because of this the term became used in such an imprecise manner as to make it virtually meaningless.

A search for a more suitable one therefore continued, and some of the now outmoded synonyms employed during this century included nodular fibromyositis (Telling 1911), myofascitis (Albee 1927), myofibrositis (Murray 1929), perineuritis (Clayton & Livingstone 1930), idiopathic myalgia (Gutstein-Good 1940), rheumatic myalgias (Good 1941) and even myodysneuria (Gutstein 1955).

Much of this terminological confusion arose because of attempts to give a single name to what are now recognised to be two separate, albeit closely related, musculoskeletal pain disorders.

Controversial physical signs

Although the syndromes discussed in this book are extremely common and cause a considerable amount of disability they have not until recently started to receive the attention they deserve. One reason for this is the considerable controversy that has raged over the years concerning the significance of some of their clinical manifestations (Simons 1975, 1976, Reynolds 1983).

Nodules and palpable bands

In 1816 the Edinburgh physician William Balfour reported the presence of nodules in the muscles of patients suffering from what he called muscular rheumatism, having felt these during the course of employing massage to help relieve its pain.

It was similarly because the 19th century Dutch physician Johan Mezger (Fig. 1.2) (Haberling 1932) taught a large number of his students how to use massage for the treatment of this disorder that one of them, the Swedish physician Uno Helleday (1876), found them to be present in what he called *chronic rheumatic 'myitis'*. And why another, the German physician Strauss (1898), was eventually able to distinguish between nodules which he described as being small, tender and apple-sized and palpable bands which he described as being painful, pencil-sized to little-finger-sized elongated structures.

The detection of these nodules and bands requires more than a cursory examination and, as the German physician Müller pointed out in 1912, they are liable to be overlooked because doctors tend not to search for them in a systematic and skilful manner. Moreover, as will be discussed at some length in Chapter 4, the main reason why the medical profession for all too

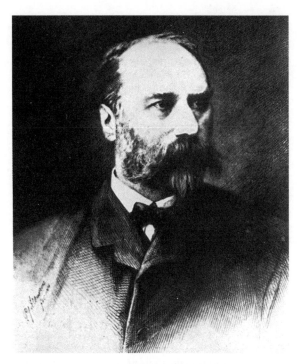

Figure 1.2 Johan Georg Mezger (1838–1900). (Reproduced by permission of The Wellcome Trust.)

long failed to show any particular interest in them is because until recently there has been no general agreement as to their diagnostic significance.

Localised points of tenderness

William Balfour (1824) also reported the presence of focal points of tenderness in the muscles of patients suffering from what was then termed muscular rheumatism, but the first person to write at length about these points was the French physician François Valleix.

In his *Traité des Néuralgies; ou Affections Douloureuses des Nerfs* published in 1841, Valleix described how pain of a shooting nature may develop when nerve endings at localised tender points in various parts of the body became hyperactive. He realised that these points are the source of the pain for he called them *'les points douloureux'* and stated:

If, in the intervals of the shooting pains, one asks (a patient with neuralgia) what is the seat of his pain, he replies then by designating limited points. ... It is only with the aid of pressure ... that one discovers exactly the extent of the painful points. ... (They) are found placed in four principal points of the trajectory of different nerves. 1st at the point of emergence of a nerve trunk ... 2nd in the points where a nerve fibre traverses the muscles, in order to approach the skin into which it will pass ... 3rd in the points where the terminal branches of a nerve come to ramify in the integument ... 4th in places where the nerve trunks ... become quite superficial.

It was unfortunate that he confused the tender points found in disorders such as trigeminal neuralgia with those found in muscles affected by what he called rheumatism for this erroneously led him to believe that the latter is a form of neuralgia (Valleix 1848), as shown by his statement:

I conclude that pain, capital symptom of neuralgia expresses itself ... in different ways. If it remains concentrated in the nerves one finds characteristic, isolated, painful points; this is *neuralgia in the proper sense*. If the pain spreads into the muscles ... this is *muscular rheumatism* ... an obvious muscular rheumatism can transform itself into a true neuralgia.

Despite his belief that neuralgia and rheumatism are different forms of the same disorder he must be given credit for being one of the first physicians to recognise that the pain in the latter emanates from tender points in muscle where nerve endings are in a state of hyperactivity. He was wrong, however, concerning the referral of pain from these points as it was his belief that this was due to it being 'propagated along neighbouring nerves'.

He was not alone, however, in thinking this as many other physicians over the years have subscribed to this view, although differing as to how they thought it might occur. Stockman's (1904) explanation was that 'a branch of a nerve may be pressed upon by a nodule, or may even pass through it, and because of this he said 'the pain radiates over a wide area perhaps far from a nodule'. Others thought it occurred as a result of pressure on a nerve when a muscle goes into spasm. A third hypothesis, and one which was widely held well into the 20th century, was that it is due to rheumatic inflammation of connective tissue in and around nerves, and it was for this reason that the terms neurofibrositis and peri-

neuritis were introduced (Clayton & Livingstone 1930, Gowers 1904, Llewellyn & Jones 1915). Those who put forward such ideas seem to have been oblivious of the fact that the British physician Thomas Inman, as long ago as 1858, had shrewdly noted that the radiation of the pain 'is independent entirely of the course of nerves'. They also seem to have ignored the observation made by the German physician Cornelius in 1903 that 'this radiation often enough absolutely does not keep to the individual nerve trunks' and is bound 'to no anatomical law'.

Cornelius moreover clearly understood that the localised points of tenderness present in the muscles of patients suffering from rheumatism contain nerve endings for he called them nerve points (*nervenpunkte*). He concluded that these nerve endings are in a state of hyperactivity because of the effect on them of external factors such as alterations in weather conditions, physical exertion and emotional upsets.

In view of all this it has to be admitted that Valleix was not as far off the mark as at first sight might be thought when he called muscular rheumatism a form of neuralgia. In retrospect it is also clear that Sir William Osler (1849–1919) was equally perceptive when during the course of discussing muscular rheumatism in the 1909 edition of his textbook *The Principles and Practice of Medicine* he stated:

It is by no means certain that the muscular tissues are the seat of the disease. Many writers claim, perhaps correctly, that it is a neuralgia of the sensory nerves of the muscles.

Regional 'rheumatism'

It is thus apparent that by the beginning of the 20th century some of the more enlightened physicians had come to appreciate that the pain in the disorder which at that time was variously called either muscular rheumatism or fibrositis is not due to some pathological process affecting the muscle fibres themselves or the fibrous tissue enveloping them but rather occurs as a result of the development of increased activity in nerve endings at specific points of tenderness in the muscles.

They also realised that it may be either generalised or restricted to one particular region of the body. However, it was not until the 1930s that clinicians started to take a particular interest in cases with localised 'rheumatic' pain. One of the first was Hunter, a physician in Canada, who in 1933 described cases in which pain localised to the abdominal region emanated from tender points in the anterior abdominal wall muscles.

Others who also did this included Edeiken & Wolferth at the University of Pennsylvania who, in 1938, reported that among patients with coronary thrombosis under their care some had developed pain in the shoulder during the course of prolonged bed rest and that of those there were two in whom they had located focal points of exquisite tenderness in the muscles around the scapula. They stated that they had decided to call these points trigger zones in view of the fact that it had proved possible to reproduce the spontaneously occurring shoulder pain by applying firm pressure to them. They furthermore found that one of the patients had noticed for himself that pressure over one of these so-called trigger zones caused pain to be referred to the left shoulder, up the left side of the neck and down the left arm.

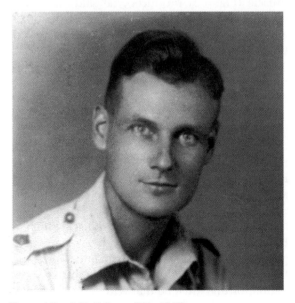

Figure 1.3 J. H. Kellgren (Italy 1943).

The physician, however, who during the 1930s made the greatest contribution to our knowledge concerning the pathogenesis, diagnosis and treatment of what are now known as the myofascial trigger point pain syndromes was John Kellgren (Fig. 1.3), who was later to become Professor of Rheumatology at Manchester University, but who at that time was working as a young research assistant under Sir Thomas Lewis, the director of Clinical Research at University College Hospital, London.

JOHN KELLGREN'S OBSERVATIONS

In a paper entitled *Suggestions Relating to the Study of Somatic Pain*, Sir Thomas Lewis (1938) stated:

As an experimental method of producing muscle pain the injection of a minute quantity of a salt solution is the most satisfactory ... In these observations I have noted that muscle pain is referred to a distance. Thus pain arising from the lower part of the triceps is often referred down the inner side of the forearm to the little finger and from the trapezius it is usually referred to the occiput. I have been fortunate in interesting Dr Kellgren in this matter. In a long series of very careful researches carried out in my laboratory he has formulated some very striking principles underlying the reference of pain from muscles – principles which appear to have an important practical bearing.

Kellgren, having learnt from Sir Thomas's experiments that pain arising from a muscle as a result of injecting a noxious substance into it is frequently referred to an area some distance away from the injection site, decided to investigate whether this pain referral occurs not only when the muscle is traumatised by this means but also when a noxious substance is injected into the fascia enveloping it.

In order to do this Kellgren (1938a) carried out a series of laboratory experiments on healthy volunteers. These experiments involved injecting variable amounts (0.1–0.3 cc) of 6% solution of sodium chloride into the belly of and into the fascia enveloping each of a number of different muscles.

His first choice was the gluteus medius muscle because of the tough well-developed fascia which covers it. After the skin over the muscle had been anaesthetised three needles were inserted through the tissues until they could be felt to impinge upon the resistant fascial layer. The fascia was then traumatised by pecking at it with each needle in turn and this produced a pain localised to a well-defined small area a few centimetres distal to the needle concerned. Then 0.1 cc of 6% hypertonic saline was injected through each needle and this also produced pain localised in a similar manner close to the injection site.

The needles were then advanced into the substance of the muscle itself. Traumatisation of the muscle by means of vigorous movements of a needle only produced a slight pain, but one, nevertheless that was felt widely over most of the buttock. However, when 0.2 cc of 6% saline was injected into the muscle a diffuse pain of greater severity was felt not only in the buttock but also down the back of the thigh and occasionally as far as the knee (Fig. 1.4). Kellgren carried out this experiment on three people and obtained similar findings with each of them.

He then carried out a similar experiment on the tibialis anterior muscle in 14 volunteers.

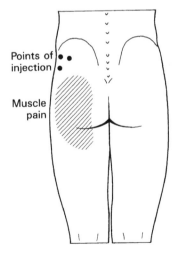

Figure 1.4   The distribution of diffuse referred pain (hatched area) produced by injecting 6% saline into three points in the gluteus muscle. (Reproduced with permission from Kellgren, J H 1938 *Clinical Science*, vol. 3, pp. 175–190. © the Biochemical Society and the Medical Research Society.)

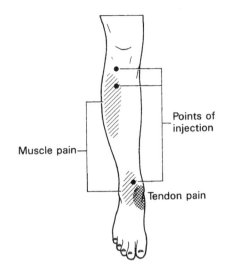

Figure 1.5   The distribution of referred pain (hatched area) from injecting 6% saline into points in the tibialis anterior muscle. Also, the pattern of locally referred pain (stippled area) from injecting saline into the tendon of this muscle at the ankle. (Reproduced with permission from Kellgren, J H 1938 *Clinical Science*, vol. 3, pp. 175–190. © the Biochemical Society and the Medical Research Society.)

Again, scratching the fascia overlying this muscle with a needle or injecting hypertonic saline into it invariably only produced a localised pain in the vicinity of the needle. In contrast to this, an injection of hypertonic saline into the belly of the muscle (Fig. 1.5) produced, he said, 'a diffuse pain felt by most subjects in front of the ankle and in the outer and middle part of the front of the leg'.

He was therefore able to demonstrate that in the case of these two muscles pain arising as a result of traumatising the overlying fascia remains localised around the site where the noxious stimulus is applied, and that in contrast to this, pain arising as a result of traumatising the muscle itself spreads diffusely and is often referred to an area some considerable distance away from the noxious stimulation site.

He next found that injecting hypertonic saline into the bellies of certain other muscles such as the pectoralis major, deltoid and vastus medialis gave rise both to a localised pain and a more diffuse referred pain. He concluded that the explanation for this must be that with these particular muscles the muscle tissue is permeated by fascial septa and that the noxious stimulus must stimulate nerve endings in both muscle and fascia simultaneously.

Another important observation made by him was that pain which develops as a result of traumatising a muscle may not appear to be muscular in origin but rather seem to be arising from some other type of structure. For example, he found that an injection of hypertonic saline into the infraspinatus muscle causes pain to be referred to the shoulder joint; that an injection into the vastus medialis muscle causes pain to be referred to the knee joint; that an injection into the masseter muscle causes pain to be felt predominately in the region of the upper jaw and because of this is liable to be described as 'toothache'. And that an injection into the multifidus muscle at the level of the first and second lumbar spines is referred to the scrotum.

Once Kellgren had completed his laboratory experiments he turned his attention to eight patients suffering from pain of muscular origin localised to specific regions of the body. These included the neck, the shoulder girdle, the arm, the leg, or lower back (Fig. 1.6). In his account of these cases (Kellgren 1938b) he clearly had difficulty in knowing what to call this regional disorder for in some places he referred to it as fibrositis and in others he called it myalgia.

He stated that whilst palpation of the area affected by the pain showed it to be only slightly tender, palpation of muscles some distance from the painful area revealed the presence of localised points, or what he chose to call tender spots, where the tenderness was so exquisite that pressure applied to them caused the patient to wince. He also noted that the application of sustained pressure to them led to an exacerbation of the spontaneously occurring pain, and that an injection of 1% procaine (Novocain) into them relieved it. He deduced from these observations that the reason why these localised points in muscles, or what are now called trigger points, are so exquisitely tender is that they are loci where nerve endings are in a state of hyperactivity and that it is because of this that the pain develops.

The only other physician in Britain who wrote about this type of muscle pain during the 1930s was Gutstein, a Polish refugee. Gutstein (unlike Kellgren, who in 1938 published his clinical observations in the *British Medical Journal*), published his findings that year in the less widely read *British Journal of Physical Medicine*, and that is possibly one of the reasons why it did not receive the attention it deserved. Nevertheless, in an attempt to get the medical profession to take notice of what he had to say about musculoskeletal pain, he wrote a number of papers on the subject over the next 10 years. Confusingly, however, during the course of this he changed his name three times and kept giving the regional musculoskeletal pain disorder he was discussing a different name. Thus in 1938 and again in 1940, under the name of M. Gutstein, he wrote about what he called muscular or common rheumatism. In 1940, under the name of Gutstein-Good, he called the disorder idiopathic myalgia. A year later, by which time he had changed his name yet again to Good, he wrote about rheumatic myalgias! Then in 1950 he called it fibrositis, and in 1951 non-articular rheumatism. To add to the confusion, there was at about the same time an R. R. Gutstein (1955) calling this disorder myodysneuria!

Despite all this Good made the valuable observation that pressure applied to tender points, or what he called myalgic spots in muscle or tendon, gives rise to both local and referred pain, and he must be given the credit for being the first person to stress that the patterns of pain referral from tender points in individual muscles are the same in everyone and illustrated these in well-executed drawings. Like Kellgren, his method of alleviating the pain that emanates from these 'myalgic spots' was by injecting a local anaesthetic into them.

Sadly, the medical profession in Britain largely ignored Kellgren's and Good's valuable observations. One reason for this was that by the 1950s many of its leading rheumatologists had come to the conclusion that fibrositis, or non-articular rheumatism as it was by that time more commonly called, is not an organic disorder and that psychogenic rheumatism was a more appropriate name for it. They were led to believe this because of doubts concerning the significance of

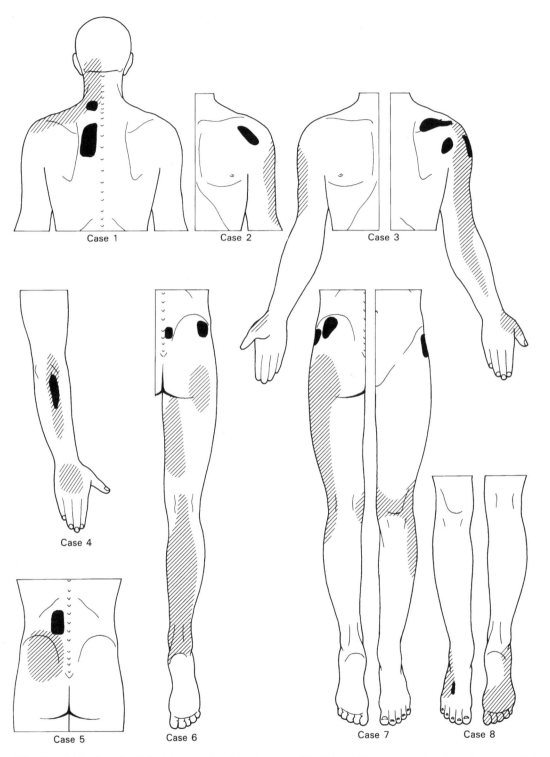

Case 1

Case 2

Case 3

Case 4

Case 5

Case 6

Case 7

Case 8

Figure 1.6 The distribution of pain (hatched area) and tender spots (black) in eight cases in which the pain was abolished by injecting Novocain into the tender spots. (Reproduced with permission from Kellgren 1938b, p. 326.)

its physical signs, the absence of any characteristic histological appearances and the lack of any specific laboratory tests. Typical of this view was the one expressed by Ellman & Shaw (1950) who, during the course of discussing patients with this disorder stated:

From the striking disparity between the gross nature of their symptoms and the poverty of the physical findings ... it seems clear that the nature of this often very prolonged *incapacity* is psychiatric in the majority of cases ... the patient aches in his limbs because in fact he aches in his mind.

Another reason was that specialists in the field of physical medicine in Britain at that time were of the opinion that the pain which Kellgren and others considered to be of muscular origin develops instead as the result of disorders in the vertebral column and, in particular, because of the impingement of degenerative discs upon nerve roots (de Blecourt 1954, Christie 1958, Cyriax 1948).

Fortunately there were physicians in other parts of the world who were sufficiently perspicacious to recognise the merits of Kellgren's observations. One of these was Michael Kelly in Australia. Kelly not only adopted Kellgren's methods of diagnosing and relieving referred pain from points of maximal tenderness in muscles but recorded his clinical observations in a series of valuable papers published over a period of 21 years from 1941 onwards. References to the majority of these are to be found in his last paper (Kelly 1962).

MYOFASCIAL TRIGGER POINT PAIN SYNDROMES

It was, however, the American physician Janet Travell (1901–1997) (Fig. 1.7) who, from the 1940s onwards, contributed the most to our understanding of the type of muscle pain Kellgren and others had been investigating. She first began to take an interest in it after reading how Edeiken & Wolferth (1936) had been able to reproduce spontaneously occurring shoulder pain by applying pressure to tender points in muscles around the scapula.

She read Edeiken & Wolferth's report at a time when she herself was suffering from a painful

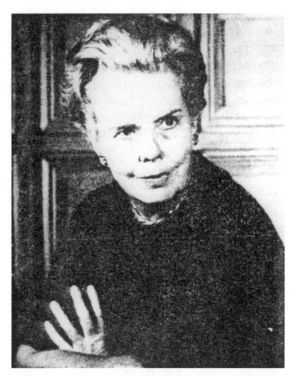

Figure 1.7 Janet Travell (1901–1997).

shoulder as a result of having strained some muscles during the course of her work. As she said in her autobiography *Office Hours: Day and Night* (1968):

Poking around at night in the muscles over my shoulder blade, trying to give some 'do it yourself' massage, I was astonished to touch some spots that intensified, or reproduced my pain, as though I had turned on an electric switch. It was my first introduction to the enigmatic trigger area. No nerve existed, I knew, to connect those firing spots directly with my arm. I was baffled, but I did not discard the observation on the grounds that I could not explain it.

Following this she decided to study the subject further and the opportunity to do this arose almost immediately when in 1936 she was appointed to work under Dr Harry Gold at Sea View Hospital on Staten Island, New York. At this hospital, which specialised in the treatment of tuberculosis, a large number of patients, having been kept in bed for long periods, suffered severe pain in their shoulders and arms. As she says in her autobiography, 'When I examined them by systematic palpation of the scapula and chest muscles, I easily uncovered the presence of trigger areas. I knew what to look for'.

Her interest in the referral of pain from trigger areas in muscles having been aroused in this manner, she was prompted to read what others, including Kellgren (1938b), Steindler & Luck (1938) and Steindler (1940) had to say on the subject.

Following this, Travell persuaded Dr Myron Herman, the medical resident at Sea View Hospital, to inject procaine into tender points present in the chest wall muscles of patients with painful shoulders. And it was because this proved to be so successful that she and her cardiologist colleague, Seymour Rinzler, decided to treat a number of patients with chest pain of muscular origin under their care in the medical wards at the Beth Israel Hospital in a similar manner (Travell et al 1942).

Travell and Rinzler then published two other outstanding papers on the subject. In one of these (Rinzler & Travell 1948) they drew attention to the fact that tender points, or what by that time they were calling trigger areas, may develop in the muscles of the chest wall as a secondary event in patients with cardiac pain and reported that it is possible to relieve the pain either by injecting procaine into them, or by spraying the overlying skin with ethyl chloride. In the other (Travell & Rinzler 1948) they showed how closely the pattern of pain referral from trigger areas in muscles of the chest wall may simulate that of ischaemic heart disease.

They were not, however, the first to recognise this, as Gutstein (1938), Kelly (1944) and Mendlowitz (1945) had previously described how pain from 'tender spots' in the muscles of the chest wall may have a similar pattern of distribution to that of coronary heart disease pain.

Arthur Steindler, Professor of Orthopaedic Surgery at the State University of Iowa, was the first to give the name trigger points to the points of maximal tenderness in muscles from which pain is referred to distant sites and the first to employ the adjective myofascial when describing the referral of pain from points of this type in the

gluteus maximus muscle in a disorder he called the gluteal myofascial syndrome (Steindler 1940).

This notwithstanding it is only right that Janet Travell should be given the credit for bringing the term myofascial pain into general use. She did this during the early 1950s after having observed, whilst doing an infraspinatus muscle biopsy, that the pain pattern evoked by stretching or pinching the fascia enveloping the muscle is similar to that when the same is done to the muscle itself. She also popularised the use of the term myofascial trigger point (MTrP), confirmed that each muscle in the body has its own specific pattern of MTrP pain referral, drew attention to various individual MTrP pain syndromes and showed that when only one syndrome is present, the pain is localised to a single region of the body and that when several syndromes develop concomitantly the pain is generalised.

By 1951 Travell and Rinzler had recognised a large number of these syndromes and gave a detailed description of them at that year's meeting of the American Medical Association. In the following year they published an account of

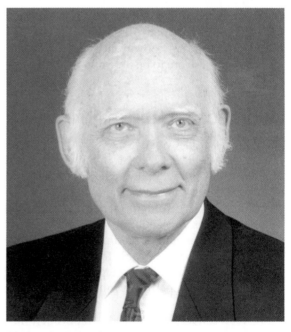

Figure 1.8 David Simons.

them in a classic contribution to the subject entitled *The Myofascial Genesis of Pain* that was particularly notable for the clarity of its illustrations (Travell & Rinzler 1952). And then 31 years later Travell and her colleague David Simons (Travell & Simons 1983) had gained such considerable experience in the diagnosis and management of these syndromes that they were able to publish the first authoritative textbook on the subject.

Since that time considerable progress has been made concerning our understanding of the pathophysiology of MTrP pain (see Ch. 4) and much of this has been due to pioneer work initiated by David Simons (Simons 1999) (Fig. 1.8).

FIBROMYALGIA

In 1965 Smythe, a rheumatologist, and Moldofsky (Fig. 1.9), a psychiatrist in Toronto, Canada, decided to carry out electroencephalographic studies on a group of patients with generalised muscle pain and disturbed sleep. They found that the latter was due to the 8–10 c/s (cycles per second) alpha rhythm normally found in rapid eye movement (REM) light sleep intruding into the slow 1–2 c/s delta rhythm of non-REM deep sleep (Moldofsky 1986, Moldofsky et al 1975, Smythe 1986).

Following on from this it became apparent that such patients, predominantly female, suffer from a specific syndrome that is characterised by persistent generalised muscle pain, non-restorative sleep, early morning stiffness, marked fatigue and a large number of tender points at certain specific sites in the body (Ch. 16).

When Smythe & Moldofsky (1977) first drew attention to this disorder they somewhat confusingly called it the fibrositis syndrome. But

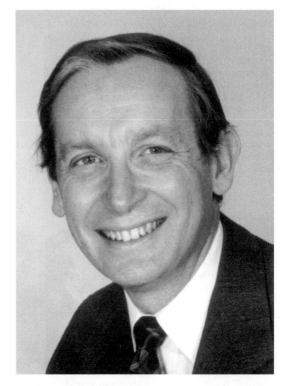

Figure 1.9 Harvey Moldofsky.

for the same reason that made this term unacceptable earlier in the century it was soon abandoned and in 1981 it was re-named fibromyalgia (Yunus et al 1981), a term that has since been officially included in the World Health Organization's 10th revision of its International Classification of Diseases where it has been given the number M79.0.

In addition to this the American College of Rheumatology (Wolfe et al 1990) has now laid down specific criteria for its diagnosis (see Ch. 16, Box 16.1).

REFERENCES

Albee F H 1927 Myofascitis. A pathological explanation of many apparently dissimilar conditions. American Journal of Surgery 3:523–533

Baldry P E 1971 The battle against heart disease. University Press, Cambridge

Balfour W 1815 Observations on the pathology and cure of rheumatism. Edinburgh Medical and Surgical Journal 11:168–187

Balfour W 1816 Observations with cases illustrative of new simple and expeditious mode of curing rheumatism and sprains. Adam Black, Edinburgh

Balfour W 1824 Illustrations of the efficacy of compression and percussion in the cure of rheumatism and sprains. The London Medical and Physical Journal 51:446–462, 52:104–115, 200–208, 284–291

Christie B G 1958 Discussion on non-articular rheumatism. Proceedings of the Royal Society of Medicine 51:251–255

Clayton E G, Livingstone J L 1930 Fibrositis. Lancet i:1420–1423

Cornelius A 1903 Narben und Nerven. Deutsche Militärärztlische Zeitschrift 32:657–673

Cyriax J 1948 Fibrositis. British Medical Journal ii:251–255

de Blecourt J J 1954 Screening of the population for rheumatic diseases. Annals of Rheumatic Diseases 13:338–340

Edeiken J, Wolferth C C 1936 Persistent pain in the shoulder region following myocardial infarction. American Journal of Medical Science 191:201–210

Ellman P, Shaw D 1950 The chronic 'rheumatic' and his pains. Psychosomatic aspects of chronic non-articular rheumatism. Annals of Rheumatic Diseases 9:341–357

Good M G 1941 Rheumatic myalgias. Practitioner 146:167–174

Good M G 1950 The role of skeletal muscle in the pathogenesis of diseases. Acta Medica Scandinavica 138:285–292

Good M G 1951 Objective diagnosis and curability of non-articular rheumatism. British Journal of Physical Medicine and Industrial Hygiene 14:1–7

Gowers W R 1904 Lumbago: its lessons and analogues. British Medical Journal i:117–121

Gutstein M 1938 Diagnosis and treatment of muscular rheumatism. British Journal of Physical Medicine 1:302–321

Gutstein M 1940 Common rheumatism and physiotherapy. British Journal of Physical Medicine 3:46–50

Gutstein R R 1955 A review of myodysneuria (fibrositis). American Practitioner 6:570–577

Gutstein-Good M 1940 Idiopathic myalgia simulating visceral and other diseases. Lancet ii:326–328

Haberling W 1932 Johan Georg Mezger of Amsterdam. The founder of scientific massage (translated by Emilie Recht). Medical Life 39:190–207

Helleday U 1876 Nordiskt medicinskt arkiv 6 and 8 Nr 8. P A Norstedtosöner, Stockholm

Hunter C 1933 Myalgia of the abdominal wall. Canadian Medical Association Journal 28:157–161

Inman T 1858 Remarks on myalgia or muscular pain. British Medical Journal 407–408; 866–868

Kellgren J H 1938a Observations on referred pain arising from muscle. Clinical Science 3:175–190

Kellgren J H 1938b A preliminary account of referred pain arising from muscle. British Medical Journal i:325–327

Kelly M 1944 Pain in the chest: observations on the use of local anaesthesia in its investigation and treatment. Medical Journal of Australia 1:4–7

Kelly M 1962 Local injections for rheumatism. Medical Journal of Australia 1:45–50

Lewis Sir Thomas 1938 Suggestions relating to the study of somatic pain. British Medical Journal i:321–325

Llewellyn L J, Jones A B 1915 Fibrositis. Rebman, New York

Mendlowitz M 1945 Strain of the pectoralis minor, an important cause of praecordial pain in soldiers. American Heart Journal 30:123–125

Moldofsky H 1986 Sleep and musculoskeletal pain. American Journal of Medicine 81(suppl 3A):85–89

Moldofsky H, Scarisbrick P, England R, Smythe H 1975 Musculoskeletal symptoms and non-REM sleep disturbance in patients with fibrositis syndrome and healthy subjects. Psychosomatic Medicine 371:341–351

Müller A 1912 Untersuchungsbefund am rheumatisch erkranten muskel. Zeitschrift Klinische Medizin 74:34–73

Murray G R 1929 Myofibrositis as a simulator of other maladies. Lancet i:113–116

Osler W 1909 The principles and practice of medicine, 7th edn. S. Appleton & Co, New York, p 396

Reynolds M D 1983 The development of the concept of fibrositis. Journal of the History of Medical and Allied Sciences 38:5–35

Rinzler S, Travell J 1948 Therapy directed at the somatic component of cardiac pain. American Heart Journal 35:248–268

Ruhmann W 1940 The earliest book on rheumatism. British Journal of Rheumatism II(3):140–162 [This paper includes an original translation of de Baillou's *Liber de Rheumatismo* which, originally written in medieval Latin, was first published by a descendant, M J Thevart in 1736, i.e. 120 years after the author's death.]

Scudamore C 1827 A treatise on the nature and cure of rheumatism. Longman, London, p 11

Simons D G 1975 Muscle pain syndromes – Part I. American Journal of Physical Medicine 54:289–311

Simons D G 1976 Muscle pain syndromes – Part II. American Journal of Physical Medicine 55: 15–42

Simons D G 1999 General overview. In: Simons D G, Travell J G, Simons L S (eds) Travell & Simons myofascial pain and dysfunction, vol. 1, 2nd edn. Williams & Wilkins, Baltimore, pp 11–93

Smythe H 1986 Tender points. Evolution of concepts of the fibrositis/fibromyalgia syndrome. American Journal of Medicine 81 (suppl 3A):2–6

Smythe H A, Moldofsky H 1977 Two contributions to understanding of the 'fibrositis' syndrome. Bulletin of Rheumatic Diseases 28:928–931

Steindler A 1940 The interpretation of sciatic radiation and the syndrome of low-back pain. Journal of Bone and Joint Surgery 22:28–34

Steindler A, Luck J V 1938 Differential diagnosis of pain low in the back. Journal of the American Medical Association 110:106–113

Stockman R 1904 The causes, pathology and treatment of chronic rheumatism. Edinburgh Medical Journal 15:107–116, 223–225

Strauss H 1898 Über die sogenannte 'rheumatische muskelschwiele'. Klinische Wochenschrift 35:89–91, 121–123

Sydenham Thomas 1676 Observationes Medicae. The works of Thomas Sydenham translated by R G Latham in 1848. Sydenham Society, London.

Telling W H 1911 Nodular fibromyositis, an everyday affliction, and its identity with so-called muscular rheumatism. Lancet i:154–158

Travell J 1968 Office hours: day and night. World Publishing Company, New York

Travell J, Rinzler S 1948 Pain syndromes of the chest muscles. Resemblance to effort angina and myocardial infarction, and relief by local block. Canadian Medical Association Journal 59:333–338

Travell J, Rinzler S H 1952 The myofascial genesis of pain. Postgraduate Medicine 11:425–434

Travell J, Simons D G 1983 Myofascial pain and dysfunction. The trigger point manual. Williams and Wilkins, Baltimore

Travell J, Rinzler S, Herman M 1942 Pain and disability of the shoulder and arm: treatment by intramuscular infiltration with procaine hydrochloride. Journal of the American Medical Association 120:417–422

Valleix F 1841 Traité des néuralgies: ou, affections douloureuses des nerfs. Baillière, Paris

Valleix F 1848 Eétudes sur le rheumatisme musculaire, et en particulier sur son diagnostic et sur son traitement.

Bulletin général de thérapeutique médicale et chirurgicale 35:296–307

Wolfe F, Smythe H A, Yunus M B, Bennett R M et al 1990 The American College of Rheumatology 1990 criteria for the classification of fibromyalgia: report of the Multicenter Criteria Committee. Arthritis and Rheumatism 33:160–172

Yunus M, Masi A T, Calabro J J, Miller K A, Feigenbaum S L 1981 Primary fibromyalgia (fibrositis) clinical study of 50 patients with matched controls. Seminars in Arthritis and Rheumatism 11:151–171

2

Relevant neurophysiological mechanisms

INTRODUCTION

In this chapter it will be shown that our present understanding of pain stems from important discoveries made during the past fifty years.

Following a brief review of some of the earlier ideas on the subject, current views concerning the neural mechanisms involved in the production, modulation, persistence and alleviation of the type of pain that arises as a result of the stimulation of nociceptors (nociceptive pain) will be discussed. It will then be explained how present-day knowledge of these has provided insight into the ones involved in the production of myofascial trigger point (MTrP) pain and has led to the development of neurophysiologically based methods of alleviating it.

ORIGINAL BELIEFS

For centuries there has been much controversy as to the manner in which pain arises. One of the first to ponder upon this was the French mathematician and philosopher René Descartes (1596–1650) in the post-Renaissance period. In his famous treatise *L'homme*, which was published posthumously in 1664 and which Foster translated into English in 1901, Descartes concluded from philosophical reflections rather than from the carrying out of experiments, that pain is felt because of the existence of a direct line of communication between the peripheral tissues and the brain. He likened the system to the bell-ringing mechanism in a church tower with the bell sounding in the belfry as a result of a rope being pulled some distance below it. He illustrated how he thought the mechanism worked in practice by means of his now famous drawing depicting a boy receiving a burn to his foot, and feeling pain from this as a result of signals passing uninterruptedly up the spinal column to the brain.

This simplistic view of events continued to be accepted until pain began to be investigated experimentally two hundred years later. The first to do this was the outstanding German physiologist Johannes Müller (1801–1858), who considered that not only sensory organs like the eyes and the ears, but also all other structures in the body such as the skin, are connected to the brain by sensory nerves. And that the type of sensation experienced when nerves of this type in any particular structure are stimulated is dependent on the specific form of energy this creates in them. This concept became enshrined in his well-known law of specific nerve energies.

Although Müller recognised the existence of the five classical senses of hearing, seeing, tasting, smelling and touching, he somewhat confusingly considered that pain and other sensations arising from a structure such as the skin are variants of touch, for he wrote in his *Elements of Physiology* published in 1842:

Sensation is a property common to all the senses, but the kind of sensation is different in each: thus, we have the sensation of light, of sound, of taste, of smell and of feeling or touch. By feeling and touch we understand the peculiar kind of sensation of which ordinary sensitive nerves generally . . . are susceptible. The sensations of itching, of pleasure and pain, of heat and cold, and those excited by the act of touch in its more limited sense, are varieties of this mode of sensation.

Müller not only believed that the reason why each of these senses, including pain, have their own specific characteristics is because the sensory nerves attached to each of the different structures from which they arise have their own particular special form of energy but also because this energy is conveyed to one or other of a number of different, highly specialised parts of the brain. Once he had reached this conclusion

the hunt for special cortical centres, already started earlier that century in London by the famous surgeon, artist and anatomist Charles Bell, continued and it was not long before the visual and auditory centres in the brain were located by means of identifying the nerves leading to these areas from the eye and ear.

Sensory receptors

The next major advance in unravelling the complexities of pain perception was made by the German physician Max von Frey (1852–1932) as a result of carefully investigating the sensory receptors in the skin. He did this with the aid of various ingenious devices including a pin on a string to map out 'pain spots' and a type of hairbrush to map out 'touch spots'. From these and other investigations he identified four separate types of sensory receptors in the skin for cold, warmth, touch and pain. Moreover, he concluded that the end bulbs which had already been described by Krause are cold receptors, that the end organs previously located by Ruffini are warmth receptors, that the corpuscles Meissner had found are touch receptors; and that the free nerve endings identified by himself are pain receptors (Boring 1942).

Whilst von Frey correctly identified pain receptors or what today are called nociceptors (tissue damage receptors), the assumption made by both him and his contemporaries that the intensity with which pain arising from these is felt is in direct proportion to the strength of stimulus applied to them was soon to be proved wrong.

Central pain-summation mechanisms

As Melzack & Wall (1988a) have pointed out, one of the first to challenge this assumption was the German physician Alfred Goldscheider (1858–1935), as a result of some sensory tests carried out by a contemporary compatriot, Bernard Naunyn, on patients with tabes dorsalis, a late-onset neurological manifestation of syphilis. In that disorder a warm test-tube applied to the skin initially gives rise to an appropriately warm sensation but repeated brief applications of it produces an increasingly hot sensation until, eventually, this takes the form of an unbearable burning. Also the insertion of a needle into the skin, which in a normal person gives rise to no more than a very transitory sharp sensation, in a patient with tabes dorsalis produces a diffuse prolonged burning type of pain.

This build-up and prolongation of the pain experience, often after an interval of time, led Goldscheider to postulate that there may be some form of pain-summation mechanism in the spinal cord, but he offered no conjecture as to how it might work. He, nevertheless, caused others to think about the possibility and eventually, Livingston, in his classic monograph *Pain Mechanisms*, published in 1943, put forward the suggestion that this phenomenon might possibly be due to the initiation of activity in closed self-exciting neuronal loops called by him reverberatory circuits.

There is no evidence that reverberatory circuits such as envisaged by Livingston actually exist. Nevertheless, by putting forward this idea at a time when physicians were increasingly becoming aware that the amount of pain suffered by people in response to noxious stimuli of similar intensity varies widely and also that, in certain circumstances, even innocuous ones may be pain-producing, he encouraged his contemporaries to put aside the long-held view that pain signals pass uninterruptedly to the brain and to explore the possibility that they may be either augmented or suppressed by various means during the course of their transmission through the peripheral and central nervous systems.

CURRENT CONCEPTS

Pain – a physico-emotional experience

Pain, unlike other sensory experiences such as seeing or hearing, has both an emotional and a physical component. The definition of pain put forward by the International Association for the Study of Pain Subcommittee on Taxonomy is that it is 'an unpleasant sensory and emotional experience associated with actual or potential tissue damage, or described in terms of such damage' (Merskey 1979).

As Hannington-Kiff (1974) has pointed out, pain has three main components: physical, rational and emotional. The physical component is determined by the responsiveness of an individual's nociceptive system to a given stimulus; the rational component is derived from an objective interpretation of pain in the cerebral cortex; and the emotional component is determined by the responsiveness of an individual's limbic system to any particular noxious stimulus.

It therefore follows that for a given noxious stimulus, the intensity with which pain is felt varies from person to person, and with regard to this it is important to distinguish between the pain perception threshold and the pain tolerance threshold. The pain perception threshold is the least stimulus intensity at which a subject perceives pain. This, contrary to popular belief, is much the same in everyone so that, for example, a thermal stimulus applied to the skin is invariably around 44–45°C. However, the pain tolerance threshold, defined as the maximum amount of pain which an individual is prepared to tolerate, varies widely from person to person.

This, of course, is of considerable practical importance when attempting to assess pain and the effect of any particular form of treatment on it, for it is not changes in pain threshold that have to be measured but rather changes in pain tolerance.

Pain tolerance depends on a person's emotional response to a noxious stimulus. And it is of interest with respect to this to note that the 17th century Dutch philosopher Benedict Spinoza (1632–1677) referred to pain as 'a localised form of sorrow'.

The reaction of individuals to pain throughout their lives is liable to be influenced by a number of factors. These include their psychological make-up, cultural background, ethnic origin and the attitude of parents towards it during their childhood (Bond 1979, Zborowski 1952).

Pain tolerance is also dependent on changes in mood, with anxiety or depression reducing it, and on the circumstances in which the pain develops. Thus, for example, the pain from a severe wound sustained in the heat of battle may hardly be noticed, whereas pain from a similar injury incurred in a less stressful environment is liable to cause considerable suffering (Beecher 1959). Moreover, the intensity with which pain is felt is diminished by anything which distracts attention from it. This is why some people find background music helpful whilst undergoing a painful experience such as at the dentist (Gardner & Licklider 1959). Also why those who suffer chronic pain are able to tolerate it better if their minds are kept occupied by carrying out absorbing tasks (Wynn Parry 1980).

Furthermore, the perception of, and reaction to, noxious stimuli is also influenced by past experiences. This has been demonstrated in ingenious experiments carried out on various animals, including dogs (Melzack 1969, Melzack & Scott 1957) and monkeys (Lichstein & Sackett 1971).

Pain is occasionally entirely psychogenic. More often it is a complex physico-emotional experience occurring either as a result of the stimulation of nociceptors, and therefore called nociceptive pain, or as a result of damage to either the peripheral or central nervous system and therefore called neuropathic (neurogenic) pain. Nociceptive pain may be either physiological or pathological. Neuropathic pain is invariably pathological (Woolf 1991).

Physiological nociceptive pain

Physiological nociceptive pain is the sensation experienced when nociceptors in structures such as the skin or muscle are subjected to transient non-tissue-damaging noxious mechanical, thermal or chemical stimulation. Pain of this type has a protective role because of the flexion withdrawal reflex it invariably evokes, and because the memory of it serves to ensure that, as far as possible, future similarly potential tissue-damaging circumstances are avoided. Such pain, as Woolf (1989) states:

... is something we all experience frequently in our daily lives by touching hot or cold objects or by exposure to intense external mechanical stimuli that may scratch or prick our skin and, indeed, such pain

occurs frequently in the clinical context with interventions such as injections.

Pain of this type has to be distinguished from pathological nociceptive pain that develops when tissues become damaged.

Pathological nociceptive pain

The tissue damage responsible for the development of pathological nociceptive pain may be readily apparent. This, however, is not always so, as, for example, when such pain arises as a result of MTrP nociceptor activity (Ch. 4).

Recent studies have shown that the behavioural and physical responses to pathological nociceptive pain are dependent on a number of facilitatory and inhibitory modulating mechanisms in various parts of the peripheral and central nervous systems. The structures involved in this complex process include nociceptors, their associated afferent nerve fibres, spinal cord dorsal horns, ascending and descending transmission pathways, the reticular formation in the midbrain and medulla, the thalamus, the limbic system and the cerebral cortex.

As this book is primarily concerned with pain that arises as a result of nociceptive activity developing at TrP sites in muscles, the structures just mentioned which are involved in its production and modulation will be considered in some detail, but before doing so, it is necessary to discuss pain that develops as a result of the stimulation of nociceptors in the skin.

SKIN NOCICEPTORS

Nociceptors in the skin are of two types, A-delta and C-polymodal.

Cutaneous A-delta nociceptors

A-delta nociceptors in the skin are high-threshold mechanoreceptors that become active in response to any intense potentially tissue-damaging mechanical stimulus. In addition, approximately 20–50% of them are mechanothermal receptors that respond not only to mechanical stimuli but also to suddenly applied heat in the noxious range from 45°C upwards.

The receptive field of these high threshold A-delta nociceptors in the skin consists of a number of sensitive spots about 1 mm in diameter grouped together in a cluster covering on average a total of 5 mm^2 (Georgopoulos 1974).

A-delta nociceptor activity gives rise to pain which takes the form of an immediate, sharp, relatively brief pricking sensation – the so-called first or fast pain (Fig. 2.1). This sensation serves to provide a warning of impending tissue damage and is accompanied by reflex flexion withdrawal movements designed to avoid or minimise such damage.

The pain develops as a result of noxiously generated information being conveyed from these nociceptors to the dorsal horn in the spinal cord via medium diameter (1–5 μm) myelinated nerve fibres (Perl 1968) at a conduction velocity of 5–15 metres per second (m/s) (11–33.5 miles per hour) (Table 2.1). From there, it is equally rapidly transmitted up the contralateral laterally situated neospinothalamic pathway to the somatosensory cortex in the parietal lobe (Fig. 2.2).

Cutaneous C-polymodal nociceptors

When skin is damaged as a result of trauma or some disease process, the first physiological type

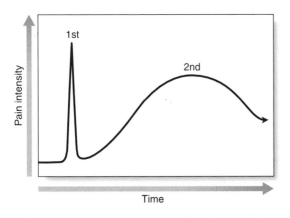

Figure 2.1 Diagrammatic representation of the comparative durations of the first transient physiological pain produced by potentially damaging stimulation of A-delta skin nociceptors and of the second longer lasting pain produced by tissue-damage-induced stimulation of C-polymodal skin nociceptors.

of pain just described is followed by a slower onset, more diffuse, dull aching, persistent, treatment-demanding type of pain – the second pain (Fig. 2.1). This second pain arises as a result of activity developing in unmyelinated C-polymodal nociceptors (C-PMNs). These receptors are termed polymodal because they are capable of responding to either thermal, mechanical or chemical noxious stimuli applied to the skin.

The receptive field of a C-PMN in the skin is smaller than that of a myelinated A-delta nociceptor and usually consists of a single area rather than a cluster of spots (Fields 1987a).

Noxious information generated as a result of high intensity stimulation of cutaneous C-PMNs is conveyed along small diameter (0.25–1.5 μm) non-myelinated afferent fibres (Table 2.1) at a conduction velocity rate of 0.5–2 m/s (1–4.5 mph) to the dorsal horn. Wide dynamic range neurons in the dorsal horn then transmit this information up the contralateral medially situated paleo-spino-diencephalic pathway to the frontal cortex (Fig. 2.2).

MUSCLE NOCICEPTORS

The nociceptors in skeletal muscle mostly take the form of free nerve endings in the walls of arterioles and the surrounding connective tissue (Stacey 1969).

As Mense (1993) has pointed out, 'The marked sensitivity of these free nerve endings to chemical stimuli, particularly to those associated with disturbances of the microcirculation, may be related to their location in or close to the walls of blood vessels'.

Skeletal muscle contains two types of nociceptors – group III and group IV.

Group III muscle nociceptors

Group III nociceptors in muscle are connected to the dorsal horn by medium-sized myelinated afferent fibres.

It has for long been known that pain may be produced by squeezing a muscle between the finger and thumb (Lewis 1942a). And Paintal

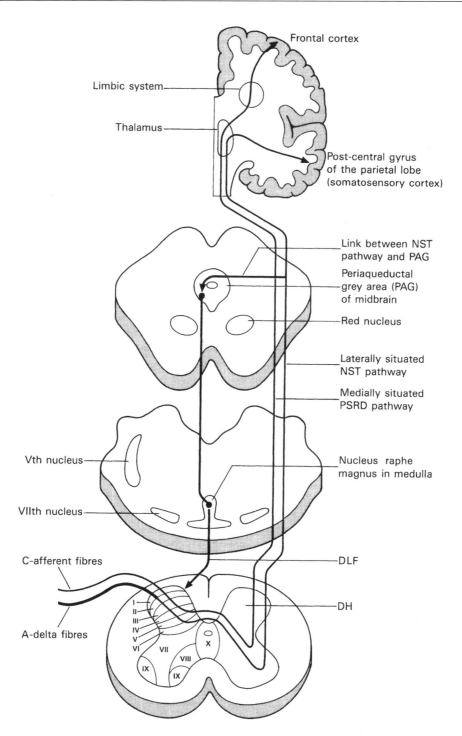

Figure 2.2   Diagrammatic representation of the course taken by the two ascending 'pain' pathways – the neospinothalamic (NST) pathway carrying A-delta 'pin prick' information, and the paleo-spino-diencephalic pathway carrying C 'tissue damage' information. It also shows the descending inhibitory pathway – the dorsolateral funiculus (DLF) which links the periaqueductal grey area (PAG) and the nucleus raphe magnus (NRM) with the dorsal horn (DH).

Table 2.1 Nerve fibre conduction velocities

Nerve fibre	Diameter	Conduction velocity	Function
A-beta (myelinated)	5–15 µm	30–100 m/s (67–223 mph)	Mechanoreception
A-delta (myelinated)	1–5 µm	5–15 m/s (11–33.5 mph)	Nociception (first transient pain)
C (unmyelinated)	0.25–1.5 µm	0.5–2 m/s (1–4.5 mph)	Nociception (second long-term pain)

(1960), from experiments on cats, came to the conclusion that this pressure-induced pain develops as a result of the stimulation of these group III nociceptors. The majority of these pressure receptors (56%) have high thresholds for mechanical stimulation and their activation therefore requires firm noxious squeezing of the muscle, although some respond to light pressure (Raja et al 1988).

Animal experiments have shown that group III nociceptors may also be activated by intra-arterial injections of endogenous substances, such as bradykinin and serotonin, normally released from damaged muscle (Kumazawa & Mizumura 1977), and by the intramuscular injection of hypertonic saline (Paintal 1960).

In addition to this, Mense & Meyer (1988), in experiments on animals, have shown that by infiltrating these nociceptors' receptive fields with bradykinin it is possible to sensitise them and that by lowering their pain threshold in this way they then become responsive to stimuli that would normally be innocuous.

Group III muscle ergoreceptors (non-nociceptive mechanoreceptors)

Experiments on skeletal muscles and tendons in the cat have revealed that a high proportion of group III afferents are attached to low-threshold non-nociceptive mechanoreceptors. Their thresholds, whilst above those of muscle spindles and tendon organs, are nevertheless well within the physiological range so that as a consequence they can be activated by such stimuli as innocuous deformation of the muscle and forceful stretching of it (Mense & Meyer 1985). They therefore tend to be activated during exercise and have an ergoreceptive role.

Group IV muscle nociceptors

Group IV nociceptors in muscle are situated at the peripheral terminals of small diameter unmyelinated afferent fibres and therefore correspond to the C-polymodal nociceptors in the skin. And as will be discussed in Chapter 4, there are grounds for believing that the nociceptors involved in the production of MTrP pain are of this type.

Activation of muscle group IV nociceptors

When a muscle becomes traumatised, either as a result of a direct injury or because of it becoming overloaded, one of the reasons why pain is liable to develop is the consequent tissue damage causing various algesic substances to be liberated that activate group IV nociceptors at MTrP sites in it.

These nociceptor-activating substances include bradykinin, 5-hydroxytryptamine (5-HT; also called serotonin) and potassium ions.

Bradykinin, one of the most potent pain-producing substances present in inflammatory exudates and damaged tissues (Fock & Mense 1976), is produced by enzymatic cleavage from its precursor molecule kallidin present in plasma proteins (Mense 1993).

5-HT is released from platelets and mast cells. And potassium ions are liberated when the sarcoplasm of muscle cells becomes damaged.

Sensitisation of group IV muscle nociceptors

Bradykinin not only activates nociceptors but also sensitises them with, as a consequence, a lowering of their pain threshold so as to make them responsive not only to high intensity noxious stimuli but also to low intensity, mildly noxious or innocuous ones (Mense 1993). In addition, it has the effect of releasing prostaglandins of the E-type (particularly E_2) from damaged tissue cells (Jose et al 1981). And these in turn also have a powerful nociceptor-sensitising effect. By this means therefore bradykinin is capable of potentiating its own sensitising action.

It is because of the sensitisation of its nociceptors that a MTrP is so exquisitely tender, and why the patient involuntarily flinches and utters an expletive when firm pressure is applied to it (Ch. 4).

Neurogenic inflammation

Bradykinin and 5-HT have a strong vasodilatory effect that leads to the development of oedema. Because of this, Sicuteri (1967) calls them vasoneuroactive substances.

In addition to this, when unmyelinated skin C-polymodal and muscle group IV nociceptors become activated and sensitised, they release from their peripheral terminals a number of neuropeptides. These include substance P, calcitonin gene-related peptide, vasoactive intestinal polypeptide and neurokinins. These neuropeptides also give rise to vasodilatation with increased permeability and the development of tissue oedema (Rang et al 1991).

It may be seen therefore that, due to the release of vasoneuroreactive substances and neuropeptides, a sterile neurogenic inflammatory reaction develops with, as a consequence, augmentation of nociceptive pain. In discussing this, Fields (1987b) states:

In a sense, then, nociceptor activity is not merely a passive signal indicating that tissue damage has occurred, but may play an active role in body defences by participating in the inflammatory process ... although the clinical significance of this neurogenic component of inflammation has yet to be determined, there is no doubt that it exists.

Central sensitisation

The activation and subsequent sensitisation of a MTrP's group IV nociceptors together with the neurogenic inflammatory changes just described account for the development of MTrP pain and the exquisite tenderness (primary hyperalgesia) at a MTrP site.

The pain that emanates from a MTrP is not felt locally but is referred to a site some distance away (zone of pain referral). And although the tissues at this distant site are healthy, the application of a mildly noxious stimulation to them, such as that provided by firm pressure, stretching, or the carrying out of movements, shows them to be hyperalgesic (secondary hyperalgesia).

The reason for this secondary hyperalgesia developing is that the sensory afferent barrage set up by the activated and sensitised MTrP nociceptors causes neurons in the dorsal horn to develop a marked increase in the excitability of their sensory processing mechanisms, a phenomenon known as central sensitisation and one which allows them to respond in an abnormal manner to A-beta proprioceptive sensory afferent stimulation with, as a consequence, the development of A-beta sensory afferent-mediated pain.

The biochemical mechanisms responsible for central sensitisation developing are complex and as Coderre et al (1993) and Mense (1997), in comprehensive reviews of the subject have pointed out, there is still much to be learned about them.

Basically, however, it would seem that the sensory afferent barrage set up as a result of the activation and sensitisation of group IV nociceptors on reaching the dorsal horn leads to the release of neuropeptides and glutamate and aspartate excitatory amino acids. These chemicals then have a depolarising effect on N-methyl-D-aspartate (NMDA) receptor ion channels in the cell membranes of dorsal horn neurons.

Under normal conditions these ion channels are held closed by magnesium ions which prevent calcium ions from entering these neurons. The effect of this intense depolarisation, however, is to remove the magnesium ions with the result that their calcium ion content rises (Woolf 1991). And it is because of this that that their excitability becomes increased (MacDermott et al 1986) with the consequent development of the neuroplastic changes known as central sensitisation.

Intracellular second messengers

Recent evidence suggests that this elevation in the calcium ion content of dorsal horn neurons is also promoted by the effects of phospholipase-produced intracellular second messengers. These include inositol triphosphate (IP3) and diacylglycerol (DAG). IP3 is thought to stimulate the release of calcium ions from intracellular stores whilst the role of DAG is to activate protein kinase C (PKC). Chen & Huang (1992) have demonstrated that PKC increases NMDA-activated currents in isolated trigeminal cells by reducing the voltage-dependent magnesium block of NMDA-receptor channels, and by this means increases the calcium ion influx to neurons. Also, that this in turn, by raising the intracellular calcium ion content, increases PKC activity and its effects on NMDA receptor channels. Coderre et al (1993) are of the opinion that this positive feedback loop may make an important contribution to the production and maintenance of central sensitisation.

Effects of central sensitisation

From animal experiments (Mense 1997) there are grounds for believing that the sensitisation of dorsal horn neurons brought about as a result of the sensory afferent barrage which develop in response to the activation and sensitisation of group IV nociceptors at MTrP sites has the following effects: (i) an increase in the receptive fields of dorsal horn neurons leads to the spread and referral of MTrP pain; (ii) the development of A-beta-mediated pain with, as a consequence, the development of secondary hyperalgesia in the zone of MTrP pain referral; and (iii) the perpetuation of dorsal horn neuronal activity with, as a consequence, the persistence of the pain.

It should be noted that for some unknown reason this dorsal horn neuronal hyperexcitability is more readily produced by the sensory afferent barrage arising from activity in muscle group IV nociceptors than by one arising from activity in skin C-polymodal nociceptors (Wall & Woolf 1984).

The referral of pain from myofascial trigger points

Lewis (1942b) was one of the first to point out that pain which develops as a result of the application of a noxious stimulus to the skin is accurately located by the brain but that pain which develops as a result of injury to muscle is perceived by the brain as arising some distance away from the affected site.

The pain referral theory currently accepted as being the most credible is the convergence-facilitation concept first put forward by Mackenzie in 1909, reintroduced by Ruch in 1949, and more recently modified by Mense.

An integral part of the hypothesis put forward by Mense (1991) is the assumption that afferent fibres from a muscle's nociceptors make synaptic contact not only with dorsal horn neurons responsible for conducting rostrally nociceptive information from that muscle but also with neighbouring neurons that normally transmit centripetally sensory information from other muscles and/or from the skin.

Noordenbos (1987) would certainly have considered such an assumption to be justified for he said, 'one to one synaptic transmission is the exception rather than the rule in the CNS. A neuron is acted upon by many other neurons and it in turn, by virtue of the ramification, acts upon many other neurons'.

In the light of Mense's hypothetical circuitry depicted in Figure 2.3, it would seem reasonable to suggest with respect to MTrP pain that when nociceptors at a MTrP site in a proximally situated muscle become activated and sensitised (p. 23), the afferent barrage which develops in their sensory afferents (A), not only activates and sensitises the dorsal horn neurons (1) primarily responsible for transmitting, rostrally, nociceptive information conveyed to them by these afferents, but because of the synaptic link (B) it also activates and sensitises dorsal horn neurons (2) that are primarily responsible for transmitting centripetally sensory information from a distal muscle. Thus because of this the brain receives confusing messages and as a result mislocates the pain and perceives it as coming from the distal muscle.

Theoretically, according to Mense's hypothesis, excitation of dorsal horn neurons (3) concerned with transmitting information from the skin should also take place because of activity developing in pathway C (Fig. 2.3) with, as a result of this, the referral of MTrP pain to the skin. In practice, however, this does not happen.

Mense also expressed the opinion that path D (Fig. 2.3) in his diagram offers an explanation for the experimental finding that after strong stimulation of muscle nociceptors, dorsal horn neurons with input from muscle sometimes exhibit new receptive fields in a distal muscle. And since then he has added two new components to the convergence-projection theory. These are that 'convergent connections from deep tissues to dorsal horn neurones are not present from the beginning but are opened by nociceptive input from skeletal muscle', and that 'referral to myotomes outside the lesion is due to spread of central sensitisation to adjacent spinal segments' (Mense 1994).

The development of muscle pain as a consequence of visceral disease

When nociceptive sensory afferent fibres innervating a visceral organ and those innervating a somatic structure enter the spinal cord at the same segmental level, they converge on the same dorsal horn transmission neurons. The consequence of this is that the brain, because it has no way of telling from which of these two sites the noxious stimulus has arisen and because the transmission neurons are more frequently activated by somatic stimuli than they are by visceral ones, tends to mislocate the pain of visceral origin and erroneously perceive it as coming from a somatic structure such as muscle.

The convergence of visceral and somatic afferent fibres on to the same transmission neurons is particularly common in the thoracic region (Cervero 1983, Foreman et al 1984).

A good example of this is the pain of myocardial ischaemia. The afferent input from the heart, together with the sensory input from somatic structures on the left side of the chest and from the ulnar aspect of the left arm, all enter the

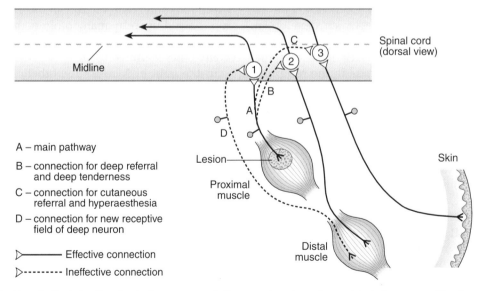

A – main pathway

B – connection for deep referral and deep tenderness

C – connection for cutaneous referral and hyperaesthesia

D – connection for new receptive field of deep neuron

▷——— Effective connection

▷----- Ineffective connection

Figure 2.3 Hypothetical circuitry of spinal neurons mediating muscle pain and associated phenomena. The figure is largely based on the convergence-facilitation concept of Mackenzie (1909). (Reproduced with permission from the *Canadian Journal of Physiology and Pharmacology* (1990) 69: 610–616.)

dorsal horn at the level of the first thoracic segment, with the result that the brain erroneously locates the pain in the praecordium and inner side of the left arm.

It also helps to explain why, when coronary heart disease pain is referred down the left arm, the tissues in the arm, despite being healthy, become tender.

Melzack and Wall (1988b), in discussing this, state:

The tenderness of the arm suggests that nerve impulses from the heart and from the region where pain is referred must converge and summate and thereby increase the pain.

Finally, it remains to be said that the convergence-facilitation hypothesis helps to explain why the nociceptive input from internal organs appears to augment the excitation of transmission neurons primarily concerned with receiving inputs from muscle nociceptors. It is this mechanism that probably accounts for the clinical observation that muscle tenderness and pain often develop in association with visceral diseases.

Despite the various hypotheses and anatomical observations just described, there is still much work to be done before there can be any certainty as to exactly how pain referral from MTrPs, or for that matter from any other source, takes place. After discussing the matter at some length, Simons (1990) concluded:

We see that there is much evidence for many mechanisms that refer pain, tenderness and autonomic phenomena . . . the fact that at this time we are unable to identify which mechanism(s) contribute to the clinical pain phenomena with which we are concerned does not mean that their recognition is unimportant. It does suggest that this is one of the important gaps in our knowledge that must be filled before we can hope to truly understand muscle pain syndromes.

TRANSMISSION OF NOCICEPTIVE INFORMATION TO THE BRAIN

The spinal cord's dorsal and ventral horn laminae

The Swedish anatomist, Bror Rexed (1952) established that the cells in the spinal cord are arranged in layers or laminae (Fig. 2.2). There are six laminae in the dorsal horn (laminae I–VI); three in the ventral horn (laminae VII–IX); and an additional column of cells clustered around the central canal known as lamina X (Fields 1987c).

At the outer part of the dorsal horn there is a clear zone visible to the naked eye to which the Italian anatomist Luigi Rolando (1773–1831) first drew attention. It is now known to be made up of a marginal layer (lamina I) and the substantia gelatinosa (lamina II). The latter will be considered in some detail when discussing the pain-modulating gate control theory.

Transmission neurons

There are three types of transmission neurons responsible for projecting sensory information to the brain.

(1) Non-nociceptive neurons

These are found mainly in laminae III and IV and their function is to transmit proprioceptive information to the brain.

(2) Nociceptive specific neurons

These are present principally in lamina I but to a lesser extent in lamina V (Christensen & Perl 1970) and transmit A-delta nociceptive inputs from the skin to the brain.

(3) Wide dynamic range neurons

These are present in all the laminae but are mainly concentrated in laminae V, VII and VIII. They have been given this name because they respond to a wide range of stimuli including both noxious and innocuous ones that are conveyed to them via sensory afferent fibres. The information that they project to the higher centres therefore varies according to the particular type of stimulus applied to receptors in either skin, muscle or a viscus.

Trigeminal brainstem nociceptive transmission neurons

Orofacial sensory information is conveyed to the higher centres by transmission neurons in the trigeminal brainstem complex. This complex consists of a main sensory nucleus and a spinal descending tract nucleus which, from its upper to its lower part, is divided into the subnuclei oralis, interpolaris and caudalis (see Fig. 11.5). Although electrophysiological and behavioural studies have implicated the subnuclei oralis and interpolaris in orofacial pain mechanisms, it is the subnucleus caudalis which is considered to be of particular importance with respect to the transmission of nociceptive information (Sessle 1990). And it is because this structure has such close morphological and physiological similarities with the spinal cord's dorsal horns that the alternative name that has now been given to it is the medullary dorsal horn (Bonica 1990).

There is therefore reason to believe that it is principally neurons in the subnucleus caudalis that are involved in the centripetal transmission of information generated in nociceptors in the craniofacial region including those present at MTrP sites. And, as will be discussed in Chapter 11, in the case of migraine and tension-type headaches it serves to integrate vascular and myofascial nociceptive inputs prior to their transmission to the cerebral cortex (Olesen 1991).

PATHWAYS FOR CENTRIPETAL TRANSMISSION OF NOCICEPTIVE INFORMATION

The long-held belief that nociceptive information is transmitted centripetally via a single contralateral spinothalamic tract had to be revised in the 1950s when it was shown that the transmission is through two separate pathways with each of these having its own conduction velocity and termination in the brain (Kerr et al 1955).

It is now recognised that these pathways have developed over the course of time as part of an evolutionary process (Melzack & Wall 1988c) and their relative importance varies from one species to another (Willis 1989).

The phylogenetically younger tract is the neospinothalamic pathway and the older one is the paleo-spino-reticulo-diencephalic pathway (spinoreticular tract) (Bowsher 1957).

Neospinothalamic pathway

The neospinothalamic pathway (Fig. 2.2) arises from the dorsal horn's laminae I and V, where the majority of the small myelinated A-delta nociceptive fibres terminate. It ascends in the contralateral anterolateral tract to reach the ventrobasal nucleus in the lateral part of the thalamus, from where it projects to the somatosensory cortex in the post-central gyrus. This topographically organised lateral pathway subserves the sensory-discriminative process responsible for the localisation and identification of a noxious stimulus (Melzack & Casey 1968) and for determining when such a stimulus reaches the pain threshold.

Paleo-spino-reticulo-diencephalic pathway (syns: spinoreticular tract, paramedian pathway)

This pathway, which Melzack & Casey (1968) call the paramedian pathway, arises mainly from laminae VII and VIII of the dorsal horn and to a lesser extent from lamina V (Fig. 2.2). As this pathway carries noxiously generated information that is conveyed to the dorsal horn by nonmyelinated C and group IV sensory afferents which terminate in neurons in laminae I and II, it follows that electrical impulses from these neurons have to pass through several internuncial relays before reaching laminae V, VII and VIII. From the dorsal horn, it ascends in the contralateral anterolateral tract alongside the neospinothalamic pathway until it reaches the base of the brain, where it separates from this by passing medially into the brainstem's reticular tissue. And from there, it ascends to the cerebral cortex via medially situated intralaminar nuclei in the thalamus.

BRAINSTEM'S RETICULAR FORMATION

The reticular formation which ramifies throughout the medulla and midbrain is so called because its dense mass of neurons with overlapping and intertwining dendrites give it a net-like appearance.

As Casey (1980) has pointed out, it is because neurons in the reticular formation have bifurcating axons which project downwards to the spinal cord and upwards to the thalamus and hypothalamus that this structure is so extremely well adapted to playing a major integrating role in pain experience and behaviour.

It is because the reticular formation has descending axons which project to ventral horn motor neurons that when, because of anxiety, this brainstem structure becomes hyperactive, motor neuronal stimulation leads to increased motor efferent activity in muscles. As a consequence of this there is an increase in muscle tone (Nathan 1982) and, for reasons to be discussed in Chapters 3 and 4, the development of MTrP pain. As Mense (1990) has succinctly stated, 'skeletal muscle is a tool for expressing emotional states in higher mammals and, thus, psychogenic changes of muscle tone may become a source of pain'.

The reticular formation contains several nuclei which make important contributions to the experience of pain and the behavioural activities associated with this. One of these is the nucleus reticularis gigantocellularis situated in the medulla. This nucleus, which receives a large input from the paramedian pathway and which has an upwards projection to the intralaminar part of the thalamus, contains neurons whose discharge in response to a noxious stimulus sets off aversive escape behaviour (Casey 1971a, 1971b; Casey et al 1974). In addition, serotonin-containing cells in this nucleus and the adjacent nucleus raphe magnus, together with neurons in the periaqueductal grey area of the midbrain from which they receive an excitatory input, form the upper part of the opioid peptide-mediated descending inhibitory system that is of such considerable importance in the control of pain.

Most of the fibres in the paramedian pathway terminate at the reticular formation but some continue upwards to the medially situated intralaminal nuclei of the thalamus. There are also separate ascending projections from the reticular formation that reach both these thalamic nuclei and the hypothalamus. It is because of this link between the reticular formation and the hypothalamus that tissue-damage-induced, noxiously generated information conveyed centripetally in the paramedian pathway has autonomic concomitants.

From the intralaminal nuclei of the thalamus there are projections to a number of structures clustered around the thalamus which collectively form the limbic system. In addition, there are projections to other parts of the brain including, in particular, the frontal lobe.

Limbic system

The limbic system consists of a group of structures clustered around the thalamus. These include the hypothalamus, the hippocampus (Greek, 'sea horse'), the amygdala (Latin, 'almond'), the cingulate gyrus and the cingulum bundle which connects the hippocampus with the frontal cortex.

There is evidence to show that the limbic structures control the motivational or behavioural responses to pain together with the emotional (affective) response to it.

Therefore, it is the extent to which the limbic system becomes activated in response to any given noxious stimulus that determines how much any particular individual suffers from it – in other words, the degree to which it hurts that person. Thus it is activity in the limbic system which governs a person's pain tolerance.

Frontal cortex

As pain is a physico-emotional experience it is considerably influenced by cognitive activities such as memories of past experiences, mood and prevailing circumstances. By virtue of the frontal cortex having a two-way communication system not only with all sensory cortical areas but also with the limbic and reticular structures, it controls both these cognitive activities and the paramedian system's motivational-affective ones (Melzack & Casey 1968).

In the past, extensive resections of the frontal lobes were performed as a last resort for intractable pain. Patients who underwent this, because the sensory component of pain subserved by the somatosensory cortex was still present, remained aware of the pain and often said it was as intense as before, but they were no longer worried about it and no longer needed medication for it. The effect of a lobotomy, therefore, was to reduce the motivational-affective and aversive dimensions of the pain experience. As Freeman & Watts (1950) remarked, 'prefrontal lobotomy changes the attitude of the individual towards his pain, but does not alter the perception of pain'.

PAIN-MODULATING MECHANISMS

Fast blocks slow concept

Henry Head's (1920) identification of an epicritic system which suppresses a protopathic one; Zotterman's (1933) discovery that the speed with which nociceptive information is conducted along small diameter unmyelinated sensory afferents is much slower than the speed with which proprioceptive information is conducted along large diameter myelinated fibres; and Bishop's (1946) observations concerning what he called the fast and slow sensory systems led Noordenbos (1959) to consider the possibility that one of the ways in which pain modulation may be brought about is by activity in the rapidly conducting large diameter myelinated system having an inhibitory effect on activity in the slower conducting small diameter unmyelinated system. This is an interaction which he pithily described as 'fast blocks slow'. This concept so impressed Wall (1960) that he decided to investigate it experimentally and in a series of ingenious recordings from single dorsal horn cells was able to confirm that pain suppression does occur as a result of this fast–slow sensory nerve interaction. Prior to this it had been discovered that

pain suppression may also be brought about by the development of activity in a descending inhibitory system situated in the spinal cord.

Discovery of a descending inhibitory system

In 1954 Hagbarth and Kerr found that stimulation of either the reticular formation, the cerebellum or the cerebral cortex has a controlling influence on the flow of nociceptive impulses up the anterolateral tract, and concluded that this must be because each of these structures is capable of exerting a descending inhibitory effect on dorsal horn transmission cells. Then, in 1958, Melzack, Stotler and Livingston quite unexpectedly discovered, during the course of experiments on cats, that damage to a small area of reticular tissue known as the central tegmental tract situated near the midbrain's periaqueductal grey area markedly enhances pain perception in these animals. It was presumed that this must be because tissue damage at this site interferes with a naturally occurring inhibitory system. The presence of such a system has since been confirmed and it is now known that it is serotonergically mediated (see p. 37).

Gate-control theory

The gate-control theory put forward by Melzack and Wall in 1965 has profoundly influenced present ideas concerning the transmission of noxious impulses from the periphery to the cortex and how the sensation of pain may be modulated by various physicochemical mechanisms in the peripheral and central nervous systems. Admittedly, this theory has had to be revised over the years in the light of further knowledge. Nevertheless it remains a remarkably useful hypothesis, for as Liebskind & Paul (1977) said when discussing reasons for the current interest in pain research,

Probably the most important was the appearance in 1965 of the gate-control theory of pain by Melzack and Wall. This theory, like none before it, has proved enormously heuristic. It continues to inspire basic research and clinical applications.

Melzack and Wall were led to formulate their hypothesis because of various important discoveries made during the 1950s, but as Wall (1990) has since admitted, what influenced their thinking most of all was Noordenbos's ideas concerning the interaction between large and small diameter sensory afferent fibres and Wall's ability to provide experimental confirmation of this.

The theory as originally propounded by them stated that in each dorsal horn there is a gate-like mechanism which inhibits or facilitates the flow of afferent impulses into the spinal cord. The opening or closing of the 'gate' is dependent on the relative activity in large diameter (A-beta) and small diameter fibres (A-delta and C), with activity in the large diameter fibres tending to close the 'gate' and activity in the small diameter fibres tending to open it. In addition, the position of the 'gate' is influenced by the brain's descending inhibitory system.

Substantia gelatinosa

From the start, Melzack and Wall envisaged the 'gate' as being the dorsal horn's lamina II, or what is known as the substantia gelatinosa, where inhibitory interneurons are situated. They also premised that the interaction between the large and small diameter fibres influences activity in these interneurons and also in the dorsal horn transmission cells (T cells). It was thought, and subsequently confirmed, that the large diameter myelinated afferents excite the inhibitory interneurons, and that the effect of this is to reduce presynaptically the input to the T cells and thereby to inhibit pain. They further postulated that activity in small diameter unmyelinated fibres, by inhibiting activity in the inhibitory interneurons, facilitates the flow of noxious impulses to the T cells and thereby enhances pain.

By the time that Melzack and Wall introduced their theory, there was already good evidence to support their belief that it is the substantia gelatinosa (lamina II) which acts as the 'gate'. Szentagothai (1964) and Wall (1964) had shown that it receives axons directly and indirectly from large and small diameter fibres, that it has connections with cells in deeper laminae, and that its cells connect with one another and are connected to similar cells at distant sites – on the ipsilateral side by means of Lissauer's tract and on the opposite side by means of fibres that cross the cord.

Although it remains reasonable to assume that it is the substantia gelatinosa which acts as the spinal gating mechanism, Melzack and Wall (1982a) have found it necessary to emphasise that there is still no absolute proof of this. They also posed the rhetorical question – 'If the substantia gelatinosa is a gate control, why is it so complex?' – and answered this by saying it would be wrong to consider that this structure is only concerned with the modulation of nociceptive impulses, but rather that it has to monitor all forms of incoming information and that it is likely to have 'to control and emphasise different aspects of the arriving messages with the emphasis changing from moment to moment'.

There can be no doubt, therefore, that the substantia gelatinosa has the properties of a complex computer and, the greater the detail in which its structure and function are studied, the more intricate the mechanisms contained in it are found to be. There is now experimental evidence to show that the cells in it, together with those in the underlying laminae, are somatotopically organised (Melzack & Wall 1982b) in the same way as are cells in the dorsal column's medial lemniscus system (Millar & Basbaum 1975) and cells in midbrain structures (Soper & Melzack 1982).

It is now also known that the afferent nociceptive input to the substantia gelatinosa is influenced by several descending inhibitory systems linking cortical and brainstem structures with the dorsal horn via the dorsolateral funiculus. At the present time it would seem that of the various descending inhibitory systems, it is the opioid peptide mediated one which is the most important and for this reason a detailed account of it will be given later in this chapter.

It is obvious from the number of peptides found in the substantia gelatinosa in recent years that its function must be extremely complicated.

These include vasoactive intestinal peptide, somatostatin, angiotensin, cholecystokinin and substance P (Jessell 1982). Endogenous opioids are also found in the dorsal horn of the spinal cord in the same areas as small diameter primary pain afferents containing substance P neurons and opiate receptors (Clement-Jones 1983). And once it became known that morphine inhibits the release of substance P, a primary afferent nociceptive transmitter, it became clear that, in addition to there being an opioid peptide-mediated descending inhibitory system, opioid-containing interneurons presynaptically control the afferent nociceptive input to the spinal cord (Jessell & Iversen 1977).

There are thus strong arguments in support of Melzack and Wall's original idea that the substantia gelatinosa acts as a complicated 'gating' mechanism which modulates the input of noxiously generated information to the spinal cord and its onward transmissions to the brain. For a more detailed account of the evidence in support of the substantia gelatinosa's role as a controlling 'gate', reference should be made to Wall's (1980a, 1980b, 1989) comprehensive reviews of the subject.

Revision of the gate-control theory

Advances in knowledge since 1965 have inevitably led to the theory being revised. For example, Melzack and Wall soon came to the conclusion that there are excitatory as well as inhibitory interneurons in the substantia gelatinosa and that the inhibition not only occurs presynaptically, as originally thought, but also takes place postsynaptically.

Furthermore, when the gate-control theory was first put forward, it was considered that the flow of centripetal impulses into the dorsal horn, and from there up to the brain, was influenced partly by descending inhibitory mechanisms and partly by the relative activity in small diameter and large diameter afferent nerve fibres, and that it is always the net result of these various facilitatory and inhibitory effects which control the activation of T cells.

When Wall, however, re-examined the theory in 1978, he pointed out that the situation was not as straightforward as might have appeared at first, and that large diameter fibre activity is, in certain circumstances, capable of firing T cells, so that the inputs from large and small fibres may at times summate with each other. He also admitted that their original ideas concerning the inhibitory effects of large diameter fibres was much influenced by Noordenbos (1959) who, having shown that in post-herpetic neuralgia there is a loss of large myelinated fibres, generalised from this observation by proposing that pain in general is due to a loss of inhibition normally provided by large fibres. However, as Wall (1978) said,

> We now know that loss of large fibres is not necessarily followed by pain. In Friedreich's ataxia there is just such a preferential large-fibre deficit without pain... and ... the polyneuropathy of renal failure in adults is not associated with complaints of pain although there is a preferential destruction of large fibres.

He then cites many other examples to show that 'Any attempt to correlate the remaining fibre diameter spectrum with the symptomatology of neuropathies is no longer possible'.

This notwithstanding, it would seem that when the central nervous system is intact and unaffected by disease, the balance between the large and small diameter fibres in determining the output of T cells remains an acceptable hypothesis. The theory has also been subjected to criticism by Nathan (1976) for neglecting the known facts about stimulus specificity of nerve fibres which have emerged since von Frey first developed his theory about this in the closing years of the 19th century.

For all these various reasons and others, including advances in knowledge concerning the relative functions of A-delta and C nerve fibres, Melzack and Wall have had to subject their theory to certain modifications (Wall 1978, Melzack & Wall 1982c, 1988d). Nevertheless, it remains remarkably useful and has been considerably enriched by subsequent biochemical discoveries. Much, however, remains to be explained. For example, the descending control system has turned out to be not one system but a number of systems involving a complexity of chemical substances. And when enkephalin-containing terminals and opiate receptor-bearing axons were discovered, it was assumed that they must make contact, but, surprisingly, this apparently is not so (Hunt et al 1980).

Despite all this, 25 years after Melzack and Wall first put forward their gate-control theory, Verrill (1990), during the course of reviewing its influence on current ideas concerning pain modulation was led to conclude that,

Despite continuing controversy over details, the fundamental concept underlying the gate theory has survived in a modified and stronger state accommodating and harmonizing with, rather than supplanting specificity and pattern theories. It has stimulated multidisciplinary activity, opened minds and benefited patients.

ENDOGENOUS PAIN-SUPPRESSING SUBSTANCES

Opiate receptors

During the 1970s, biochemists and pharmacologists were becoming increasingly convinced that the reason why morphine is such a powerful analgesic is that there are highly specific pharmacological receptors in the central nervous system on which this substance can readily act. In 1973, Solomon Snyder of the Johns Hopkins School of Medicine, Baltimore, and Candice Pert of the US National Institute of Mental Health discovered during the course of basic research on drug addiction that there are clusters of cells in certain parts of the brain, including the brainstem nuclei, the thalamus and hypothalamus, which serve as opiate receptors (Pert & Snyder 1973). A number of cells in the dorsal horn were then also found to have the same function (Atweh & Kuhar 1977). The finding of opiate receptors in the midbrain perhaps was not so surprising as it had already been shown that an injection of only a small amount of morphine into the area has a considerable analgesic effect (Tsou & Jang 1964). However, of particular interest was the discovery that there are also cells with the same function in the substantia

gelatinosa of the dorsal horn and that a local injection of a small amount of morphine into this structure has a markedly inhibitory effect on the response of lamina V transmission cells to afferent nociceptive stimuli (Duggan et al 1976). This lent considerable support to the idea that the substantia gelatinosa has an important pain-modulating function. It is now known that there are at least three distinct types of opioid receptors termed mu, kappa and delta (Paterson et al 1983).

The distribution of opiate receptors in the central nervous system (CNS) is of considerable interest. There are numerous ones in the paramedian system's intralaminal (medial) thalamic nuclei, the reticular formation and limbic structures. In contrast, however, there are only a few in the neospinothalamic system's ventrobasal thalamus and post-central gyrus. This explains why a micro-injection of morphine into structures in the paramedian system has a powerful analgesic effect but not when injected into the ventrobasal thalamus. It also explains why morphine has no effect on the first, rapid onset, transitory type of pain which develops when A-delta nociceptors in the skin are stimulated, as for example, by a pinprick, and yet is capable of suppressing the second, slow onset, more prolonged type of pain which may arise when damage to the skin is of such severity as to activate its C-polymodal nociceptors. Also, why it is capable of suppressing the similar type of widespread dull aching pain which arises when group IV muscle nociceptors are subjected to trauma-induced activation.

In the dorsal horn there are large numbers of opiate receptors situated postsynaptically on the intraspinal part of C-afferent nerve fibres, but at present the biological significance of these remains unknown (Fields & Basbaum 1989). In addition, there is evidence to suggest that they may also be present at the peripheral ends of these fibres (Schaible & Grubb 1993).

It is because of a particularly high concentration of opiate receptors in the substantia gelatinosa that a micro-injection of morphine into this structure has a marked pain-suppressing effect. It is also why lumbar intrathecal injections of opiates produce profound analgesia in animals (Yaksh & Rudy 1976) and man (Wang et al 1979).

In addition, there is a high concentration of opiate receptors in the corpus striatum. Their function there, however, is unknown. They are also extremely numerous in the brainstem's respiratory centre. This explains why morphine is such a powerful respiratory depressant.

Opioid peptides

Once these opiate receptors had been located, it was argued that nature was hardly likely to have provided animals, including humans, with them for the sole purpose of having somewhere for opium and its derivatives to latch on to should they happen to be introduced into the body. It was considered far more probable that they are present because morphine-like substances (opioid peptides) are produced endogenously.

A search for physiologically occurring morphine-like substances was therefore instituted. Many scientists took part in this including Snyder and his colleagues at Baltimore; Terenius and Wahlström in Uppsala; and Hughes, Kosterlitz and their co-workers in Aberdeen.

The big breakthrough occurred in 1975 when Hughes, Kosterlitz and their colleagues in the Unit for Research on Addictive Drugs at Aberdeen University, in collaboration with a research team at Reckitt & Colman, isolated a substance from the brains of pigs which appeared to act like morphine and which latched on to opiate receptors in the brain. They named it enkephalin ('in the head'). It was a major discovery, and Lewin (1976) showed considerable prescience by commenting:

With the structure of enkephalin now at hand ... we are now poised for an exciting breakthrough in the complete understanding of opiate analgesia, addiction and tolerance. Probably the most intriguing aspect of all this is the inescapable implication of the existence of an unexpected chemical transmitter system in the brain, a system which may have something to do with dampening pain, but almost certainly has more general effects also.

Linda Fothergil at Aberdeen University and Barry Morgan at Reckitt & Colman attempted to analyse its structure and soon established that it was a peptide, but came up against certain technical difficulties in discovering the exact sequence of its amino acids. Therefore, they enlisted the help of a spectroscopist, Howard Morris, at Imperial College, London. Morris was able to show that in fact there are two enkephalin polypeptides – leucine (leu) and methionine (met) enkephalin – but for a time the chemical source from which these substances are made in the body remained a mystery.

By a strange chance, about the time that Morris was considering this, he attended a lecture at Imperial College given by Derek Smythe of the National Institute for Medical Research on beta-lipotrophin, a 91 amino acid peptide which had been isolated from the pituitary glands of sheep 10 years previously (Li et al 1965). Smythe showed a series of slides illustrating its chemical structure and as Morris sat there looking at these, he suddenly saw to his amazement the amino acid sequence of met-enkephalin hidden away in the 61–65 position of the beta-lipotrophin structure. It subsequently became apparent, however, that met- and leu-enkephalin are derived by enzyme cleavage not from this substance but from the precursor proenkephalin A. Since the discovery of the enkephalins, opioid bioactivity has been found in various beta-lipotrophin fragments with the most potent of these being one in the 61–91 position known as beta-endorphin (Fig. 2.4).

It is now known that beta-endorphin, together with beta-lipotrophin and ACTH (corticotrophin), are all derived by enzyme cleavage from a large precursor peptide called pro-opiomelanocortin but that, of these three polypeptides, only beta-endorphin has known analgesic activity, and also that ACTH acts as a physiological antagonist of this (Smock & Fields 1980).

More recently two other opioid peptides with N-terminals identical to that of leu-enkephalin have been isolated. These are dynorphin, a 17 amino acid peptide (Goldstein et al 1979), and the decapeptide alpha-neoendorphin (Weber et al 1981), both of which are cleaved from yet another precursor, pro-enkephalin B (pro-dynorphin).

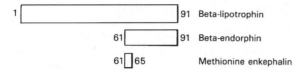

Figure 2.4 Schematic representation of the 91 amino acid peptide beta lipotrophin and other peptides structurally related to it.

These various substances are sometimes referred to collectively as endorphins (endogenous morphine-like substances) but as there are three distinct families of these peptides – enkephalins, dynorphins and endorphins – it is better simply to call them opioid peptides (Thompson 1984).

Distribution of endogenous opioid peptides

Studies using radioimmunoassays and immunohistochemical techniques have demonstrated high levels of enkephalins and dynorphins in the limbic structures, the periaqueductal grey area, the nucleus raphe magnus and the substantia gelatinosa of the dorsal horn. From these sites, opioid peptides spill over into the cerebrospinal fluid. In addition, opioid peptides are released from the anterior pituitary and adrenal medulla into the plasma.

By means of radioimmunoassays and gel filtration techniques, it has been possible to demonstrate the presence of beta-endorphin and met-enkephalin in human plasma (Clement-Jones 1983). Beta-endorphin is found there in association with beta-lipotrophin and ACTH. And each of these shows the same pattern of circadian secretion from the anterior pituitary (Shanks et al 1981). Plasma levels of met-enkephalin, however, show no relationship to those of these other three peptides during circadian studies and corticosteroid suppression tests. This is because unlike them, it is not derived from the pituitary (Clement-Jones & Besser 1983) but rather from a number of other structures including the adrenal glands (Clement-Jones et al 1980), the gut, sympathetic ganglia and peripheral autonomic neurons (Smith et al 1981).

MYOFASCIAL TRIGGER POINT PAIN-SUPPRESSING TECHNIQUES

Deep dry needling

Muscle proprioceptive sensory afferents

A MTrP is made up of a number of dysfunctional motor end plates, juxtapositional contraction knots and closely related neurovascular bundles that contain blood vessels, contiguous sympathetic fibres, group IV small diameter nociceptive sensory afferent fibres and group IA, IB and II large diameter proprioceptive sensory afferents (see Fig. 4.2). The function of the latter fibres is to transmit to the brain information about the change in the length of muscle fibres and the rate at which this takes place.

Dry needle-evoked local twitch response

One of the effects of rapidly inserting a needle into the substance of an active MTrP (see Ch. 4) is to produce a local twitch response (LTR). This LTR causes alterations to take place in the length and tension of the muscle fibres. And one of the outcomes of this is the arousal of proprioceptive activity with the development of a large diameter sensory afferent input to the dorsal horn. This is because a change in total length of the muscle fibres and the rate of this change is detected by group IA fibres, and the total change in length is sensed by group II fibres.

Chu (1995) has therefore expressed the belief that when a needle is rapidly thrust into a MTrP with its group IV nociceptors in an active pain-producing state, the local twitch response evoked leads to the development of a large diameter sensory afferent proprioceptive input to the spinal cord and this, for reasons previously discussed (see p. 30), has the 'gate-controlling' effect of blocking the intra-dorsal horn passage of noxious information generated in the MTrP's nociceptors with, as a consequence, alleviation of the pain (Box 2.1).

This, however, would only seem to be one of the mechanisms involved, for a controlled trial carried out by Fine et al (1988) has shown that any pain alleviation brought about by a local anaesthetic injection into a TrP is reversed by the specific opioid receptor antagonist naloxone. There are therefore grounds for believing that the pain-relieving effect of needling a TrP is due not only to the proprioceptive gate-controlling effect just described but also to a needle-induced activation of an endogenous opioid system.

This MTrP deactivating technique has been termed intramuscular stimulation (Gunn 1996) but in my view is best called deep dry needling in order to distinguish it from what has come to be known as superficial dry needling.

Lewit (1979), a physician in Czechoslovakia, was the first to draw attention to the use of deep dry needling (DDN) for the deactivation of MTrPs. Since then Gunn (1996) has written extensively and enthusiastically about it. And Hong (1994), from carrying out comparative clinical trials, has concluded that in order to obtain the best results with this procedure, it is necessary to evoke a series of LTRs by rapidly inserting the needle into a number of separate loci in the MTrP (see Chs 4 and 7).

One considerable disadvantage of the technique is that inserting a needle into an active MTrP gives rise to a considerable amount of pain and this is markedly increased when the needle is repeatedly thrust into it for the purpose of evoking a number of LTRs in quick succession.

Superficial dry needling

The stimulation of A-delta nerve fibres such as, for example, may be brought about by inserting a needle into the skin is capable of suppressing cutaneous C-polymodal and muscle group IV nociceptive pain by several means (Bowsher 1991). These include its direct action on enkephalinergic inhibitory interneurons in the dorsal horn and indirect action on them via the serotonergic descending inhibitory system, and also its stimulating effect on a descending noradrenergic system and bringing into action diffuse noxious inhibitory controls.

Enkephalinergic inhibitory interneurons (Fig. 2.5)

The dorsal horn terminals of cutaneous A-delta sensory afferents not only project to Waldeyer cells in lamina I which transmit noxiously generated information conveyed in these afferents up the contralateral neospinothalamic tract to the somatosensory cortex, with, as a consequence, the development of a transitory 'first' pain. They have also been shown, both in the cat (Bennett et al 1982) and in humans (Abdel-Maguid & Bowsher 1984), to project to enkephalinergic inhibitory interneurons (stalked cells) situated along the border separating lamina I (marginal layer) from lamina II (substantia gelatinosa).

Box 2.1   Deep dry needling's MTrP-pain relieving mechanisms

1. Insertion of a needle into an active pain-producing MTrP
↓
Activation of pain-suppressing endogenous opioid system
ALSO
2. Repeated rapid insertions of needle into active MTrP
↓
Local twitch responses
↓
Alterations in length of muscle fibres
↓
Mechanoreceptive large diameter sensory afferent input to dorsal horn
↓
Blockade of intra-dorsal horn passage of the MTrP's nociceptive information
↓
Alleviation of the MTrP pain

And A-delta sensory afferent-induced activity in these interneurons causes them to release opioid peptides which then block the intra-dorsal horn passage of noxiously generated information conveyed to the spinal cord in C-polymodal and group IV sensory afferents by suppressing activity in cells to which these afferents project.

Serotonergic descending inhibitory system (Fig. 2.5)

Melzack et al's (1958) observations, during the course of experiments on cats, that damage to a small area of rectangular tissue known as the central tegmental tract situated near to the midbrain's periaqueductal grey area markedly enhances pain perception (see p. 30), prompted David Reynolds, a young psychologist at the University of Windsor, Ontario, to investigate whether, by electrically stimulating this tract, it might be possible to increase the effects of any inhibitory system that might be present there to such an extent as to bring about pain suppres-sion. And in 1969 he reported that the effect of doing this is to produce such a profound degree of analgesia that it is possible to carry out sur-gical operations on conscious rats and other animals (Reynolds 1969).

Unfortunately, although Reynolds' observa-tions were clearly of the utmost importance, they were regrettably viewed with considerable scep-

ticism and largely ignored. And it was not until Mayer et al (1971), with no knowledge of Reynolds' contributions to the subject, independ-ently carried out similar experiments on rats, that any notice was taken of the remarkable phenom-enon, now generally referred to as stimulation-produced analgesia.

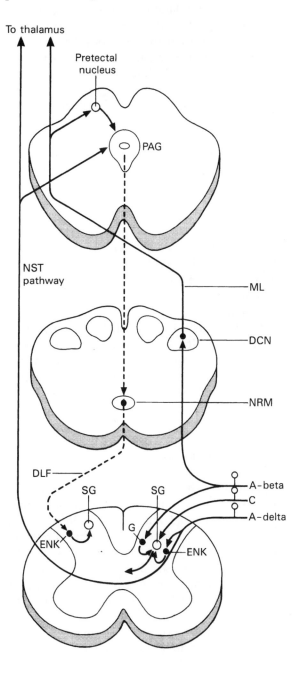

Figure 2.5   Tissue damage nociceptive information reaches the substantia gelatinosa (SG) via C-afferent fibres. The onward transmission of this information is inhibited by enkephalinergic interneurons (ENK) which are activated via A-delta 'pin prick' fibres as they enter the cord and via serotonergic inhibitory fibres that descend in the dorsolateral funiculus (DLF) from the nucleus raphe magnus (NRM) in the medulla and periaqueductal grey area (PAG) in the midbrain (the descending inhibitory system). The descending inhibitory system is brought into action either via collaterals which link the neospinothalamic 'A-delta pin prick' ascending pathway (NST) with the PAG, or via collaterals which form a link between the PAG and the medial lemniscus (ML), which arises from dorsal column nuclei (DCN) connected to A-beta fibres in the dorsal column. The onward transmission of tissue damage nociceptive information in C-afferent fibres is also inhibited by inhibitory GABA-ergic interneurons (G) which are activated by A-beta fibres that enter the substantia gelatinosa. (Based on Bowsher (1991), with permission.)

It has been found possible to produce analgesia by electrically stimulating óne or other of several sites in the brain, but the most consistently effective manner of doing this is to place electrodes either on the periaqueductal grey area in the midbrain or on the nucleus raphe magnus in the medulla (Liebeskind & Paul 1977).

Although stimulation-produced analgesia was first demonstrated in experimental animals, it was quickly shown to have considerable therapeutic value in relieving humans of persistent severe pain. Moreover, humans have been shown to obtain more lasting analgesia using this method than do many types of animals (Adams 1976, Hosobuchi et al 1977).

Electrical stimulation of the brainstem for the purpose of suppressing pain had not been in use for long before it was discovered that its analgesic effect could be abolished by the morphine antagonist naloxone (Akil et al 1976) and that the injection of a small amount of morphine directly into the periaqueductal grey area produces analgesia (Herz et al 1970, Mayer & Price 1976, Mayer & Watkins 1981). It was therefore concluded that morphine must activate neurons in a descending inhibitory system situated in the brainstem.

Mayer & Liebeskind (1974) have shown that this pain inhibitory system arises in the periaqueductal grey area (PAG) in the midbrain, has a pathway that projects to the nucleus raphe magnus (NRM) in the medulla, and from there axons descend in the dorsolateral funiculus of the spinal cord to terminate on the stalked enkephalinergic inhibitory interneurons present in dorsal horns (Basbaum et al 1977).

It is now known that serotonin (5-hydroxy-tryptamine) is the main transmitting agent in this system (Basbaum & Fields 1978), and that para-chlorophenylalanine, a serotonin inhibitor, suppresses the analgesia brought about by electrical stimulation of either the PAG or the NRM, and suppresses the analgesia produced by the micro-injection of morphine into either of these two structures (Anderson & Proudfit 1981).

The PAG at the upper end of this system has fibres projecting to it from the hypothalamus which in turn is under the control of the pre-frontal cortex. Therefore, its function is influenced by activity in the higher centres.

This inhibitory system is also brought into action when A-delta nerves in the skin are stimulated as this sets up activity in the neospinothalamic ascending pathway, which at the midbrain level gives off a collateral to the PAG (Mantyh 1982).

Noradrenergic descending inhibitory system

Stimulation of A-delta nerve fibres also brings this system into action because the neospinothalamic tract up which A-delta nociceptive information is transmitted has collaterals which connect with the locus coeruleus at its upper end in the pons (Craig 1992). And from there axons descend down the spinal cord with activity in them exciting a noradrenergic-mediated inhibitory effect on the various dorsal horn cells with which they make synaptic contact, including those involved in the intra-dorsal horn transmission from C-polymodal skin and group IV muscle nociceptors.

Diffuse noxious inhibitory controls

Le Bars et al (1979) have identified a pain-modulating system called by them diffuse noxious inhibitory controls (DNIC).

DNIC is brought into action when A-delta nerve fibres are stimulated such as, for example, by inserting a needle into the skin, because there are collaterals which link the neospinothalamic pathway with the subnucleus reticularis dorsalis in the medulla (Villaneuva et al 1988). And from there axons descend in the dorsolateral funiculus to make contact with and have an opioidergic inhibitory effect on neurons responsible for transmitting noxiously generated information to the brain (Bernard et al 1990).

These direct and indirect pain-modulating systems just described are the ones that are brought into action when a needle is inserted into the skin and subcutaneous tissues immediately overlying a MTrP in order to bring about A-delta sensory afferent-induced suppression of pain arising as a result of the development of activity in its group IV nociceptors – a procedure known as superficial dry needling.

For reasons to be explained at length in Chapter 7, this has for long been used by the author and is now being increasingly widely employed by physicians and physiotherapists throughout the world in the routine treatment of the MTrP pain syndrome.

Its effectiveness is dependent on whether it is carried out heterosegmentally or segmentally.

Heterosegmental superficial dry needling

Descending serotonergic, noradrenergic and DNIC pain inhibitory systems are brought into action when dry needle stimulation of A-delta fibres is carried out anywhere in the body.

Segmental superficial dry needling (Box 2.2)

For dry needle stimulation of A-delta fibres to have the maximum MTrP pain-suppressing effect, as will be emphasised again when discussing various MTrP deactivating techniques in Chapter 7, it is essential for the needle to be inserted into the skin and subcutaneous tissues immediately overlying the intramuscularly situated TrP.

The reason for this is that it ensures that the intra-dorsal horn passage of noxiously generated information from the MTrP's group IV nociceptors is blocked by the needle-induced A-delta sensory afferent input to the spinal cord, having both a direct action on the dorsal horn's enkephalinergic inhibitory interneurons at that segmental level and an indirect one on them via the serotonergic and noradrenergic descending inhibitory systems.

Transcutaneous electrical nerve stimulation

Low-threshold mechanoreceptors in the skin (Table 2.1) transmit mechanoreceptive information to the spinal cord in large diameter (5–15 μm) A-beta myelinated sensory afferents at a conduction velocity of 30–100 m/s (67–223 mph).

These mechanoreceptors in the skin are stimulated when it is stretched or lightly touched, and also when the hairs on it are bent.

As previously stated, Melzack & Wall (1965) based their gate-control theory on the supposition that stimulating large diameter A-beta sensory afferents has the effect of blocking the intra-dorsal horn transmission of noxious information arising from small diameter non-myelinated skin C and group IV muscle nociceptors.

It was this hypothesis that led Wall & Sweet (1967) to deduce that because large diameter A-beta fibres have a lower electrical resistance than small diameter C fibres it should be possible to suppress the transmission of noxious information along these latter fibres by electrically stimulating A-beta fibres – a deduction which led

---

Box 2.2   Segmental superficial dry needling's MTrP pain-relieving mechanisms

Insertion of needle into tissues immediately overlying active pain-producing MTrP
↓
Stimulation of A-delta sensory afferents
↓
Direct arousal of activity in dorsal horn-situated enkephalinergic inhibitory interneurons
PLUS
indirect stimulation of these as a result of creation of activity in a serotonergic descending inhibitory system
AND
the creation of activity in the descending noradrenergic system
↓
Blockade of intra-dorsal horn passage of MTrP's nociceptive information
↓
Alleviation of MTrP pain

them to introduce the type of therapy known as transcutaneous electrical nerve stimulation (TENS).

There are two main forms of this, conventional TENS and acupuncture-like TENS.

Conventional TENS

With conventional continuous TENS A-beta sensory afferents are stimulated by passing a high frequency (40–150 Hz), low intensity current between electrodes attached to the skin.

Experimental work carried out by Duggan & Foong (1985) has provided evidence to suggest that A-beta sensory afferent stimulation brought about by this means causes the release of gamma-aminobutyric acid (GABA), an inhibitory neurotransmitter that blocks the intra-dorsal horn transmission of noxious information generated in C and group IV nociceptors (Thompson 1989).

Acupuncture-like TENS

With acupuncture-like pulsed TENS a low frequency (1–5 Hz), high intensity current is employed. Unlike with conventional TENS, this produces an analgesia that is abolished by the opioid antagonist naloxone (Sjölund & Eriksson 1979). And, for this reason, the analgesia must develop as a result of a current of this type stimulating A-delta sensory afferents with the consequent development of activity in opioid peptide-mediated pain-modulating mechanisms (see p. 36).

A disadvantage of acupuncture-like TENS as originally employed was that it was not well tolerated due to it giving rise to unacceptably painful muscle contractions (Andersson et al 1976, Melzack 1975). This, however, has been circumvented by Eriksson et al (1979) introducing a technique in which trains of high frequency stim-

uli are repeated at a low frequency. Also, by stimulators now having been made available in which the pulse duration (width) and/or frequency can be modulated or the pulse simply randomised.

Indications for use of conventional and acupuncture-like TENS

A large survey carried out by Johnson et al (1991) has shown that the only way of deciding which form of TENS gives the optimum relief from any particular type of pain is by trial and error.

This notwithstanding, it has to be said that in general conventional TENS tends to be better for musculoskeletal and visceral nociceptive pain. And acupuncture-like TENS is preferable for neuropathic (neurogenic) pain (Thompson 1998), especially where hyperaesthesia and/or dysaesthesia are prominent features (Sjölund et al 1990).

TENS has been shown to alleviate MTrP pain (Graff-Radford et al 1989). A disadvantage, however, is that any pain relief obtained with it disappears within 30 minutes of the stimulator being switched off. Stimulation therefore has to be continued for several hours every day and over the course of time there is liable to be a declining response, a phenomenon known as TENS analgesia tolerance (Johnson et al 1991).

For this reason TENS cannot be recommended for the routine treatment of the MTrP pain syndrome, but it is helpful in providing short-term symptomatic relief such as, for example, when severe acute musculoskeletal pain develops in the low back immediately following the prolapse of an intervertebral disc.

Comprehensive reviews of the use of this form of therapy have been provided by Thompson (1986, 1994, 1998) and Thompson & Filshie (1993).

REFERENCES

Abdel-Maguid T E, Bowsher D 1984 Interneurons and proprioneurons in the adult human spinal grey matter and general somatic afferent cranial nerve nuclei. Journal of Anatomy 139:9–20

Adams J E 1976 Naloxone reversal of analgesia produced by brain stimulation in the human. Pain 2:161–166

Akil H, Mayer D J, Liebeskind J C 1976 Antagonism of stimulation produced analgesia by naloxone, a narcotic antagonist. Science 191:961–962

Anderson E G, Proudfit H K 1981 The functional role of the bulbospinal serotonergic system. In: Jacobs B L, Gelperin A (eds) Serotonin neurotransmission and behaviour. MIT Press, Cambridge, MA, pp 307–338

Andersson S A, Hansson G, Holmgren E, Renberg O 1976 Evaluation of the pain suppressant effect of different frequencies of peripheral electrical stimulation in chronic pain conditions. Acta Orthopaedica Scandinavica 47:149–157

Atweh S F, Kuhar M J 1977 Autodiographic localization of opiate receptors in rat brain 1. Spinal cord and lower medulla. Brain Research 22:471–493

Basbaum A I, Fields H L 1978 Endogenous pain control mechanisms: review and hypothesis. Annals of Neurology 4:451–462

Basbaum A I, Marley J J E, O'Keefe J, Clanton C H 1977 Reversal of morphine and stimulus-produced analgesia by subtotal spinal cord lesions. Pain 3:43–56

Beecher H K 1959 Measurements of subjective responses. Oxford University Press, Oxford

Bennett G J, Ruda M A, Gobel S, Dubner R 1982 Enkephalin-immunoreactive stalked cells in Lamina IIb islet cells in cat substantia gelatinosa. Brain Research 240:162–166

Bernard J F, Villaneuva L, Carroue J, Le Bars D 1990 Efferent projections from the sub-nucleus reticularis dorsalis (SRD): A Phaseolus vulgaris leucoagglutinin study in the rat. Neuroscience Letters 116:257–262

Bishop G H 1946 Neural mechanisms of cutaneous sense. Physiological Reviews 26:77–102

Bond M R 1979 Pain. Its nature, analysis and treatment. Churchill Livingstone, Edinburgh

Bonica J J 1990 Anatomic and physiologic basis of nociception and pain. In: Bonica J J (ed) The management of pain, 2nd edn. Lea & Febiger, Philadelphia, PA, ch 3

Boring E G 1942 Sensation and perception in the history of experimental psychology. Appleton-Century-Crofts, New York

Bowsher D 1957 Termination of the central pain pathway in man: the conscious appreciation of pain. Brain 80:606–622

Bowsher D 1991 The physiology of stimulation-produced analgesia. Journal of the British Medical Acupuncture Society IX(2):58–62

Calimlim J F, Wardell W M, Sriwatanakue K et al 1982 Analgesic effect of parenteral metkephamid acetate in treatment of post-operative pain. Lancet i: 1374–1375

Casey K L 1971a Somatosensory responses of bulboreticular units in awake cat: relation to escape-producing stimuli. Science 173:77–80

Casey K L 1971b Responses of bulboreticular units to somatic stimuli eliciting escape behaviour in the cat. International Journal of Neuroscience 2:15–28

Casey K L 1980 Reticular formation and pain: towards a unifying concept. In: Bonica J J (ed) Pain. Raven Press, New York, pp 93–105

Casey K L, Keene J J, Morrow T 1974 Bulboreticular and medial thalamic unit activity in relation to aversive behaviour and pain. In: Bonica J J (ed) Pain, advances in neurology. Raven Press, New York, vol 4, pp 197–205

Cervero F 1983 Somatic and visceral inputs to the thoracic spinal cord of the cat. Journal of Physiology (London) 337:51–67

Chen L, Huang L 1992 Protein kinase C reduces Mg^{2+} block by NMDA-receptor channels as a mechanism of modulation. Nature 356:521–523

Christensen B N, Perl E R 1970 Spinal neurons specifically excited by noxious or thermal stimuli: marginal zone of the dorsal horn. Journal of Neurophysiology 33:293–307

Chu J 1995 Dry needling (intramuscular stimulation) in myofascial pain related to lumbosacral radiculopathy. European Journal of Physical Medicine and Rehabilitation 5(4):106–121

Clement-Jones V 1983 Role of the endorphins in neurology. Practitioner 227:487–495

Clement-Jones V, Besser G M 1983 Clinical perspectives in opioid peptides. British Medical Bulletin 39(1):95–100

Clement-Jones V, Lowry P J, Rees L H et al 1980 Metenkephalin circulates in human plasma. Nature 283:295–297

Coderre T J, Katz J, Vaccarino A L, Melzack R 1993 Contribution of central neuroplasticity to pathological pain: review of clinical and experimental evidence. Pain 52:259–285

Craig A D 1992 Spinal and trigeminal lamina I input to the locus coeruleus anterogradely labeled with Phaseolus vulgaris leucoagglutinin (PHA-L) in the cat and the monkey. Brain Research 584:325–328

Duggan A W, Foong F W 1985 Bicuculline and spinal inhibition produced by dorsal column stimulation in the cat. Pain 22:249–259

Duggan A W, Hall J G, Headley P M 1976 Morphine, enkephalin and the substantia gelatinosa. Nature 264:456–458

Eriksson M B E, Sjölund B H, Nielzen S 1979 Long-term results of peripheral conditioning stimulation as an analgesic measure in chronic pain. Pain 6:335–347

Fields H L 1987a–c Pain. McGraw-Hill, New York, p 22 (a), p 35 (b), pp 44–56 (c)

Fields H L, Basbaum A I 1989 Endogenous pain control mechanisms. In: Wall P D, Melzack R (eds) Textbook of pain, 2nd edn. Churchill Livingstone, Edinburgh, pp 206–220

Fine P G, Milano R, Hare B D 1988 The effects of myofascial trigger point injections are naloxone reversible. Pain 32:15–20

Fock S, Mense S 1976 Excitatory effects of 5-hydroxytryptamine, histamine, and potassium ions on muscular group IV afferent limits: a comparison with bradykinin. Brain Research 105:459–469

Foreman R D, Blair R W, Weber R N 1984 Viscero-somatic convergence onto T_2–T_4 spinoreticular, spinoreticular-spinothalamic and spinothalamic tract neurons in the cat. Experimental Neurology 85:597–619

Foster M 1901 Translation of Descartes R, L'homme (1664). In: Lectures on the history of physiology during the 16th, 17th and 18th centuries. Cambridge University Press, Cambridge

Freeman W, Watts J W 1950 Psychosurgery in the treatment of mental disorders and intractable pain. C C Thomas, Springfield, IL

Gardner W J, Licklider J C R 1959 Auditory analgesia in dental operations. Journal of the American Dental Association 59:1144–1149

Georgopoulos A P 1974 Functional properties of primary afferent units probably related to pain mechanisms in primate glabrous skin. Journal of Neurophysiology 39:71–83

Goldstein A, Tachibana S, Lowney L I, Hunkapiller M, Hood L 1979 Dynorphin (1–13) an extraordinarily potent opioid peptide. Proceedings of the National Academy of Sciences of the United States of America 76:6666–6670

Graceley R H, Dubner R, Wolskee P J, Dector W R 1983 Placebo and naloxone can alter post-surgical pain by separate mechanisms. Nature 306:264–265

Graff-Radford S B, Reeves J L, Baker R L, Chiu D 1989 Effects of transcutaneous electrical nerve stimulation on myofascial pain and trigger point sensitivity. Pain 37:1–5

Gunn C C 1996 The Gunn approach to the treatment of chronic pain. Churchill Livingstone, Edinburgh

Hagbarth K E, Kerr D I B 1954 Central influences on spinal afferent conduction. Journal of Neurophysiology 17:295–307

Hannington-Kiff J F 1974 Pain relief. Heinemann Medical, London

Head H 1920 Studies in neurology. Kegan Paul, London

Herz A, Albus K, Metys J, Schubert P, Teschemacher H 1970 On the sites for the anti-nociceptive action of morphine and fentanyl. Neuropharmacology 9:539–551

Hong C-Z 1994 Lidocaine injection versus dry needling to myofascial trigger point. American Journal of Physical medicine and Rehabilitation 73:256–263

Hosobuchi Y, Adams J E, Linchitz R 1977 Pain relief by electrical stimulation of the central grey matter in humans and its reversal by naloxone. Science 177:183–186

Hughes J, Smith T W, Kosterlitz H W, Fothergill L A, Morgan B A, Morris H R 1975 Identification of two related pentapeptides from the brain with potent opiate agonist activity. Nature 258:577–579

Hunt S P, Kelly J S, Emson P C 1980 The electron microscope localization of methionine enkephalin within the superficial layers of the spinal cord. Neuroscience 5:1871–1890

Jessell T W 1982 Neurotransmitters and CNS disease – pain. Lancet ii:1084–1087

Jessell T W, Iversen L L 1977 Opiate analgesics inhibit substance P release from rat spinal trigeminal nucleus. Nature 268:549–551

Johnson M I, Ashton C H, Thompson J W 1991 An in-depth study of long-term users of transcutaneous electrical nerve stimulation (TENS). Implications for clinical use of TENS. Pain 44:221–229

Jose P J, Page D A, Wolstenholme B E, Williams T J, Dumonde D C 1981 Bradykinin-stimulated prostaglandins E2 production of endothelial cells and its modulation by antiiflammatory compounds. Inflammation 5:363–378

Kerr D I B, Haughen F P, Melzack R 1955 Responses evoked in the brain stem by tooth stimulation. American Journal of Physiology 183:252–258

Kumazawa T, Mizumura K 1977 Thin-fibre receptors responding to mechanical, chemical and thermal stimulation in the skeletal muscle of the dog. Journal of Physiology 273:179–194

Le Bars D, Dickenson A H, Besson J M 1979 Diffuse noxious inhibitory controls (DNIC). I: Effects on dorsal horn convergent neurones in the rat. II: Lack of effect on non-convergent neurones, supraspinal involvement and theoretical implications. Pain 6:283–304, 305–327

Levine J D, Gordon N C, Jones R T, Fields H L 1978 The narcotic antagonist naloxone enhances clinical pain. Nature 272:826–827

Levine J D, Gordon N C, Fields H L 1979 Naloxone dose dependently produces analgesia and hyperalgesia in postoperative pain. Nature 278:740–741

Lewin R 1976 The brain's own opiate. New Scientist 69:13

Lewis J W, Cannon J T, Liebeskind J E 1980 Opioid and non-opioid mechanisms of stress analgesia. Science 208:623–625

Lewis J W, Sherman J E, Liebeskind J C 1981 Opioid and non-opioid stress analgesia: assessment of tolerance and cross tolerance with morphine. Journal of Neuroscience 1:358–363

Lewis J W, Tordoff M G, Sherman J E, Liebeskind J C 1982 Adrenal medullary enkephalin-like peptides may mediate opioid stress analgesia. Science 217:557–559

Lewis T 1942a,b Pain. Macmillan, New York, p 3 (a), pp 118–122 (b)

Lewit K 1979 The needle effect in the relief of myofascial pain. Pain 6:83–90

Li C H, Barnafi L, Chrétien M, Chung D 1965 Isolation and amino-acid sequences of beta-LPA from sheep pituitary glands. Nature 208:1093–1094

Lichstein L, Sackett G P 1971 Reactions by differentially raised rhesus monkeys to noxious stimulation. Developmental Psychobiology 4:339–352

Liebeskind J C, Paul L A 1977 Psychological and physiological mechanisms of pain. American Review of Psychology 28:41–60

Livingston W K 1943 Pain mechanisms. Macmillan, New York

MacDermott A B, Mayer M L, Westbrook G L, Smith S J, Barker J L 1986 NMDA-receptor activation increases cytoplasmic calcium concentration in cultured spinal cord neurons. Nature 321:519–522

Mackenzie J 1909 Symptoms and their interpretation. Shaw & Sons, London

Mantyh P W 1982 The ascending input to the midbrain periaqueductal gray of the primate. Journal of Comparative Neurology 211:50–64

Mayer D J, Liebeskind J C 1974 Pain reduction by focal electrical stimulation of the brain. An anatomical and behavioral analysis. Brain Research 68:73–93

Mayer D J, Price D D 1976 Central nervous system mechanisms of analgesia. Pain 2:379–404

Mayer D J, Watkins L R 1981 The role of endorphins in endogenous pain control systems. In: Emrich H M (ed) Modern problems in pharmopsychiatry: The role of endorphins in neuropsychiatry. S Karger, Basel

Mayer D J, Wolfle T H, Akil H, Carder B, Liebeskind J C 1971 Analgesia from electrical stimulation in the brainstem of the rat. Science 174:1351–1354

Melzack R 1969 The role of early experience in emotional arousal. Annals of the New York Academy of Sciences 159:721–730

Melzack R 1975 Prolonged relief of pain by brief transcutaneous somatic stimulation. Pain 1:357–373

Melzack R, Casey K L 1968 Sensory, motivational and central control determinants of pain: a new conceptual model. In: Kenshalo D (ed) The skin senses. C C Thomas, Springfield, IL, pp 423–443

Melzack R, Scott T H 1957 The effects of early experience on the response to pain. Journal of Comparative Physiology and Psychology 50:155–161

Melzack R, Wall P D 1965 Pain mechanisms. A new theory. Science 150:971–979

Melzack R, Wall P D 1982a–c The challenge of pain. Penguin, Harmondsworth, Middlesex, p 236 (a), p 237 (b), p 260 (c)

Melzack R, Wall P D 1988a–d The challenge of pain, 2nd edn. Penguin, Harmondsworth, Middlesex, p 157 (a), p 56 (b), p 125 (c), pp 170–175 (d)

Melzack R, Stotler W A, Livingston W K 1958 Effects of discrete brainstem lesions in cats on perception of noxious stimulation. Journal of Neurophysiology 21:353–367

Mense S 1990 Physiology of nociception in muscles. In: Fricton J R, Awad E (eds) Advances in pain research and therapy. Raven Press, New York, vol 17

Mense S 1991 Considerations concerning the neurobiological basis of muscle pain. Canadian Journal of Physiology and Pharmacology 69:610–616

Mense S 1993 Nociception from skeletal muscle in relation to clinical muscle pain. Pain 54:241–289

Mense S 1994 Referral of muscle pain. New aspects. American Pain Society Journal 3(1):1–9

Mense S 1997 Pathophysiologic basis of muscle pain syndromes. An update. Physical Medicine and Rehabilitation Clinics of North America 8(1):23–53

Mense S, Meyer H 1985 Different types of slowly conducting afferent units in cat skeletal muscle and tendon. Journal of Physiology 363:403–417

Mense S, Meyer H 1988 Bradykinin-induced modulation of the response behaviour of different types of feline Group III and IV muscle receptors. Journal of Physiology 398:49–63

Merskey H 1979 Pain terms: a list with definitions and notes on usage. Recommended by the IASP sub-committee on taxonomy. Pain 6:249–252

Millar J, Basbaum A I 1975 Topography of the projection of the body surface of the cat to cuneate and gracile nuclei. Experimental Neurology 49:281–290

Müller J 1842 Elements of physiology, Taylor, London

Nathan P W 1976 The gate-control theory of pain. A critical review. Brain 99:1123–1158

Nathan P 1982 The nervous system, 2nd edn. Oxford University Press, Oxford, p 119

Noordenbos W 1959 Pain. Elsevier, Amsterdam

Noordenbos W 1987 Some historical aspects. Pain 29:141–150

Olesen J 1991 Clinical and pathophysiological observations in migraine and tension-type headache explained by integration of vascular, supraspinal and myofascial inputs. Pain 46:125–132

Oyama T, Jin T, Yamaya R 1980 Profound analgesic effects of beta-endorphin in man. Lancet i:122–124

Paintal A S 1960 Functional analysis of Group III afferent fibres of mammalian muscles. Journal of Physiology 152:250–270

Paterson S J, Robson L E, Kosterlitz H W 1983 Classification of opioid receptors. British Medical Bulletin 39:31–36

Perl E R 1968 Myelinated afferent fibres innervating the primate skin and their response to noxious stimuli. Journal of Physiology (London) 197:593–615

Pert C D, Snyder S H 1973 Opiate receptor: demonstration of nervous tissue. Science 179:1011–1014

Raja S N, Meyer R A, Campbell J N 1988 Peripheral mechanisms of somatic pain. Anesthesiology 68:571–590

Rang H P, Bevan S, Dray A 1991 Chemical activation of nociceptive peripheral neurones. British Medical Bulletin 47(3):534–548

Rexed B 1952 The cytoarchitectonic organization of the spinal cord in the cat. Journal of Comparative Neurology 96:415–495

Reynolds D V 1969 Surgery in the cat during electrical analgesia induced by focal brain stimulation. Science 164:444–445

Ruch T C 1949 Visceral sensation and referred pain. In: Fulton J (ed) Howell's textbook of physiology, 16th edn. Sanders, Philadelphia, pp 385–401

Schaible H-G, Grubb B D 1993 Afferent and spinal mechanisms of joint pain. Pain 55:5–54

Sessle B J 1990 Central nervous system mechanisms of muscular pain. In: Fricton J R, Awad E (eds) Advances in pain research and therapy. Myofascial pain and fibromyalgia. Raven Press, New York, vol 17, pp 91–97

Shanks M F, Clement-Jones V, Linsell C J et al 1981 A study of 24 hour profiles of plasma mentenkephalin in man. Brain Research 212:403–409

Sicuteri F 1967 Vasoneuroactive substances and their implications in vascular pain. In: Friedman A P (ed) Research and clinical studies in headache. Karger, Basel, vol 1, pp 6–45

Simons D 1990 Muscular pain syndromes. In: Fricton J R, Awad E (eds) Advances in pain research and therapy. Myofascial pain and fibromyalgia. Raven Press, New York, vol 17, p 12

Sjölund B H, Eriksson M B E 1979 Endorphins and analgesia produced by peripheral conditioning stimulation. In: Bonica J J, Albe-Fessard D, Liebeskind J C (eds) Advances in pain research and therapy 3. Raven Press, New York, pp 587–599

Sjölund B H, Eriksson M B E, Loeser J D 1990 Transcutaneous and electrical stimulation of peripheral nerves. In: Bonica J J (ed) The management of pain, 2nd edn. Lea & Febiger, PA, vol 2, pp 1852–1861

Smith R, Grossman A, Gaillard R et al 1981 Studies on circulating mentenkephalin and beta-endorphin: normal subjects and patients with renal and adrenal disease. Clinical Endocrinology 15:291–300

Smock T, Fields H L 1980 ACTH (1–24) blocks opiate-induced analgesia in the rat. Brain Research 212:202–206

Soper W Y, Melzack R 1982 Stimulation-produced analgesia. Evidence for somatotopic organization in the midbrain. Brain Research 251:301–311

Stacey M J 1969 Free nerve endings in skeletal muscle of the cat. Journal of Anatomy 105:231–254

Szentogathai J 1964 Neuronal and synaptic arrangement in the substantia gelatinosa rolandi. Journal of Comparative Neurology 122:219–239

Thompson J W 1984 Opioid peptides. British Medical Journal 288(6413):259–260

Thompson J W 1986 The role of transcutaneous electrical nerve stimulation (TENS) for the control of pain. In: Doyle D (ed) International symposium in pain control. Royal Society of Medicine Services International Congress and Symposium Series 123. Royal Society of Medicine, London

Thompson J W 1989 Pharmacology of transcutaneous nerve stimulation (TENS). Journal of the Intractable Pain Society of Great Britain and Ireland 7(1):33–40

Thompson J W 1994 Neuropharmacology of the pain pathways. In: Wells P E, Frampton V, Bowsher D (eds) Pain management and physiotherapy, 2nd edn. Butterworth Heinemann, Oxford.

Thompson J W 1998 Transcutaneous electrical nerve stimulation (TENS). In: Filshie J, White A (eds) Medical acupuncture. A western scientific approach. Churchill Livingstone, Edinburgh, ch 11

Thompson J W, Filshie J 1993 Transcutaneous electrical nerve stimulation (TENS) and acupuncture. In: Doyle D, Hanks G, MacDonald N (eds) Oxford textbook of palliative medicine. Oxford University Press, Oxford

Tsou K, Jang C S 1964 Studies in the site of analgesic action of morphine by intra cerebral microinjection. Scientia Sinica 113:1099–1109

Verrill P 1990 Does the gate theory of pain supplant all others? British Journal of Hospital Medicine 43:325

Villaneuva L, Bouhassira B, Bing Z, Le Bars D 1988 Convergence of heterotopic nociceptive information on to subnucleus reticularis dorsalis neurons in the rat medulla. Journal of Neurophysiology 60:980–1009

Wall P D 1960 Cord cells responding to touch, damage and temperature of skin. Journal of Neurophysiology 23:197–210

Wall P D 1964 Presynaptic control of impulses at the first central synapse in the cutaneous pathway. Progress in Brain Research 12:92–118

Wall P D 1978 The gate-control theory of pain mechanisms. A re-examination and a re-statement. Brain 101:1–18

Wall P D 1980a The role of substantia gelatinosa as a gate control. In: Bonica J J (ed) Pain. Raven Press, New York, pp 205–231

Wall P D 1980b The substantia gelatinosa. A gate control mechanism set across a sensory pathway. Trends in Neurosciences (Sept): 221–224

Wall P D 1989 The dorsal horn. In: Wall P D, Melzack R (eds) Textbook of pain, 2nd edn. Churchill Livingstone, Edinburgh, ch 5

Wall P D 1990 Obituary – William Noordenbos (1910–1990). Pain 42:265–267

Wall P D, Sweet W H 1967 Temporary abolition of pain. Science 155:108–109

Wall P D, Woolf C J 1984 Muscle but not cutaneous C-afferent input produces prolonged increases in the excitability of the flexion reflex in the rat. Journal of Physiology (London) 356:443–458

Wang J K, Nauss L A, Thomas J E 1979 Pain relief by intrathecally applied morphine in man. Anesthesiology 50:149–151

Weber E, Roth K A, Barchas J 1981 Colocalisation of alpha-neo-endorphin and dynorphin immunoreactivity in hypothalamic neurons. Biochemical and Biophysical Research Communications 103:951–958

Willis W D 1989 The origin and destination of pathways involved in pain transmission. In: Wall, P, Melzack R (eds) Textbook of pain, 2nd edn. Churchill Livingstone, Edinburgh, ch 6

Woolf C J 1989 Recent advances in the pathophysiology of acute pain. British Journal of Anaesthesia 63:139–146

Woolf C J 1991 Central mechanisms of acute pain. In: Bond M R, Charlton J E, Woolf C J (eds) Pain research and clinical management vol. 4. Proceedings of the VIth World Congress on Pain, Elsevier, Amsterdam, pp 25–34

Woolf C J, Wall P D 1983 Endogenous opioid peptides and pain mechanisms: a complex relationship. Nature 306:739–740

Wynn Parry C B 1980 Pain in avulsion lesions of the brachial plexus. Pain 9:41–53

Yaksh T L, Rudy T A 1976 Analgesia mediated by a direct spinal action of narcotics. Science 192:1357–1358

Zborowski M 1952 Cultural components in responses to pain. Journal of Social Issues 8:16–30

Zotterman Y 1933 Studies in the peripheral nervous mechanisms of pain. Acta Medica Scandinavica 80(3):185–190

3

The emotional aspects of pain

INTRODUCTION

Because pain which develops as a result of the activation and sensitisation of myofascial trigger point (MTrP) nociceptors in the MTrP pain syndromes, like all other types of organic pain, is a complex physico-emotional experience it is first necessary in this chapter to discuss the following topics – the emotional reactions to acute and chronic organic pain; anxiety-induced MTrP pain; pain-induced behaviour; and methods of assessing the emotional component of organic pain.

Consideration will then be given to various psychiatric disorders in which pain may at times be the presenting feature. Clearly it is essential to be able to differentiate between these and MTrP pain syndromes because for reasons to be discussed the latter are all too frequently erroneously assumed to be psychogenic.

Finally, because MTrP pain is liable to develop as a result of injury caused by industrial and road traffic accidents, various aspects of the compensation process will be considered, including the adverse psychological effects on claimants of protracted litigation.

EMOTIONAL REACTIONS TO PAIN

Acute organic pain

Before discussing factors that influence an individual's response to acute pain it is first necessary to point out that, unlike chronic pain, this particular sensory experience serves a useful purpose. For example, by evoking a flexor withdrawal reflex, it may either prevent tissues subjected to trauma from becoming damaged or limit the extensiveness of the damage. In addition, it may serve to draw attention to some serious internal disorder which requires urgent medical attention. Moreover, as Wall (1979) has pointed out, by causing an injured part to be kept at rest it frequently assists with the healing process.

For these reasons people born with an inability to feel pain are at a serious disadvantage as this is liable to lead to considerable delay in the diagnosis of potentially life-threatening conditions such as, for example, acute appendicitis or the perforation of a peptic ulcer. As a result of this they tend to die prematurely (Comings & Amromin 1974, Sternbach 1963).

Although acute pain therefore has a protective role and is normally felt as soon as tissues become injured, under stressful circumstances it may not be experienced until some time after the injury. Thus, for example, a soldier wounded in the heat of battle may not feel pain until the fighting is over (Beecher 1959). And an athlete, injured on the sports field, may not experience pain until after the game is finished (Craig 1989).

This phenomenon is also not infrequently observed in patients seen in casualty departments. Melzack et al (1982) studied 138 patients arriving at one hospital's emergency department with various major injuries and found there was a delay in the onset of pain in 51 of them (37%). The interval ranged from several minutes in some cases to several hours in others. Similarly, Norris & Watt (1983) reported that 23% of a group of patients with car accident-induced whiplash injuries to the neck did not develop pain for periods ranging from 2 to 48 hours.

The reason for the delay in the onset of pain in circumstances such as these is not certain. Possibly it is simply due to the emotional shock of a sudden severe injury serving to distract attention from the pain. The explanation, however, may be far more complex than this. One suggestion (Frenk et al 1986) is that it may be because stress activates endogenous painsuppressing systems in the hypothalamic-pituitary-adrenal axis.

The principal emotional reaction to acute pain is anxiety. Some of the factors which influence this include ethnic attitudes towards pain and parental reactions towards it.

That the emotional response to pain is markedly influenced by a person's cultural background is exemplified by those of Anglo-Saxon stock tending in the main to react to acute pain in a stoical and undemonstrative manner in contrast to those of Italian origin who in general react to it in a far more vociferous and attention-seeking manner (Zborowski 1952). And, as Melzack & Wall (1988a) have pointed out, whether parents respond to pain in an anxious or calm manner very much influences how their offspring cope with it, not only during their childhood but for the rest of their lives. The temperament of an individual also has an influence on pain tolerance so that emotionally stable people cope with pain better than those, who, because of neuroticism, overreact to the stresses imposed upon them by everyday events. It is for this reason that people of an anxious temperament suffer more pain following surgical operations than do those of a more phlegmatic nature (Taenzer et al 1986).

Chronic organic pain

Chronic pain, in contrast to acute pain, serves no useful purpose. And, over the course of time, it is liable to cause anyone suffering from it to become anxious, depressed, irritable, angry and resentful (Krishnan et al 1985). With respect to MTrP pain such reactions are therefore prone to develop when, for a number of different reasons including the setting-up of various self-perpetuating MTrP nociceptor activating mechanisms (see Chs 2 and 4), it has persisted for an appreciable period of time.

Biochemical changes would seem to contribute to these emotional reactions.

Messing & Lytle (1977) have shown that persistent pain leads to a decrease in the central nervous system's serotonin activity and have suggested that this may be one of the reasons for the development of insomnia, depression and a lowering of the pain tolerance.

Terenius (1980) has expressed the opinion that this lowering of the pain tolerance may also be due to a fall in the cerebrospinal fluid's endorphin level. And, after having reviewed a number of studies, he concluded that what distinguishes organic pain from psychogenic pain is a lowering of endorphin and serotonin levels with the former but not with the latter.

ANXIETY-INDUCED MTrP PAIN

MTrP pain most commonly develops as a result of trauma-induced nociceptor activity. And, as previously stated, should such pain become chronic, anxiety is liable to arise as a secondary event. Conversely, there are grounds for believing that people who suffer from long-term anxiety are prone to develop MTrP pain. When they do so it is liable to arise in any region of the body, but three of the commoner ones are the head (Ch. 11), the chest (Ch. 14) and the lower back (Ch. 12).

The manner in which anxiety causes MTrP activity to develop is far from clear. This is shown by the controversy that has for long existed concerning the cause of tension-type headache (T-TH). It was originally believed that it was due to anxiety-induced tension in the scalp and neck muscles compressing blood vessels and that the ischaemia produced in this manner was responsible for the activation of MTrP nociceptors. This theory, however, had to be abandoned once electromyographic studies had shown that neck and head muscle activity in T-THs is never more than moderately increased and that in many cases there is no increase (Bakal & Kaganov 1977, Olesen & Jensen 1991). Also, it was soon realised that any increase in muscle tension that may be present is never sufficient to constrict blood vessels (Olesen & Bonica 1990). And it has since become evident that muscle has to contract at approximately 30% of its maximal contraction force before this is liable to happen (Mense 1997).

There are, however, two possible reasons why anxiety is liable to lead to the development of TrP activity.

One is that emotionally induced arousal of the brain's reticular system (Ch. 2) creates activity in the descending reticulo-spinal tract with, as a consequence, stimulation of dorsal-horn-situated motor neurons and a resultant increased activity in muscles' motor nerves (Nathan 1982). The effect of this on MTrPs' dysfunctional motor endplates (Ch. 4) may then be such as to cause MTrP activity to develop.

The other is that McNulty et al's (1994) needle electromyographic evaluation of a TrP's response to a psychological stress has provided grounds for believing that stress may be capable of causing TrP activity to develop as a result of it giving rise to autonomic nervous system hyperexcitability.

A practical implication of all this is that when MTrP pain develops in someone of an anxious disposition deactivation of MTrPs is only likely to provide short-term relief from the pain unless, at the same time, measures are taken to reduce the anxiety. My personal preference is to include amongst these hypnotherapy and to teach the patient to practise autohypnosis on a regular daily basis (Hilgard & Hilgard 1994). Benzodiazepines should not be employed for reducing anxiety now that there is evidence to show that they are liable to exacerbate anxiety, depression, anger and hostility in chronic pain patients (Aronoff et al 1986).

PAIN-INDUCED BEHAVIOUR

Pain influences the manner in which a person behaves. Forms of behaviour adopted as a result of pain include the use of body language to indicate the suffering it causes. There may be changes in lifestyle with, in particular, the curtailment of physical activities for the purpose of minimising the suffering.

The reactions of others to this pain-induced behaviour is liable to reinforce it (Fordyce 1976, 1990). For example, the use of forms of body language such as groaning, crying and wincing may have the effect of making normally uncaring members of the family attentive and sympathetic and the satisfaction the patient derives from this may encourage the continuance of this type of behaviour. Material advantages obtained by a physical disability also tend to influence behaviour. For example, the discovery that pain-induced restriction of movements leads to the avoidance of certain unpleasant or arduous tasks is liable to encourage a patient to continue to adopt a restricted lifestyle long after the need for this has passed.

This subconscious employment of pain behaviour long after the primary cause for its development has ceased to exist is referred to by Bonica (1990) as a 'pain habit'. And efforts on the part of a doctor to break this habit not infrequently cause the patient to become hostile, resentful and uncooperative.

ASSESSING THE EMOTIONAL COMPONENT OF ORGANIC PAIN

It is because organic pain has an emotional component that patients when describing it are liable to employ not only adjectives such as aching, tingling or burning, but also adjectives like depressing, horrible or excruciating to convey the suffering caused by it. It follows therefore that because all types of pain experience have an emotional component it must never be assumed that pain is necessarily psychogenic simply because a patient uses a predominance of affective terms to describe it.

Melzack & Torgerson (1971) in recognising that there are three main categories of pain experience – sensory, evaluative and affective (emotional) – drew up the McGill Pain Questionnaire and this, together with a more recently introduced shortened version (Melzack 1987), has been shown to be of considerable value in its assessment. The emotional component of organic pain may also be evaluated by the use of the more complex Minnesota Multiphasic Personality Inventory (MMPI).

Sternbach et al (1973) used this inventory to compare the relative incidence of psychological disorders in patients with acute (i.e. less than 6 months' duration) and chronic low-back pain. They found that although people with acute pain had elevated scores for depression, anxiety, hysteria and hypochondriasis, they were significantly higher in those with chronic pain. The MMPI was also employed by Sternbach &

Timmermans (1975) in a study of 113 patients with low-back pain of at least 6 months' duration. An assessment was made before and after either surgery followed by rehabilitation or rehabilitation only. From these assessments it was found that there was a significant decrease in the hysteria, depression, anxiety and hypochondriasis scores following successful alleviation of the pain.

Melzack & Wall (1988b), in discussing these findings, stated:

It is evident from studies such as these that it is unreasonable to ascribe chronic pain to neurotic symptoms. The patients with the thick hospital charts are all too often prey to the physicians' innuendoes that they are neurotic and that their neuroses are the cause of the pain. Whilst psychological processes contribute to pain, they are only part of the activity in a complex nervous system. All too often, the diagnosis of neurosis as the cause of pain hides our ignorance of many aspects of pain mechanisms.

PSYCHOGENIC PAIN

Psychogenic pain is relatively rare but as it is essential to be able to distinguish it from somatic pain such as that which emanates from MTrPs some of the psychiatric disorders in which it is liable to arise will now be considered.

Breuer & Freud (1895) were among the first to draw attention to the possibility that pain may at times be a manifestation of hysteria. Since then it has become generally agreed that pain may arise as a direct result of a number of different disorders of the mind and over the past hundred years the psychodynamics responsible for this in what Engel (1959) has called 'the pain-prone patient' have been extensively studied both by him and by other psychoanalysts (Blumer 1975, Violon-Jurfest 1980)

Psychiatric disorders that may occasionally be a primary cause for pain developing include schizophrenia, the endogenous and reactive forms of depression, the somatisation disorder, hypochondriasis, and the conversion disorder or what was formerly known as conversion hysteria.

Schizophrenia

Pain arising as a result of schizophrenic hallucinations is very rare. In a series of 78 patients Watson et al (1981) found only one case in which the pain appeared to be entirely delusional.

Depression

Depression of the endogenous (psychotic) and reactive (neurotic) types has the effect of lowering the patient's pain tolerance so that a noxious stimulus which normally would cause no more than mild discomfort gives rise to pain. Fields (1987) has suggested that this may be because depressives have low levels of pain-inhibiting neurotransmitters such as serotonin, noradrenaline (norepinephrine) and endogenous opioid peptides; or alternatively, because depressed patients, as a result of their affective disorder, worry that even mild pain is the harbinger of some serious illness.

The somatisation disorder

A disorder which was originally considered to be a form of hysteria but was later separated from this and referred to as Briquet's syndrome (Purtell et al 1951, Guze 1967, 1985) is currently known as the somatisation disorder. And the criteria for its diagnosis have now been laid down in the 3rd edition of the American Psychiatric Association's *Diagnostic and Statistical Manual of Mental Disorders* – DSM III (1980).

The disorder, which is severely disabling, begins before the age of 30 and is characterised by the development over the years of a number of different psychologically determined symptoms including pain that affects in turn various systems of the body so that patients suffering from it may, over the course of time, come under the care of a number of different specialists, such as neurologists, gastroenterologists, urologists, gynaecologists, cardiologists and rheumatologists. Patients suffering from this disorder become so convinced that their symptoms are indicative of serious organic disease and are so unwilling to be reassured this is not so, even after carefully conducted clinical examinations and routine investigations, that doctors find themselves forced, often against their better judgement, to carry out large numbers of unnecessary, highly sophisticated and expensive diagnostic procedures, to prescribe much inappropriate medication, and even to carry out unwarranted surgical operations. No wonder Quill (1985) has referred to it as 'one of medicine's blind spots'.

Low-back pain is one of the commonest complaints of those with this disorder and its persistence despite various forms of conservative treatment all too often leads to the carrying out of equally unrewarding surgical procedures.

Because of the nature of the disorder its diagnosis is one which perforce has invariably to be made retrospectively. And because of this it is likely to be recognised more readily in countries like Britain, where general practitioners control the referral of their patients to consultants and collate the reports received from them, than it is in countries like the USA, where patients take it upon themselves to consult one specialist after another in a somewhat haphazard and uncoordinated manner (Murphy 1989). And yet, despite this, it is apparently less prevalent in Britain than it is in the United States (Deighton & Nicol 1985, Lloyd 1986).

It should be made clear that patients with the somatisation disorder are not fabricating their symptoms. This is in direct contrast to patients with Munchausen's syndrome – the syndrome named after Baron Munchausen, the 18th century fictional character who recounted highly fanciful stories during the course of his travels. Patients with that disorder get themselves admitted to one hospital after another, often under assumed names, by virtue of presenting themselves to casualty departments complaining of carefully selected fictitious symptoms for the sole purpose of either persuading physicians to give them opiates or surgeons to perform operations on them.

Hypochondriasis

The term hypochondriasis (Greek – hypo + khondros – (cartilage)) was introduced by the ancient

Greeks for the depressive disorder melancholia (Greek – melas (black) + khole (bile)) because of their belief that the upper part of the abdomen just below the costal cartilages is the region from which it arises. Its current usage, however, is for a disorder in which the patient misinterprets normal physiological sensations or inconsequential pathological ones that may develop in any part of the body as being indicative of the presence of some much feared life-threatening disease.

The obsessional preoccupation with these symptoms is such that even repeated and extensive investigations may fail to provide reassurance. For example, it is not uncommon for a hypochondriac to become convinced that discomfort occurring as a result of trauma to muscles in the left anterior chest wall is due to heart disease and in such a case, no matter how many tests are carried out, it may prove impossible to dispel the patient's anxiety. In addition, both the anxiety and the trauma may cause MTrP nociceptors to become activated with the pain which develops as a result only serving to make the fear of heart disease worse.

Conversion disorder

The American Psychiatric Association *Diagnostic and Statistical Manual of Mental Disorders* DSM III (1980) defines conversion disorder (formerly known as conversion hysteria) as a disturbance in physical functioning suggestive of organic disease but which in reality is an expression of psychological conflict or need.

Psychological factors are judged to be aetiologically involved on the basis that invariably an emotional conflict either initiates or exacerbates this disorder and because it is one which serves to provide the patient with an excuse for avoiding distressing circumstances or tasks and has the effect of arousing sympathy and attention from family and friends.

The disorder may manifest itself in a variety of different ways including paralysis of a limb, aphonia, fits, blindness, and bizarre forms of sensory loss. Such manifestations, however, appear to be less common now than formerly and the most frequent one at the present time would seem to be pain (Ziegler et al 1960, Ziegler & Imboden 1962).

A patient with the conversion disorder invariably reacts to any physical disability it may give rise to in a remarkably detached, unemotional and resigned manner or what the 19th century physician Pierre Janet referred to as 'la belle indifference'.

It is because the pain is characteristically confined to one particular part of the body that Walters (1961) decided to call it psychogenic regional pain. The diagnosis and management of this has been comprehensively reviewed by Feinmann (1990).

TRAUMA-INDUCED MTrP PAIN ERRONEOUSLY DIAGNOSED AS EMOTIONAL IN ORIGIN

Trauma-induced MTrP pain is very often considered erroneously to have a psychological cause. There would seem to be two main reasons for this. One is that the type of trauma that is likely to lead to the activation of MTrP nociceptors rarely causes overt tissue damage and, as a result, is liable to be overlooked. The other is that all too frequently MTrPs are not looked for when pain of uncertain origin is being investigated.

From having served on a medical appeal tribunal for many years it has become apparent to me that a disturbingly large number of people who suffer from MTrP pain as a result of an industrial injury, on seeking compensation for this are unjustly considered to be neurotic and are erroneously informed that their pain has no organic basis simply because the physical examination carried out on them has not included a search for MTrPs.

It would seem that it was also because of a failure to look for these that reports appeared in the early 1980s (Biering-Sorensen 1984, Roland & Morris 1983) stating that up to 30% of patients with chronic back and neck pain show no evidence of organic disease and led Crue & Pinskey (1984) to introduce the diagnostic term chronic intractable benign pain (CIBP). They defined this as being non-neoplastic pain, of six months or more duration, that develops in the absence of objective physical signs. And in view of the latter they concluded that pain of this type must be a 'central' phenomenon – or in other words 'all in the mind'.

Doubts as to the validity of this concept, however, were soon to arise when Fishbain et al (1986) carried out a psychiatric assessment and a physical examination that included a search for MTrPs in 283 chronic pain patients consecutively admitted under their care to the University of Miami School of Medicine. For they found that only 0.3% of these patients fulfilled the DSM III criterion for psychogenic pain which requires for its diagnosis that 'no organic pathology can be found to account for the pain'. They found that the pain in 85% of them emanated from MTrPs, an observation which led them to remark:

We believe that a significant number of patients receiving a diagnosis of psychogenic pain disorder may actually be suffering from the myofascial pain syndrome. Until this diagnosis is routinely excluded in chronic pain patients' physical examinations, it will be difficult to compare chronic pain patient populations for the incidence of psychogenic pain disorder.

The aptness of the term CIBP was further challenged when Rosonoff et al (1989) at the University of Miami studied a group of 90 patients with chronic low-back pain and 34 patients with chronic neck pain, for in all of these patients the criteria laid down by Crue and Pinskey for its employment were met and yet clinical examination revealed the presence of MTrPs in 96.7% of those with low-back pain and 100% of those with neck pain. In view of this they concluded that:

CIBP patients do have abnormal physical findings indicative of musculoskeletal disease: probably fibrositis and/or specific myofascial syndromes as a source of peripheral nociception. These findings question the validity of the CIBP concept and point to a need for a carefully conducted all-inclusive physical examination as a basic initial requirement in the classification of chronic pain patients.

It is therefore clear that until the importance of examining muscles for TrPs is more widely recognised, the error of considering that the pain which emanates from them is psychogenic will continue to be made.

PSYCHOLOGICAL EFFECTS OF COMPENSATION-SEEKING ON PAIN

As persistent pain, including MTrP pain, incurred as a result of industrial injuries and road traffic accidents commonly leads sufferers to seek financial redress, it is necessary to discuss at some length the psychological stresses imposed upon compensation claimants and the adverse effects these may have on them.

Many injustices are committed as a result of it being too readily assumed that the persistence of pain in accident compensation cases is due to a superimposed neurosis or even malingering. Accidents undoubtedly give rise to much psychological distress (Muse 1985, 1986) but this does not mean that post-accident pain which does not respond readily to treatment is necessarily psychological in origin and in some way associated with an unconscious or even at times conscious desire for compensation. Such an assumption, however, has tended to be made ever since the Workmen's Compensation Act was introduced in Great Britain in 1897 and in other countries shortly after this (Mendelson 1992). Jones & Llewellyn, for example, committed this error in a book published in 1917 entitled Malingering or the Simulation of Disease. In 1932 Collie even stated that 'fraud is a product of the age of the workman's compensation act, of trade unions and allied clubs. There are no malingerers in countries where there is no workman's compensation act'.

Whilst Kennedy (1946) did not go so far as to say that compensation seekers whose pain persists long after an accident and which fails to respond to conventional treatment are malingerers, he did, however, believe that they suffer from a compensation neurosis, a disorder which, according to him is 'a state of mind, born out of fear, kept alive by avarice, stimulated by lawyers and cured by a verdict!'

Miller (1961) was also of this opinion for he said that the persistence of pain in compensation seekers is due to the development of a superimposed accident neurosis and that the pain in such cases invariably starts to improve once compensation has been awarded.

Such views, however, have since been challenged. Two separate surveys of injured workers in Australia (Balla & Moraitis 1970, Ellard 1970) have shown that patients do not necessarily improve and return to work once compensation has been awarded. Also, Mendelson (1982, 1984, 1986), after having extensively studied compensation cases in that country, has concluded that 'patients are not cured by the verdict' and that the pain usually remains as intense after the financial settlement as before. Others who have confirmed that patients continue to experience symptoms and require treatment following the settlement of their compensation claims include Hohl (1974), Encel & Johnston (1978), Kelly & Smith (1981), Tarsh & Royston (1985) and Melzack et al (1985).

Melzack et al (1985), in commenting both on Mendelson's findings and on their own psychological studies of accident compensation cases state:

. . . the phrase 'compensation neurosis' is an unwarranted biased diagnosis. Not only are the disability and the pain not cured by the verdict but compensation patients do not exaggerate their pain or show evidence of neurosis or other psychopathological symptoms greater than those seen in pain patients without compensation.

Although it is now generally accepted that neither subconscious amplification of symptoms as a result of a neurosis, nor conscious indulgence in wilful fabrication of symptoms, is a major problem among industrial and road traffic accident compensation claimants, it is nevertheless becoming increasingly recognised that the adversarial nature of the compensation systems used in many countries may well tend to have adverse physico-emotional effects on claimants. It is believed (Guest & Drummond 1992, Mendelson 1992) that these adverse effects result from the anxiety created by protracted litigation, by uncertainties concerning the outcome of claims and by feelings of insecurity that are brought about by the long-term unemployment such systems encourage.

The idea that long-term unemployment has a deleterious effect on the treatment and rehabilitation of compensation seekers was first mooted by White (1966, 1969) as a result of his studies in a group of workers suffering from low-back pain in Canada. He concluded his initial report by stating:

Perhaps effective placement of these unfortunate workmen in jobs which are within the limitations imposed by the pain would maintain morale, avoid concentration of their attention on their complaints and, while keeping up reasonable bodily activities, allow passage of sufficient time for the condition to subside. A scientific study of such a plan might be enlightening and rewarding.

Support for this view has subsequently come from Beals & Hickman (1972) who showed that the longer patients with injuries of the back and extremities are kept unemployed, the less likelihood there is of them returning to work. Dworkin et al (1985), in a survey carried out in the USA, found that the response to treatment of chronic pain in a group of patients who had been awarded compensation, or who were waiting settlement of their compensation claims, was not significantly different from that of another group who had either not received compensation or had not applied for it. However, what did influence the response to treatment in both groups was the employment status of the patients, with the employed responding better than the unemployed. This finding led them to suggest 'that it would be valuable to redirect attention away from the deleterious effects of the "compensation neurosis" and towards the roles of activity and employment in the treatment and rehabilitation of chronic pain patients'.

Leaver (1988), who carried out a study of patients with industrial injuries in Australia, also emphasised the importance of finding work for injured employees as soon as possible, having established that a quick return to work following injury alleviates financial worries and by so doing favourably influences the response to treatment.

With respect to this, Carron et al's (1985) comparison of the effects on workers of two very different industrial accident compensation systems operating in the USA and New Zealand is particularly enlightening. In this study information obtained from questionnaires completed by a group of employees with low-back pain given treatment in a clinic in New Zealand was compared with information obtained in a similar manner from a group of employees treated for the same disorder in a clinic in the USA.

In America claims are processed slowly and the claimant is required to have work-related disability. This not infrequently gives rise to protracted litigation and whilst this is going on it is in the compensation seeker's interest to remain off work. In New Zealand, however, because of a 'no fault' type of compensation system the employee is not required to prove that the injury is work-related in order to receive compensation. As a consequence of this and because claims are dealt with expeditiously, conflict between employers, insurers and claimants is reduced to a minimum. Moreover during the time that claims are being settled, claimants are provided with treatment and rehabilitation programmes designed to get them back to whatever type of work is suitable to their individual needs as quickly as possible. This is considered to be of such importance that employees who refuse to accept work within their capacity are liable to incur substantial penalties.

In view of these differences it is hardly surprising that when Carron and his colleagues came to analyse the questionnaires, they found that although the pain initially suffered by the New Zealand and the US group was similar, there were nevertheless more psychological disturbances, a higher intake of medication and a greater degree of social, recreational and vocational dysfunction both before and after treatment amongst the Americans. They also confirmed that compensation is sought less often and claims are settled more quickly in New Zealand and that as a result, accident-induced low-back pain employees in that country have a better quality of life than their counterparts in America.

Similar findings obtained by Guest & Drummond (1992) in a study of industrial chronic back pain sufferers in Australia led them to conclude that:

Rehabilitation, incorporating methods of coping with pain and emotional distress, should begin as soon as possible after injury. Since many compensation systems are probably a major source of stress, advice on how to deal with these aspects should be included in rehabilitation programmes. In the longer term compensation systems should be modified to direct their emphasis away from financial settlement and towards finding suitable employment for injured workers.

REFERENCES

American Psychiatric Association Committee on Nomenclature and Statistics 1980 Diagnostic and statistical manual of mental disorders. American Psychiatric Association, Washington DC.

Aronoff G M, Wagner J M, Spangler A S 1986 Clinical interventions for pain. Journal of Consulting and Clinical Psychology 54:769–775

Bakal D A, Kaganov J A 1977 Muscle contraction and migraine headache: psychological concepts. Headache 17:208–215

Balla J I, Moraitis 1970 Knights in armour: a follow-up study of injuries after legal settlement. Medical Journal of Australia 2:355–361

Beals R K, Hickman N W 1972 Industrial injuries of the back and extremities. Journal of Bone and Joint Surgery 54A:1593–1611

Beecher H K 1959 Measurement of subjective responses. Oxford University Press, New York

Biering-Sorensen F 1984 Physical measurements as risk indicators for low-back trouble over a one year period. Spine 9:106–119

Blumer D 1975 Psychiatric considerations in pain. In: Rothman R H, Simeone F A (eds) The spine. W B Saunders, Philadelphia

Bonica J J 1990 General considerations of chronic pain. In: Bonica J J (ed) The management of pain, 2nd edn. Lea & Febiger, Philadelphia, p 189

Breuer J, Freud S 1895 Studies on hysteria. Reprinted in complete psychological works of Freud. Hogarth Press, London, 1955

Carron H, De Good D E, Tait R 1985 A comparison of low back patients in the United States and New Zealand: Psychosocial and economic factors affecting severity of disability. Pain 21:77–89

Collie J 1932 Fraud in medico-legal practice. Edward Arnold, London, p 1

Comings D E, Amromin G D 1974 Autosomal dominant insensitivity to pain with hyperplastic myelinopathy and autosomal dominant indifference to pain. Neurology 24:838–848

Craig K D 1989 Emotional aspects of pain. In: Wall P A, Melzack R (eds) Textbook of pain, 2nd edn. Churchill Livingstone, Edinburgh, pp 220–230

Crue B L, Pinskey J J 1984 An approach to chronic pain of nonmalignant origin. Postgraduate Medical Journal 60:858–864

Deighton C M, Nicol A R 1985 Abnormal illness behaviour in young women in a primary care setting: is Briquet's syndrome a useful category? Psychological Medicine 15:515–520

Dworkin R H, Handlin D S, Richlin D M, Brand L, Vannucci C 1985 Unravelling the effects of compensation, litigation, and employment on treatment response in chronic pain. Pain 23:49–59

Ellard J 1970 Psychological reactions to compensable injury. Medical Journal of Australia 2:349–355

Encel S, Johnston C E 1978 Compensation and rehabilitation. A survey of workers' compensation cases involving back injuries and lump sum settlements. New South Wales University Press, Sydney

Engel G 1959 'Psychogenic' pain and the pain-prone patient. American Journal of Medicine 26:899–918

Feinmann C 1990 Psychogenic regional pain. British Journal of Hospital Medicine 43:123–127

Fields H 1987 Pain. McGraw Hill, New York, p 80

Fishbain D A, Goldberg M, Meagher R, Steele R, Rosonoff H 1986 Male and female chronic pain patients categorised by DSM-111 psychiatric diagnostic criteria. Pain 26:181–197

Fordyce W 1976 Behavioral methods in chronic pain and illness. Mosby, St Louis

Fordyce W 1990 Learned pain: pain as behavior. In: Bonica J (ed) The management of pain, 2nd edn. Lea & Febiger, Philadelphia, PA, pp 291–299

Frenk H, Cannon J T, Lewis J W, Liebeskind J C 1986 Neural and neurochemical mechanisms of pain inhibition. In: Sternbach R A (ed) The psychology of pain, 2nd edn. Raven Press, New York, pp 25–48

Guest G H, Drummond P D 1992 Effect of compensation on emotional state and disability in chronic back pain. Pain 48:125–130

Guze S B 1967 The diagnosis of hysteria: what are we trying to do? American Journal of Psychiatry 124:491–498

Guze S B 1985 The validity and significance of the clinical diagnosis of hysteria (Briquet's syndrome). American Journal of Psychiatry 132:138–141

Hilgard E R, Hilgard J R 1994 Hypnosis in the relief of pain. Brunner/Mazel, New York

Hohl M 1974 Soft-tissue injuries of the neck in automobile accidents: factors influencing prognosis. Journal of Bone and Joint Surgery 56A:1675–1682

Jones A B, Llewellyn L J 1917 Malingering or the simulation of disease. Heinemann, London

Kelly R, Smith B N 1981 Post-traumatic syndrome: another myth discredited. Journal of the Royal Society of Medicine 74:275–277

Kennedy F 1946 The mind of the injured worker: its effect on disability periods. Compensation Medicine 1:19–24

Krishnan K R R, France R D, Pelton S, McCann U D, Davidson J, Urban B J 1985 Chronic pain and depression.

(11) symptoms of anxiety in chronic low back patients and their relationship to subtypes of depression. Pain 22:289–294

Leaver R 1988 Workers' compensation and rehabilitation: an employer's perspective. Technical report, Workers Compensation and Rehabilitation Commission of Western Australia

Lloyd G G 1986 Psychiatric syndromes with a somatic presentation. Journal of Psychosomatic Research 30:113–129

McNulty W H, Gevirez R N, Hubbard D R et al 1994 Needle electromyographic evaluation of trigger point response to a psychological stressor. Psychophysiology 31(3):313–316

Melzack R 1987 The short-term McGill Pain Questionnaire. Pain 30:191–197

Melzack R, Torgerson W S 1971 On the language of pain. Anesthesiology 34:50–59

Melzack R, Wall P 1988a,b The challenge of pain, 2nd edn. Penguin Books, Harmondsworth, p 20 (a), p 32 (b)

Melzack R, Wall P, Ty T C 1982 Acute pain in an emergency clinic: latency of onset and descriptor patterns. Pain 14:33–43

Melzack R, Katz J, Jeans M E 1985 The role of compensation in chronic pain. Analysis using a new method of scoring the McGill Pain Questionnaire. Pain 23:101–112

Mendelson G 1982 Not 'cured by a verdict': effect of legal settlement on compensation claimants. Medical Journal of Australia 2:132–134

Mendelson G 1984 Compensation, pain complaints and psychological disturbance. Pain 20:169–177

Mendelson G 1986 Chronic pain and compensation: a review. Journal of Pain Symptomatic Management 1:135–144

Mendelson G 1992 Compensation and chronic pain. Pain 48:121–123

Mense S 1997 Pathophysiologic basis of muscle pain syndromes. Physical Medicine and Rehabilitation Clinics of North America 8(1):23–53

Messing R B, Lytle L D 1977 Serotonin-containing neurons: their possible role in pain and analgesia. Pain 4:1–21

Miller H 1961 Accident neurosis. British Medical Journal 1:919–925; 992–998

Murphy M 1989 Somatization: embodying the problem. British Medical Journal 298:1331–1332

Muse M 1985 Stress-related post-traumatic chronic pain syndrome: criteria for diagnosis and preliminary report on prevalence. Pain 23:295–300

Muse M 1986 Stress-related post-traumatic chronic pain syndrome: behavioral treatment approach. Pain 25:389–394

Nathan P 1982 The nervous system, 2nd edn. Oxford University Press, Oxford, p 119

Norris S H, Watt I 1983 The prognosis of neck injuries resulting from rear-end vehicle collisions. Journal of Bone and Joint Surgery 65B:608–611

Olesen J, Bonica J J 1990 Headache. In: Bonica J J (ed) The management of pain, 2nd edn. Lea & Febiger, Philadelphia, PA, pp 706–711

Olesen J, Jensen R 1991 Getting away from muscle contraction as a mechanism of tension-type headache. Pain 46:123–124

Purtell J J, Robins E, Cohen M E 1951 Observations on clinical aspects of hysteria. A quantitative study of 50 hysteria patients and 156 control subjects. Journal of the American Medical Association 146:902–909

Quill T E 1985 Somatisation disorder – one of medicine's blind spots. Journal of the American Medical Association 254(21):3075–3079

Roland M, Morris R 1983 A study of the natural history of back pain. Spine 8:141–150

Rosonoff H L, Fishbain D A, Goldberg M, Santana R, Rosonoff R S 1989 Physical findings in patients with chronic intractable benign pain of the neck and/or back. Pain 37:279–287

Sternbach R A 1963 Congenital insensitivity to pain: a critique. Psychological Bulletin 60:252–264

Sternbach R A, Timmermans G 1975 Personality changes associated with a reduction of pain. Pain 1:177–181

Sternbach R A, Wolf S R, Murphy R W, Akeson W H 1973 Traits of pain patients: The low-back 'loser'. Psychosomatics 14:226–229

Taenzer P A, Melzack R, Jeans M E 1986 Influence of psychological factors in postoperative pain, mood and analgesic requirements. Pain 24:331–342

Tarsh M J, Royston C 1985 A follow-up study of accident neurosis. British Journal of Psychiatry 146: 18–25

Terenius L Y 1980 Biochemical assessment of chronic pain. In: Kosterlitz H W, Terenius L Y (eds) Pain and society. Verlag Chemie, Basel, pp 355–364

Violon-Jurfest A 1980 The onset of facial pain: a psychological study. Psychotherapy and Psychosomatics 34:11–16

Wall P D 1979 On the relation of injury to pain. Pain 6:253–264

Walters A 1961 Psychogenic regional pain alias hysterical pain. Brain 84(1):1–18

Watson G D, Chandarana P C, Merskey H 1981 Relationships between pain and schizophrenia. British Journal of Psychiatry 138:33–36

White A W M 1966 Low back pain in men receiving workmen's compensation. Canadian Medical Association Journal 95:50–56

White A W M 1969 Low back pain in men receiving workmen's compensation: a follow-up study. Canadian Medical Association Journal 101:61–67

Zborowski M 1952 Cultural components in responses to pain. Journal of Social Issues 8:16–30

Ziegler F J, Imboden J B 1962 Contemporary conversion reactions. A conceptual model. Archives of General Psychiatry 6:279–287

Ziegler F J, Imboden J B, Meyer E 1960 Contemporary conversion reactions: a clinical study. American Journal of Psychiatry 116:901–909

4

Myofascial trigger point pain

INTRODUCTION

The muscle pain disorders discussed in Parts I and II of this book have traditionally been given the collective term the myofascial pain syndrome (MPS) but because this is sometimes used, as Simons et al (1999) have emphasised, 'for many conditions that cause muscle pain without reference to and in the absence of trigger points' it is my personal preference to call them the myofascial trigger point pain (MTrP) syndromes in order to emphasise that it is as a result of the activation and sensitisation of MTrP nociceptors that the pain in these disorders develops.

MTrP pain mainly affects adults but children may also develop it (Aftimos 1989, Bates & Grunwaldt 1958, Fine 1987). Its incidence is approximately the same for both sexes. This is unlike fibromyalgia, in which over four-fifths of patients are females (Yunus 1989).

There have been no large epidemiological studies but as McCain (1994) states, 'anecdotal evidence from expert examiners suggest that MPS is a very common condition, particularly in industry where it is a frequent cause of disability after trauma'.

Confirmation that the incidence of MTrP pain is high comes from Fricton et al (1985a), who found that 54.6% of a large group of patients with chronic head and neck pain had pain of this type; from Skootsky et al (1989), who found that 85% of patients presenting with low-back pain to a general internal medicine practice had MTrPs as the source of the pain; and from Schiffman et al (1990), who in an epidemiological study of orofacial pain in a young adult female population found that in 50% of them the pain was of MTrP origin.

Although it is over 60 years since John Kellgren, when working at University College Hospital, London, first showed that it is from what are now called MTrPs that the pain emanates, there continues to be a strange reluctance on the part of clinicians to confer upon these structures the importance they deserve.

In the past one of the main reasons for doubting the existence of MTrPs was that when tissues considered on clinical grounds to contain them were examined microscopically no specific histopathology could be demonstrated. Now that recent neurophysiological and histological studies have led to their structure and function becoming better understood (Gerwin 1994, Hong 1999, Hong & Simons 1998, Mense 1990, 1993a, 1993b, 1997, Simons 1996, 1999, Simons et al 1999), it is to be hoped that the importance of searching for them as part of the routine investigation of pain of uncertain origin will become more widely recognised.

In this chapter the characteristics of MTrPs will be discussed in some detail but first it is necessary to say something about the morphology of skeletal muscle and the physiological mechanisms involved in its contraction.

MORPHOLOGY OF SKELETAL MUSCLE

A skeletal muscle is made up of a large number of muscle fibres with each of these containing numerous myofibrils (1–2 μm in diameter) that lie parallel to each other along its longitudinal axis (Fig. 4.1).

PHYSIOLOGICAL MECHANISMS INVOLVED IN VOLUNTARY MUSCLE CONTRACTION

Actin–myosin sliding muscle contraction mechanism

Each myofibril contains on average approximately 1500 thick myosin filaments and 3000 thin actin filaments. These actin filaments are attached to structures known as Z bands and the portion of a myofibril that lies between two of these is called a sarcomere. It is as a result of the relative sliding movement of the actin and myosin filaments with, as a consequence, shortening of the sarcomeres, that muscle contraction takes place. This normally occurs when, in response to a nerve-induced action potential, calcium ions stored in the sarcoplasmic reticulum are released into the sarcoplasm surrounding the myofibrils and activate the actin–myosin sliding muscle contraction mechanism.

Muscle contraction energy supply

In addition to calcium, energy is required for this contractile process to take place. This is provided by the degradation of adenosine triphosphate (ATP) to adenosine diphosphate brought about as a result of the action of the enzyme ATPase present in the 'heads' of myosin filaments.

The sarcoplasmic reticulum's calcium pump effect

A muscle contraction continues only for so long as there is a high concentration of calcium in the sarcoplasm. However, calcium released from the sarcoplasmic reticulum in response to a single action potential remains in the sarcoplasm for only a brief period. This is because a pump located in the walls of the sarcoplasmic reticulum continuously drives the calcium back into it. For this reason a muscle contraction that arises in response to a single action potential has a duration of not more than 1/30th of a second. It therefore follows that for a muscle contraction to last

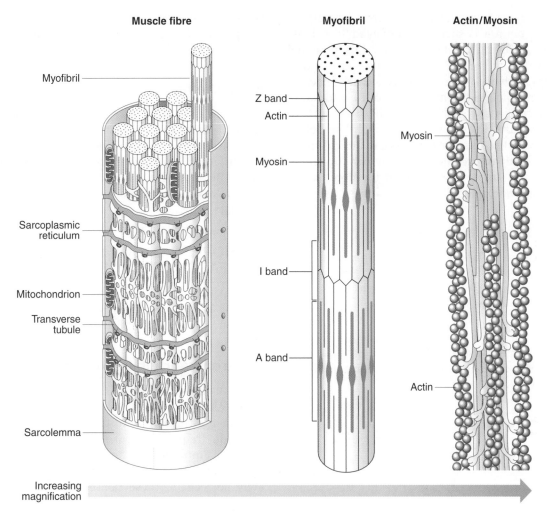

Figure 4.1   Schematic representation of the compartments of a muscle fibre. (Reproduced with permission of Professor R. Edwards.)

for any appreciable period of time there has to be a quick succession of action potentials.

Motor efferent contraction mechanism

A voluntary muscle's contraction is in response to brain-generated impulses descending in the spinal cord and setting up activity in motor units.

A motor unit

Each motor unit has an alpha-motor neuron in the spinal cord's anterior horn. From this neuron an axon passes first through the spinal nerve and then through a motor nerve which, on entering the muscle, divides into a number of branches, with each of these terminating at a motor end-plate (Fig. 4.2) in the form of a claw-like connection embedded in the surface of a muscle fibre (Salpeter 1987).

A nerve action potential initiated by an alpha-motor neuron is therefore conveyed to a large number of muscle fibres. When this potential enters an individual muscle fibre via a motor endplate there is a synchronous release of packets of acetylcholine (ACh) present in the endplate's synaptic clefts. The liberated ACh is then responsible for the development of an endplate potential and when this reaches a certain critical size it triggers off an excitatory wave which, travelling along the surface membrane of the fibre (sarcolemma), causes the fibre to contract.

Motor endplate zone

A motor endplate is most commonly located at the centre of a muscle fibre. And the area of muscle where motor endplates are to be found is known as the motor endplate zone.

A muscle usually has only one of these situated in the mid-part of its belly. There are, however, some muscles which have fascial septa dividing them into several compartments and

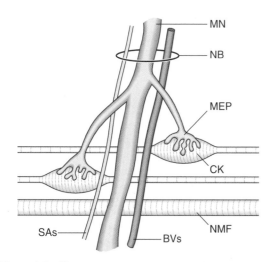

Figure 4.2 Diagrammatic representation of part of a myofascial trigger point showing two motor endplates (MEPs) and juxtapositional contraction knots (CKs); also a neurovascular bundle (NB) containing motor nerves (MNs), nociceptive and proprioceptive sensory afferents (SAs) and blood vessels (BVs) with closely associated sympathetic fibres. Note: in normal muscle fibre (NMF) the sarcomeres are of equal length. In a muscle fibre containing a contraction knot there is shortening of the sarcomeres at that site and compensatory lengthening of them on either side.

with these there is then an endplate zone in each compartment. An example of such a muscle is the rectus femoris.

Motor point

A muscle's motor point is by definition the site where a twitch can be elicited in response to the application of a minimal electrical stimulus to the surface. It was formerly said to be where the motor nerve enters the muscle but the present view is that it is located at the muscle's motor endplate zone.

PATHOPHYSIOLOGY OF MYOFASCIAL TRIGGER POINTS

Current concepts concerning the pathophysiology of MTrPs stem from recently carried out electromyographic and histological studies.

Electromyographic studies

The first to examine a MTrP's electrical activity were Weeks & Travell (1957), who observed that TrPs in the trapezius muscle exhibited a series of high frequency spike-shaped discharges with an amplitude of approximately 1000 µV and a duration of 1–3 ms, and that sites immediately adjacent to these points were electrically silent.

The next to do this were Hubbard & Berkoff (1993). In their study they included 8 pain-free people with latent MTrPs and 54 patients with active MTrPs in the trapezius muscle. With a monopolar EMG needle they recorded a continuous low amplitude potential of about 50 µV in latent MTrPs and both this and high amplitude spike activity of about 100–700 µV in active MTrPs. They found no sustained spontaneous EMG activity outside the 1–2 mm nidus of a TrP.

They decided that,

... the activity is not localised enough to be generated in an endplate, nor does it have the expected location or waveform morphology for endplate activity. We theorize that the TrP EMG activity is generated from sympathetically stimulated intrafusal muscle fibre contractions ...

and concluded that,

...a MTrP is located in the muscle spindle as the intrafusal fibres of this are sympathetically innervated.

Support for this view came from studies in which Hubbard (1996) carried out EMG-guided injections of various biochemical substances into MTrPs. For, from these, he was able to confirm that a MTrP's electrical activity is eliminated by the alpha-adrenergic blockade produced by both phentolamine and phenoxybenzamine. Also, he found that whereas the competitive alpha-blocker phentolamine, when injected either intravenously or directly into a MTrP, only eliminates the EMG-recorded electrical activity transiently, the non-competitive alpha-blocker phenoxybenzamine, when administered by either of these routes, eliminates it indefinitely. And furthermore, that it produces a significant reduction in MTrP pain for up to 24 hours.

It has to be said, however, as Hubbard himself pointed out, that these studies were both unblinded and preliminary.

Motor endplate electromyographic activity

Among the first to study motor endplate electromyographic activity were Jones et al who, in 1955, using an iron deposition technique to confirm the position of their recording needle, recorded a low amplitude activity of 50–700 µV when they inserted it into a muscle site which histologically was shown to contain a number of small nerves. Although the wave pattern was similar to the one Hubbard and Berkoff believed arose in muscle spindles, Jones and his co-workers' observations that denervation abolished the electrical activity after 24 hours, that the insertion of the needle gave rise to acute pain and that brief muscle twitches developed as the needle entered the site all strongly suggest, as Gerwin (1994) has pointed out, that the plexus of motor nerves into which the needle was inserted was a TrP site. Also, against the needle having been inserted into a muscle spindle, was that no such structure could be identified within the vicinity of its tip.

Support for the belief that MTrPs are located in the region of motor endplates rather than muscle spindles has also come from more recent studies carried out by Simons et al (1995a, 1995b, 1995c, 1995d) who, when they investigated the electrical activity described by Hubbard and Berkoff, employed a five-fold higher amplification and a ten-fold increase in sweep speed for their recordings (Simons et al 1999).

By this means they were able to identify two separate electrical waveform components when a needle is inserted into a MTrP locus (Fig. 4.3); a constantly found spontaneous electrical activity (SEA) consisting of continuous low-amplitude (10–50 µV, occasionally 80 µV) noise-like action potentials; and at times, especially from a particularly active MTrP, intermittent large-amplitude spikes (100–600 µV).

They found that in order to demonstrate the presence of SEA at a MTrP site it is essential to employ high-sensitivity recordings and to insert the needle into the MTrP very slowly.

Hong (1999), during the course of commenting on these recent electromyographic studies, states:

There is strong evidence that the SEA found in an MTrP region of human muscle . . . corresponds to an abnormal pattern of endplate electrical activity, due to excessive acetylcholine release (Liley 1956, Heuser & Miladi 1971, Ito et al 1974). Spontaneous electrical activity is not continuously dependent on spinal cord activity, since the transection of the peripheral nerve or spinal cord did not induce any obvious change in SEA in one hour in a recent animal study (Hong & Yu 1998). Recent animal studies with intra-arterial infusion of neuromuscular blocking agent or calcium blocking agent (Chen et al 1998a, 1998b) have further confirmed that active loci are abnormal endplate potentials.

Support for the belief that MTrPs lie outside the muscle spindles in the vicinity of extrafusal motor endplates also comes from Cheshire et al (1994) finding that it is possible to deactivate a MTrP by injecting the botulinum A toxin into it, for the effect of this substance is to block the release of acetylcholine from motor nerve terminals.

Gerwin (1999), after having reviewed the evidence provided by all those engaged in studying

MTrPs electromyographically, has reconciled the diverse views expressed by concluding that 'the electromyographic [EMG] activity is most consistent with activity generated by a dysfunctional motor endplate. This abnormal endplate activity is modulated by sympathetic nerve activity'.

Histological studies

When in 1976 Simons & Stolov identified points of tenderness with characteristics similar to those of human MTrPs in taut bands found to be present in the muscles of dogs, and then examined the portions of muscle containing them under the microscope, they made the following discoveries.

In cross sections of the biopsies they observed groups of darkly staining enlarged round muscle fibres. And in longitudinal sections these fibres were found to contain fusiform swellings to which they gave the name contraction knots. A contraction knot which is approximately the length of and lies in close proximity to a motor endplate is a segment of muscle fibre that has become abnormally thickened as a result of its sarcomeres having become markedly contracted. On either side of the knot the muscle fibre's sarcomeres are considerably thinner than those in a normal muscle fibre due to compensatory stretching (Fig. 4.2).

As Simons (1999) has recently pointed out, the discovery by Simons & Stolov (1976) that there are a large number of contraction knots in a low-magnification field is indicative that in any one MTrP many such knots are present. And it is the contracted sarcomeres in these knots that give a MTrP and the taut band containing it a palpable ropiness and nodularity.

From his own and other workers' studies Simons (1999) has been led to conclude that both the development of contraction knots in a MTrP and the latter's spontaneous electrical activity are due to the excessive release of acetylcholine from dysfunctional motor endplates.

Morphology

From recently carried out electromyographic and histopathological studies it is evident that structurally a MTrP is made up of a collection of dysfunctional motor endplates, juxtapositional contraction knots and neurovascular bundles with each of these containing blood vessels and contiguous sympathetic fibres; a motor axon and its nerve terminals; and sensory afferents attached to proprioceptors and nociceptors (Fig. 4.2).

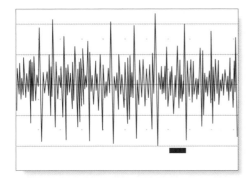 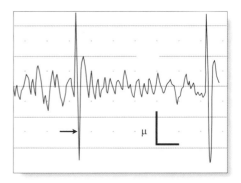

Figure 4.3 Spontaneous electrical activity (SEA) and spike characteristic of an active locus in a human trigger point. Both records are of essentially the same activity; the difference is in the recording speed. A, slow speed which presents a one-second record that shows the general pattern of activity, but little detail. B, recording at 10 times faster speed (0.1 s record) that shows the noise-like spontaneous activity of low amplitude and two superimposed, intermittent, sharp, initially negative spikes of high amplitude. Amplification is less for the slow record. (Reproduced with permission from Simons D G 1996 Clinical and etiological update of myofascial pain from trigger points. *Journal of Musculoskeletal Pain* (1996) 4(1/2): 112.)

Myofascial trigger points' sensory afferents

Proprioceptive sensory afferents

The proprioceptive afferents in the neurovascular bundle at a MTrP site include group IA attached to annulospiral muscle spindles, group IB attached to Golgi tendon organs and group II attached to flower spray muscle spindles.

The rapid insertion of a needle into a MTrP leads to the development of a local twitch response (see p. 66). This causes changes to take place in a muscle fibre's length and tension which in turn lead to the stimulation of these large diameter proprioceptive afferents. There is reason to believe that it is because of the ability of these stimulated afferents to block the intra-dorsal horn passage of noxiously generated information from a MTrP's group IV nociceptors (see Ch. 2, Box 2.1) that it is possible to relieve MTrP pain employing the deep dry needling technique discussed in Chapters 2 and 7.

Nociceptive sensory afferents

There is no certainty at the present time whether pain which arises from a MTrP does so as a result of activity developing in both the muscle's group III and IV nociceptor nerve endings or only in the latter. It is only possible to hypothesise about this and in doing so the following considerations will be taken into account.

As stated in Chapter 2, group III muscle nociceptors are the peripheral terminals of thin myelinated sensory afferents with a conduction velocity in the cat of 2.5–20 m/s and group IV muscle nociceptors are the peripheral terminals of even thinner unmyelinated sensory afferents with a conduction velocity of less than 2.5 m/s. Structurally therefore these group III and group IV sensory afferents are the counterparts of the skin's A-delta and C-polymodal nociceptive sensory afferents.

As also discussed in Chapter 2, trauma-induced stimulation of cutaneous A-delta nociceptors gives rise to the production of an immediate onset transient sensation known as the 'first' pain. And

in those cases, where the trauma is of such severity as to give rise to tissue damage, this 'first' pain is quickly replaced by a persistent dull aching type of discomfort known as the 'second' pain which is produced as a result of activity developing in C-polymodal nociceptors.

Much less, however, is known about the relative contributions of group III and group IV nociceptors to the development of muscle pain, for as Raja et al (1988) have stated, 'The differential role, if any, of the myelinated and unmyelinated muscle nociceptors is not clear at the present time'. And as Bowsher (personal communication, 1992) has stated, 'nobody knows what is felt when human muscle group III afferents are stimulated'.

It is necessary therefore to see what may be learnt from animal experiments, and with respect to these, it should be noted that when recordings have been made of the electrical activity in single muscle afferent units it has been found that those muscle receptors which are true nociceptors (i.e. those that are able to distinguish between noxious and innocuous stimuli) are not responsive to a low intensity stimulus such as that provided by weakly applied pressure or stretching within the physiological range but are responsive to high intensity noxious ones such as those which, in humans, cause MTrP nociceptor activity to develop. Furthermore, it has been shown that the conduction velocity of these nociceptors' sensory afferents is below 2.5 m/s and that they are therefore of the non-myelinated group IV type (Bessou & Laporte 1961, Mense 1993a, Mense & Meyer 1985, 1988, Paintal 1967).

There are therefore grounds for believing that MTrP pain develops as a result of the activation and sensitisation of group IV nociceptors (see Chs 2 and 7).

Factors responsible for development of MTrP nociceptor activity

MTrP nociceptors become activated and sensitised (see Ch. 2) in response to high intensity noxious stimulation brought about by one or other of the following means.

Trauma to muscle

The commonest reason for TrP activity developing is trauma. This may take the form of direct injury to a muscle or the acute or chronic overloading of it. Alternatively, the muscle may be subjected to repeated episodes of microtrauma such as, for example, may happen with a repetitive strain injury (Ch. 10).

Muscle ischaemia

As Simons & Mense (1998) have pointed out, the long-held belief that pain in a muscle leads to the development of spasm in it and that this in turn leads to the production of more pain is a misconception, for physiological studies have shown that muscle pain tends to inhibit, not facilitate, reflex contractile activity of the same muscle (Simons et al 1999). Nevertheless, should a muscle for one reason or another go into spasm severe enough to render it ischaemic then the ischaemia is liable to cause MTrP nociceptors to become activated (Mense 1993b).

Muscle ischaemia brought about by arterial obstruction of sufficient severity to lead to the development of intermittent claudication may also cause TrP activity to develop (Ch. 13).

Visceral-somatic reflex

MTrPs are liable to develop activity should they lie within a zone of visceral pain referral. An example of this is the development of TrP activity in muscles of the chest wall to which pain has been referred as a result of coronary heart disease (Ch. 14). Another is MTrP activity developing in the epigastric region when pain is referred there from a peptic ulcer (Ch. 15).

Radiculopathic compression of motor nerves

From electromyographic studies carried out on paraspinal muscles by Chu (1995) there is evidence to show that entrapment of a nerve root, because of the effect motor nerve compression has on dysfunctional motor endplates at TrP sites, leads to the development of TrP activity in muscles innervated by it.

Anxiety

When, because of chronic anxiety, a person holds a group of muscles in a persistently contracted state, TrPs in them are liable to become activated. McNulty et al (1994) have provided evidence to show that one possible cause for this is the development of autonomic nervous system activity (see Ch. 3).

Another possible reason is anxiety-induced hyperactivity in the reticular system having a stimulating effect on spinal cord alpha-motor neurons and this in turn causing activity to develop in motor nerves that terminate on dysfunctional motor endplates at MTrP sites (see Chs 2 and 3).

Other possible causes

Other possible reasons for MTrP nociceptors becoming activated include exposure of muscle to adverse environmental conditions such as excessive cold, extreme heat, damp and draughts. It may also happen as a result of a rise in body temperature during the course of a febrile illness (Melzack & Wall 1988).

MTrP activity usually develops in muscles that are otherwise normal. It does so even more readily, however, in muscles that have become weakened or wasted by some underlying disease (Ch. 5), or when they have been kept immobile for some time, such as, for example, may happen during the course of a chronic illness, or following a stroke (Ch. 5), or when a limb is encased in a plaster cast.

Myofascial trigger point activity

An active MTrP is one whose nociceptors have undergone sufficient activation and sensitisation to cause pain to be referred to a site some distance from it (a zone of pain referral). Active MTrPs are of three types – primary, secondary and satellite.

Primarily activated MTrPs

These are TrPs in a muscle or group of muscles whose nociceptor activity is primarily responsible for the development of the MTrP pain syndrome. They may be the only ones to undergo activity but in some cases secondary MTrP activity takes place.

Secondarily activated MTrPs

Secondary TrP activity may take place either in the initially affected muscles' synergists or in their antagonists or both. TrP activity in the synergists develops when these muscles become overloaded as a result of compensating for the weakened primarily affected ones. TrP activity in the antagonists develops when these muscles become strained as a result of counteracting the tension in and shortening of the primarily affected ones.

Satellite MTrPs

Satellite TrPs are ones which develop activity when the muscle in which they are situated is in another muscle's zone of TrP pain referral.

From these satellite MTrPs pain is then referred to even yet more distant sites. It is as a consequence of this that pain initially emanating from one MTrP may eventually affect a wide area. For example, it is not uncommon for pain arising from a MTrP in the lower part of the posterior chest wall to be referred to the buttock; satellite TrPs in the gluteal muscles may then become active and pain from there may be referred down the back of the leg, with the development of activity in satellite TrPs in the calf muscles.

For the successful treatment of MTrP pain it is essential that all the primary, secondary and satellite MTrPs are systematically located and deactivated.

Latent MTrPs

A latent MTrP is one whose nociceptors have undergone a limited amount of activation and sensitisation but not sufficient to cause pain to develop. The sensitisation of the nociceptors, however, is enough to cause the TrP to be as exquisitely tender on firm palpation as an active pain-producing one is. For this reason latent MTrPs are liable to be discovered during the course of routine examinations of healthy people.

Sola & Kuitert (1955), in a survey of 200 fit young people serving in the American Air Force (100 males, age range 17–27; and 100 females, age range 18–35), found that 54 of the females and 45 of the males had MTrPs which, whilst exquisitely tender, were not causing pain and therefore were considered to be in a latent phase.

MTrP-related taut bands

A MTrP which itself is only a few millimetres in diameter is located at the centre of a taut cord-like band of muscle fibres several centimetres in length.

In addition to this constantly-sited central TrP, TrPs may also in some cases be located at a taut band's terminal attachments. It has been suggested that the reason these attachment TrPs become active is because the sustained tension exerted by a taut band on its insertion sites leads to the development of an enthesopathy (Simons et al 1999).

There is considerable controversy concerning the reasons for the development of taut bands. There is no evidence to suggest that they develop simply because of the laying down of fibrous tissue or because of localised accumulations of fluid. Also, not as the German physician Schade (1919) postulated, because of the gelling of muscle proteins (myogelose).

Because a band of this type disappears once the MTrP present in it has been deactivated by one or other of the methods described in Chapter 7, its development must be due to muscle fibres in the vicinity of the MTrP undergoing some type of readily reversible contracture.

Simons (1988) originally put forward the hypothesis that a taut band arises because sarcomeres in the region of a MTrP undergo shortening as a result of calcium being released when the trauma responsible for the development of MTrP activity causes the muscle's sarcoplasmic reticulum to rupture.

Simons (1996) has since postulated that the muscle fibre shortening produced in this manner gives rise to an energy crisis as a result of it impairing the local circulation with, as a consequence, the development of tissue hypoxia and a diminished nutrient supply, whilst it at the same time producing an increased metabolic demand. This lack of energy, by compromising recovery of the calcium by the sarcoplasmic reticulum, perpetuates the cycle.

Measurements made by Brückle et al (1990) showing that there is an extremely low oxygen tension inside a taut band adds credence to this hypothesis.

Simons et al (1999), as a result of integrating recently discovered electrophysiological and histological findings at MTrP sites, have now hypothesised,

that a TrP is essentially a region of many dysfunctional endplates and that each dysfunctional endplate is associated with a section of muscle fiber that is maximally contracted (a contraction knot).

And that,

. . . the taut band of a TrP would be caused by the increased tension of involved muscle fibres both because of the tension produced by the maximally shortened sarcomeres in the contraction knot and also because of the increased (electric) tension produced by all the remaining elongated (and therefore thin) sarcomeres.

When considering the pathogenesis of taut bands it is necessary to bear in mind that two recent surveys have shown them to be present in the muscles of healthy people.

Wolfe et al (1992) examined the muscles of a group of patients with fibromyalgia, a group with the MTrP pain syndrome and a group of people with no disease. They found taut bands to be present as frequently in this latter group as they were in the other two groups. Njoo & Van der Does (1994), in a prospective comparative study to determine the incidence of MTrPs in patients with non-specific low-back pain and healthy controls, found taut bands to be present in 6 of the 63 people (approx. 10%) in the control group.

As, therefore, taut bands are found in pain-free individuals, Simons (1996) has been led to conclude that although it was previously assumed that MTrP activity is the cause of them developing, it is more likely that they develop first and are a necessary precursor for the development of latent MTrPs.

Moreover, there are grounds for believing that the propensity to form palpable bands and to

develop MTrP pain is genetically determined (Pellegrino et al 1989).

Local twitch response

It is only possible to palpate taut bands that lie close to the surface in superficially placed muscles. And if a palpable band is 'snapped' by drawing the examining finger sharply across it at a TrP site in a manner similar to that employed when plucking a violin string, it is possible to evoke a transient contraction of the muscle fibres. This local twitch response (LTR) may be either visible or felt under the examining finger. And in some cases it is both seen and felt.

It is also possible to elicit a LTR by means of rapidly inserting a needle into a MTrP. And from doing this Hong (1994a) has shown that a MTrP is made up of a number of separate loci and that by needling each of these in turn it is possible to produce a succession of LTRs. Furthermore, from the results of a trial carried out by him (Hong 1994b), he has been led to conclude that when deactivating a MTrP by means of inserting a needle into it (deep dry needling) or injecting a local anaesthetic into it, the evocation of a series of LTRs is essential (see Ch. 7).

As evoking a LTR by rapidly inserting a needle into a MTrP is an extremely painful procedure there is reason to believe that the response is initiated by the stimulation of the latter's sensitised nociceptors and that the twitch develops as a result of the sensory afferent barrage set up by this giving rise to reflex motor efferent activity on reaching the spinal cord.

Support for the concept that a LTR is essentially a spinal reflex and is not dependent on supraspinal influences comes from experiments on rabbits carried out by Hong and his co-workers (Hong & Torigoe 1994, Hong et al 1995). In these they showed that the local twitch response cannot be evoked should the nerve supplying the muscle be either anaesthetised or severed. Also, that no twitch response is obtainable immediately following spinal cord transection but is once the cord has recovered from any surgically induced shock.

Simons (1976), Fricton et al (1985b) and Simons & Dexter (1995) have recorded the electromyographic activity which takes place when a local twitch response is evoked by 'plucking' a taut band at a MTrP site. Simons & Dexter (1995) also recorded this when local twitch responses were evoked by means of rapidly inserting a monopolar EMG needle repeatedly into a MTrP. The local twitch responses produced by this latter means have also been visualised by means of ultrasound imaging (Gerwin & Duranleau 1997).

Fibrositic nodules

Fibrositic nodules are curiously enigmatic structures that develop in the muscles of patients with the MTrP pain syndrome. And what is particularly puzzling about them is that they only develop in the lumbar region and, but far less commonly, in the region of the neck and shoulders.

The first person to examine fibrositic nodules under the microscope was Ralph Stockman, Professor of Medicine at Glasgow University. In 1904 he published a report stating that he had found evidence of inflammatory changes in the connective tissue of these structures and that he was of the opinion that the pain caused by them is due to this inflamed connective tissue infiltrating the walls of nerves. Subsequent 20th century investigators, including Schade (1919), who was the next to carry out a detailed examination of them, were unable to confirm Stockman's findings.

Schade carried out his study of fibrositic nodules on soldiers in a German field hospital during the First World War. He made two important observations. One was that fibrositic nodules discovered in the muscles of a number of soldiers continued to be palpable when these men, for a variety of different reasons, had to be deeply anaesthetised. Another was that fibrositic nodules present in the muscles of soldiers who subsequently died continued to be palpable following death up to the time that rigor mortis set in. These observations led him to conclude that fibrositic nodules do not develop as a result of localised muscle spasm. And his failure to confirm the presence of inflammatory changes described by Stockman caused him to refute the

idea that they develop as a result of an inflammatory hyperplasia of muscle connective tissue. He therefore came to the conclusion that nodules and palpable bands, both of which cause localised areas of muscle to feel abnormally hard (muskelharten), develop as a result of a change in the colloidal state of muscle cytoplasm so as to transform it from a colloid in liquid solution (sol) to a colloid in a gelatinous form (gel). This led him to coin the term myogelose for this assumed chemical change and for English writers when subsequently discussing it to call it either muscle gelling or myogelosis.

The German orthopaedic surgeon Glogowski and the pathologist Wallraff were the first to carry out a detailed study of the histological changes associated with so-called myogelose. In 1951 they reported the results of examining 24 biopsies of muscle hardening (muskelharten), but despite the use of no less than nine tissue stains, they were unable to demonstrate any significant abnormalities and concluded that myogelosis must occur at the sarcoplasmic level beyond reach of the light microscope.

In the meantime, in Britain, Copeman and Ackerman (1944) added to the confusion by concluding erroneously that nodules felt in the muscles of patients with low-back pain are nothing more than herniated fat lobules.

It was not until Brendstrup et al (1957) carried out the first controlled biopsy and biochemical study of fibrositic nodules that their true nature became apparent. In this study, the microscopic appearances of biopsies of paraspinal muscles containing palpable fibrositic nodules were compared with those of biopsies taken from normal contralateral paraspinal muscles in 12 patients undergoing operations for prolapsed intervertebral discs. The authors stressed that, as the subjects were fully anaesthetised and the muscles relaxed with curare, neither painfulness nor muscle spasm could have been factors in choosing the areas for biopsy, and that the selection of sites was done entirely by feeling for fibrositic nodules.

They found a striking difference between the microscopic appearances of the nodules, and those of the controls. By staining sections with toluidine blue, they were able to demonstrate in the 'fibrositic' specimens interstitial mucinous oedema containing acid mucopolysaccharides and an accumulation of mast cells. In addition, biochemical analysis of these specimens showed a much higher concentration of hexosamine and hyaluronic acid than in the controls. Hyaluronic acid has a strong water-binding capacity and therefore, not surprisingly, the extracellular fluid content of the fibrositic specimens was considerably more than that of the controls and constituted, in effect, an oedema of the connective tissue. At that time it was thought that oedema of this type, by distorting the peripheral nerve endings, might be an important contributory factor in the development of pain (Wegelius & Absoe-Hansen 1956).

Knowledge concerning the structure of fibrositic nodules was advanced still further by Awad (1973), who took from 10 patients biopsies of muscle in which these nodules could be felt and examined them with the electron microscope. The skin overlying each nodule to be biopsied was carefully marked with an indelible pen. Muscle fascicles approximately 1 cm wide and 2 cm long were then dissected out at these sites after they had been grasped firmly between the opposing jaws of a modified chalazion clamp. The reason for doing this was partly to prevent the development of muscle contraction artefacts but also to ensure that the fluid content of the muscle remained trapped within the biopsy material.

When examined under the light microscope, the muscle fibres appeared normal except that in every case there seemed to be an increase in the number of interstitial nuclei. However, what was of much greater significance was the discovery in 8 out of the 10 cases of a large amount of amorphous material in between the muscle fascicles which, when stained with toluidine blue, was shown to consist of acid mucopolysaccharides. This substance, which is known to have enormous water-binding properties, under normal conditions is only present in small amounts in muscle extracellular tissue.

On electron microscopic examination, it was noted that this amorphous material

distended the spaces between muscle fibres which were themselves of normal appearance. In addition, large clusters of platelets were observed and mast cells were seen to be discharging mucopolysaccharide-containing granules into the extracellular space. The next most common finding of any significance was an increased amount of connective tissue (5 cases).

It was concluded that this water-retaining mucopolysaccharide amorphous substance in fibrositic nodules is what causes them to be space-occupying structures that stretch the surrounding muscle tissue. It was also concluded that the accumulation of this substance in the extracellular tissues is what impairs the oxygen flow to muscle fibres and increases their acidity, and that it is this increased acidity which sensitises muscle sensory nociceptors and converts them into pain-producing trigger points.

However, as Awad (1990) has pointed out, several questions remain to be answered, including, does the accumulation of mucopolysaccharides in fibrositic nodules occur as a result of an increased production of this normally occurring substance, or a decrease in its degradation, or a change in its quality?

Sympathetic changes associated with myofascial trigger point activity

As there are sympathetic fibres in the neurovascular bundles that lie in close proximity to dysfunctional motor endplates at a MTrP site it is hardly surprising that nociceptor activity sometimes causes sympathetically mediated changes to take place.

It is, for example, because of the setting up of sympathetic overactivity that the skin temperature of the extremity of a limb affected by MTrP pain is not infrequently considerably reduced and that reversal of this temperature change takes place once the MTrP has been deactivated.

In keeping with this clinical observation are the results of thermographic studies carried out both by Diakow (1992) and by Kruse & Christiansen (1992) for these showed that the skin temperature over a diffuse area distal to a MTrP becomes lowered following the application of firm pressure to the MTrP.

With reference to this it is of interest that Hubbard (1996) observed that the effect of injecting the alpha-adrenergic blocking drug phentolamine either intravenously or locally into a MTrP was to reduce significantly the number of spikes recorded electromyographically; and that Hong et al (1997) confirmed this in a similar study carried out on rabbits.

When considering the sympathetic innervation of MTrPs, it is pertinent to recall that Travell as long ago as 1954, from observations made during the course of inserting a needle thermocouple into a MTrP, came to the conclusion that it is a region of increased metabolism and/or decreased circulation. And to recall that histological studies at MTrP sites led Fassbender (1975) to a similar conclusion. It would seem therefore that one of the reasons for impairment of the circulation at a MTrP site is sympathetically mediated vasoconstriction.

It is possible that these vasoconstrictive changes at a MTrP site may lead to the development of venous congestion in the skin overlying it with, as a consequence, an increase in its temperature. Thermographic studies carried out by Fischer (1984) showed that an area of skin 5–10 cm in diameter directly overlying a MTrP was 0.5–1.0°C warmer than the adjacent skin. He referred to this area of increased heat as a discoid 'hot spot'. There is, however, no general agreement as to the location of these thermographically demonstrable 'hot spots' for both Fischer (1986a) and Weinstein (1986) have since described them as being in zones of pain referral. Furthermore, a thermographic study carried out by Swerdlow & Dieter (1992) on 365 patients with clinically demonstrable MTrPs, found that whilst 'hot spots' could be demonstrated in the majority of these patients, the sites at which they were identified did not correspond with those at which MTrPs were located. They concluded therefore that more research was required in order 'to determine the physiology responsible for these common and persistent thermal phenomena'.

PERPETUATION OF MYOFASCIAL TRIGGER POINT PAIN

MTrP pain may disappear spontaneously once the trauma-induced inflammatory reaction responsible for releasing MTrP nociceptor-activating and -sensitising chemical substances into the tissues has resolved. Not infrequently, however, the pain persists long after tissue healing has taken place. The reasons for this happening are not certain and in our present state of knowledge current concepts concerning possible mechanisms are no more than working hypotheses (Mense 1990).

The three possibilities that will be considered are the perpetuation of the pain brought about by the arousal of (1) dorsal horn neuronal plasticity, (2) the development of self-perpetuating ischaemic changes at MTrP sites and (3) the setting up of self-perpetuating circuits between MTrPs and the spinal cord.

Spinal dorsal horn plasticity
(Box 4.1a,b,c)

There are grounds for believing that the sensory afferent barrage set up by activated and sensitised MTrP nociceptors causes the intra-dorsal horn release of neuropeptides (e.g. substance P, calcitonin gene-related peptide). And that these neuropeptides encourage the release of

---

Box 4.1a   Dorsal horn neuronal plasticity

Trauma-induced tissue damage
↓
MTrP nociceptive activation and sensitisation of MTrP nociceptors
↓
Sensory afferent barrage
↓
Release from group IV sensory afferents' dorsal horn terminals
of
neuropeptides (substance P, calcitonin gene-related peptide etc.)
and
Excitatory amino acids (glutamate, aspartate)

Box 4.1b Dorsal horn neuronal plasticity

Neuropeptides and excitatory amino acids
↓
Changes in N-methyl-D-aspartate receptors
↓
Setting up of state of excitability in dorsal horn
nociceptive neurons
i.e. central sensitisation

---

excitatory amino acids such as glutamate and aspartate which act at dorsal horn nociceptive neuron N-methyl-D-aspartate (NMDA) receptor sites.

The co-release of these neuropeptides and excitatory amino acids has the effect of bringing about a state of excitability in dorsal horn nociceptive neurons (Dubner & Basbaum 1994). That is to say it causes them to undergo the phenomenon known as central sensitisation (see Ch. 2).

The effects of this central sensitisation are to increase the receptive fields of these neurons; to bring about the development of A-beta-mediated hyperalgesia; and to ensure the persistence of the nociceptor-mediated pain (Mense 1993b).

Development of self-perpetuating ischaemic changes at MTrP sites

(Box 4.2a,b)

MTrP nociceptor-sensitising substances such as bradykinin and prostaglandins, which are released into the tissues as a result of a trauma-induced inflammatory reaction, cause both vasodilatation and an increase in vascular permeability. This results in the development of oedema which, by compressing veins, causes the tissues to become ischaemic. Once this happens a

vicious circle is created because the ischaemia encourages the release of yet more MTrP-sensitising chemical substances. Moreover, any ischaemia produced in this manner is liable to be self-perpetuating by virtue of it depleting the muscle of adenosine triphosphate with, as a result, a failure of the muscle's calcium pump mechanism; so that as a consequence, the muscle goes into spasm and causes still further ischaemia-producing blood vessel compression to take place.

This persistent ischaemia accounts for the reduced oxygen tension found to be present at MTrP sites (Brückle et al 1990) and as hypoxia is a potent stimulator of bradykinin release it encourages the perpetuation of MTrP sensitisation and, as a consequence, the persistence of pain.

It seems likely that this circulatory stasis and hypoxia at MTrP sites is responsible for the presence of the so-called ragged red fibres found in the vicinity of MTrPs (Bengtsson et al 1986a). Such fibres can certainly be produced in response to experimentally induced ischaemia (Heffner & Barron 1978). Found in both the MTrP pain syndrome and fibromyalgia, they are considered to be the hallmark of any mitochondrial disorder and are believed to arise as a result of hypoxic-induced alterations in mitochondrial adenosine triphosphate production (Henriksson & Mense 1994).

Self-perpetuating circuits between MTrPs and the spinal cord

Motor efferent activity (Box 4.3)

The sensory afferent barrage produced by activated and sensitised MTrP nociceptors, on reaching the spinal cord, project not only to transmission neurons in the dorsal horn but also to motor neurons in the ventral horn with, as a

---

Box 4.1c Dorsal horn neuronal plasticity

Dorsal horn nociceptive neuronal sensitisation
↓   ↓   ↓
Increase in receptive fields   Development of A-beta-mediated pain   Persistence of MTrP nociceptor-mediated pain

---

Box 4.2a Self-perpetuating ischaemic changes at MTrp sites

Trauma
↓
Tissue damage
↓
Release of TrP nociceptor-activating substances
↓
followed by
Release of nociceptor-sensitising substances (NSSs)
such as bradykinin and prostaglandins
↓
Vasodilatation and oedema
↓
Compression of veins
↓
Ischaemia
↓
Encourages further release of NSSs

Box 4.2b Self-perpetuating ischaemic changes at MTrp sites

Nociceptor-sensitising substance (NSS)-induced
ischaemia
↓
Muscle adenosine triphosphate depletion
↓
Calcium pump mechanisms break down
↓
Muscle spasm
↓
Ischaemia with reduced oxygen tension at MTrP sites
↓
Further release of NSSs
↓   ↓
Perpetuation of nociceptor   Persistence of pain
sensitisation

Box 4.3 Motor efferent activity

Trauma-induced MTrP nociceptor activation and
sensitisation
↓
Sensory afferent barrage
↓
Activity in ventral horn motor neurons
↓
Motor efferent activity
↓
Perpetuation of dysfunction at MTrP's motor endplates
↓
Perpetuation of MTrP nociceptor activity

Box 4.4 Sympathetic efferent activity

MTrP nociceptor-induced sensory afferent barrage
↓
Activates sympathetic preganglionic neurons
↓
Activates noradrenergic postganglionic neurons
↓
Increased sympathetic efferent activity
↓
Release of noradrenaline (norepinephrine)
↓
Perpetuation of MTrP nociceptor activation

---

result, the setting up of activity in motor axons. It was originally thought that it was the consequent development of muscle spasm, which in turn caused the muscle containing a TrP to become ischaemic, that led to the perpetuation of MtrP activity and the persistence of pain (Fields 1987).

It requires, however, a considerable amount of spasm to render a muscle ischaemic. And in the light of recent knowledge concerning the structure of MTrPs, the more likely explanation is that it is the effect of the motor efferent activity on a MTrP's dysfunctional motor endplates that is responsible for the perpetuation of its nociceptor activation and sensitisation and, as a consequence, persistence of the pain.

Sympathetic efferent activity (Box 4.4)

Another possibility is that the sensory afferent barrage produced by activated and sensitised MTrP nociceptors, on reaching the spinal cord, activates sympathetic preganglionic neurons in the intermediolateral column present in the tissues separating the dorsal and ventral horns. This, in turn, would cause noradrenergic postganglionic neurons in the sympathetic chain to become activated with, as a result, the development of activity in sympathetic efferents and, as a consequence, the release of noradrenaline (norepinephrine). The latter would then help to maintain the MTrP nociceptors in an activated and sensitised state.

This hypothesis, which was first put forward by Livingston (1943) as a result of observations on patients with reflex sympathetic dystrophy, has since received support from in vitro experimental rat muscle receptor studies carried out by Kieschke et al (1988).

MYOFASCIAL TRIGGER POINT PAIN REFERRAL

Physiological mechanisms

Current concepts concerning the mechanisms responsible for the referral of pain from MTrPs were discussed in some detail in Chapter 2.

Pain referral patterns

During her lifetime Janet Travell made a special study of MTrP pain referral patterns (see Ch. 1). She found that each muscle in the body has its own specific pattern and that for most of them it is in a caudal direction.

Simons (1993) has estimated that in 48% of muscles it is in a downwards direction; that in 5% of them it is an upwards direction; that in 10% of them it is locally around the MTrP; that in 17% it is both locally and downwards; and that in 20% it is in an upwards and downwards direction.

THE SEARCH FOR MYOFASCIAL TRIGGER POINTS

It cannot be stressed too strongly that in the investigation of persistent pain it is essential for the physical examination to include a methodical search for TrPs. Guidance as to which muscles may contain them is obtained by paying careful attention to the distribution of the pain and observing whether any movements of the body are restricted as a result of the pain and if so which ones.

Each muscle under suspicion should then be put slightly on the stretch and systematically palpated. Some authorities state that for muscles which overlie bone this should be done by means of flat palpation with the tips of the fingers drawn firmly across the muscle in a manner similar to that employed when kneading dough. For those which do not overlie bone pincer palpation should be used with the muscle firmly squeezed between the thumb and fingers.

The difficulty about employing this latter technique, however, is that normal healthy muscle is extremely tender when firmly squeezed (Lewis 1942). Because of this it is my personal preference to use flat palpation for all muscles.

It is necessary to emphasise how important it is to apply firm pressure when attempting to locate MTrPs for one of the commonest reasons for overlooking them is palpation carried out too gently. Firmly applied flat palpation over a healthy muscle causes no discomfort. When carried out over muscle situated in a MTrP's zone of pain referral and over muscle in close proximity to a MTrP it causes no more than slight discomfort. In contrast to this, firm pressure applied to the tissues directly overlying a MTrP gives rise to such considerable discomfort as to cause the patient involuntarily to flinch. This flexion withdrawal reflex is known as the jump sign. In addition, the discomfort may cause the patient to utter an expletive.

It is because of these two reactions that it is my practice to refer to MTrPs as 'jump and shout' points when teaching students.

Pressure threshold measurements at MTrP sites

Because of the sensitisation of its nociceptors a MTrP is so exquisitely tender that its pressure threshold, i.e. the minimal amount of pressure required to induce pain, is considerably reduced. Measurements made with the pressure threshold meter devised by Fischer (1986b) show that the mean normal pressure threshold at healthy muscle sites is in the range 5.4–9.0 kg/cm^2 for males and 3.7–6.8 kg/cm^2 for females. In contrast to this, pressure threshold measurements at MTrP sites may be as low as 0.5–1.5 kg/cm^2. And following successful deactivation of a MTrP there may be a three- to six-fold increase in these pressures.

There is in my view little or nothing to be gained from employing a pressure threshold meter in everyday clinical practice. The semi-objective measurements made with it are mainly of use during the carrying out of clinical trials and medico-legal work.

A detailed account of pressure algometry (dolorimetry) can be found in Fischer's comprehensive review of the subject (Fischer 1994).

DIAGNOSIS OF THE MTrP PAIN SYNDROME

As there are no electrophysiological, histological, biochemical or imaging techniques available for the routine diagnosis of MTrP pain syndrome it necessarily follows that this can only be made from its symptoms and characteristic physical signs.

Symptoms

Pain

The pain is most often described as taking the form of a dull ache. In most cases there is an intermittent mild to moderate discomfort aggravated by the carrying out of certain movements. In some, however, the pain is both severe and constant.

With a single MTrP pain syndrome the pain is localised to one region of the body but should several syndromes develop concomitantly the pain is generalised.

Restricted range of movements

A muscle containing an active TrP and its associated taut band develops increased tension and shortening. There is also enthesopathic tenderness in the region of the terminal attachments of the taut band. This combination of increased muscle tension, muscle shortening, enthesopathic tenderness and TrP-induced pain is liable to lead to the restriction of movements.

These restricted movements may be either a symptom complained of by the patient or a physical sign elicited by the clinician.

Muscle weakness

A patient with MTrPs is liable to complain of difficulty in carrying out certain movements as a result of the development of muscle weakness. Careful observation by the clinician as to which movements are affected as a result of this gives an indication as to where the active MTrPs are likely to be located.

Sleep disturbance

Sleep is liable to be disturbed by pain when pressure is exerted on TrPs as a result of the muscle or muscles containing them being lain upon, and also when TrP activity is increased as a result of muscles containing them being kept in a persistently shortened state.

The sleep disturbance experienced by patients with the MTrP pain syndrome is, however, never as profound or as disabling as that experienced by fibromyalgia sufferers who, because it is of such poor quality, wake up feeling exhausted.

Peripheral hypothermia

A person with active MTrPs in an arm or leg is liable to complain of the limb's extremity being extremely cold. This autonomic dysfunction disappears once the MTrPs have been successfully deactivated and is never as severe as that which is responsible for development of the Raynaud's phenomenon in fibromyalgia.

Physical signs

'Jump' and 'shout' reactions

A MTrP is by definition a point of maximum tenderness, with firm pressure (approx. 4 kg) applied to the tissues immediately overlying it causing a flexion withdrawal reflex to take place, the 'jump' sign, and in some cases the utterance of an expletive, the 'shout' sign. These reactions are obtained with both active and latent MTrPs.

Pain reproduction

When pressure is applied for about 10–15 seconds to an active MTrP it is possible to reproduce the patient's spontaneously experienced pain. As Gerwin (1999), however, has pointed out, the reliability of this test is dependent on the patient's ability to provide relevant information concerning what is felt.

An added confusion, as Hong et al (1996) have shown, is that whilst referred pain can invariably be reproduced when sustained pressure is applied to an active MTrP, this may also at times happen when it is applied to latent MTrPs. Furthermore, both Nice et al (1992) and Njoo & Van der Does (1994) found out, there was a low level of concordance with this test amongst those taking part in their inter-rater reliability MTrP diagnosis studies. It therefore cannot be used as a standard for the diagnosis of the MTrP pain syndrome.

Palpable taut bands

It is generally accepted that a MTrP located somewhere along the length of a taut palpable band is in an active phase. However, not only does the palpation of a taut band require skill and experience but it is only possible to do this providing the muscle containing it is superficially placed. Moreover, it has to be remembered that the presence of a taut band without an accompanying MTrP is not of any diagnostic significance as bands of this type have been located in pain-free healthy people (Wolfe et al 1992).

Local twitch response

The eliciting of a local twitch response by sharply 'plucking' a palpable taut band at a MTrP site confirms that the MTrP is in an active phase but it is only possible to do this when the muscle containing the MTrP is superficially placed. Furthermore, a practical difficulty is that to obtain such a response by this means or by the rapid insertion of a needle into an active MTrP (see p. 66) requires a certain amount of manual dexterity.

Peau d'orange cutaneous and subcutaneous tissue thickening

Some patients with the MTrP pain syndrome develop a peau d'orange thickening of the skin and subcutaneous tissues. No pitting oedema is present but pressure applied to the skin with a blunt instrument such as the end of a matchstick produces a persistent clean-cut indentation. Gunn & Milbrandt (1978) originally called this disorder trophoedema and more recently Simons et al (1999) have termed it panniculosis.

The tissue thickening makes it difficult to roll the skin between the thumb and forefingers and in a severe case it is not possible to pick up the skin.

This tissue change occurs even more frequently and extensively in fibromyalgia. This has led Zohn & Clauw (1999) to devise a skin rolling test which they hope may prove to be a valuable objective diagnostic procedure in this disorder.

Intertester reliability of physical signs

Four studies (Gerwin et al 1995, Nice et al 1992, Njoo & Van der Does 1994, Wolfe et al 1992) have been carried out for the purpose of determining the concordance reached by a number of examiners when eliciting these various active MTrP-related physical signs. In all except the first of these studies the kappa statistic derived by Cohen (1960) was employed prospectively for the purpose of estimating the degree of agreement reached by a number of observers after correcting for chance agreement. In the trial carried out by Wolfe et al (1992) this statistical measurement was determined retrospectively by Simons and Skootsky (Simons 1996).

In the study carried out by Wolfe et al (1992) four physicians with extensive experience of diagnosing the MTrP pain syndrome, examined muscles in three groups of patients (8 with MTrP syndrome, 7 with fibromyalgia and 8 healthy people) for MTrP tenderness, pain recognition, pain referral, taut bands and local twitch responses. Concordance was low and it was considered that the most likely explanation for this result was that the clinicians concerned were not permitted to agree a uniform examination technique prior to the carrying out of the study (Simons 1996).

In the same year Nice at al (1992) reported the results of a study in which thoracolumbar paraspinal muscles of 50 patients with low-back pain were examined in turn by 12 physiotherapists. In this trial a MTrP was considered to be present when the application of firm pressure to the tissues overlying it for a maximum of 10 seconds caused the patient to report the onset of pain at a distant site or an increase in the intensity of the pain already present at the site. Reliability of this test was found to be poor as evidenced by a low kappa coefficient and it has been suggested that a possible reason for this was inadequate training of the examiners (Simons 1996).

In 1994 Njoo & Van der Does reported the findings obtained by a general medical practitioner in Holland with long experience of locating MTrPs and by four final year Dutch medical students trained in doing this by the practitioner. In their study the quadratus lumborum and gluteus medius muscles were examined in 61 cases of non-specific low-back pain and in 63 controls.

An attempt was made to elicit all of the physical signs Wolfe and his co-workers looked for with, in addition to these, an assessment of limited stretch range.

It was found that of these only localised tenderness, jump sign and pain recognition were reliable criteria for the presence of MTrPs. Because of the amount of training each of the examiners had received concordance among them was high.

That inter-rater agreement can be increased as a result of training is evident from two studies carried out by Gerwin et al (1995). In the first of these, 4 physicians examined 25 subjects for muscle tenderness, taut bands, local twitch response and referred pain. Twenty-one months later the same clinicians attempted to elicit these physical signs in 10 new subjects following a 3-hour training session.

Agreement among them was poor in the first trial but in the second one, carried out following a period of intensive training, a high degree of inter-examiner concordance was achieved.

The MTrP pain syndromes and the fibromyalgia syndrome – an overlapping spectrum?

The diagnosis of a single MTrP pain syndrome, because it is confined to one region of the body, is relatively straightforward but when, as not infrequently happens, several syndromes of this type develop concomitantly in various regions, the widespread pain that ensues has to be distinguished from that present in the fibromyalgia syndrome (FS).

One difficulty in doing this is that patients with FS may have not only this disorder's characteristic tender points (TPs) which, by definition, are points of maximal tenderness at specified sites with pressure applied to them causing pain to be felt locally, but also TrPs with pressure applied to them causing pain to be referred some distance from them.

Bengtsson et al (1986b) were among the first to report the presence of both TPs and TrPs in FS, having found that 83.6% of their patients with this disorder had one or more TrPs. Others who have observed this include Granges & Littlejohn (1993), who in a musculoskeletal pain disorders comparative study found that out of a group of 60 patients with FS, 41 (68.3%) had TrPs, and Gerwin (1995), who in a study of 96 subjects with muscle pain presenting to a community pain clinic found that 25 had FS and of these 18 (72%) had TrPs.

Another reason for diagnostic confusion, as Bennett (1990) has stated, is that not uncommonly a patient with the MTrP pain syndrome ultimately ends up suffering from FS.

It may therefore be seen that there is much to support the hypothesis put forward by İnanıcı et al (1999) that these two disorders form a spectrum of overlapping musculoskeletal pain conditions.

Criteria for the diagnosis of the MTrP pain syndrome

In order to ensure the wider recognition of the MTrP pain syndrome as a clinical entity it is essential for its diagnostic criteria to be kept as simple and as non-controversial as possible.

It is generally agreed that the presence of one or more MTrPs is the hallmark of this disorder. Fortunately MTrPs are readily detectable because of the 'jump' and 'shout' reactions that are elicited immediately firm pressure is applied directly over them. And when, in the absence of any other obvious pain-producing disorder, they are found to be present in one particular region of the body that is affected by a persistent dull aching type of pain it is, in my opinion, reasonable to assume that the pain is emanating from them without putting the patient to the discomfort of having sustained pressure applied to each of the MTrP sites for the purpose of showing that this is so. Particularly as any pain relief obtained by the carrying out of a MTrP-deactivating procedure helps to confirm the diagnosis.

Although it is true that palpating a taut band and eliciting a local twitch response at a MTrP site serves to confirm that the MTrP is in an active phase, these two physical signs can never be made essential criteria for the diagnosis of the disorder as it is only possible to demonstrate their presence when the muscle containing the MTrP is superficially placed.

It must have been considerations such as these that led Yunus (1993) cogently to ask why it should not be possible for all patients with regional muscle pain to be classified as having the MTrP pain syndrome on the basis of pain and tender points alone.

Apart from clinical trials when possibly more exacting criteria may be required (Simons 1990), it would seem eminently sensible to make these two the only ones necessary for the diagnosis of this disorder in everyday clinical practice. It has to be admitted, however, that this only applies to cases of regional muscle pain. For when it comes to generalised muscle pain the finding of points of maximal tenderness can only be of limited value as by this means alone it is not possible to decide whether a patient has multiple MTrP pain syndromes or fibromyalgia. To do this other considerations have to be taken into account including whether or not the criteria for the diagnosis of fibromyalgia laid down by the American College of Rheumatology are fulfilled.

The purpose of keeping the criteria for the diagnosis of a single MTrP pain syndrome as simple and as straightforward as possible is to help ensure that this disorder becomes more readily recognised rather than, as at present, when all too frequently, it remains undiagnosed and as a consequence inadequately treated. It cannot be stressed too strongly that it is essential for doctors and physiotherapists during the course of their training to be shown how to examine muscles for MTrP activity and to be taught the importance of looking for MTrPs when investigating pain of uncertain origin.

All this notwithstanding, there is currently no consensus concerning the essential criteria for the diagnosis of the MTrP pain syndrome and in view of this the International Myopain Society is presently engaged in conducting a large-scale multi-centre study in an attempt to rectify this matter (Russell 1999).

REFERENCES

Aftimos S 1989 Myofascial pain in children. New Zealand Medical Journal 102:440–441

Awad E A 1973 Interstitial myofibrositis: hypothesis of the mechanism. Archives of Physical Medicine 54:440–453

Awad E A 1990 Histopathological changes in fibrositis. In: Fricton J R, Awad E A (eds) Advances in pain research and therapy. Raven Press, New York, vol 17, pp 249–258

Bates T, Grunwaldt E 1958 Myofascial pain in childhood. Journal of Pediatrics 53:198–209

Bengtsson A, Henriksson K G, Laarson J 1986a Muscle biopsy in primary fibromyalgia. Scandinavian Journal of Rheumatology 15:1–6

Bengtsson A, Henriksson K G, Jorfeldt L et al 1986b Primary fibromyalgia – a clinical and laboratory examination of 55 patients. Scandinavian Journal of Rheumatology 15:340–347

Bennett R M 1990 Myofascial pain syndromes and the fibromyalgia syndrome: a comparative analysis. In: Fricton J R, Awad E (eds) Advances in pain research and therapy. Raven Press, New York, vol 17, pp 43–65

Bessou P, Laporte Y 1961 Étude des récepteurs musculaires innervés par les fibres afférentes de Groupe III chez le chat. Archives of Italian Biology 99:293–321

Brendstrup D, Jespersen K, Asboe-Hansen G 1957 Morphological and chemical connective tissue changes in fibrositic muscles. Annals of Rheumatic Diseases 16:438–440

Brückle W, Suckfüll M, Fleckenstein W, Weiss C, Müller W 1990 Gewebe-po$_2$–messung in der verspannten ruckenmuskulatur (M. erector spinae). Zeitung Rheumatol 49:208–216

Chen S-M, Chen J-T, Kuan T-S, Hong C-Z 1998a Effects of neuromuscular blocking agent on the spontaneous electrical activity of active loci in a myofascial trigger spot of rabbit skeletal muscle. Journal of Musculoskeletal Pain 6(suppl 2):25

Chen S-M, Chen J-T, Kuan T-S, Hong C-Z 1998b Inhibitory effects of calcium channel blocker on the spontaneous electrical activity of myofascial trigger point. Journal of Musculoskeletal Pain 6(suppl 2):24

Cheshire W P, Abashian S W, Mann J D 1994 Botulinum toxin in the treatment of myofascial pain syndrome. Pain 59:65–69

Chu J 1995 Dry needling (intramuscular stimulation) in myofascial pain related to lumbosacral radiculopathy. European Journal of Physical Medicine and Rehabilitation 5(4):106–121

Cohen J 1960 A coefficient of agreement for nominal scales. Educational Psychology Measurements 20:37–46

Copeman W S, Ackerman W L 1944 'Fibrositis' of the back. Quarterly Journal of Medicine 13:37–51

Diakow P R 1992 Differentiation of active and latent trigger points by thermography. Journal of Manipulative Physiology and Therapeutics 15:439–441

Dubner R, Basbaum A I 1994 Spinal dorsal horn plasticity following tissue or nerve injury. In: Wall P D, Melzack R (eds) Textbook of pain, 3rd edn. Churchill Livingstone, Edinburgh, pp 225–241

Fassbender H G 1975 Pathology of rheumatic diseases. Springer-Verlag, New York

Fields H L 1987 Pain. McGraw-Hill, New York, pp 152–154

Fine P G 1987 Myofascial trigger points in children. Journal of Pediatrics 111:547–548

Fischer A A 1984 Diagnosis and management of chronic pain in physical medicine and rehabilitation. In: Ruskin A P (ed) Current therapy in physiatry. WB Saunders, Philadelphia, pp 123–145

Fischer A A 1986a The present status of neuromuscular thermography: Clinical Proceedings, Postgraduate Medicine. Custom Communications (March), pp 26–33

Fischer A A 1986b Pressure threshold meter. Its use for quantification of tender spots. Archives of Physical Medicine and Rehabilitation 67:836–838

Fischer A A 1994 Pressure algometry (dolorimetry) in the differential diagnosis of muscle pain. In: Rachin E S (ed) Myofascial pain and fibromyalgia. Mosby, St Louis, ch 6

Fricton J, Kroening R, Haley D, Siegert R 1985a Myofascial pain syndrome of the head and neck. A review of clinical characteristics of 164 patients. Oral Surgery, Oral Medicine, Oral Pathology 60(6):15–23

Fricton J R, Auvinem M D, Dykstra D, Schiffman E 1985b Myofascial pain syndrome: electromyographic changes associated with local twitch response. Archives of Physical Medicine and Rehabilitation 66:314–317

Gerwin R D 1994 Neurobiology of the myofascial trigger point. In: Masi A T (ed) Fibromyalgia and myofascial

pain syndromes. Baillière's Clinical Rheumatology 8(4):747–762

Gerwin R D 1995 A study of 96 subjects examined both for fibromyalgia and myofascial pain. Journal of Musculoskeletal Pain 3(suppl 1):121

Gerwin R D 1999 Differential diagnosis of myofascial pain syndrome and fibromyalgia. Journal of Musculoskeletal Pain 7(1/2):209–215

Gerwin R D, Duranleau D 1997 Ultrasound identification of the myofascial trigger point. Muscle and Nerve 20:767–768 [Letter]

Gerwin R D, Shannon S, Hong C-Z, Hubbard D, Gevirtz R 1995 Identification of myofascial trigger points: inter-rater agreement and effect of training. Journal of Musculoskeletal Pain 3(suppl 1) 55 (abstract)

Glogowski G, Wallraff J 1951 Ein beitrag zur Klinik und Histologie der Muskelhärten (Myogelosen). Zeitschrift für Orthopädie 80:237–268

Granges G, Littlejohn G 1993 Prevalence of myofascial pain syndrome in fibromyalgia syndrome and regional pain syndrome: a comparative study. Journal of Musculoskeletal Pain 1(2):19–35

Gunn C C, Milbrandt W E 1978 Early and subtle signs in low back sprain. Spine 3(93):267–281

Heffner R R, Barron S A 1978 The early effects of ischaemia upon skeletal muscle mitochondria. Journal of Neurological Science 38:295–315

Henrikkson K G, Mense S 1994 Pain and nociception in fibromyalgia: clinical and neurobiological considerations in aetiology and pathogenesis. Pain Reviews 1:245–260

Heuser J, Miledi R 1971 Effect of lanthanum ions on function and structure of neuromuscular junctions. Proceedings of the Royal Society of London B Biological Science 179:247–260

Hong C-Z 1994a Considerations and recommendations regarding myofascial trigger point injection. Journal of Musculoskeletal Pain 2(1):29–59

Hong C-Z 1994b Lidocaine injection versus dry needling to myofascial trigger point. The importance of a local twitch response. American Journal of Physical Medicine and Rehabilitation 73:256–263

Hong C-Z 1999 Current research on myofascial trigger points – pathophysiological studies. Journal of Musculoskeletal Pain 7(1/2):121–129

Hong C-Z, Simons D G 1998 Pathophysiologic and electrophysiologic mechanisms of myofascial trigger points. Archives of Physical Medicine and Rehabilitation 79:863–871

Hong C-Z, Torigoe Y 1994 Electrophysiological characteristics of localized twitch responses in responsive taut bands of rabbit skeletal muscle. Journal of Musculoskeletal Pain 2(2):17–43

Hong C-Z, Yu J 1998 Spontaneous electrical activity of rabbit trigger spot after transection of spinal cord and peripheral nerve. Journal of Musculoskeletal Pain 6(4):45–48

Hong C-Z, Torigoe Y, Yu J 1995 The localised twitch responses in responsive taut bands of rabbit skeletal muscle fibres are related to the reflexes at spinal cord level. Journal of Musculoskeletal Pain 3(1):15–34

Hong C-Z, Chen Y-N, Twehous D, Hong D H 1996 Pressure threshold for referred pain by compression on the trigger point and adjacent areas. Journal of Musculoskeletal Pain 4(3):61–79

Hong C-Z, Chen J-T, Chen S-M, Kuan T-S 1997 Myofascial trigger point is related to sympathetic activity (abstract). American Journal of Physical Medicine and Rehabilitation 76:169

Hubbard D R 1996 Chronic and recurrent muscle pain. Pathophysiology and treatment, and review of pharmacologic studies. Journal of Musculoskeletal Pain 4(1/2):123–143

Hubbard D R, Berkoff G M 1993 Myofascial trigger points show spontaneous needle EMG activity. Spine 18(13):1803–1807

İnanıcı F, Yunus M B, Aldag J C 1999 Clinical features and psychologic features in regional soft tissue pain: comparison with fibromyalgia syndrome. Journal of Musculoskeletal Pain 7(1/2):293–302

Ito Y, Miledi R, Vincent A 1974 Transmitter release induced by a 'factor' in rabbit serum. Proceedings of the Royal Society of London B Biological Science 187:235–241

Jones R V, Lambert E H, Sayre G P 1955 Source of a type of 'insertion activity' in electromyography with evaluation of a histologic method of localisation. Archives of Physical Medicine and Rehabilitation 35:301–310

Kieschke J, Mense S, Prebhakar N R 1988 Influence of adrenaline and hypoxia on rat muscle receptors in vitro. Progress in Brain Research 74:91–97

Kruse R A Jr, Christiansen J A 1992 Thermographic imaging of myofascial trigger points: a follow-up study. Archives of Physical Medicine and Rehabilitation 73:819–823

Lewis Sir Thomas 1942 Pain. Macmillan, New York, pp 3, 41

Liley A W 1956 An investigation of spontaneous activity at the neuromuscular junction of the rat. Journal of Physiology 132:650–666

Livingston W K 1943 Pain mechanisms. Macmillan, New York

McCain G A 1994 Fibromyalgia and myofascial pain syndromes. In: Wall P D, Melzack R (eds) Textbook of pain. Churchill Livingstone, Edinburgh, ch 26

McNulty W H, Gevirtz R N, Hubbard D R et al 1994 Needle electromyographic evaluation of trigger point response to a psychological stress. Psychophysiology 31(3):313–316

Melzack R, Wall P D 1988 The challenge of pain, 2nd edn. Penguin, Harmondsworth, Middlesex, p 186

Mense S 1990 Considerations concerning the neurobiological basis of muscle pain. Canadian Journal of Physiology and Pharmacology 69:610–616

Mense S 1993a Neurophysiology of muscle in relation to pain. In: Voeroy H, Merskey H (eds) Progress in fibromyalgia and myofascial pain. Elsevier Science, Amsterdam, pp 23–39

Mense S 1993b Nociception from skeletal muscle in relation to clinical muscle pain. Pain 54:241–289

Mense S 1997 Pathophysiologic basis of muscle pain syndromes. An update. Physical Medicine and Rehabilitation Clinics of North America 8(1):23–52

Mense S, Meyer H 1985 Different types of slowly conducting afferent units in cat skeletal muscle and tendon. Journal of Physiology 363:403–417

Mense S, Meyer H 1988 Bradykinin-induced modulation of the response behaviour of different types of feline Group III and Group IV muscle receptors. Journal of Physiology 398:49–63

Nice D A, Riddle D L, Lamb R L, Mayhew T P, Rueker K 1992 Intertester reliability of judgements of the presence of trigger points in patients.

Archives of Physical Medicine and Rehabilitation 73:893–898

Njoo H K, Van der Does E 1994 The occurrence and inter-rater reliability of myofascial trigger points in the quadratus lumborum and gluteus medius: a prospective study in non-specific low back pain patients and controls in general practice. Pain 58:317–323

Paintal A S 1967 A comparison of the nerve impulses of mammalian non-medullated nerve fibres with those of the smallest diameter medullated fibres. Journal of Physiology 193:523–533

Pellegrino M J, Waylonis G W, Somner A 1989 Familial occurrence of primary fibromyalgia. Archives of Physical Medicine and Rehabilitation 70:61–63

Raja S, Meyer J N, Meyer R A 1988 Peripheral mechanisms of somatic pain. Anesthesiology 68:571–590

Russell I J 1999 Reliability of clinical assessment measures for the classification of myofascial pain syndrome. Journal of Musculoskeletal Pain 7(1/2):309–324

Salpeter M M 1987 Vertebral neuromuscular junctions: general morphology, molecular organization and functional consequences. In: Salpeter M M (ed) The vertebrate neuromuscular junction. Alan R. Liss, New York, pp 1–54

Schade H 1919 Beiträge zur Umgrenzung and Klärung einer Lehre von der Erkältung. Zeitschrift Geselschaft Experimentaler Medizin 7:275–374

Schiffman E, Fricton J R, Haley D P, Shapiro B L 1990 The prevalence and treatment needs of subjects with temporomandibular disorders. Journal of the American Dental Association 120(3):295–303

Simons D G 1976 Electrogenic nature of palpable bands and 'jump sign' associated with myofascial trigger points. In: Bonica J J, Albe-Fessard D (eds) Advances in pain research therapy. Raven Press, New York, vol 1.

Simons D G 1988 Myofascial pain syndrome due to trigger points. In: Goodgold J (ed) Rehabilitation medicine. International rehabilitation medicine association monograph series, no. 1. Mosby, St Louis, pp 686–723

Simons D G 1990 Muscular pain syndromes. In: Fricton J, Awad E (eds) Advances in pain research and therapy. Raven Press, New York, vol 17, pp 1–41

Simons D G 1993 Referred phenomena of myofascial trigger points. In: Vecchiet L, Albe-Fessard D, Lindblom U (eds) New trends in referred pain and hyperalgesia. Elsevier Science, Amsterdam, ch 28

Simons D G 1996 Clinical and etiological update of myofascial pain from trigger points. Journal of Musculoskeletal Pain 4(1/2):93–121

Simons D G 1999 Diagnostic criteria of myofascial pain caused by trigger points. Journal of Musculoskeletal Pain 7(1/2):111–120

Simons D G, Dexter J R 1995 Comparison of local twitch responses elicited by palpation and needling of myofascial trigger points. Journal of Musculoskeletal Pain 3(1):49–61

Simons D G, Mense S 1998 Understanding and measurement of muscle tone as related to clinical muscle pain. Pain 75:1–17

Simons D G, Stolov W C 1976 Microscopic features and transient contraction of palpable bands in canine muscle. Archives of Physical Medicine and Rehabilitation 55:65–88

Simons D G, Hong C-Z, Simons L S 1995a Prevalence of spontaneous electrical activity at trigger spots and control sites in rabbit muscle. Journal of Musculoskeletal Pain 3(1):35–48

Simons D G, Hong C-Z, Simons L S 1995b Nature of myofascial trigger points, active loci. Journal of Musculoskeletal Pain 3(suppl 1):62

Simons D G, Hong C-Z, Simons L S 1995c Spontaneous electrical activity of trigger points. Journal of Musculoskeletal Pain 3(suppl 1):124

Simons D G, Hong C-Z, Simons L S 1995d Spike activity in trigger points. Journal of Musculoskeletal Pain 3(suppl 1):125

Simons D G, Travell J G, Simons L S 1999 General overview. Myofascial pain and dysfunction. The trigger point manual, 2nd edn. Williams & Wilkins, Baltimore, vol 1, ch 2

Skootsky S, Jaeger B, Oye R K 1989 Prevalence of myofascial pain in general internal medicine practice. Western Journal of Medicine 151(2):157–160

Sola A E, Kuitert J H 1955 Myofascial trigger point pain in the neck and shoulder girdle. North West Medicine 54:980–984

Stockman R 1904 The causes, pathology and treatment of chronic rheumatism. Edinburgh Medical Journal 15:107–116, 223–235

Swerdlow B, Dieter J N 1992 An evaluation of the sensitivity and specificity of medical thermography for the documentation of myofascial trigger points. Pain 48:205–213

Travell J (1954) Introductory comments. In: Ragan C (ed) Connective tissues. Transactions of the fifth conference. Josiah Macy Jr Foundation, New York, pp 12–22

Travell J G, Simons D G 1983 Myofascial pain and dysfunction. The trigger point manual. Williams & Wilkins, Baltimore, vol 1

Weeks V D, Travell J 1957 How to give painless injections. AMA Scientific Exhibits 1957. Grune & Stratton, New York, pp 318–322

Wegelius O, Absoe-Hansen G 1956 Mast cell and tissue water. Studies on living connective tissue in the hamster cheek pouch. Experimental Cell Research 11:437–443

Weinstein G 1986 The diagnosis of trigger points by thermography. Academy of Neuro-muscular Thermography: Clinical Proceedings, Postgraduate Medicine. Custom Communications (March), pp 96–98

Wolfe F, Simons D, Fricton J et al 1992 The fibromyalgia and myofascial pain syndromes – a preliminary study of tender points and trigger points in persons with fibromyalgia, myofascial pain syndrome and no disease. Journal of Rheumatology 19:944–951

Wolfe F, Smythe H A, Yunus M B et al 1990 The American College of Rheumatology 1990 criteria for the classification of fibromyalgia. Report of the multicenter criteria committee. Arthritis and Rheumatism 33(2):160–172

Yunus M B 1989 Fibromyalgia syndrome: new research on an old malady. British Medical Journal 298:474–475

Yunus M B 1993 Research in fibromyalgia and myofascial pain syndromes – current status, problems and future directions. Journal of Musculoskeletal Pain 1(1):23–41

Zohn D A, Clauw D J 1999 A comparison of skin rolling and tender points as a diagnostic test for fibromyalgia. Journal of Musculoskeletal Pain 7(3):127–136

5

Nociceptive nerve pain, neuropathic pain and myofascial trigger point pain

INTRODUCTION

It is essential to be able to distinguish between pain emanating from myofascial trigger points (MTrPs), neural pain arising either as a result of the activation of nociceptors in nerve endings (nociceptive nerve pain), and pain resulting from damage to or dysfunction of axons in the peripheral or central nervous system (neuropathic pain). Regrettably, however, diagnostic errors are all too common.

A frequent mistake is for pain referred down a limb from MTrPs to be considered to have developed as a result of nerve root compression. Diagnostic confusion also not infrequently arises when MTrP pain and neural pain of one type or another develop concomitantly, when MTrP pain develops in someone with a neurological disorder, and when muscle shortening caused by MTrP activity gives rise to nerve root entrapment.

Circumstances in which diagnostic difficulties such as these are likely to arise will therefore be considered in some detail. Before doing so, however, current views concerning the pathophysiology of neuropathic pain will be discussed. And the clinical manifestations of nociceptive nerve pain and neuropathic pain will be described.

Finally, methods employed for alleviating nociceptive nerve pain and neuropathic pain will be reviewed.

PATHOPHYSIOLOGY OF NEUROPATHIC PAIN

There is still considerable ignorance concerning the pathophysiology of neuropathic pain and it will only be possible to allude briefly to it here. More comprehensive accounts include those of Bennett (1994), Devor (1991, 1994) and Wall (1991).

Ectopic neural pacemaker nodules

Sensory afferents rely for their metabolism on proteins synthesised in the dorsal root ganglion and so when a sensory nerve becomes either traumatised or diseased, the part of it distal to the site of injury degenerates but the proximal stump in the vicinity of the ganglion survives.

The axons in the proximal part of an injured nerve, local patches of demyelination along an axon and cells in the dorsal root ganglion itself are then all liable to become sources of aberrant electrical activity which, when transmitted to the brain, are responsible for the development of neuropathic pain.

This aberrant electrical activity arises from tiny nodules that develop in injured nerve endings, neuromas and along the axons of damaged nerves (Devor 1991). As they generate repetitive firing separate from that which develops in normal axons they are called ectopic neural pacemaker nodules (ENPNs).

ENPNs not only fire spontaneously but are sensitive to a broad range of physical, chemical and metabolic stimuli and once triggered by no more than, for example, a brief mechanical stimulus, are liable to continue firing for seconds, minutes or even many hours. However, following intense bursts of this abnormal activity they have a tendency to become refractory with, as a consequence, a long interval in between each paroxysm of pain, a phenomenon not infrequently observed, for example, in patients with trigeminal neuralgia.

There is evidence to suggest that the liability to develop EPNS is genetically determined (Devor & Raber 1990).

Cross-excitation in the peripheral nervous system

Activity in a sensory axon normally has no effect on that in neighbouring axons. However, when an axon becomes damaged cross-excitation is liable to take place. Two factors would seem to be mainly responsible for this, hyperexcitability of ENPNs and the destruction of an axon's insulation.

Cross-excitation in the peripheral nervous system takes several forms. These include electrical (ephaptic) crosstalk, crossed afterdischarge at nerve injury sites, crossed afterdischarge in dorsal root ganglia and sympathetic-sensory coupling.

Electrical (ephaptic) crosstalk

It has for long been known that current from the cut end of an axon excites neighbouring axons immediately following injury. This form of ephaptic coupling only lasts for a few minutes and is therefore unlikely to be of any clinical significance (Granit & Skoglund 1945). However, it has now been shown that several weeks later there is a resurgence of this electrical crosstalk which then persists (Meyer et al 1985, Seltzer & Devor 1979).

This delayed persistent ephaptic crosstalk takes place in neuromas and in regenerating nerve distal to the site of injury (Seltzer & Devor 1979), in patches of demyelination (Rasminsky 1980) and in dorsal root ganglia infected by a virus such as the one responsible for herpes simplex (Mayer et al 1986).

Crossed afterdischarge at nerve injury sites

Crossed afterdischarge, unlike ephaptic crosstalk, develops soon after nerve injury and is less dependent on close axonal apposition. In this disorder single impulses have no effect but repetitive activity, possibly by releasing gradually increasing amounts of a chemical mediator within the nerve, has the effect of inducing repetitive autonomous firing in neighbouring axons (Lisney & Devor 1987).

With respect to this it should be noted that activity in A-beta fibres is liable to cause crossed afterdischarge in A-delta fibres but for some as yet unknown reason not so readily in C fibres (Amir & Devor 1992).

Crossed afterdischarge in dorsal root ganglia

Devor and Wall (1990), in experiments on rats, have shown that activated sensory neurons in a dorsal root ganglion (DRG) can cross-excite neurons in neighbouring ganglia. And, moreover, that this can occur when the peripheral nerve is intact or only partially damaged. It is as a consequence of this that A-beta activity evoked by stroking the skin is capable of activating A-delta DRG neurons.

Noordenbos (1959) pointed out that it is possible that DRG crossed afterdischarge may be capable of giving rise to the development of hyperpathic symptoms such as sensory spread and allodynia in the absence of any neural abnormality.

Sympathetic-sensory coupling

Sympathetic activity in a disorder such as the complex regional pain syndrome type 1 (also known as reflex sympathetic dystrophy; RSD) releases noradrenaline (norepinephrine) and it has been postulated that this chemical substance, by activating injured sensory afferents, causes neuropathic pain to develop (Devor 1983).

Deafferentation pain

Normally when a neural pathway that transmits nociceptive information becomes damaged, the intensity with which noxious stimuli are perceived is reduced. However, in cases where damage to a sensory afferent is such as to cause its dorsal root to become torn away from the spinal cord, the dorsal horn transmission neurons with which it normally connects undergo a marked increase in their excitability. There is, as a result of this, not only, as might be expected, impairment of sensibility for noxious stimuli but, in addition, the paradoxical development of spontaneous pain.

This deafferentation pain is not only very severe but is perceived by the patient as coming from tissues that are otherwise anaesthetic. Another characteristic of this kind of pain is that

there is often a delay of 1–12 weeks before it comes on.

Deafferentation pain, for example, develops whenever a brachial plexus injury is so severe as to cause avulsion of its dorsal roots (Wynn Parry 1980). With brachial plexus avulsion there is usually severe pain of a continuous burning type with, in addition, brief paroxysms of pain that have a sharp shooting electric-shock-like quality. The pain is perceived as arising from denervated tissues that are at least partially anaesthetic. However, despite this anaesthesia, paraesthesiae and in some cases dysaesthesiae are commonly experienced.

This deafferentation pain is very difficult to alleviate other than by surgically destroying the hyperactive nociceptive dorsal horn transmission neurons (Nashold & Ostdahl 1979).

Sensory afferent barrage-induced sensitisation of dorsal horn nociceptive neurons

The afferent barrage from activated and sensitised nociceptors triggers off long-lasting excitability in dorsal horn nociceptive neurons. These neurons when sensitised in this manner become responsive to inputs from A-beta fibres attached to low-threshold mechanoreceptors in the skin with, as a consequence of this, the production of A-beta-mediated pain and the development of hyperalgesia in response to mildly noxious stimuli together with allodynia in response to innocuous mechanical ones (Woolf 1989).

It is also because of this 'wind-up' phenomenon that the excitability of these central cells and their ongoing activity increases to such an extent as to cause the pain to persist on a long-term basis.

Any type of persistent pain, including neuropathic and MTrP nociceptive pain, may cause this central sensitisation to develop (see Chs 2 and 4). With regard to neuropathic pain, it has been shown by Bennett & Xie (1988), in experiments on rats, that a partial nerve lesion produced by constricting the nerve leads to the development of a massive afferent barrage from the dorsal root ganglia and that the effect of this is to set up a very prolonged hyperpathic state. Wall (1991) has suggested that the effect of a sensory afferent barrage such as this together with the decreased central inhibition brought about by a lesion of this type may give rise to such considerable excitation in the transmission neurons as to cause them to die as a result of amino acid excitotoxicity (Coderre et al 1993). And as he pointed out 'this induced degeneration would be one way in which temporary hyperexcitability could be converted to permanent and irreversible changes'.

CLINICAL MANIFESTATIONS OF PAIN OF NEURAL ORIGIN

Pain of neural origin may be either nociceptive nerve pain (nerve trunk pain) or neuropathic pain.

Nociceptive nerve pain (nerve trunk pain)

Nociceptive nerve pain, or what Asbury and Fields (1984) have called nerve trunk pain, is caused by the activation of nociceptors present in the epi-, peri- and endoneurium of a nerve root or plexus. Pain of this type develops as a result of nerve root compression caused, for example, by a neoplasm or a prolapsed intervertebral disc. It may have a shooting electric-shock-like quality or it may, like MTrP pain, take the form of a diffuse dull ache. However, unlike MTrP pain, whose pattern of pain referral never coincides with the course taken by a nerve, the radiation of nociceptive nerve pain is invariably along the length of the involved nerve. And, moreover, the latter not infrequently is found to be tender. Both nociceptive nerve pain and neuropathic pain often have accompanying neurological signs (Arner & Meyerson 1989). These, however, may also be present in patients with MTrP pain due to MTrP nociceptor activity giving rise to muscle shortening, and this, in some places in the body, causes a nerve root to become entrapped (see p. 87).

In addition, nociceptive nerve pain, such as that brought about by a ruptured intervertebral disc, may lead to the secondary development of MTrP pain (see Ch. 4 and later in this chapter).

Neuropathic pain

Neuropathic pain arises as a result of damage to or dysfunction of axons and is in part due to the activation of nociceptors. Because of this, it may have an aching quality similar to that of nociceptive pain. But more often it takes the form of either a burning sensation or shooting electric-shock-like sensations. In addition, there may be unusual non-painful sensations such as that of insects crawling under the skin or a feeling that the tissues are being ripped apart (dysaesthesiae).

Howard Fields (1987), during the course of discussing the bizarre nature of neuropathic pain, states that 'its strange quality probably results from the disruption of the sensory apparatus so that a normal pattern of neural activity is no longer transmitted to the perceptual centers. Although the message that reaches these centers is clearly unpleasant patients recognize that the sensations are not "normal" pain sensations'.

Moreover, unlike nociceptive pain which comes on at the time tissues become damaged, neuropathic pain tends to develop after a latent period.

With most neuropathic pain disorders examination of the affected area reveals the presence of a sensory disturbance with the most frequent being a thermal one.

Another common sensory abnormality is the elicitation of pain by a normally non-painful stimulus, a phenomenon known as allodynia. Allodynia is of three types, tactile, cold and movement. Tactile allodynia is the pain elicited by a phasic light tactile stimulus such as that produced by a current of cold air blowing across the skin. Cold allodynia is the pain produced in response to exposure to a normally non-painful cold stimulus. And movement allodynia is the pain produced in response to muscle contraction. Allodynia occurs as a result of the stimulation of A-beta low threshold rapidly-adapting mechanoreceptors with small receptive fields (Bowsher 1991).

Peripheral nervous system neuropathic pain disorders

These may be divided into two main groups.

One group consists of disorders in which pain of a shooting electric-shock-like character develops in conjunction with allodynia but in the absence of a sensory deficit. Examples of such disorders include trigeminal neuralgia, both in its idiopathic form and when arising as a complication of multiple sclerosis; also Morton's metatarsalgia, a disorder in which pain shoots up the leg when the sole of the foot touches the ground because of a neuroma under a metatarsal head; and, but rarely at the present time, tabes dorsalis.

The other group consists of disorders in which there is a burning pain and a sensory deficit, with or without shooting pains and allodynia. Examples of such disorders include postherpetic neuralgia, diabetic neuropathy, neuralgic amyotrophy, brachial plexus avulsion and phantom limb pain.

Central nervous system neuropathic pain

Pain which arises as a result of stroke-induced damage to the central nervous system was originally known as the thalamic syndrome. Now, however, that it is realised that the lesion is not always in the thalamus but may be in one or other of the pathways leading to or from this structure, it is referred to as central post-stroke pain (Leijon et al 1989).

SOME DIAGNOSTIC PITFALLS

Trigger point pain in muscles weakened by neurological disease

A common error is to assume that pain which develops in the presence of a neurological dis-order must necessarily be due to damage inflicted by the latter on the nervous system. This, however, is not necessarily so for sometimes the pain arises from TrPs in muscles which, weakened by the neurological disorder, become overloaded.

Poliomyelitis is an example of a disease in which this not infrequently happens. Both in this disorder and in other lower motor neuron disorders pain may emanate from MTrP nociceptors that have become activated as a result of the strain imposed upon atrophied muscles or because of postural deformities produced by these weakened muscles.

By contrast there are neurological disorders in which pain is initially neural in origin but at a later stage is due to the development of MTrP activity. Neuralgic amyotrophy is an example of this. In this condition there is a sudden onset of a severe deep aching pain in the shoulder region. This subsides in 7–10 days. However, by that time there is marked wasting of the supraspinatus, infraspinatus, the serratus anterior and deltoid muscles. These overloaded and weakened muscles then become painful due to the activation of MTrP nociceptors.

Concomitant neuropathic and myofascial trigger point pain

There are a number of disorders in which pain is due either to neural damage, or to the development of MTrP activity, or at times to the concomitant development of both.

Multiple sclerosis

Multiple sclerosis is a disorder in which pain may arise as a result of the demyelination of the trigeminal nerve or other nerves. It may also emanate from MTrP nociceptors should these become activated either because of the strain imposed upon weakened paralysed muscles or because of the ischaemia which develops in spastic muscles (Mense 1993). Sometimes both types of pain develop concomitantly.

Central post-stroke pain

Central post-stroke pain (CPSP) is the name now given to what was formerly known as the thalamic syndrome until computerised axial tomography showed that the lesion, rather than being in the thalamus itself, is in the spinothalamic pathway. This type of pain may also develop following a subarachnoid haemorrhage and with spinal lesions.

One striking feature is the relative mildness of the motor deficit. In a series of 156 patients with central pain of this type reported by Bowsher (1996) only 8% were hemi- or monoplegic.

The pain characteristically takes the form of a severe burning sensation such as is experienced when a hand is immersed in ice-cold water. Other descriptive terms sometimes employed include aching, pricking, lacerating, shooting, squeezing and throbbing. The distribution of the pain is extremely variable. It may be confined to the face and/or the proximal or distal part of a limb. In some cases the whole of one side of the body is affected.

There is often a latent interval between the onset of the stroke and the development of pain. The pain came on immediately in only 37% of the stroke patients in Bowsher's series of cases. And in well over half of all the patients there was a median onset time of 3–4 months.

Stress and noise are well known to exacerbate the pain. Allodynia brought on by touch is extremely common. In addition, Bowsher was one of the first to draw attention to movement allodynia, with several of his patients feeling no pain if they kept still but experiencing severe pain on the slightest movement. In addition, the vast majority of patients have a pinprick and thermal stimulation deficit.

Autonomic disturbances are also observed with, in particular, cutaneous vasoconstriction that can be reversed by a calcium channel blocker such as nifedipine.

Post-stroke myofascial trigger point pain

This pain is liable to develop as a result of MTrP activity developing when muscles weakened by a stroke become overloaded during attempts to restore movements to them. It may also develop in conjunction with the pain of a glenohumeral joint capsulitis when there has been a failure to put the shoulder joint repeatedly through a full range of passive movements during the time the arm remains paralysed.

When the pain, which is of a diffuse dull aching type, is referred down a limb there is liable to be accompanying sympathetically mediated vasoconstrictive changes in the hand or foot. Treatment in the form of deactivation of the MTrPs by one means or another both alleviates the pain and abolishes this sympathetic overactivity.

Prolapsed intervertebral disc

Pain that develops following the prolapse of an intervertebral disc may be one or other of several types. When the nucleus pulposus first begins to herniate through the annulus fibrosus, pain is liable to develop as a result of its impingement upon nociceptors in the dura mater. When it herniates still further, nociceptors in sciatic nerve roots become activated with, as a consequence, the development of nociceptive nerve pain in the low-back and leg.

In addition, with this radiculopathy, as with nerve root entrapment from any other cause, TrP activity is liable to develop in muscles supplied by the damaged nerve roots with, as a consequence, the development of superimposed MTrP pain. As discussed in Chapter 4, there are grounds for believing that this is because of the effect of motor nerve compression on motor end-plates at TrP sites.

Malignant disease

Malignant disease is yet another disorder in which pain may be of more than one type. Neoplastic nerve compression gives rise to nociceptive nerve pain and neoplastic infiltration of a nerve causes the development of neuropathic pain. In addition, the pain in this disease may be due to the activation of MTrP nociceptors when muscles, weakened as a result of the disease, become overloaded.

Postherpetic neuralgia

It has to be remembered that in certain neuropathic pain disorders such as postherpetic neuralgia where the pain is both severe and difficult to treat (Loeser 1986, Watson et al 1991), muscles in the vicinity of the affected area tend to be held in a persistently contracted state. When this happens, TrPs in them are liable to become active with, as a consequence, the development of superimposed myofascial pain.

Nerve entrapment as a result of MTrP muscle shortening

Finally, it is necessary to bear in mind that when MTrP nociceptors become activated and sensitised, not only does pain emanate from these nociceptors but the TrP activity causes the muscle to become shortened and this in certain parts of the body gives rise to nerve root entrapment.

The following are some common examples: entrapment of the lower trunk of the brachial plexus by taut shortened bands in a scalene or pectoralis minor muscle; the development of occipital neuralgia with numbness, tingling and a burning sensation in the scalp because of compression of the greater occipital nerve as a result of TrP-induced shortening of the semispinalis capitis muscle; hyperaesthesia or dysaesthesia arising in the paravertebral region as a result of TrP-induced shortening of paraspinal muscles causing pressure to be exerted on dorsal rami of spinal nerves; foot drop and sensory changes brought about as a result of TrP-induced shortening of the peroneus longus muscle causing entrapment of the peroneal nerve; and entrapment of the sciatic nerve occurring as a result of TrP-induced shortening of the piriformis muscle.

MANAGEMENT OF PAIN OF NEURAL ORIGIN

As those who have to deal with musculoskeletal pain disorders also at times have to treat nociceptive nerve pain and neuropathic pain, their management will be discussed briefly.

Treatment of nociceptive nerve pain

The alleviation of this type of pain may require the decompression of a nerve root but there are some cases where it may be achieved by the use of either a non-steroidal anti-inflammatory drug (NSAID), a corticosteroid or a narcotic drug.

It is worth trying a NSAID whenever the pain is in part due to inflammatory compression of a nerve root such as may happen with a radiculopathy caused, for example, by a disc protrusion or neoplastic compression of a nerve root.

Vecht (1989), in a pilot study carried out on 10 patients with radicular pain secondary to a vertebral metastasis, reported significant pain relief after one week of treatment with a high-dose NSAID regime (naproxen 1500–2000 mg/day).

Corticosteroids may also reduce inflammatory oedema responsible for the compression of a nerve root. For example, dexamethasone is considered by some (Green 1975), but not others (Haimoivic & Beresford 1986, Hedeboe et al 1982), to be helpful in the alleviation of radicular pain caused by a herniated intervertebral disc (see Ch. 12). Also, Vecht et al (1989) have found dexamethasone to be highly effective in relieving pain arising as a result of metastastic spinal cord compression. When used for this purpose it should be given in the relatively high dose of 4 mg twice a day or more (Hanks 1991).

Although narcotic drugs, as discussed later, are not particularly effective in controlling neuropathic pain, they have nevertheless been shown to be useful in the treatment of nociceptive nerve pain. Vainio & Tigerstedt (1988), for example, have reported the efficacy of them in relieving cancer-evoked radicular pain.

Treatment of neuropathic pain disorders

Because much has still to be learnt concerning the pathophysiology of neuropathic pain disorders, their treatment remains far from satisfactory. However, over the past few years there have been some significant advances both in the use of drugs and in the employment of various physical modalities for this purpose. Some of these will now be considered. More extensive reviews include those provided by Bowsher (1991) and Fields (1994).

Tricyclic antidepressants

This group of drugs has proved to have a useful pain-relieving effect in a number of different conditions such as fibromyalgia, migraine and neuropathic pain of a burning character. The one most widely employed is amitryptyline. This drug's pain-relieving effect is independent of its mood-influencing one (Feinmann 1985, Watson et al 1982) and therefore should initially be given in the relatively small dose of 15–20 mg each night, other than in the elderly when the starting dose should be not more than 10 mg nocte. With neuropathic pain, however, the dose may have to be increased gradually over the weeks up to 150 mg in younger patients or 100 mg in the elderly. It is important when determining the optimum dosage for any particular individual to bear in mind that it takes time for any pain relief to be obtained and the patient should be warned about this.

Unfortunately tricyclic antidepressants have a number of undesirable side-effects such as urinary retention, interference with memory, orthostatic hypotension, drowsiness and dryness of the mouth. Dryness of the mouth, which is one of the commonest causes of non-compliance, may be counteracted by the use of an artificial saliva spray or by the use of chewing gum. Desipramine would seem to be as effective as amitryptyline and some people tolerate it better.

The use of tricyclics should be avoided in patients with glaucoma for even a relatively small dose may precipitate an acute attack. They also should not be used in those with prostatic hypertrophy or cardiac conduction defects.

In view of these undesirable side-effects it was hoped that the better tolerated newer non-tricyclic antidepressants such as fluoxetine (Prozac) would relieve neuropathic pain but the results so far have been disappointing (Max et al 1992).

Membrane-stabilising agents

With electric-shock-like neuropathic pain, repetitive firing from ectopic pacemakers takes place as a result of an increase in the permeability of sensory endings to various ions, particularly sodium (Na^+) ions. It is therefore sometimes possible to alleviate pain of this type by the use of Na^+-channel blockers which act as membrane stabilisers. There are three classes of these: anticonvulsants such as sodium valproate, carbamazepine, phenytoin, lamotrigine and gabapentin; local anaesthetics such as lignocaine (lidocaine); and cardiac antiarrhythmic drugs such as mexiletine.

Sodium valproate Treatment with this drug should start with 200 mg at night and the dose increased each week up to a maximum of 600–800 mg a day. If no relief is obtained after a month, another anticonvulsant such as carbamazepine or phenytoin should be tried.

Unwanted side-effects of this drug may include some impairment of cognitive function and alertness. Weight gain is not uncommon. Transient alopecia may also occur and, curiously, straight hair when it regrows may be curly. In addition, a dose-related tremor may develop. And very rarely hepatic failure occurs but this in the main is only seen in children under 3 years old with some pre-existing serious disorder (Davidson 1991).

Carbamazepine Carbamazepine should be given initially in a dosage of 100 mg a night for three nights, and then increased by 100 mg increments every other day up to 100 mg three times a day. In a minority of cases this may give adequate pain relief but if not, and providing the drug is being well tolerated, it may be increased by 100 mg a week up to a maximum of 1200 mg a day in divided doses.

Side-effects such as dizziness, dry mouth, slurred speech, somnolence and ataxia may necessitate stopping the drug for 24 hours. It can then often be restarted at a lower dosage. The occasional development of leucopenia and other blood disorders makes regular blood checks essential. The appearance of an erythematous rash is an indication for discontinuing the drug.

McQuay et al (1995) systematically reviewed the various randomised controlled trials that had been carried out to assess the efficacy of anticonvulsant drugs in the management of neuropathic pain and with respect to trigeminal neuralgia concluded that approximately 70% of patients with this disorder obtained significant relief from the use of carbamazepine. After a time, however, its effectiveness tends to wear off. In cases where this happens and in those where there is a failure to obtain any significant pain relief, another anticonvulsant such as phenytoin may be tried. If this fails to give any worthwhile relief, some form of surgical intervention may be required.

Phenytoin As this drug has a long half-life, a single daily dose may be used. However, it is one of the few drugs for which the dosage has to be controlled by measurements of plasma concentrations (Brodie & Feely 1991). For trigeminal neuralgia refractory to carbamazepine a dose of 200–300 mg a day may be required.

Lamotrigine The action of this neuronal sodium channel blocker is to inhibit excessive release of glutamate, a neurotransmitter associated with the development of central sensitisation. A double-blind placebo-controlled crossover study has shown it to be effective, when used in combination with carbamazepine, in controlling refractory trigeminal neuralgia (Zakrewska et al 1997).

It would also seem to have a place when used in high dosage in the treatment of central pain (Canavera & Bonicalzi 1996).

Gabapentin This anti-epileptic drug, which is structurally related to the neurotransmitter gamma-aminobutyric acid, has been shown to be of value in the treatment of postherpetic neuralgia and diabetic neuropathy (Backonja et al 1997).

Lignocaine (lidocaine) Intravenous lignocaine has been shown to alleviate the pain in a variety of different neuropathic pain disorders (Glazer & Portenoy 1991) including postherpetic neuralgia (Rowbotham et al 1991).

Mexiletine Mexiletine, a drug originally introduced for the treatment of cardiac arrhythmias, like lignocaine, acts as a membrane stabiliser by virtue of its being a sodium channel blocker and when administered orally has been found to alleviate diabetic neuropathic pain (Dejgard et al 1988) and peripheral nerve injury pain (Chabal et al 1992).

Narcotics

The use of opioid analgesics in the treatment of neuropathic pain is highly controversial.

A controlled study carried out by Arner & Meyerson (1988) led them to conclude that narcotics are of no value in alleviating pain of this type. Portenoy et al 1990, however, from a study in which opioid infusions were employed concluded that although neuropathic pain has a reduced responsiveness to opioid drugs there is not an inherent resistance to them. For this reason it is necessary to titrate the dose until either intolerable side-effects develop or 'complete' or 'adequate' analgesia is obtained.

Support for this belief was provided by a study carried out by Rowbotham et al (1991) which showed that an infusion of morphine reduces the pain of postherpetic neuralgia, and by a study carried out by Jadad et al (1992) in patients with chronic neuropathic pain.

Arner and Meyerson (1989) and also Vecht (1989) have suggested that some of the confusion concerning this matter may have arisen because of the difficulty in distinguishing clinically between neuropathic pain and readily opioid-responsive nociceptive nerve pain or what Asbury & Fields (1984) have called nerve trunk pain. This is a diagnostic difficulty which is particularly likely to arise in any disorder such as cancer where both these types of pain may be present at the same time.

All this notwithstanding, Fields (1994), from extensive experience with the use of narcotics in the treatment of neuropathic pain disorders, is of the opinion that they are of value in patients who fail to respond to tricyclic and membrane-stabilising drugs. He recommends first giving a fentanyl infusion and, in those cases where there is a good response to this, then administering a narcotic analgesic such as methadone, levorphanol, or a sustained release morphine preparation. He nevertheless emphasises that 'clearly a long-term prospective trial of this approach needs to be carried out'.

N-methyl-D-aspartate (NMDA) receptor blockers

No discussion concerning the treatment of neuropathic pain would be complete without reference to the possible use in the future of NMDA receptor blockers.

With any type of pain, including neuropathic pain, there is hyperexcitability of dorsal horn nociceptive neurones and the development of central sensitisation (see Ch. 2). This phenomenon is responsible for various effects including persistence of the causative pain and the development of A-beta-mediated pain; and because there is evidence to show that excitatory amino acids acting at NMDA receptor sites contribute to its development, the effects of the NMDA receptor blockers magnesium chloride and ketamine have been explored.

Magnesium chloride The reason for investigating the possible use of an intravenous infusion of magnesium chloride was that Mg^{2+} ions have been shown to exert a physiological ion channel block at NMDA receptor sites and, by so doing, to prevent extracellular calcium ions from entering the cells and contributing to secondary neuronal changes. However, Felsby et al (1995), in a pilot study on 10 patients with peripheral nerve damage, found that a magnesium chloride infusion had no effect on either the neuropathic pain or the allodynia.

Ketamine Ketamine, an anaesthetic-inducing agent and NMDA receptor antagonist related to the hallucinogen phencyclidine, has been shown to relieve phantom limb pain (Stannard & Porter 1993), postherpetic neuralgia (Eide et al 1994), causalgia (Byas-Smith et al 1993) and peripheral nerve damage pain (Felsby et al 1995).

The drug has to be infused intravenously and although it has been shown to have an immediate neuropathic pain-relieving effect it remains to be seen whether it provides any worthwhile long-lasting benefit, particularly as it often leads to the development of hallucinogenic reactions and other untoward side-effects. With respect to these, it is pertinent to note that despite this drug's anti-epileptic effect it is of no value in the long-term treatment of seizures because of the development of motor and behavioural toxicity (Rogawaski & Porter 1990).

Thus, although ketamine has been shown to be helpful in alleviating acute pain such as during the changing of burn dressings (Gordon 1987), its value in relieving chronic pain has yet to be established.

The development of clinically effective NMDA receptor blockers for the alleviation of neuropathic pain and other forms of chronic pain therefore remains a challenge for the future (Dubner 1991).

Topically applied substances

In cases where hyperaesthesia and allodynia are particularly troublesome various topically applied agents are sometimes helpful.

There is evidence to suggest that capsaicin, the main ingredient of hot peppers, exerts a topical analgesic effect by depleting C-polymodal nociceptors of the neurotransmitter substance P. Applied in the form of an ointment it has been shown to be useful in alleviating postherpetic neuralgia (Watson et al 1988) and diabetic neuropathic pain (Capsaicin Study Group 1991). One disadvantage is that initially it gives rise to a burning sensation which at times may prove intolerable (Watson et al 1988) but fortunately the undesirable effect usually passes off after a few weeks.

Postherpetic neuralgia may also be relieved sometimes by a lotion consisting of 4% dispersable aspirin in chloroform (King 1988). Other alternatives include the local anaesthetic lignocaine (lidocaine) (Rowbotham & Fields 1989), lignocaine-based Emla cream (Stow et al 1989) and benzydamine cream (Coniam & Hunton 1988).

Physical modalities

Transcutaneous electrical nerve stimulation Transcutaneous electrical nerve stimulation of A-beta nerve fibres is often of value in the treatment of neuropathic pain in disorders such as postherpetic neuralgia, central post-stroke damage and brachial plexus avulsion. Care, however, has to be taken not to place the electrodes on hyperaesthetic skin as stimulation of the A-beta

sensory afferents at such a site makes the pain worse; nor should they be placed over an area of skin where the sensory loss is such that there are insufficient A-beta fibres to stimulate. It is therefore best to place them above the lesion on normally sensitive skin or over a nerve supplying the affected area (Thompson 1986).

Acupuncture The pain-relieving effect of acupuncture is opioid peptide mediated and as neuropathic pain is not readily relieved by opioid drugs it is hardly surprising that it has not proved to be particularly useful in alleviating this type of pain. Lewith et al (1983) found it to be of no value in the treatment of postherpetic neuralgia.

REFERENCES

Amir R, Devor M 1992 Axonal cross-excitation in nerve-end neuromas: comparison of A-beta and C fibres. Journal of Neurophysiology 68:1160–1166

Arner S, Meyerson B A 1988 Lack of analgesic effects of opioids on neuropathic and idiopathic forms of pain. Pain 33:11–23

Arner S, Meyerson B 1989 Reply to Dr Vecht's comments. Pain 39:245–246

Asbury A K, Fields H L 1984 Pain due to peripheral nerve damage: an hypothesis. Neurology 34:1587–1590

Backonja M, Hes M S, LaMoreaux L K, Garofalo E A, Koto E M, US Gabapentin Study Group 210. 1997 Gabapentin (GBP, Neurontin) reduces pain in diabetics with painful peripheral neuropathy: results of a double-blind, placebo-controlled clinical trial (945–210) [abstract]. In: Proceedings of the 16th annual meeting of the American Pain Society. New Orleans, 23–26 October 1997

Bennett G J 1994 Neuropathic pain. In: Wall P D, Melzack R (eds) Textbook of pain, 3rd edn. Churchill Livingstone, Edinburgh, pp 201–224

Bennett G J, Xie Y K 1988 A peripheral mononeuropathy in rat. Pain 33:87–108

Bowsher D 1991 Neurogenic pain syndromes and their management. British Medical Bulletin 47(3):15–28

Bowsher D 1996 Central pain: clinical and physiological characteristics. Journal of Neurology, Neurosurgery and Psychiatry 61:62–69

Brodie M J, Feely J R 1991 Therapeutic drug monitoring and clinical trials. In: Feely J (ed) New drugs. British Medical Journal, London, pp 15–28

Byas-Smith M G, Max M B, Gracely R G, Bennett G J 1993 Intravenous ketamine and alfentanil in patients with chronic causalgic pain and allodynia. In: Abstracts of the seventh world congress of pain, IASP publ., Seattle, WA, p 454

Canavera S, Bonicalzi V 1996 Lamotrigine control of central pain. Pain 68:179–181

Capsaicin Study Group 1991 Treatment of painful diabetic neuropathy with topical capsaicin. A multicenter, double-blind vehicle-controlled study. Archives of Internal Medicine 151: 2225–2229

Chabal C, Jacobson L. Mariano A, Chancy E, Britell C W 1992 The use of oral mexiletine for the treatment of pain after peripheral nerve injury. Anesthesiology 76:513–517

Coderre T J, Katz J, Vaccarino L, Melzack R 1993 Contribution of central neuroplasticity to pathological pain: review of clinical and experimental evidence. Pain 52:259–285

Coniam S W, Hunton J 1988 A study of benzydamine cream in post-herpetic neuralgia. Research and Clinical Forum 10:65–68

Davidson D L W 1991 Anticonvulsant drugs. In: Feely J (ed) New drugs, 2nd edn. British Medical Journal, London, p 316

Dejgard A, Petersen P, Kastrup J 1988 Mexiletine for the treatment of chronic painful diabetic neuropathy. Lancet i:9–11

Devor M 1983 Nerve pathophysiology and mechanisms of pain in causalgia. Journal of the Autonomic Nervous System 7:371–384

Devor M 1991 Neuropathic pain and injured nerve: peripheral mechanisms. British Medical Bulletin 47(3):619–630

Devor M 1994 The pathophysiology of damaged peripheral nerves. In: Wall P D, Melzack R (eds) Textbook of pain, 3rd edn. Churchill Livingstone, Edinburgh, pp 79–100

Devor M, Raber P 1990 Heritability of symptoms in an experimental model of neuropathic pain. Pain 42:51–67

Devor M, Wall P D 1990 Cross excitation among dorsal root ganglion neurons in nerve injured and intact rats. Journal of Neurophysiology 64:1733–1746

Dubner R 1991 Pain and hyperalgesia following tissue injury: new mechanisms and new treatments. Pain 44:213–214

Eide P K, Jorum E, Stubhaug A, Bremnes J, Breivik H 1994 Relief of post-herpetic neuralgia with the N-methyl-D-aspartate receptor antagonist ketamine: a double-blind, cross-over comparison with morphine and placebo. Pain 58:347–354

Feinmann C 1985 Pain relief by antidepressants: possible modes of action. Pain 23:1–8

Felsby S, Nielsen J, Arendt-Nielsen L, Jensen T S 1995 NMDA receptor blockade in chronic neuropathic pain: a comparison of ketamine and magnesium chloride. Pain 64:283–291

Fields H 1987 Pain. McGraw-Hill, New York

Fields H 1994 Peripheral neuropathic pain: an approach to management. In: Wall P D, Melzack R (eds) Textbook of pain, 3rd edn. Churchill Livingstone, Edinburgh, pp 991–996

Glazer S, Portenoy R K 1991 Systemic local anaesthetics in pain control. Journal of Pain Symptom Management 6:30–39

Gordon M D 1987 Burn care protocols: administration of ketamine. Journal of Burn Care and Rehabilitation 8:146–149

Granit R, Skoglund C R 1945 Facilitation, inhibition and depression at the 'artificial synapse' formed by the cut end of a mammalian nerve. Journal of Physiology (London) 124:84–99

Green L N 1975 Dexamethasone in the management of symptoms due to herniated lumbar disc. Journal of Neurology, Neurosurgery and Psychiatry 38:1211–1217

Haimoivic I C, Beresford H R 1986 Dexamethasone is not superior to placebo for treating lumbosacral radicular pain. Neurology 36:1593–1594

Hanks C W 1991 Opioid-responsive and opioid non-responsive pain in cancer. British Medical Bulletin 47(3):718–731

Hedeboe J, Buhl M, Ramsing P 1892 Effects of using dexamethasone and placebo in the treatment of prolapsed lumbar disc. Acta Neurologica Scandinavica 65:6–10

Jadad A R, Carroll D, Glynn C J, Moore R A, McQuay H J 1992 Morphine responsiveness of chronic pain: double-blind randomised crossover study with patient-controlled analgesia. Lancet 339:1367–1371

King R B 1988 Concerning the management of pain associated with herpes zoster and of post-herpetic neuralgia. Pain 33:73–78

Leijon G, Bovie J, Johansson I 1989 Central post-stroke pain. Neurological symptoms and pain characteristics. Pain 36:13–25

Lewith G T, Field J, Machin D 1983 Acupuncture compared with placebo in post-herpetic neuralgia. Pain 17:361–368

Lisney S J W, Devor M 1987 Afterdischarge and interactions among fibers in damaged peripheral nerve in the rat. Brain Research 415:122–136

Loeser J D 1986 Herpes zoster and post-herpetic neuralgia. Pain 25:149–164

McQuay H, Carroll D, Jadad A R, Wiffen P, Moore A 1995 Anticonvulsant drugs for management of pain: a systematic review. British Medical Journal 311:1047–1052

Max M B, Lynch S A, Muir J, Shoaf S E, Smoller B, Dubner R 1992 Effects of desipramine, amitryptyline and fluoxetine on pain in diabetic neuropathy. New England Journal of Medicine 326:1250–1256

Mayer M L, James M H, Russel R T, Kelly J S, Pasternak C A 1986 Changes in excitability induced by herpes simplex viruses in rat dorsal root ganglion neurons. Journal of Neuroscience 6:391–402

Mense S 1993 Nociception from skeletal muscle in relation to clinical muscle pain. Pain 54:241–289

Meyer R A, Raja S N, Campbell J N, Mackinnon S E, Dellon A L 1985 Neural activity originating from a neuroma in the baboon. Brain Research 25:255–260

Nashold B S, Ostdahl R H 1979 Dorsal root entry zone lesions for pain relief. Journal of Neurosurgery 51:59–69

Nathan P W, Wall P D 1974 Treatment of post-herpetic neuralgia by prolonged electrical stimulation. British Medical Journal iii:645–647

Noordenbos W 1959 Pain. Elsevier, Amsterdam

Portenoy R K, Foley K M, Inturrisi C E 1990 The nature of opioid responsiveness and its implications for neuropathic pain: new hypotheses derived from studies of opioid infusions. Pain 43:273–286

Rasminsky M 1980 Ephaptic transmission between single nerve fibres in the spinal nerve roots of dystrophic mice. Journal of Physiology (London) 305:151–169

Rogawaski M A, Porter R J 1990 Antiepileptic drugs: pharmacological mechanisms and clinical efficiency with consideration of promising developmental stage compounds. Pharmacological Reviews 42(3):223–286

Rowbotham M C, Fields H L 1989 Topical lidocaine reduces pain in post-herpetic neuralgia. Pain 38:297–302

Rowbotham M C, Reisner L M, Fields H L 1991 Both intravenous lidocaine and morphine reduce the pain of post-herpetic neuralgia. Neurology 41:1024–1028

Seltzer Z, Devor M 1979 Ephaptic transmission in chronically damaged peripheral nerves. Neurology 29:1061–1064

Stannard C F, Porter G E 1993 Ketamine hydrochloride in the treatment of phantom limb pain. Pain 54:227–230

Stow P J, Glynn C J, Minor B 1989 EMLA cream in the treatment of post-herpetic neuralgia. Efficacy and pharmacokinetic profile. Pain 39:301–306

Thompson J W 1986 The role of transcutaneous electrical nerve stimulation (TENS) for the control of pain. In: Doyle D (ed) International symposium in pain control. Royal Society of Medicine Services. International Congress and Symposium, series 123. Royal Society of Medicine Services Ltd, London, pp 27–47

Vainio A, Tigerstedt Z 1988 Opioid treatment of radiating cancer pain: oral administration versus epidural techniques. Acta Anaesthesiologica Scandinavica 32:179–185

Vecht C J 1989 Nociceptive nerve pain and neuropathic pain. Pain 39:243–244

Vecht C J, Haaxma-Reiche H, Van Putten W L T, Visser M et al 1989 Conventional versus high-dose dexamethasone in metastatic spinal cord compression. Neurology 39(suppl 1):220

Wall P D 1991 Neuropathic pain and injured nerve: central mechanisms. British Medical Bulletin 47(3):631–643

Watson C P, Evans R J, Reed D K, Merskey H et al 1982 Amitryptyline versus placebo in post-herpetic neuralgia. Neurology (NY) 32:671–673

Watson C P, Evans R J, Watt V R 1988 Post-herpetic neuralgia and topical capsaicin. Pain 33:333–340

Watson C P, Watt R V, Chipman M, Birkett N, Evans R J 1991 The prognosis with post-herpetic neuralgia. Pain 46:195–199

Woolf C J 1989 Recent advances in the pathophysiology of acute pain. British Journal of Anaesthesia 63:139–146

Wynn Parry C B 1980 Pain in avulsion lesions of the brachial plexus. Pain 9:41–53

Zakrewska J, Chaudry Z, Nurmikkot T, Patton D, Mullens E 1997 Lamotrigine (lamietal) in refractory trigeminal neuralgia: results from a double-blind placebo controlled cross-over study. Pain 73:223–230

6

Concomitant complex regional pain and myofascial trigger point pain syndromes

INTRODUCTION

It is over fifty years since Livingston (1943), in his classic monograph *Pain Mechanisms*, stated that myofascial trigger points (MTrPs) are liable to become active and contribute to the pain of reflex sympathetic dystrophy (RSD) – now called complex regional pain syndrome (CRPS type 1). Nevertheless this observation is still not sufficiently well recognised, for there is no reference to it in standard textbook accounts of this disorder. However, now that at least three recent studies have confirmed the veracity of Livingston's observation, it is to be hoped that at last it will begin to receive the attention it deserves.

One study was carried out by Filner (1989) who looked specifically for MTrPs in 40 patients with RSD and found active pain-producing ones to be present in 36 of them. In another study, Lin et al (1995) searched for MTrPs in 84 patients with RSD and located active pain-producing ones in 82% of them. And a third, by Inamura et al (1997), also found myofascial pain to be present in 82% of a series of cases with RSD.

Therefore in view of this confirmation that complex regional pain and MTrP pain frequently coexist, the following topics will be discussed in this chapter: aetiological factors and pain-producing mechanisms common to the myofascial trigger point (MTrP) pain syndrome and CRPS type 1 (RSD); current views concerning the pathophysiology of the latter; and methods of treating it including where necessary the deactivation of MTrPs.

Firstly, however, it is necessary to clear up any confusion that may exist concerning terminology.

TERMINOLOGY

Sudeck's atrophy

At the beginning of the 20th century the collective term Sudeck's atrophy (Sudeck 1900, 1902) was introduced for the two related disorders that until recently were called causalgia and reflex sympathetic dystrophy.

Causalgia

This term, derived from the Greek kausis (burning) and algos (pain), was first introduced by Weir Mitchell (1867) for a disorder which he and his colleagues (Mitchell et al 1864) had encountered three years previously in soldiers with bullet-induced nerve damage incurred during the American Civil War.

During World War I Leriche (1939) found that he was able to relieve the pain in this disorder by carrying out a sympathectomy and thus was able to show that it is sympathetically mediated.

This disorder, which develops as a complication of partial nerve damage, has clinical manifestations that include severe diffuse burning, allodynia, hyperalgesia and hyperpathia in the distal part of a limb. The pain is liable to be aggravated by various physical and emotional factors. In addition, there are vasomotor and sudomotor disturbances. Also, trophic changes eventually develop in the area affected by the pain.

Reflex sympathetic dystrophy

It was subsequently realised that a sympathetically mediated disorder of a similar type may develop when tissues other than nerves are damaged and in 1946 Evans called this reflex sympathetic dystrophy (RSD). The taxonomy subcommittee of the International Association for the Study of Pain (IASP) (1986) subsequently

defined it as 'continuous pain in a portion of an extremity after trauma which may include fracture but does not involve a major nerve associated with sympathetic hyperactivity'.

Complex regional pain syndrome

The appropriateness of the term RSD has, however, recently been questioned. This is because, as Stanton-Hicks et al (1995) have pointed out, any dystrophy that may be present in this disorder refers to changes in soft tissues which are not invariably due to postganglionic sympathetic activity, which may or may not be the consequence of a reflex, and which, when present, only arise at a late stage of the disorder.

It was because of increasing doubt as to the usefulness and aptness of the term RSD that a consensus workshop was held in Orlando, Florida in the autumn of 1993. The goals of this workshop were to examine the terms RSD, causalgia, sympathetically maintained pain and sympathetically independent pain and to consider the need for updating the taxonomy adopted by the IASP. The outcome of this was a nosological revision (Stanton-Hicks et al 1995), with the disorders previously known as RSD and causalgia called collectively the complex regional pain syndrome (CRPS) and CRPS subdivided into two types – CRPS type 1 (RSD) and CRPS type 2 (formerly causalgia).

This revised terminology has now been included in the second edition of the IASP *Classification of Chronic Pain* (Merskey & Bogduk 1994).

AETIOLOGICAL FACTORS COMMON TO CRPS TYPE 1 (RSD) AND THE MTrP PAIN SYNDROME

That CRPS type 1 (RSD) and the MTrP pain syndrome may be present concomitantly is hardly surprising considering that the aetiological factors responsible for their development are the same, trauma being by far the commonest one. It may be of such severity as to fracture a bone but often is no more than a relatively minor soft-tissue injury. Livingston (1943), when discussing the sympathetically mediated syndrome's causation stated:

The onset of symptoms may follow the most commonplace of injuries. A bruise, a superficial cut, the prick of a thorn or a broken chicken bone, a strain or even a post-operative scar may act as the causative lesion. The event which precipitates the syndrome may appear both to the physician and the patient as of minor consequence, and both have every reason to anticipate the same prompt recovery that follows similar injuries. This anticipation is not realised and the symptoms tend to become progressively worse.

Both syndromes may also develop following a myocardial infarction or a cerebrovascular accident.

PAIN-PRODUCING MECHANISMS COMMON TO BOTH THE MTrP PAIN SYNDROME AND CRPS TYPE 1 (RSD)

The main aetiological factor in both the MTrP pain syndrome and CRPS type 1 (RSD) is trauma of sufficient intensity to damage the tissues. As a result of this tissue damage, various chemical substances, including bradykinin, serotonin and potassium ions are liberated that activate nociceptors with, as a consequence, the development of nociceptive pain.

Bradykinin and other substances, including prostaglandins, then sensitise these nociceptors. The effect of this sensitisation process is to lower the nociceptors' pain threshold so as to make them responsive to low-intensity stimuli with, as a consequence, the development of exquisite tenderness at the site of injury (primary hyperalgesia).

With both syndromes the sensory afferent barrage set up by these activated and sensitised nociceptors causes nociceptive neurons in the dorsal horn to become sensitised. And when this happens pain develops as a result of the latter responding in an abnormal and exaggerated manner to A-beta proprioceptive inputs from tissues some distance from the injury site. The effect of this is for secondary hyperalgesia to develop with tenderness elicited when firm pressure is applied to this otherwise healthy tissue.

COMPLEX REGIONAL PAIN SYNDROME TYPE 1 (RSD)

Pathophysiology

There is much controversy concerning the pathophysiology of this syndrome (McMahon 1991). Campbell et al (1992) have put forward the hypothesis that in people genetically predisposed to developing this disorder the sensory afferent barrage set up by nociceptors which have undergone trauma-induced activation and sensitisation has three effects.

The first is for it to cause a phenotypic change to take place at some unspecified site, possibly the dorsal root ganglion, with the synthesis of alpha-1-adrenoceptors which, on being transported to the periphery, become incorporated within the walls of these nociceptors. The second is for it to bring about the sensitisation of the dorsal horn's wide dynamic range transmission neurons with, as a result, the persistence of sympathetically mediated pain and the development of A-beta-mediated pain in the absence of cutaneous stimulation (Roberts 1986). And the third is for it to cause the responsiveness of neighbouring sympathetic preganglionic neurons to become modified with, as a consequence, the development of aberrant sympathetic efferent activity.

It is believed that it is because of this aberrant sympathetic efferent activity that noradrenaline (norepinephrine) is released from postganglionic sympathetic terminals. This then binds to these alpha-1-adrenoreceptors at nociceptor sites and by so doing augments the initial nociceptor activation and sensitisation and ensures that the pain and hyperalgesia persist.

In support of this hypothesis was the discovery that intravenous phentolamine, a short-acting alpha-adrenergic antagonist, relieves the pain. This observation incidentally led Arner (1991) and Raja et al (1991) to introduce the phentolamine test for both diagnosing CRPS and predicting the outcome of treating it with some form of sympathetic blockade.

Also in favour of this hypothesis is that an anaesthetic block of a sympathetic ganglion, by eliminating the sympathetic efferent drive, relieves the pain; that the topical application of clonidine does this by reducing the release of noradrenaline (norepinephrine) from sympathetic terminals; that the systemic administration of the alpha-adrenergic receptor antagonists phenoxy-benzamine (Ghostine et al 1984) and prazosin (Abram & Lightfoot 1981) do this by blocking the activation of nociceptors; and that regionally administered intravenous guanethidine does this because of its ability to eliminate noradrenaline (norepinephrine) stores in sympathetic terminals.

It would also seem that it is this aberrant sympathetic efferent activity which brings about the vasomotor changes responsible for the skin becoming abnormally warm or cold and for the tissues ultimately becoming dystrophic. And which brings about the sudomotor changes responsible for the development of either anhidrosis or hyperhidrosis.

Before concluding this discussion it has to be said that against the idea that the sensitisation of dorsal horn transmission neurons causes sympathetically mediated pain to persist is that although these neurons are markedly sensitive to the analgesic effect of morphine, pain of this type is abnormally resistant to the action of opiates (Roberts & Kramis 1992).

From these brief comments it may be seen that the pathophysiology of this syndrome is both complex and highly controversial. And those who wish to study it in greater detail should consult more comprehensive reviews such as those provided by McMahon (1991) and Blumberg & Janig (1994).

Clinical manifestations

As those who deal with the MTrP pain syndrome also have to be able to diagnose the less frequently occurring CRPS type 1 (RSD), it is necessary to give a detailed account of its clinical manifestations.

This syndrome affects either an upper or lower extremity. Although the trauma responsible for it developing may give rise to tissue damage anywhere along the length of the limb, it invariably manifests itself at the distal part. A good example of this is the so-called shoulder–hand syndrome in which trauma-induced tissue damage in the shoulder region is followed by sympathetically mediated pain developing in the hand (see Ch. 10).

Its development is traditionally divided into three stages (Bonica 1990).

In the first stage, which may last from a few weeks to a few months, the main features are pain, swelling of the tissues (non-pitting oedema) and changes in the skin temperature. In the second stage, which may last for a similar period of time, trophic changes take place. These include disordered nail growth, increased hair growth, palmar or plantar fibrosis and either thinning of the skin or, alternatively, hyperkeratosis. In the third stage, which is liable to last indefinitely, muscle atrophy and joint contracture develop.

Osteoporosis, a well-known complication of this disorder, develops so gradually that although its presence can be demonstrated during the second stage by the use of technetium isotope scintigraphy, it is not until the third stage that it is sufficiently well advanced to be seen in plain radiographs.

For the successful treatment of CRPS type 1 (RSD) its diagnosis at an early stage is essential. It was for this reason that Hannington-Kiff (1974) suggested naming the disorder the sympathetic overdrive syndrome in the hope that the acronym SOS might serve to emphasise the urgency of diagnosing and treating it as quickly as possible. The presenting features of the disorder will therefore be discussed at some length.

Blumberg & Janig (1994) carried out a detailed analysis in 190 patients. The commonest presenting feature was distal generalised swelling (96% of the patients). The next two most frequent were diminished muscle strength (92%) and reduced movements (88%).

Somewhat surprisingly, only 75% of patients complained of pain. Moreover, it was not always of a burning type. In some cases it was either throbbing, shooting or even aching in character. However, when present it was nearly always felt deep inside the distal part of the affected extremity.

The vasomotor changes were variable with the extremity being either initially warm or cold in 54% and 21% respectively. The sudomotor changes were similarly variable with these giving rise to hypohidrosis or hyperhidrosis in 17% and 25% respectively.

The sensory changes were also variable – hypoalgesia and hyperalgesia being present in 58% and 29% respectively; hypoaesthesia in 79% and hyperaesthesia in only 0.4%. Moreover, allodynia was absent early on in the disorder and its presence could only be demonstrated in 8% of the patients at a later stage. Hyperpathia was also not observed in this series of patients. This was particularly surprising as both of these sensory changes are usually considered to develop frequently in this disorder (Bonica 1990).

From the results of their survey Blumberg & Janig (1994) have questioned the appropriateness of staging this syndrome. They concluded that it is of far greater value to grade patients according to whether the sensory, autonomic, motor and trophic changes are mild, moderate or severe.

Veldman et al (1993) have also studied the early symptoms and signs in 829 patients referred to them over an 8-year period. Their findings were broadly similar to those of Blumberg and Janig with the noticeable exception that pain was present in 93% of their patients, an incidence which more closely accords with the sine qua non for this disorder and one which led to the recently introduced terms complex regional pain syndrome type 1 (RSD) and type 2 (causalgia).

Veldman et al also queried the validity of the conventional method of staging this disorder and suggested that its development might be more appropriately divided into two phases, a 'warm' one and a 'cold' one from having observed that the longer the disorder is present the more likely it is for the affected limb to be cold. However, this is not invariable as 13% of their patients had cold extremities at the onset of the disorder and some still had warm limbs after 8–12 years.

In summary therefore the essential features of CRPS type 1 (RSD) at an early readily treatable stage include pain, which may or may not be burning in type, and generalised swelling (non-pitting oedema) in the distal part of an extremity. In addition, there are also various vasomotor, sudomotor and sensory changes, and restricted movements due to pain and muscle weakness.

Treatment

As the main purpose of this book is to discuss the diagnosis and management of myofascial pain disorders, the treatment of CRPS type 1 (RSD) will only be discussed briefly. More detailed reviews can be found in Charlton (1991) and Hannington-Kiff (1994).

Physiotherapy

There is widespread agreement as to the need for physiotherapy to be carried out with the aim of ensuring that the painful limb is kept mobile and the range of its movements increased. In addition to this the application of heat in various forms such as short wave diathermy or interferential therapy is considered to be helpful. It has to be said, however, that no placebo-controlled studies of physiotherapy in the treatment of this disorder have as yet been carried out (Paice 1995).

Sympathetic blockade

A long-established means of carrying this out is to inject a local anaesthetic into either the stellate ganglion in the neck or the sympathetic chain in the lumbar region, depending on the site of the lesion (Wang et al 1985).

The efficacy of this form of treatment has, however, been recently challenged. Kozin (1992), after reviewing 500 patients subjected to it, concluded that 'the majority of patients have transient or no significant pain relief'. And Carr et al (1996), having carried out a meta-analysis of randomised clinical trials and controlled studies involving 1144 patients, concluded that the effect of a sympathetic blockade of this type is similar to that of a placebo.

An alternative technique, first introduced by Hannington-Kiff (1974), is to inject a catecholamine-depleting drug such as guanethidine into the affected limb after its arterial blood supply has been cut off by means of the application of a tourniquet. This, too, is widely employed but recent trials (Jadad et al 1995, Ramamurthy & Hoffman 1995) have shown it to be no more effective than a placebo.

The value of anaesthetic and chemical blocks in the routine treatment of this disorder is therefore far from certain. Nevertheless, until such a time as a better understanding of the pathogenesis of this disorder leads to the development of a more effective therapeutic approach, their continued use would seem to be justified even though, as so often happens, treatment of this type has to be repeated at short intervals over a long period of time; and even though, as Schott (1998) has pointed out, their frequent employment is both expensive and not without risk.

Pharmacotherapy

There are several drugs available for the treatment of this disorder. These include alpha-adrenergic blocking agents such as phenoxybenzamine and phentolamine; beta-adrenergic blocking ones such as propranolol; calcium-channel blocking drugs such as nifedipine; corticosteroids; and the serotonin antagonist ketanserin. Of these, the two most helpful seem to be nifedipine and phenoxybenzamine.

Both Prough et al (1985) and Muizelaar et al (1997), in a much larger series of patients, have reported obtaining significant pain relief with nifedipine.

Muizelaar and his co-workers recommend that at an early stage of CRPS nifedipine should be administered in a dose of 10 mg t.i.d. for 2 days, then 20 mg t.i.d. for 2 days, and if this is not successful, yet well tolerated, the dosage can be increased to 30 mg t.i.d. or 20 mg q.i.d. And then, if after 5–7 days on this dose no improvement is noted, a switch to phenoxybenzamine should be made (10 mg at night increased to a maximum of 10 mg q.i.d. over a period of 8–11 days). For the most severe cases, however, these authors recommend administering phenoxybenzamine from the outset.

The commonest side-effect with nifedipine is headache aggravated by bending accompanied by photophobia and phonophobia. The headaches, however, are usually mild and rarely are they severe enough to necessitate discontinuing the drug. Other, but less frequent, side-effects include dizziness, light-headedness and nausea.

Phenoxybenzamine is much more toxic. In Muizelaar et al's series of patients it caused dizziness, general malaise, orthostatic hypotension and erectile dysfunction (in men) in varying degrees in practically all cases. Some, in addition, complained of nausea and diarrhoea; 22% of their patients had to stop taking the drug because of side-effects.

Both Muizelaar et al (1997) and Paice (1995) have pointed out that in order to decide the relative efficiency of the various drugs currently being used in the treatment of this disorder there is a need for large-scale multi-centre prospective controlled trials to be carried out.

Deactivation of MTrPs

In all cases of CRPS type 1 (RSD) it is vital to search for pain-producing MTrPs and when these are found to be present to deactivate them (see Ch. 7).

The importance of this has recently been stressed by Sola (1994) when discussing how the MTrP pain syndrome and CRPS not infrequently coexist in the upper extremity; by Filner (1989), who stated that the MTrP pain syndrome *must* be treated in order to fully resolve RSD, and by Lin et al (1995), who were led to conclude that the MTrP pain syndrome is very common in patients with RSD and that its treatment is essential.

REFERENCES

Abram S E, Lightfoot R W 1981 Treatment of long-standing causalgia with prazocin. Regional Anaesthesia 6:79–81

Arnér S 1991 Intravenous phentolamine test: diagnostic and prognostic use in reflex sympathetic dystrophy. Pain 46:17–22

Blumberg H, Janig W 1994 Clinical manifestations of reflex sympathetic dystrophy and sympathetically maintained pain. In: Wall P D, Melzack R (eds) Textbook of pain, 3rd edn. Churchill Livingstone, Edinburgh, pp 685–698

Bonica J J 1990 Causalgia and other reflex sympathetic dystrophies. In: Bonica J J (ed) The management of pain, 2nd edn. Lea and Febiger, Philadelphia, pp 220–243

Campbell J, Meyer R A, Raja S N L 1992 Is nociceptor activation by α_1-adrenoreceptors the culprit in sympathetically maintained pain? American Pain Society Journal 1(1):3–11

Carr D B, Celeda M S, Lau J 1996 What is the evidence for the therapeutic role of local anaesthetic sympathetic blockade in RSD or causalgia? An attempted meta-analysis [abstract]. In: Eighth World Congress on Pain, Vancouver, 17–22 August 1996. IASP Press, Seattle, p 406.

Charlton J E 1991 Management of sympathetic pain. British Medical Bulletin 47(3):601–618

Evans J A 1946 Reflex sympathetic dystrophy. Surgical Clinics of North America 26:780–790

Filner B E 1989 Role of myofascial pain syndrome treatment in the management of reflex sympathetic dystrophy syndrome. Communication to the 1st international symposium on myofascial pain and fibromyalgia. Minneapolis

Ghostine S Y, Comair Y G, Turner D M et al 1984 Phenoxybenzamine in the treatment of causalgia. Journal of Neurosurgery 60:1263–1268

Hannington-Kiff J G 1974 Intravenous regional sympathetic block with guanethidine. Lancet i:1019–1020

Hannington-Kiff J G 1994 Sympathetic nerve blocks in painful limb disorders. In: Wall P D, Melzack R (eds) Textbook of pain, 3rd edn. Churchill Livingstone, Edinburgh, pp 1035–1054

Inamura S T, Lin T Y, Teitaria M J, Fischer A A et al 1997 The importance of myofascial pain syndrome in reflex sympathetic dystrophy. Physical Medicine and Rehabilitation Clinics of North America 8:207–211

International Association for the Study of Pain subcommittee on taxonomy 1986 Classification of chronic pain. Description of chronic pain syndromes and definition of pain terms. Pain (suppl 3)

Jadad A R, Carroll D, Glynn C J, McQuay H J 1995 Intravenous regional sympathetic blockade for pain relief in reflex sympathetic dystrophy: a systematic review and a randomized double-blind crossover study. Journal of Pain Symptom Management 10:13–20

Kozin F 1992 Reflex sympathetic dystrophy: a review. Clinical and Experimental Rheumatology 10:401–409

Leriche R 1939 The surgery of pain. Williams & Wilkins, Baltimore, MD

Lin T Y, Teixeira M J, Kaziyama H H S, Pai H J et al 1995 Myofascial pain syndrome (MPS) associated with reflex sympathetic dystrophy (RSD). Journal of Musculoskeletal Pain 3(suppl 1):150

Livingston W K 1943 Pain mechanisms: a physiological interpretation of causalgia. Macmillan, New York

McMahon S B 1991 Mechanisms of sympathetic pain. British Medical Bulletin 47(3):584–600

Merskey H, Bogduk N (eds) (1994) Classification of chronic pain. Description of chronic pain syndromes and definition of pain terms, 2nd edn. IASP Press, Seattle, WA.

Mitchell S W 1867 On the diseases of nerves resulting from injuries. In: Flint A (ed) Contributions relating to causation and prevention of disease and to camp diseases. US Sanitary Commission Memoirs, New York

Mitchell S W, Morehouse G R, Keen W W 1864 Injuries of nerves and their consequences. J B Lippincott, Philadelphia

Muizelaar J P, Kleyer M, Hertogs I A M, De Lange D C 1997 Complex regional pain syndrome (reflex sympathetic dystrophy and causalgia): management with the calcium channel blocker nifedipine and/or the alpha-sympathetic blocker phenoxybenzamine in 59 patients. Clinical Neurology and Neurosurgery 99:26–30

Paice E 1995 Reflex sympathetic dystrophy. British Medical Journal 310:1645–1648

Prough D S, McLeskey C H, Poehling G G, Koman L A, Weeks D B, Whitworth T, Semble E L 1985 Efficacy of oral nifedipine in the treatment of reflex sympathetic dystrophy. Anesthesiology 62:796–799

Raja S N, Treede R-D, Davis K D, Campbell J N 1991 Systemic alpha-adrenergic blockade with phentolamine: a diagnostic test for sympathetically maintained pain. Anesthesiology 74:691–698

Ramamurthy S, Hoffman J 1995 The guanethidine study group. Intravenous regional guanethidine in the treatment of reflex sympathetic dystrophy/causalgia: a randomized double-blind study. Anaesthesia and Analgesia 81:718–723

Roberts W J 1986 A hypothesis on the physiological basis for causalgia and related pain. Pain 24:297–311

Roberts W J, Kramis R C 1992 Adrenergic mediation of SMP: via nociceptive or non-nociceptive afferents or both? American Pain Society Journal 1(1):12–15

Schott G D 1998 Interrupting the sympathetic outflow in causalgia and reflex sympathetic dystrophy. British Medical Journal 316:792–793

Sola A E 1994 Upper extremity pain. In: Wall P D, Melzack R (eds) Textbook of pain, 3rd edn. Churchill Livingstone, Edinburgh, p 466

Stanton-Hicks M, Janig W, Hassenbusch S, Haddox J D, Boas R, Wilson P 1995 Reflex sympathetic dystrophy: changing concepts and taxonomy. Pain 63:127–133

Sudeck P 1900 Uber die akute enzudliche knockenatrophie. Archive für Klinike Chirurgie 62:147–157

Sudeck P 1902 Uber die akute (trophoneurotische) knockenatrophie nach entzündungen und trauma der extremitäteps. Deutsche Medizinische Wochenschrift 28:336–338

Veldman P H Jr, Reynen H M, Arntz I E, Goris R J A 1993 Signs and symptoms of reflex sympathetic dystrophy: prospective study of 829 patients. Lancet 342:1012–1016

Wang J R, Johnson K E, Istrup D M 1985 Sympathetic blocks for reflex sympathetic dystrophy. Pain 23:13–17

7

Methods of treating myofascial trigger point pain

INTRODUCTION

Management of the myofascial trigger point (MTrP) pain syndrome includes firstly finding all of the MTrPs from which the pain is emanating. This can only be done by means of a systematically carried out examination, with guidance as to where to search for them being obtained from the distribution of the pain and by observing which movements aggravate it. It is essential not only to locate MTrPs in the primarily affected muscles, and in these muscles' synergists and antagonists (secondary MTrPs), but also to locate any satellite MTrPs that may be present in the primary and secondary MTrPs' zones of pain referral (Ch. 4).

These MTrPs then need to be deactivated by one or other of several currently available methods. The principal ones include deeply applied techniques such as injecting a local anaesthetic into the MTrP, injecting saline into it, and inserting a dry needle into it. Also important are superficially applied techniques, such as stimulating nerve endings in the subcutaneous tissues immediately overlying the muscle containing the MTrP either by injecting water into these tissues or by inserting a needle into them. Reasons will be given as to why this latter superficial dry needling technique is the one recommended for use in the vast majority of cases.

Having deactivated all of the MTrPs found during the course of the initial examination, the affected region of the body should once again be put through its range of movements because any restriction of these, together with any pain experienced whilst carrying them out, helps to determine whether any MTrPs have been overlooked.

When all of the MTrPs from which the pain is emanating have been deactivated, appropriate muscle stretching exercises should be taught.

It is also necessary to identify and correct any structural abnormalities that may perpetuate MTrP activity; to identify and correct any faulty postures adopted either in the home or workplace which, by overloading muscles may cause MTrPs to become reactivated; and to identify and correct any biochemical disorders that are now recognised to cause MTrP activity to persist.

DEACTIVATING MYOFASCIAL TRIGGER POINTS

Deeply applied techniques

Injection of a local anaesthetic into a MTrP

When John Kellgren, whilst working with Sir Thomas Lewis in the 1930s at University College Hospital, London, found that the pain of what he called myalgia emanates from what are now known as MTrPs, his method of alleviating it was to inject a 1% solution of procaine (Novocain) into these points (Kellgren 1938).

His rationale for doing this was presumably procaine's nerve-blocking effect. He therefore must have been surprised to find that by this means he could often relieve the pain for at least 24 hours, and often considerably longer, considering that the nerve blockade produced by this local anaesthetic usually only lasts for a few hours.

Janet Travell, the American physician who from the 1940s onwards took over the study of MTrP pain from where Kellgren left off (see Ch. 1), was quick to realise that the prolonged analgesia produced by injecting procaine into a MTrP must be due to some mechanism other than its nerve-blocking effect, once it had become evident to her that pain relief of a similarly long duration could be obtained by simply inserting a needle into the MTrP (Travell 1960, Travell & Rinzler 1952).

Travell, however, found that needling a MTrP is a painful procedure and that the pain often lasts for several minutes after withdrawal of the needle. She therefore decided to continue to use Kellgren's method of injecting a local anaesthetic through the needle for the sole purpose of helping to suppress this treatment-induced pain.

Kellgren (1938) had used a 1% solution of procaine in normal saline but Travell found that a 0.25–0.5% solution is sufficiently strong to suppress the ephemeral pain that arises when a needle impinges upon a MTrP and that it is less likely to give rise to side-effects.

The following succinct description of her technique appeared in the classic paper 'The myofascial genesis of pain' (Travell & Rinzler 1952).

By pressing on trigger area, demonstrate pain reference to patient.

Ask patient to announce when pain radiation is felt during infiltration. When needle hits trigger area, pepper region by moving it in and out of muscle, injecting 1 to 2 cc continuously.

Use 0.25 to 0.5 per cent procaine hydrochloride in physiologic saline (unless history of procaine allergy).

Use a sharp 22 to 24 gauge needle, 1 to 3 inches long, depending on site of trigger area.

Apply hemostasis promptly.

Check success of injection. If trigger area is still tender, reinfiltrate at different depths and angles.

Recent modifications

The technique described above has recently been modified.

It has for long been known that when procaine is injected or a dry needle inserted into a MTrP a visible contraction, the so-called local twitch response (LTR), can be evoked. Hong (1994a) has observed that either by injecting procaine into or by inserting a needle into various parts of a MTrP it is possible to produce a succession of LTRs. From this he has concluded that a MTrP is made up of a number of individual loci and that for its successful deactivation each of these loci has to be penetrated with, as a consequence, the production of numerous LTRs. This necessitates pushing a needle in and out of the MTrP several times. And in order to avoid damaging the muscle whilst doing this, Hong advises using a thin needle and for its movements to be carried out at a very fast speed of approximately 100–200 mm/s, a technique which clearly requires considerable manual dexterity and practice.

Following the development of this technique Hong (1994b) carried out a trial to compare the pain-relieving effectiveness of either injecting lignocaine (Lidocaine) into a MTrP in the upper part of the trapezius muscle or inserting a dry needle into it. Another purpose of the trial was to determine whether or not eliciting a succession of LTRs during the course of deactivating a MTrP by one or other of these two procedures is of importance.

In this study 58 patients with MTrP pain were divided up into four groups. Group I (26 patients) had 0.5% lignocaine (Lidocaine) injected into their MTrPs. Group II (15 patients) had dry needles inserted into their MTrPs. LTRs were elicited during multiple needle insertions in both of these groups.

There were also two subgroups. Group IA (9 patients) received injections of 0.5% lignocaine (Lidocaine) into MTrPs and group IIA (8 patients) had dry needles inserted into MTrPs *without* LTRs being elicited.

Response to treatment was assessed by measuring, before and after treatment, subjective changes in pain intensity on a visual analogue scale, changes in pain threshold with an algometer, and changes in the range of motion of the cervical spine on lateral bending with a goniometer.

The results were that 15 (55%) of the 26 patients in group I treated with a lignocaine (Lidocaine) injection and 7 (47%) of the 15 patients in group II treated with dry needling reported complete pain relief immediately following treatment; 11 patients (42%) in group I and 6 patients (40%) in group II reported that the pain was considerably improved immediately following these two types of treatment.

In contrast to this, no patients in group IA or group IIA, in which LTRs were not elicited, were pain-free immediately following treatment.

These results led Hong to conclude that the insertion of a dry needle and the injection of a local anaesthetic into a MTrP are equally effective deactivating procedures provided that with both forms of treatment successions of LTRs are elicited.

With both of these procedures he found that the multiple insertions of the needle required to obtain these LTRs gave rise to appreciable post-treatment soreness. This soreness developed within the first 2–8 hours following treatment in 42% of the patients given local anaesthetic injections and in 100% of the patients in which dry needling was carried out. Furthermore, the soreness in these latter patients was considerably more intense and of a longer duration.

It is generally accepted that this post-treatment soreness is due to needle-induced bleeding into the tissues. And because Hong and his co-workers (Hong 1994b, Hong & Torigoe 1991, Hong et al 1992) have found that in order to deactivate a MTrP successfully using his multiple LTR-eliciting technique the needle, for some as yet unexplained reason, has to be inserted more often when using dry needling than when injecting a local anaesthetic, he concluded that the higher incidence of post-treatment soreness in the dry needling group (group II) must have been due to a greater amount of damage to blood vessels. He therefore decided that injecting a local anaesthetic into a MTrP is preferable to inserting a dry needle into it. Others who have provided reviews of this local anaesthetic technique in recent years include Gerwin (1993), Rachlin (1994) and Simons et al (1999).

Pre-injection nerve block Although injecting a local anaesthetic into a MTrP is less painful than inserting a dry needle into it, the injection can still cause a considerable amount of discomfort. To obviate this, Fischer (1995a, 1995b) has recommended carrying out a pre-injection nerve block.

Choice of local anaesthetic

As the purpose of injecting a local anaesthetic into a MTrP, as opposed to simply inserting a dry needle into it, is to reduce the amount of needle-induced pain and post-treatment soreness, and is not for any nerve blocking effect it may have, there is clearly no advantage in using a long-acting agent such as bupivacaine. Furthermore, bupivacaine is likely to give rise to muscle necrosis and tends to mask activity in MTrPs close to the one being treated. It has also been shown that there is nothing to be gained by using a strong solution of a short-acting agent. For these reasons, a 0.5% solution of either procaine (Novocain) or lignocaine (lidocaine) is recommended.

Undesirable effects of local anaesthetics

These include toxic effects, hypersensitivity reactions, damage to muscle and damage to nearby structures.

Toxic effects The toxic effects liable to be produced by injecting a large amount of a local anaesthetic into the tissues include tremors, convulsions, cardiovascular collapse and respiratory failure. Vandam (1960) found that such effects are not likely to develop until 200 ml of a 0.5% procaine solution has been injected. Therefore, as the amount that has to be injected into a MTrP is not more than 0.5–1 ml, and it would be unusual for more than 10–15 MTrPs to be deactivated at any one time, the chances of a toxic reaction developing during the course of injecting it for this purpose are minimal.

Hypersensitivity reactions Mild allergic reactions that may occasionally develop include palpitations, vasovagal attacks and hypotensive episodes. These cardiovascular complications, however, far more commonly develop as a result of apprehension. Anaphylactic shock may also develop with respiratory and cardiovascular collapse similar to that produced by drug toxicity. Although this life-threatening complication is extremely rare, it is nevertheless clearly essential that intravenous diazepam, intramuscular adrenaline (epinephrine) 0.5–1.0 mg (0.5–1 ml of 1 in 1000), equipment for artificial respiration and a cardiac defibrillator are readily available whenever this MTrP-deactivating procedure is being carried out.

Muscle damage With Hong's multiple penetration MTrP deactivating technique the needle through which the anaesthetic is injected should be thin and sharp as the damage caused by repeatedly thrusting a needle through muscle during the course of this procedure is liable to lead to the development of scar tissue. And this in turn may promote further MTrP activity.

Muscle necrosis is liable to occur when a long-acting agent such as bupivacaine or mepivacaine is used (Benoit & Belt 1972). The risk of this happening is very much less with a shorter-acting local anaesthetic, such as procaine, provided that it is not mixed with adrenaline (epinephrine) for the purpose of slowing its absorption (Benoit 1978).

Muscle paralysis The injection of a local anaesthetic into muscle is capable of producing a curare-like effect with an alarming, albeit temporary, loss of power.

Damage to neighbouring structures The injection of either a local anaesthetic or the insertion of a dry needle into a MTrP is perforce an invasive procedure and in certain parts of the body the risk of damaging neighbouring structures is particularly high. For example, when carrying this out in the supraclavicular region or chest wall care has to be taken not to puncture the lung with the development of a pneumothorax.

The risk of either of these two procedures damaging vessels with bleeding into the tissues taking place has already been discussed. In addition, the insertion of a needle into a nerve may cause transient pain or tingling. However, serious long-lasting nerve damage as a result of this has up to now been rare but it is possible that the incidence may increase if Hong's rapid multiple injection technique becomes more widely used.

Injection of normal saline into MTrPs

In the mid 1950s the American physician Anders Sola decided to see whether it is possible to deactivate MTrPs by simply injecting normal saline into them. His reasons for trying this were because the injection of a local anaesthetic for this purpose which, up to then, had been the technique most widely used, may at times lead to the development of undesirable side-effects. Furthermore, Martin (1952), a physician at the Royal Free Hospital in London, had reported satisfactorily alleviating the pain of what he called fibrositis by injecting a somewhat complex mixture of benzyl salicylate and camphor in arachis oil into what, from his description of them, were clearly MTrPs.

Sola & Kuitert (1955) first injected normal saline into the MTrPs of several individuals known to be sensitive to procaine and, on finding the results to be extremely promising, proceeded to do this in 100 consecutive patients with neck and shoulder girdle MTrP pain treated by them at a United States Air Force hospital in Texas. Their conclusion was that 'the use of normal saline has none of the disadvantages often associated with the use of a local anaesthetic but appears to have the same therapeutic value'.

A year later Sola & Williams (1956) reported similarly good results in over 1000 patients with MTrP pain in various regions of the body treated at the same hospital, a finding which led them to state that 'in patients in whom hypersensitive TrPs are found, the use of saline injections into the area both for diagnostic and therapeutic purposes is recommended'.

Despite these encouraging results no further interest seems to have been taken in this MTrP deactivating technique until 1980 when Frost et al reported the results of a double-blind study comparing the effect of injecting the long-acting local anaesthetic mepivacaine (0.5%) into 28 patients' MTrPs with that of injecting physiological saline into 25 patients' MTrPs.

They decided to use physiological saline because they assumed that it would have no more than a placebo effect and that the patients treated with it would serve as a control group. They were therefore surprised to find that 76% of the patients in this group had pain relief in contrast to only 57% of the group treated with mepivacaine. From this they concluded that:

... the more favourable effect of physiological saline may be due to the longer duration of irritation since nerve impulses are not blocked by saline ... the study therefore raises questions about the mechanism by which local injections into muscles relieve pain, since there is a possibility that a similar effect might also be achieved by merely inserting a needle into the trigger point.

One year later Hameroff et al (1981) published the results of a randomised double-blind crossover study comparing the relative effectiveness of injecting 0.5% bupivacaine, 1% etidocaine and physiological saline into the MTrPs of 15 patients.

In this small trial the two local anaesthetic agents were found to be more effective than normal saline. However, as discussed in Chapter 2, there are grounds for believing that the pain suppression brought about by injecting any substance into a MTrP is due to neurophysiological mechanisms brought into action by the needle through which it is injected rather than to any pain-relieving property the injected material may possess. The results obtained in this pilot study may well have been influenced by the small number of patients in it and had the trial had a larger intake there is reason to believe that the local anaesthetic and physiological saline injections would have been shown to be equally effective.

Injection of corticosteroids into MTrPs

Bourne (1979, 1984) compared the effect of injecting a corticosteroid/local anaesthetic mixture with that of injecting a local anaesthetic into a MTrP and found that the mixture gave better results. This, however, could not have been due to the steroid's ability to combat inflammation as there is no such reaction at a MTrP site. Moreover, as a corticosteroid when repeatedly injected into the tissues is liable to damage them, its use for the deactivation of MTrPs cannot be recommended. As Travell & Simons (1983) pointed out, the only justification for its employment so far as musculoskeletal pain disorders are concerned, is in the treatment of an inflammatory lesion such as a rotator cuff tendinitis or lateral epicondylitis.

Injection of a non-steroidal anti-inflammatory drug into MTrPs

Because the non-steroidal anti-inflammatory group of drugs have an inhibitory effect on cyclooxygenase and as a result depress the production of prostaglandins that sensitise MTrP nociceptors, Frost (1986) carried out a trial to compare the pain-relieving effectiveness of injecting diclofenac (Voltarol) with that of injecting lignocaine (lidocaine) into MTrPs. In this study 24 patients with MTrP pain were divided into two groups with 11 having 1% lignocaine and 13 diclofenac injected into a MTrP.

The results tended to favour diclofenac. However, the number of patients in the trial was small and assessment of the analgesic effects was limited to measurements made on a visual analogue scale at half-hourly intervals for 5 hours. In view of this it is difficult to draw any firm conclusion and, as Frost himself said, 'only an increase in the number of patients could establish whether diclofenac gives a significantly better result . . . but the result is promising and calls for continued investigations'.

Since then, Drewes et al (1993) have carried out a double-blind study to compare the pain-relieving effectiveness of injecting either prednisolone or diclofenac into MTrPs. Thirty-eight patients completed the study and in these both forms of treatment were found to be equally effective with 84% being significantly improved. Despite this the authors felt it necessary to point out that an injection of a steroid into a muscle is liable to damage its fibres and one given into the superficial tissues is liable to cause the skin to become pitted and depigmented. Furthermore, an injection of diclofenac, particularly if it is inserted into the superficial tissues, may produce skin necrosis. Therefore, for these reasons alone, the injection of a corticosteroid or a non-steroidal anti-inflammatory drug into MTrPs cannot be recommended.

Injection of botulinum A toxin (Botox) into MTrPs

It was the discovery by Tsui et al (1986) that an injection of the botulinum A toxin, because of its ability to relax muscle, is of use in the treatment of dystonia that prompted Cheshire et al (1994) to explore the possibility of employing it in the treatment of MTrP pain. In their small double-blind study, 4 out of 6 patients with MTrP pain experienced reduction of this by at least 30% following injections of botulinum A toxin (Botox) but not following injections of normal saline.

Yue (1995) has also carried out a retrospective study of 112 patients who had botulinum toxin injected into MTrPs during the period July 1992 to November 1994; 86% of patients reported fair to excellent results with an average pain reduction of 35.6%, but 17% reported moderate to severe side-effects.

The main side-effects of this toxin are muscle weakness sufficient to impair motor function and the eventual development of muscle atrophy and because of these there is no place for its use in the treatment of MTrP pain.

There is nevertheless considerable theoretical interest in the employment of the toxin for this purpose. This is because it is known to paralyse muscles as a result of it blocking the release of acetylcholine from motor nerve terminals at the neuromuscular junction. As Simons (1996) has pointed out, 'the fact that Botox quickly inactivates MTrPs is a strong indicator that the MTrP mechanism is intimately associated with the neuromuscular junction.'

Deep dry needling

The insertion of needles into MTrPs for the relief of pain emanating from them is currently widely practised. It is not, however, some new form of treatment, for as long ago as the 6th century AD the Chinese physician Sun Ssu-Mo described how he alleviated pain of muscular origin by inserting needles into points which, from his description, were clearly what are now known as MTrPs but which he called ah shi points (Lu & Needham 1980).

News about the Chinese practice of inserting needles into the body for therapeutic purposes reached Europe 300 years ago (Baldry 1993) but as the principles upon which it was based proved unacceptable to 17th century physicians trained in Western medicine, no interest was shown in it until the beginning of the 19th century when, somewhat surprisingly, an English physician named Churchill decided to employ Sun Ssu-Mo's needling technique for the treatment of what he called rheumatalgia. He eventually published books describing his method and the results obtained with it (Churchill 1821, 1828).

These books were clearly widely read for over the next hundred years a number of physicians in England and North America employed Churchill's method of treatment. The most famous of these was Sir William Osler who, in the eighth edition of his book *The Principles and Practice of Medicine* published in 1912, at a time when he was Regius Professor of Medicine at Oxford University, described how in the treatment of lumbago he inserted 'needles of from three to four inches in length (ordinary bonnet needles, sterilized, will do) . . . into the lumbar muscles at the seat of the pain'.

Despite Osler's high standing in the medical profession nothing further was written about treatment of this type until 1952 when Travell & Rinzler made brief reference to dry needling TrPs during the course of describing their less painful technique of injecting local anaesthetic into them.

Eventually, however, interest in the dry needling of MTrPs was rekindled when Karel Lewit, a Czech physician, wrote enthusiastically about it in the late 1970s. Lewit, unlike Travell & Rinzler, was in no way deterred by it being a painful procedure, but on the contrary stated that 'the effectiveness of treatment is related to the intensity of pain produced at the trigger zone and to the precision with which the site of maximum tenderness is located by the needle'.

In his classic paper 'The needle effect in the relief of myofascial pain', Lewit (1979) describes the results of treating 241 patients with chronic myofascial pain during the years 1975–1976. The treatment consisted of inserting a needle into what he variously called sites of maximal tenderness, trigger zones and pain spots; or what, from his description of them, would currently be called MTrPs. He called the immediate analgesia produced by needling such a point the 'needle effect' and found that he was able to obtain this in 86.8% of cases.

He concluded from this that the pain-relieving effect 'previously ascribed to local anaesthetics may in fact be due to needling'.

Support for this belief has since come from Chan Gunn in Vancouver, who over the years has written extensively about the pain-relieving effect of inserting needles into MTrPs (Gunn 1989, 1996), a procedure he calls intramuscular stimulation but which, in my opinion, is better termed deep dry needling (DDN) in order to distinguish it from superficial dry needling (SDN), which will be discussed later in this chapter.

Gunn (1998) uses a solid 30 gauge acupuncture needle with a pointed tip, as this is less traumatic than the bevelled cutting edge of a hollow needle used for injections. He has pointed out that when an acupuncture needle of this type is inserted into a shortened contracted muscle the latter may relax quickly and allow the needle to be withdrawn without any difficulty, but more often, the spasm persists and when that happens the needle becomes firmly grasped and has to be left in situ for 10–30 minutes before it is possible to withdraw it.

The neurophysiological mechanisms responsible for DDN's ability to relieve MTrP pain will not be reiterated here as they have already been discussed at length in Chapter 2 (see Box 2.1).

The technique is widely used but one of its main disadvantages is that it is a very painful procedure, with Gunn (1989) himself stating that when a needle is inserted into a tight contracted band of muscle, 'the patient experiences a peculiar cramp-like sensation as the needle is grasped

. . . the intensity of the cramp parallels that of spasm: it can be excruciatingly painful, but gradually resolves as the spasm eases'.

Other disadvantages of deep dry needling and other deeply applied techniques are the risks of damaging nerves, blood vessels and other structures. And it is because of bleeding into the tissues that there is a high incidence of post-treatment soreness. Gunn (1998), however, is not deterred by this as he is of the opinion that local bleeding paradoxically promotes tissue healing by releasing substances such as platelet-derived growth factor (Ross & Vogel 1978) which stimulate collagen and protein formation.

A prospective randomised double-blind evaluation of the comparative efficacy of various deeply applied MTrP deactivating techniques, carried out by Garvey et al (1989), has confirmed the belief that inserting a needle into a MTrP is as effective as injecting lignocaine (lidocaine) or lignocaine plus a steroid into it.

Experience over the past twenty years has led me to conclude that the only absolute indication for DDN is in those cases where a very strong stimulus is required.

One example of when this is necessary is for the deactivation of MTrPs in individuals who, for some as yet unexplained reason, have a relatively poor responsiveness to needle-evoked neural stimulation (see slow reactors, p. 114).

Another is when the muscle in which the TrP to be deactivated is situated is in a state of considerable spasm such as not uncommonly happens when TrP activity arises as a secondary event following the development of a radiculopathy (Chu 1995).

Chu, like Hong (see p. 105), is of the opinion that the evoking of local twitch responses increases the effectiveness of this deep dry needling TrP deactivating technique. She calls the procedure twitch-obtaining intramuscular stimulation (TOIMS), and has provided evidence to suggest that TOIMS is particularly indicated for the alleviation of MTrP pain that develops secondary to cervical radiculopathy (Chu 1997) and lumbosacral radiculopathy (Chu 1999).

Superficially applied techniques

Vapocoolant spray applied to skin at MTrP sites

Kraus (1941) was the first to describe how spraying ethyl chloride on to the skin is capable of relieving musculoskeletal pain. It was initially used for combating the pain of joint sprains. It was then found that it is possible to use it for deactivating MTrPs. Travell & Rinzler (1952) summarised the technique adopted by them when employing it for this purpose as follows:

> Guard against fire hazards.
> Raise patient's head above level sprayed.
> Hold container 2 feet away.
> Start stream at trigger area, carry over reference zone.
> Apply stream at acute angle.
> Spray in one direction, with slow sweeping motion.
> Repeat sweeps in rhythm of a few seconds on and off.
> Lengthen interval between sweeps if aching develops.
> Do *not* frost skin.
> Stretch muscle by gentle movement.
> Continue until pain disappears and tenderness at trigger area is less.
> Stop if no effect in five minutes.

Ethyl chloride is a rapidly acting local anaesthetic and because of this has been responsible for accidental deaths. It is also potentially explosive. For these reasons, the patient must not be allowed to inhale the vapour and fire hazards must be eliminated.

It was because of these dangers that Travell (1968) helped to develop the safer alternative, fluori-methane, a mixture of two fluorocarbons. Unfortunately, this is not universally available.

Physicians who currently include the use of a vapocoolant spray in their treatment of MTrP pain mostly employ it in combination with exercises designed to stretch muscles that continue to be shortened, despite having first carried out a MTrP deactivating procedure (Rachlin 1994).

Travell & Simons (1983) gave a detailed account of the indications for and the manner of carrying out this stretch and spray technique.

Intradermal injections of water

Byrn et al (1991), in a preliminary uncontrolled study carried out at the University of Gothenburg, Sweden, found that pain was relieved for significant periods of time by injections of sterile water into the skin overlying MTrPs in the necks and shoulder girdles of patients suffering from whiplash injury.

One important disadvantage of this technique, however, is that water injected into the skin gives rise to an intense and very distressing burning sensation.

They therefore decided to compare the effectiveness of injecting 0.3–0.5 ml of sterile water with that of injecting a similar amount of normal saline into the subcutaneous tissues overlying each of a number of active MTrPs present in 40 patients with whiplash injuries of 4–6 years' standing (Byrn et al 1993). Randomisation led to 10 women and 20 men receiving injections of sterile water and 11 women and 9 men receiving injections of saline.

Neck mobility was measured with a goniometer and minimum and maximum pain levels were estimated on a visual analogue scale before and after the first treatment and at 1, 3 and 8 months. Each patient, depending on their response, received up to three treatments during the first 2 months.

At the end of 3 months, the mean total mobility of the cervical spine had increased by 39° in the sterile water group but by only 6° in the saline group ($P < 0.05$); the minimum pain level had fallen from 2.2 to 1.4 in the sterile water group but remained unchanged in the saline group ($P < 0.02$); and the maximum pain level had fallen from 8.1 to 3.8 in the sterile water group but only from 8.3 to 7.5 in the saline group ($P < 0.001$). Also, at the end of this time 19 out of 20 patients in the sterile water group assessed their condition as generally improved but only 6 in the saline group felt they had got better.

Byrn et al concluded from these results that injecting water into the subcutaneous tissues overlying MTrPs is an effective method of deactivating them.

The only drawback to injecting water into the subcutaneous tissues in the same way as injecting it into the skin is that it gives rise to an intense burning pain similar to that experienced following a wasp sting. And although this only lasts for about 30 seconds, it is extremely unpleasant. Despite this, Byrn and his co-workers considered that 'most patients tolerate it because the treatment works' and they have since used this method extensively in the treatment of patients referred to them with myofascial pain in various parts of the body.

Superficial dry needling

It was my practice to inject a local anaesthetic into MTrPs until Lewit's reported success with deep dry needling (DDN) in 1979 (see p. 109) persuaded me to adopt that technique.

From then onwards this continued to be my preferred method of deactivating them until the early 1980s, when a patient was referred to me with pain down the arm from a MTrP in the scalenus anterior muscle. In view of the proximity of the apex of the lung it was considered prudent not to push the needle into the muscle but rather to insert it into the subcutaneous tissues immediately overlying the MTrP. This proved to be sufficient for after leaving the needle in situ for a short time and then withdrawing it, the exquisite tenderness at the MTrP site had been abolished and the spontaneously occurring pain in the arm had been alleviated.

This superficial dry needling (SDN) technique was then used to deactivate MTrPs elsewhere in the body and proved to be equally effective even when the muscle containing them was deep lying. Also, any palpable bands found to be present before the treatment disappeared after it.

About the same time, Macdonald et al (1983) confirmed the efficacy of SDN by showing, in a carefully conducted trial, that myofascial pain in the lumbar region could be successfully alleviated by inserting needles into the subcutaneous tissues at MTrP sites.

In this trial, carried out at Charing Cross Hospital, London, 17 consecutive patients with chronic lumbar MTrP pain were divided into two groups. One group was treated with SDN, the other with a placebo.

In the SDN group, needles were inserted to an approximate depth of 4 mm in the skin and subcutaneous tissues immediately overlying MTrPs. Particular care was taken to avoid penetrating the muscles or their fasciae. The needles were left in situ for 5 minutes during the first treatment and, if this failed to produce a beneficial result, the length of time was doubled at the next treatment one week later, until the needles were left in situ for 20 minutes. If this failed, electrical stimulation of skin electrodes was carried out. The maximum number of treatments given was 10.

In the placebo group, electrodes applied to the skin overlying MTrPs were attached by non-current carrying wires to a purposely impressive apparatus with numerous dials and lights, and a cooling system that made a 'whirring' sound. This non-functioning machine was also initially applied for 5 minutes and if this failed to produce a beneficial result the length of time was doubled. Moreover, if the patient reported that the pain had been exacerbated, as happened in 3 cases immediately following the use of this placebo device, the treatment time was reduced.

A series of measurements made by unbiased clinical observers at the beginning and end of each course of treatment in both the active treatment group and the control group were such as to lead to the conclusion that the effectiveness of SDN is significantly superior to that of a placebo.

Since then SDN has been my preferred method of deactivating MTrPs in all patients other than a minority of them who, for reasons discussed on p. 110, require DDN.

It is easier and safer to carry out than more deeply applied ones. Also, unlike them, it is entirely painless other than for a momentary pricking sensation as the needle penetrates the skin. In addition, bleeding into the tissues only occasionally occurs and when it does, firm pressure quickly brings it under control so that post-treatment soreness is rarely complained of.

Simons & Hong (1995) have suggested that a trial should be carried out to compare the effectiveness of SDN and DDN. Whilst this would be of considerable interest there are, in my opinion, grounds for believing that both techniques have their place in the deactivation of MTrPs.

A detailed account of the procedure adopted by me when carrying out SDN will therefore be given but firstly it is necessary to amplify what was said in Chapter 2 concerning the neurophysiological mechanisms responsible for its MTrP pain-relieving ability.

The pain-suppressing effect of stimulating A-delta nerve fibres David Bowsher, Research Director of the Pain Research Institute at Walton Hospital, England, has explained that the effect of inserting a needle into the skin is to activate A-delta nerve endings (Bowsher 1976). And there are reasons for believing (Bowsher 1998) that MTrP pain suppression brought about by SDN is principally due to needle-induced stimulation of these small myelinated sensory afferent fibres creating activity in enkephalinergic inhibitory interneurons situated in the dorsal horn (Fig. 7.1).

In support of the concept that SDN's MTrP pain-alleviating effect is opioid peptide mediated is the discovery that it is possible to abolish this by administering the opioid peptide antagonist naloxone (Mayer et al 1977, Sjölund & Eriksson 1979). In addition, Fine et al (1988) found that the pain relief obtained by injecting procaine into a MTrP is reversed by naloxone.

Nevertheless, it has to be admitted that whatever contribution opioid peptides make to the suppression of MTrP pain it cannot be dependent on the liberation of a large amount of them by means of the application of a strong stimulus as usually it requires no more than a lightly applied one to deactivate a MTrP successfully.

One possibility is that the transitory effect of releasing a relatively small quantity of them is sufficient to set in motion some other as yet unidentified longer-acting pain-modulating mechanism such as the one proposed by Han.

Han (1987) has suggested that possibly one of the effects of needle-evoked neural stimulation is to cause the setting up of a serotonin- and metenkephalin-mediated circuit in a neuronal

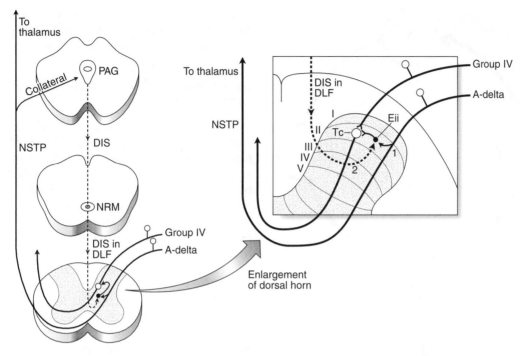

Figure 7.1   Diagram to show mechanisms considered to be responsible for the blocking of intra-dorsal horn transmission of MTrP group IV nociceptive information as a result of segmental superficial dry needling of A-delta nerve fibres. Enkephalinergic inhibitory interneurons (Eii) in the dorsal horn become activated as a result of A-delta nerves having a direct link with them (1). And an indirect link with them (2) as a result of the neospinothalamic pathway (NSTP) up which A-delta sensory information is transmitted having a collateral which projects to the periaqueductal grey area (PAG) in the midbrain at the upper end of the serotonergic descending inhibitory system (DIS) which, from the nucleus raphe magnus (NRM) in the medulla, descends in the dorsolateral funiculus (DLF) and which on reaching dorsal horns projects to Eiis. Opioid peptides produced by these Eiis then inhibit activity in group IV sensory afferents intra-dorsal horn's terminal cells (Tc).

loop made up of the arcuate nucleus of the hypothalamus, the nucleus accumbens, the amygdala, the habenula and structures in the upper part of the descending inhibitory system including the periaqueductal grey area in the midbrain and the nucleus raphe magnus in the medulla. His hypothesis is that because of the circuit set up in this mesolimbic loop of analgesia, the descending inhibitory system is enabled to block any noxious input to the spinal cord for an appreciable period of time (Fig. 7.2).

Superficial dry needling's electrically generated stimulation of A-delta nerve fibres The effect of inserting a dry needle into the skin and subcutaneous tissues is to stimulate A-delta nerve fibres both mechanically and by the setting up of an electric current.

This latter effect is due to the difference in electrical potential that exists between the needle and the skin creating a low-intensity galvanic current of injury. This electrically produced microenergy continues to be generated not only for as long as the needle is kept in situ but also for some time after it has been taken out. This sustained effect occurs because, as Karavis (1997) has stated, 'after withdrawing the needle, the unequal distribution of electrical potential (because of the high concentration of K^+ ions) round the edges of the injury creates an electrical flux potential field which acts as a stimulator of the free nerve endings of the skin for 72 hours'.

It therefore follows that when a needle is inserted into the skin and subcutaneous tissues overlying a MTrP for the purpose of de-activating the latter, A-delta nerve fibres are

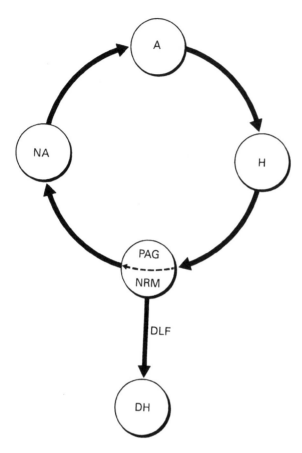

Figure 7.2   Han's proposed mesolimbic loop of analgesia. A neuronal circuit involving the nucleus accumbens (NA), the amygdala (A), the habenula (H) and the upper parts of the descending inhibitory system, the periaqueductal grey (PAG) and the nucleus raphe magnus (NRM), which are connected to the dorsal horn (DH) by the dorsolateral funiculus (DLF).

briefly stimulated mechanically and more long-lastingly by the development of an electrical current.

Strong, average and weak responders The optimum amount of stimulation required when carrying out SDN varies from one person to another. This is because people are either strong, average or weak responders. Whereas a strong responder only requires a light stimulus to deactivate a MTrP and any more than this may temporarily exacerbate the pain, a weak responder requires a much more powerful stimulus.

It follows from this that when using SDN the optimum strength of stimulus has to be determined for each individual patient.

Determination of optimum superficial dry needling stimulus

When using SDN to deactivate a MTrP it is my current practice (Baldry 1993, 1995, 1998) when treating a patient for the first time to insert an acupuncture needle (0.3 × 30 mm) into the tissues overlying the MTrP to a depth of about 5–10 mm and to leave it there without any form of manipulation for about 30 seconds. This is because the amount of neural stimulation required is the minimum necessary to abolish the exquisite tenderness, which before needling had made the patient wince involuntarily (the 'jump sign'). Therefore, on withdrawing the needle, pressure equal to that applied before needling is applied to the MTrP site to see whether this has been achieved. One 30-second period of needling is sometimes all that is required, but when it is not the needle should be replaced and left in situ for up to 2–3 minutes. Very occasionally this proves to be insufficient and the needle has to be re-introduced and left in place for an even longer period. Also the amount of neural stimulation may have to be increased by gently twirling the needle.

The purpose of adopting this step-by-step approach when determining a patient's individual responsiveness to SDN is to reduce the risk of causing a temporary but nevertheless distressing exacerbation of pain as a result of exceeding that person's optimum needle-stimulation requirement.

For those who respond particularly strongly even a 30-second period of stimulation may prove to be too much. It is therefore necessary to inform every patient undergoing SDN for the first time of the possibility that the initial treatment may temporarily exacerbate the pain. It is important to do this for, should it happen without warning, it may be the cause of much unnecessary alarm and despondency. Admittedly any such flare-up usually only lasts for 12–24 hours, but occasionally it persists for several days.

When this happens, great care must be taken to ensure that only light stimulation is applied on all subsequent occasions, and even in some cases to increase the interval in between treatments.

Provided there has not been a flare-up of pain following the first treatment, and this should be in the majority of cases where the graduated approach described above is followed, the time for which needles are left in situ at subsequent treatment sessions should either be kept the same as on the initial occasion or increased if the pain relief has not been as good as might be expected.

Following successful SDN, any palpable band and local twitch response that may have been present at a MTrP site prior to treatment should disappear.

Terminology

Before leaving the subject it is necessary to explain why the terms MTrP DDN and MTrP SDN are now widely employed rather than referring to them as deeply applied and superficially applied acupuncture. Because acus is Latin for needle this would be etymologically correct, but the reason for not doing so is to make it clear that the difference between SDN and DDN carried out at MTrP sites and traditional Chinese acupuncture is that whereas the latter is based on archaic and esoteric principles, the two needling techniques have evolved as a result of the application of present-day neurophysiological concepts.

Response to MTrP deactivating techniques

The pain relief obtained when a MTrP is first deactivated, no matter what method is used, usually lasts for 2–3 days.

In the case of acute pain, treatment should be repeated every other day. With longer-standing pain it is customary for treatment to be repeated once a week. And in some cases, an average of three treatments at weekly intervals may be sufficient to abolish the pain. In others, however, where MTrP activity persists because of, for example, some underlying irreversible structural disorder, or the development of dorsal horn neuroplasticity (central sensitisation, see Ch. 4), treatment may have to be repeated at 4–8 week intervals on a long-term basis.

Factors responsible for the persistence of MTrP activity

Irrespective of which method is employed for deactivating a MTrP, any initial pain relief obtained with it will not be maintained if causative mechanical or biochemical disorders are not identified and steps taken to correct them.

Mechanical factors

Structural disorders for which corrective measures may have to be taken include leg length inequality and relative shortness of the upper arms (see Ch. 12). Also, asymmetry of the two halves of the pelvis with a consequent functional scoliosis may need to be corrected by placing a pad under the ischial tuberosity on the smaller side when sitting.

The possibility that a faulty posture may have been adopted in the home or at the workplace also has to be considered. For if found to be so it may prove necessary, for example, to adjust the height of a stool, chair, desk or workbench.

Biochemical factors

Gerwin (1992) has drawn attention to the importance of recognising the presence of either subclinical hypothyroidism, folic acid deficiency or iron inadequacy in patients with the myofascial pain syndrome, as, in his experience, a failure to correct any one of these may cause MTrP activity to persist.

Muscle stretching exercises

After MTrPs have been deactivated, the patient should be taught how to carry out muscle stretching exercises on a regular basis.

CLINICAL TRIALS

At present there is no consensus concerning the advantages, disadvantages and efficacy of the currently available methods of deactivating MTrPs. Therefore, clinicians working in institutions with research facilities who are skilled in the use of both deeply applied and superficially applied techniques need to carry out large-scale comparative trials for the purpose of evaluating, in an objective manner, their relative safety, simplicity, patient acceptability, and in particular, their pain-relieving effectiveness.

That there has been a dearth of such trials up to now is largely because of difficulties in carrying them out. One of the main problems is a lack of reliable methods of measuring the pain-relieving effectiveness of a MTrP-deactivating technique objectively.

One of the best ways of determining the immediate efficacy of any particular procedure is to assess its nociceptor desensitising effect by measuring the change in the pressure pain threshold (minimum pressure that induces pain) at the MTrP site with a pressure algometer before and after treatment (Fischer 1987, 1994). However, even this has its shortcomings, for as Fischer (1998) has pointed out, measurements obtained with this instrument depend on a patient's subjective responses and are therefore capable of being manipulated.

Unfortunately, other assessment measures are equally subjective, a state of affairs that has led Fine (1995) to comment:

The hurdle to overcome is the ability to monitor change, without the monitor itself inducing change or introducing bias. For instance, as important as patient self-reports of pain, examiner ratings of tissue suppleness, range of motion and other functional variables are, these endpoints in and of themselves are never going to be definitive or conclusive. The heterogeneity of patients, examiners, environments and so on is far too great. We must put hope, then, into the efforts of our physiologist and instrumentation colleagues to develop tools for measuring nociceptive and myo(patho)-physiological processes in real time without disturbing these processes.

REFERENCES

Baldry P E 1993 Acupuncture, trigger points and musculoskeletal pain, 2nd edn. Churchill Livingstone, Edinburgh

Baldry P E 1995 Superficial dry needling at myofascial trigger points sites. Journal of Musculoskeletal Pain 3(3):117–126

Baldry P E 1998 Trigger point acupuncture. In: Filshie J, White A (eds) Medical acupuncture. A western scientific approach. Churchill Livingstone, Edinburgh, ch 4

Benoit P W 1978 Reversible skeletal muscle damage after administration of local anaesthetics with and without epinephrine. Journal of Oral Surgery 36:198–201

Benoit P W, Belt W D 1972 Some effects of local anaesthetic agents on skeletal muscle. Experimental Neurology 34:264–278

Bourne I H J 1979 Treatment of backache with local injections. The Practitioner 222:708–711

Bourne I H J 1984 Treatment of chronic back pain comparing corticosteroid–lignocaine injections with lignocaine alone. The Practitioner 228:333–338

Bowsher D 1976 Role of the reticular formation in response to noxious stimulation. Pain 2:361–378

Bowsher D 1998 Mechanisms of acupuncture. In: Filshie J, White A (eds) Medical acupuncture. A western scientific approach. Churchill Livingstone, Edinburgh, pp 69–82

Byrn C, Borenstein P, Linder L-E 1991 Treatment of neck and shoulder pain in whiplash syndrome with intracutaneous sterile water injections. Acta Anaesthetica Scandinavica 35:52–53

Byrn C, Olsson I, Falkheden L et al 1993 Subcutaneous sterile water injections for chronic neck and shoulder pain following whiplash injuries. Lancet 341:449–452

Cheshire W P, Abashian S W, Mann J D 1994 Botulinum toxin in the treatment of myofascial pain syndrome. Pain 59:65–69

Chu J 1995 Dry needling (intramuscular stimulation) in myofascial pain related to lumbrosacral radiculopathy. European Journal of Physical Medicine and Rehabilitation 5(4):106–121

Chu J 1997 Twitch-obtaining intramuscular stimulation (TOIMS): effectiveness for long-term treatment of myofascial pain related to cervical radiculopathy. Archives of Physical Medicine and Rehabilitation 78:1042

Chu J 1999 Twitch-obtaining intramuscular stimulation. Observations in the management of radiculopathic chronic low back pain. Journal of Musculoskeletal Pain 7(4):131–146

Churchill J M 1821 A treatise on acupuncturation being a description of a surgical operation originally peculiar to the Japanese and Chinese, and by them denominated zinking, now introduced into European practice, with directions for its performance, and cases illustrating its success. Simpkins & Marshall, London (German trans 1824, French trans 1825)

Churchill J M 1828 Cases illustrative of the immediate effects of acupuncturation in rheumatism, lumbago, sciatica, anomalous muscular diseases and in dropsy of the cellular tissue, selected from various sources and intended as an appendix to the author's treatise on the subject. Callow & Wilson, London

Drewes A M, Andreasen A, Poulsen L H 1993 Injection therapy for treatment of chronic myofascial pain: a double-blind study comparing corticosteroid versus diclofenac injections. Journal of Musculoskeletal Pain 1(3/4):289–294

Fine P G 1995 Treating myofascial pain and trigger points. Journal of Musculoskeletal Pain 3(4):87–89

Fine P G, Milano R, Hare B D 1988 The effects of trigger point injections are naloxone reversible. Pain 32:15–20

Fischer A A 1987 Pressure threshold measurement for diagnosis of myofascial pain and evaluation of treatment results. Clinical Journal of Pain 2:207–214

Fischer A A 1994 Pressure algometry (dolorimetry) in the differential diagnosis of muscle pain. In: Rachin E S (ed) Myofascial pain and fibromyalgia. Trigger point management. Mosby, St Louis, pp 121–141

Fischer A A 1995a Trigger point injections can be performed painfree using preinjection block (PIB). Journal of Musculoskeletal Pain 3(suppl 1):140

Fischer A A 1995b Local injections in pain management: trigger point needling with infiltration and somatic blocks. Physical Medicine and Rehabilitation Clinics of North America 6(4):851–870

Fischer A A 1998 Algometry in diagnosis of musculoskeletal pain and evaluation of treatment outcome: an update. Journal of Musculoskeletal Pain 6(1):5–32

Frost A 1986 Diclofenac versus Lidocaine as injection therapy in myofascial pain. Scandinavian Journal of Rheumatology 15:153–156

Frost P A, Jessen B, Siggaard-Andersen J 1980 A controlled double-blind comparison of mepivacaine injection versus saline injection for myofascial pain. Lancet i:499–501

Garvey T A, Marks M R, Wiesel S W 1989 A prospective randomized double-blind evaluation of trigger point injection therapy for low-back pain. Spine 14(9):962–964

Gerwin R 1992 The clinical assessment of myofascial pain. In: Turk D C, Melzack R (eds) Handbook of pain assessment. Guildford Press, New York, ch 5

Gerwin R D 1993 The management of myofascial pain syndromes. Journal of Musculoskeletal Pain 1(3/4):83–94

Gunn C C 1989 Treating myofascial pain – intramuscular stimulation (IMS) for myofascial pain syndromes of neuropathic origin. Health Science Center for Educational Resources, University of Washington, Seattle

Gunn C C 1996 The Gunn approach to the treatment of chronic pain. Churchill Livingstone, Edinburgh

Gunn C C 1998 Acupuncture and the peripheral nervous system. In: Filshie J, White A (eds) Medical acupuncture. A western scientific approach. Churchill Livingstone, Edinburgh, pp 137–150

Hameroff S R, Crago B R, Blitt C D, Womble J, Kanel J 1981 Comparison of bupivacaine, etidocaine and saline for trigger point therapy. Anesthesia and Analgesia 60:752–755

Han J S 1987 Mesolimbic neuronal loop of analgesia. In: Tiengo M, Eccles J, Cuello A C, Ottoson D (eds) Advances in pain research and therapy. Raven Press, New York, vol 10.

Hong C-Z 1994a Considerations and recommendations regarding myofascial trigger point injections. Journal of Musculoskeletal Pain 2(1):29–59

Hong C-Z 1994b Lidocaine injection versus dry needling to myofascial trigger point. American Journal of Physical Medicine and Rehabilitation 73:256–263

Hong C-Z, Torigoe Y 1991 Electromyographic findings of local twitch responses in the rabbit skeletal muscles. Society for Neuroscience Abstracts 17:642

Hong C-Z, Torigoe Y, Simons D G 1992 Failure of local twitch responses in rabbit skeletal muscles with repetitive needling. Scandinavian Journal of Rheumatology Supplement 94:25

Karavis M 1997 The neurophysiology of acupuncture: a viewpoint. Acupuncture in medicine. Journal of the British Acupuncture Society 15(1):33–42

Kellgren J 1938 A preliminary account of referred pains arising from muscles. British Medical Journal i:325–327

Kraus H 1941 The use of surface anesthesia in the treatment of painful motion. Journal of the American Medical Association 116:2582–2583

Lewit K 1979 The needle effect in the relief of myofascial pain. Pain 6:83–90

Lu G-D, Needham J 1980 Celestial lancets. Cambridge University Press, Cambridge

Macdonald A J R, Macrae K D, Master B R, Rubin A P 1983 Superficial acupuncture in the relief of chronic low-back pain. Annals of the Royal College of Surgeons of England 65:44–46

Martin A J 1952 Nature and treatment of fibrositis. Archives of Physical Medicine 33:409–413

Mayer D J, Price D D, Rafii A 1977 Antagonism of acupuncture analgesia in man by the narcotic antagonist naloxone. Brain Research 121:368–372

Osler W 1912 The principles and practice of medicine, 8th edn. Appleton, New York, p 1131

Rachlin E S 1994 Trigger point management. In: Rachlin E S (ed) Myofascial pain and fibromyalgia. Mosby, St Louis, pp 173–195

Ross R, Vogel A 1978 The platelet-derived growth function. Cell 14:203–210

Simons D G 1996 Clinical and etiological update of myofascial pain from trigger points. Journal of Musculoskeletal Pain 4(1/2):93–121

Simons D G, Hong C-Z 1995 Comment to Dr Baldry's dry needling technique. Journal of Musculoskeletal Pain 3(4):81–85

Simons D G, Travell J G, Simons L S 1999 Travell & Simons myofascial pain and dysfunction, the trigger point manual, 2nd edn. Williams & Wilkins, Baltimore, vol 1.

Sjölund B H, Eriksson M B E 1979 The influence of naloxone on analgesia produced by peripheral conditioning stimulation. Brain Research 173:295–302

Sola A E, Kuitert J H 1955 Myofascial trigger point pain in the neck and shoulder girdle. North West Medicine 54:980–984

Sola A E, Williams R L 1956 Myofascial pain syndromes. Neurology (Minneapolis) 6:91–95

Travell J 1960 Temporomandibular joint pain referred from muscles of the head and neck. Journal of Prosthetic Dentistry 10:745–763

Travell J 1968 Office hours: day and night. The World Publishing Company, New York

Travell J, Rinzler S H 1952 The myofascial genesis of pain. Postgraduate Medicine 11:425–434

Travell J G, Simons D G 1983 Myofascial pain and dysfunction. The trigger point manual. Williams & Wilkins, Baltimore

Tsui J K E, Stoessal A J, Eisen A, Calne S, Calne D B 1986 Double-blind study of botulinum toxin in spasmodic torticollis. Lancet ii:245–246

Vandam L D 1960 Local anesthetics. New England Journal of Medicine 263:748–750

Yue S K 1995 Initial experience in the use of botulinum toxin A for the treatment of myofascial related muscle dysfunctions. Journal of Musculoskeletal Pain 3(suppl 1):22

PART 2

Regional myofascial trigger point pain syndromes

8

The neck

INTRODUCTION

The commonest reason for the onset of stiffness of the neck, together with pain in the head, neck, shoulder girdle and arm in an otherwise fit person is the development of myofascial trigger point (MTrP) activity in the neck and shoulder girdle muscles (Fricton et al 1985, Gerwin 1995, Grosshandler et al 1985, Long 1956, Michele et al 1950, Michele & Eisenberg 1968, Simons et al 1999a, Sola & Kuitert 1955, Sola & Williams 1956).

Attention will therefore first be drawn to the pathogenesis, clinical manifestations and treatment of this cervical MTrP pain syndrome. Following this a separate section will be devoted to considering the physical and psychological complexities of this syndrome when it develops as a consequence of a whiplash injury. And then MTrP activity that arises secondary to the development of nerve root entrapment in cervical spondylosis and cervical disc prolapse will be discussed.

CERVICAL MYOFASCIAL TRIGGER POINT PAIN SYNDROME

Factors responsible for its development

The factors responsible for the primary activation of TrP nociceptors in the muscles of the neck and shoulder girdle include postural disorders, sagging of the shoulder girdle, tilting of

A

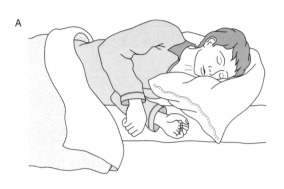

B

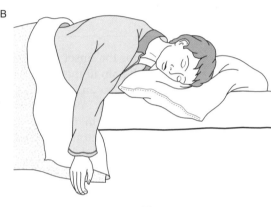

C

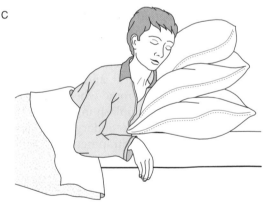

Figure 8.1   Pillow arrangement. A patient with TrPs in muscles of the neck must ensure that the pillow arrangement is such as to avoid it becoming kinked during sleep. A: Correct pillow arrangement. B and C: Incorrect pillow arrangement.

the shoulder girdle, indirect overloading of the neck muscles, direct overloading of them, acute trauma to the neck and anxiety. Each of these will be considered in turn.

Postural disorders

Muscles in the neck and shoulder girdle are liable to become overloaded when, for example, a desk, chair or workbench is not properly adjusted to an individual's body build. It may also happen when the neck muscles are held in one particular position for a long time such as, for example, may happen during the course of typing, operating a computer, driving a car or painting a ceiling. It may also occur during sleep as a result of resting the head on pillows which are either too high or too low (Fig. 8.1).

Sagging of the shoulder girdle

TrP activity may develop in the muscles of the neck and shoulder girdle of anyone who, because of occupational strains, obesity, or even laziness, has become round shouldered with drooping of the shoulder girdle – the so-called syndrome of the sagging shoulder. It my also develop when these muscles become wasted as a result of some neurological disorder such as, for example, neuralgic amyotrophy, in which transient very severe pain in the muscles of the shoulder girdle is followed by long-term wasting and weakness.

Tilting of the shoulder girdle

Tilting of the shoulder girdle with, as a consequence, the imposition of strain upon the neck muscles and the activation of TrP nociceptors in them is liable to take place as a result of a scoliosis which develops when one leg is shorter than the other. This may be a congenital defect when, in addition, there is likely to be slight facial asymmetry, a shorter upper limb and a smaller hemipelvis on the affected side. Or alternatively it may be an acquired one due, for example, to a malunited fracture or a poorly fitting joint prosthesis.

Should this lower limb equality be 6 mm or less the scoliosis takes the form of a C-shaped curve with tilting of the shoulder to the side opposite to that of the shorter leg. Should it

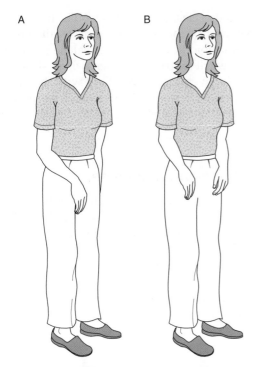

Figure 8.2   A: Person whose arms are of sufficient length in relation to the height of the torso for the elbows to reach the level of the iliac crest. B: Person with abnormally short arms so that in the relaxed standing position the elbows do not reach the level of the iliac crest.

be 10 mm or more the scoliosis takes the form of an S-shaped curve with tilting of the shoulder to the same side as that of the shorter leg (see Figs 12.14 and 12.15).

Indirect overloading of the neck muscles

There are two ways in which this may be brought about.

The first is when a painful lesion in a lower limb leads to the development of a limp. This may cause the low-back muscles to become over-loaded with, as a consequence, the development of MTrP pain. This may then lead to postural changes taking place which, in turn, have the effect of overloading muscles in the neck and causing TrP activity to develop in them.

Secondly, a person whose upper arms are so short in relation to the height of the torso that, in

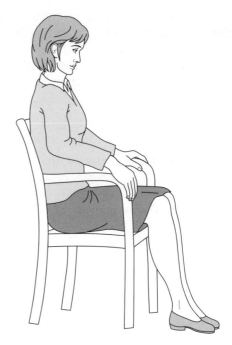

Figure 8.3   Person with abnormally short upper arms (see Fig. 8.2B) may, because of this, be unable to place elbows on the arm rest of a chair.

the relaxed standing position, the elbows do not reach the level of the iliac crest (Fig. 8.2) is liable to find that on sitting it is not possible to place the elbows on the arm rests of a chair (Fig. 8.3). The effect of this is to overload various shoulder girdle muscles such as the trapezius and levator scapulae with, as a consequence, the development and perpetuation of MTrP activity in them.

Direct overloading of the neck muscles

TrP activity may develop in the neck muscles when they become overloaded as a result of wearing unsuitable clothes, such as an overcoat which is too heavy or shoulder straps which are too tight.

Acute trauma to the neck

There are clearly many possible causes for this but one of the commonest is a whiplash injury and, because the importance of TrP activity as a major contributor to the pain in this disorder is not well recognised, its pathophysiology, clinical manifestations and management will be considered at some length later in this chapter (p. 134).

Anxiety

Finally, holding the muscles of the neck and shoulder girdle in a persistently contracted state because of anxiety not infrequently causes MTrP pain to develop. The mechanism by which this is brought about is not certain but possible ones were discussed in Chapter 3.

Clinical manifestations

The pain, which is of a dull aching character, may be confined to the neck or, in addition, may be referred either down the arm, or up to the head, or to both of these sites.

Unlike when pain in the neck and arm arises as a result of nerve root entrapment, for example because of cervical spondylosis (p. 145) or disc prolapse (p. 147), clinical examination in this disorder reveals no evidence of a neurological deficit.

Because of the pain and the shortening of the muscles that occur as a result of MTrP activity there is usually some restriction of the neck movements on the affected side. In those cases where the muscles have been subjected to particularly severe overloading the muscle spasm may be so considerable as to draw the neck sharply over to the affected side with the production of a so-called acute wry neck, which has to be distinguished from spasmodic torticollis. This, however, should present no difficulty as with this latter condition there is not only pain in the neck and severe spasm of the muscles but also clonic rotatory movements of the head and neck.

Location of myofascial trigger points

TrPs from which the pain emanates are liable to be found in one or more of the following structures – the ligamentum nuchae, the posterior cervical muscles, the levator scapulae muscle, the upper part of the trapezius muscle, the sternocleidomastoid muscle and the scalene muscles.

The search for trigger points in these structures is most conveniently carried out with the patient sitting on a chair and the tissues of the neck on the side being examined placed slightly on the stretch.

The ligamentum nuchae

One cause for pain on extending or flexing the neck is the development of trigger point activity in the ligamentum nuchae, a fibrous membrane homologous with the thoracic and lumbar supraspinous ligaments, which covers the cervical spinal processes from the external occipital protuberance above to the seventh cervical vertebra below.

Posterior cervical group of muscles

Anatomical relationships

These paravertebrally situated muscles are arranged in three layers. In descending order of depth the muscles in these three layers are the splenius capitis and cervicis; the semispinalis capitis and cervicis; and the multifidi and rotatores.

Trigger point sites and patterns of pain referral

The depth at which MTrPs are liable to be found and therefore the muscle or muscles in which they are situated varies. There are three sites in particular, however, where they are commonly found (Fig. 8.4).

From TrP 1, at the upper part of the neck just below the occiput, pain is referred along the side of the head to the temporal region and eye (Fig. 8.5). It may occasionally be accompanied by blurring of the vision (Simons et al 1999b).

From TrP 2, situated midway between the occiput and the base of the neck, pain is referred to the vertex of the head (Fig. 8.6).

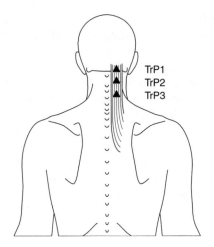

Figure 8.4   TrP 1, 2 and 3 – three common trigger point sites in the posterior cervical group of muscles.

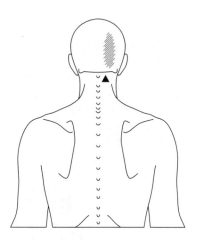

Figure 8.6   The pattern of pain referral from a trigger point (TrP 2) midway between the occiput and base of the neck in a posterior cervical muscle.

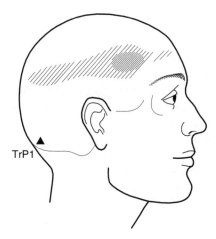

Figure 8.5   The pattern of pain referral from a trigger point (TrP 1) just below the occiput in a posterior cervical muscle.

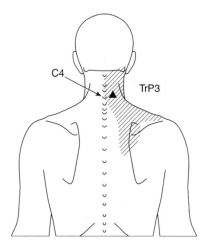

Figure 8.7   The pattern of pain referral from a trigger point (TrP 3) at the base of the neck at the level of the C4 vertebra in a posterior cervical muscle.

From TrP 3, at the base of the neck at the level of the C4–C5 vertebrae, pain is referred to the back of the neck and shoulder girdle (Fig. 8.7).

Restriction of movements

TrP activity in the posterior cervical muscles gives rise to stiffness of the neck with restricted flexion and rotation of the head and neck. This restriction of neck movements becomes even more marked when TrP activity is also present in the levator scapulae and trapezius muscles.

Levator scapulae muscle

Anatomical attachments

This muscle arises from tendinous slips attached to the transverse processes of the first four cervical vertebrae. And its lower end it is inserted into the scapula at a site close to this bone's superior angle.

Trigger point sites

TrPs may be found at two separate sites in this muscle. One is at the angle of the neck where the muscle emerges from beneath the anterior border of the trapezius muscle. The other is situated lower down the back at the site where the muscle attaches to the scapula in the vicinity of its superior angle (Fig. 8.8).

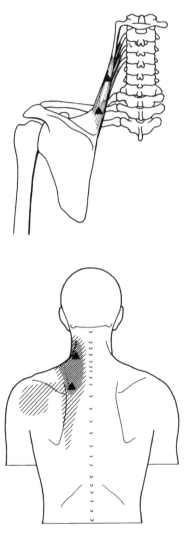

Figure 8.8 The pattern of pain referral to the neck, shoulder and inner border of the scapula from a trigger point or points (▲) in the levator scapulae muscle. Pain in this distribution occurs as a result of activity in either a trigger point at the angle of the neck or one near to the insertion of this muscle into the superior angle of the scapula, or in both.

The TrP at the angle of the neck is best palpated with the patient sitting comfortably with the elbows supported on arm rests. This helps to relax both the levator scapulae and trapezius and allows the clinician to pull the trapezius out of the way. Once the levator scapulae muscle has been identified, the TrP is most readily located by gently turning the head to the opposite side as this puts the muscle on stretch. The lower TrP may also be located with the patient in the sitting position. This TrP and its associated taut band are best identified by rolling the fingers across the muscle fibres just above the superior angle of the scapula.

Trigger point pain referral

The pain from TrP activity in this muscle is mainly felt at the base of the neck, but it may also extend upwards towards the occiput; outwards to the back of the shoulder and downwards along the inner border of the scapula (Fig. 8.8).

The pain may also radiate anteriorly around the chest wall along the course of the fourth and fifth intercostal nerves when it may erroneously be diagnosed as being either anginal or pleural, or even more frequently as being due to intercostal nerve root entrapment. In addition, it quite commonly extends down the arm along the posteromedial aspect of the upper arm and the ulnar border of the forearm and hand to terminate in the ring and little fingers, a pattern of referral that coincides with the cutaneous areas of distribution of spinal segments C8, T1 and T2 (Fig. 8.9).

Of those patients in whom levator scapulae trigger point pain is referred to these distant parts of the body, some only experience it down the arm; some only feel it around the chest wall; whilst others are aware of it at both sites simultaneously.

Restriction of movements

TrP activity in this muscle leads to the development of a painful 'stiff neck'. With this there is an inability to turn the head fully not only to the affected side because of the pain but also

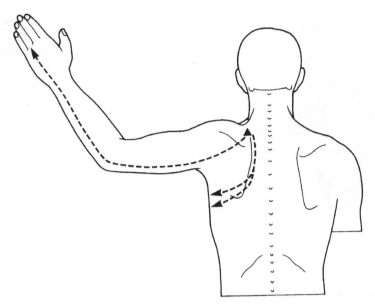

Figure 8.9 Some other patterns of pain referral from a trigger point (▲) in the levator scapulae near to its insertion into the superior angle of the scapula. These include referral down the inner side of the arm to the ring and little fingers. And referral down around the chest wall along the course of the fourth and fifth intercostal nerves.

to the opposite side because of a pain-induced increase in muscle tension.

Scapulocostal and scapulohumeral syndromes

Michele et al (1950), Russek (1952) and Michele & Eisenberg (1968), in describing the condition in which pain is referred down the arm and around the chest wall from TrP activity in the levator scapulae muscle, call it the scapulocostal syndrome. Long (1956) more appropriately divides it into the scapulocostal and scapulohumeral syndromes for, as he states, trigger point pain around the chest wall and down the arm, although commonly occurring in consort, does not always do so. However, it has to be remembered that when pain is referred down the arm from TrPs around the scapula, these trigger points may be in either the levator scapulae, the supraspinatus muscle or the infraspinatus muscle, with each of these three muscles having its own specific pattern of pain referral. Therefore, the terms scapulocostal and scapulohumeral syndromes are liable to cause confusion and are better avoided.

Trapezius muscle

Anatomical attachments

The two trapezius muscles together take the form of a diamond. They extend in the midline from the occiput above, to the twelfth thoracic vertebra below, and fan out on both sides to be attached to the clavicle in front and the spine of the scapula behind (Fig. 8.10).

For descriptive purposes the muscle may therefore be conveniently divided into an upper part extending from the occiput down to the fifth cervical spine, a middle part extending from the sixth cervical spine to the third dorsal vertebra, and a lower part extending from the fourth to the twelfth dorsal vertebra.

Trigger point sites and patterns of pain referral

Upper part of the muscle The most frequently occurring TrP (TrP 1) in the trapezius muscle is to be found along the upper border of the shoulder girdle about half way between the spine and the tip of the shoulder (Fig. 8.10).

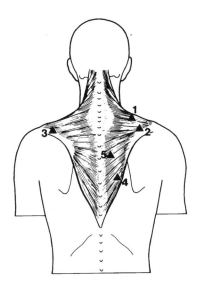

Figure 8.10   Trigger points (▲) in the trapezius muscle.

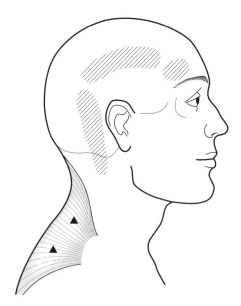

Figure 8.11   Pattern of pain referral from trigger points (▲) in the upper free border of the trapezius muscle.

TrP activity at this site is the cause of pain being referred up the side of the neck to the base of the skull, and on occasions around the side of the head to reach the temple and back of the eye (Fig. 8.11).

Sometimes there is also another TrP in the same part of the muscle situated immediately below the one already described (TrP 2, Fig. 8.10). This also causes pain to be referred up the side of the neck.

Middle part of the muscle   A TrP (TrP 3, Fig. 8.10) near the acromion may be responsible for pain being referred to the posterior part of the shoulder.

Lower part of the muscle   A TrP (TrP 4, Fig. 8.10) may be found in the outer border of the lower part just above the level of the inferior angle of the scapula. Also another one may occur just below the inner end of the scapular spine (TrP 5, Fig. 8.10). These two TrPs are not often involved but when they are, they may cause pain to be referred to the upper scapula and neck region. They are therefore always worth looking for if neck pain persists after activity in the other TrPs already described has been adequately suppressed.

Associated trigger point activity

TrP activity in the trapezius muscle may develop alone or in conjunction with TrP activity in other muscles including the levator scapulae (see p. 125), the supraspinatus (see Ch. 9) and the rhomboid muscles (see Ch. 14).

Sternocleidomastoid muscle

Anatomical attachments

This muscle, as its name implies, has a sternal and clavicular division. The tendinous, medially situated sternal division arises from the upper part of the anterior surface of the manubrium sterni. And from there it is directed upwards, laterally and backwards.

The fleshy laterally situated clavicular division arises from the medial one-third of the clavicle and from there is directed almost vertically upwards. Initially the two heads are separated by a triangular space but as they ascend the clavicular division blends with the deep surface of the sternal division about the middle of the neck to form a thick rounded belly. At its upper end

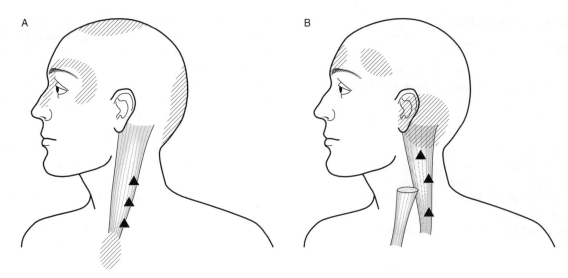

Figure 8.12 A: Patterns of pain referral from TrPs (▲) in the upper, middle and lower part of the sternal division of the sternocleidomastoid muscle. B: Patterns of pain referral from TrPs (▲) in its clavicular division.

the muscle is attached by a strong tendon to the mastoid process.

TrP activity may develop in this muscle in either its sternal or clavicular division or both.

Sternal division (Fig. 8.12A)

TrPs at the upper part of the sternal division near to the insertion of this muscle into the mastoid process are responsible for pain being referred to the occipital region and to the top of the head. There is often marked tenderness of the area of the scalp affected (Travell 1955).

TrPs in the mid-part of this division refer pain along the supraorbital ridge, around the eye and into the cheek.

TrPs at the lower end of this division near to its attachment to the sternum refer pain in a downward direction over the upper part of the sternum.

TrP activity in this division of the muscle is liable to be accompanied by various autonomic concomitants including conjunctival redness and watering of the eye and nose similar to those which develop with migrainous neuralgia (Travell 1960).

Clavicular division (Fig. 8.12B)

TrPs in the deeper clavicular part of this muscle are liable to refer pain either into the ear and post-auricular region or across the front of the forehead.

Trp activity in this division may lead to the development of episodic dizziness, unsteadiness, a sensation of veering to one side in walking and nausea. These concomitants are considered to be due to this muscle being one of the chief muscular sources of proprioceptive orientation of the head (Simons et al 1999c).

Associated trigger point activity

TrP activity in the sternocleidomastoid muscle may be accompanied by similar activity developing in other neck muscles such as the levator scapulae and scalene muscles. When this happens the patient complains not only of having a persistent headache but also of having pain in the arm and restricted movements of the neck.

Scalene muscles (Fig. 8.13)

Anatomical attachments

The scalenus anterior muscle, which lies behind the sternocleidomastoid muscle, arises above from the transverse processes of the third, fourth, fifth and sixth cervical vertebrae and, descending almost vertically, is inserted by a narrow flat tendon into the first rib.

The scalenus medius, the largest of these three muscles, arises above from the transverse processes of the lower six cervical vertebrae and is also inserted into the first rib. Anteriorly it is separated from the scalenus anterior by the subclavian artery and the brachial plexus.

The scalenus posterior, the smallest and the most deeply situated of these three muscles, arises above from the transverse processes of the fourth, fifth and sixth cervical vertebrae and is inserted by a thin tendon into the second rib.

Trigger point sites and patterns of pain referral

In order to locate TrPs in the scalenus anterior muscle palpation of it has to be carried out behind the posterior border of the clavicular division of the sternocleidomastoid muscle. To facilitate this search it is useful to apply pressure just above the clavicle in order to distend the external jugular vein, as TrPs in this muscle tend to be situated in the vicinity of where this vein crosses it (Simons et al 1999d).

In order to locate TrPs in the scalenus medius muscle it is necessary to carry out deep palpation against the transverse processes to which it is attached.

The scalenus posterior muscle is far more difficult to palpate but fortunately this is rarely necessary as the development of TrP activity in it is far less common than in the other two scalene muscles.

The referral of pain from TrPs in either the scalenus anterior, medius or posterior (Fig. 8.14) is anteriorly over the pectoral region, posteriorly along the medial border of the scapula, and laterally across the front of the shoulder and down the arm. When the latter occurs it is felt in both the front and back of the arm and extends to the thumb and index finger.

Pain from TrP activity in one or other of these muscles on the left side may closely simulate that

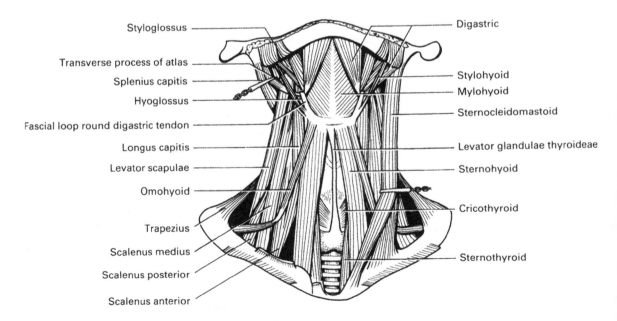

Figure 8.13 Muscles of the front of the neck. On the right the sternocleidomastoid has been removed.

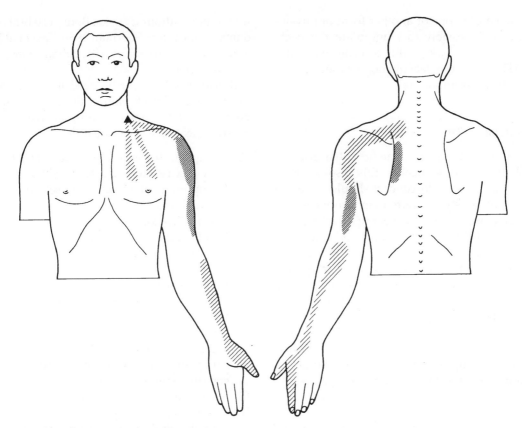

Figure 8.14 The pattern of pain referral from a trigger point or points (▲) in a scalene muscle.

of coronary heart disease both because of its distribution and because it is liable to be made worse by exertion.

In differentiating between these two sources of pain it is helpful to remember that referred pain from the scalenus anterior is relieved when both the arm and clavicle are elevated by placing the forearm on the affected side across the forehead (Ochsner et al 1935); and it is aggravated by contracting the muscle by rotating the head as far as possible to the side of the pain whilst pulling the chin down into the supraclavicular fossa.

Restriction of neck movements

It should be noted that scalene TrP activity alone causes minimal restriction of neck movements, unlike TrP activity in the levator scapulae and splenius cervicis which markedly limits this (Simons et al 1999e).

Cervical myofascial pain syndrome's differential diagnosis

Other disorders which have to be taken into account when considering this syndrome's differential diagnosis include polymyalgia rheumatica; infective, neoplastic and rheumatoid arthritic disease of the cervical spine; and trauma-induced damage to vertebrae, intervertebral discs and facet joints.

Treatment of cervical myofascial pain syndrome

The traditional approach to the management of this disorder is to splint the neck with a cervical collar, to employ one or another form of physio-therapy, and possibly to manipulate the neck. As, however, the pain in this disorder emanates from MTrPs it is the deactivation of these that is clearly the most important.

Orthopaedic collars

The wearing of an orthopaedic collar for the immobilisation of the neck in this disorder is of very limited value. Moreover it should never be worn continuously for more than two weeks. as prolonged use causes weakening, wasting and shortening of the neck muscles. In addition, the patient may become unduly reliant on it and is then reluctant to leave it off. Therefore, after two weeks of continuous use the patient should only be allowed to wear it on particular occasions such as when sleeping, and during the course of carrying out any task which places a persistent strain on the neck muscles as, for example, when operating a computer for any length of time, or travelling an appreciable distance in a car.

Physiotherapy

Short wave diathermy, interferential stimulation or ultrasound may be employed. The application of heat by any of these methods, however, only provides non-specific temporary symptomatic pain relief.

Mechanically applied traction is liable to damage the tissues and may for this reason increase the pain. Its use therefore cannot be recommended (Weinberger 1976). Manually applied traction is preferable, for it often provides a certain amount of pain relief, but is not as effective as exercises designed to stretch individual muscles.

Manipulation

This is an increasingly popular, highly specialised technique which should only be used by practitioners well trained in its use.

High velocity/low amplitude thrust, which is perhaps the most widely used form of manipula-tion, is not without its risks. Both vertebral artery damage (Easton & Sherman 1986, Fast et al 1987) and cervical cord injury (Kleynhans 1980) have been reported.

It also should never be used indiscriminately for the relief of neck pain of uncertain aetiology. Wells (1994) provides a comprehensive list of contraindications. These include:

1. Malignant disease of the bone or soft tissues.
2. Bone disease such as osteomyelitis, osteoporosis (of whatever cause), and tuberculosis.
3. Spinal cord compression.
4. Cauda equina compression.
5. Recent fractures.
6. Vertebrobasilar insufficiency.
7. Inflammatory arthritis such as rheumatoid arthritis and ankylosing spondylitis.
8. Bony or ligamentous instability of whatever cause, e.g. spondylolisthesis, fractures, cranio-cervical and lumbosacral anomalies.
9. Severe degenerative changes and long standing spinal deformity.
10. Severe nerve root irritation or compression.
11. Pregnancy; generally all vigorous procedures to the lower thoracic and lumbar spine are to be avoided after the third month.
12. Pain of unknown origin.
13. Recent whiplash trauma to the neck.
14. Anticoagulant therapy and current or recent steroid therapy.
15. Certain psychological states where there is clear evidence that the patient has developed an obsessional dependence on 'having his spine clicked back'.

From this it is clear that manipulation should only be employed by highly trained diagnosticians with access to a wide range of investigatory procedures.

It is not known for certain how manipulation relieves pain. One possibility is that it has the effect of stretching the muscles and by so doing deactivating MTrPs. Those who wish to know more about this technique should consult either Wells's (1994) relatively short but otherwise excellent review of it or a more extensive treatise on the subject such as that provided by Grieve (1986).

Deactivation of cervical myofascial trigger points

Because all muscles in the neck are in close proximity to large vessels and nerves, and those in the anterior part of it are covered by the apex of the lung, out of all the superficial and deep MTrP deactivating procedures described in Chapter 7 superficial dry needling (SDN) is by far the simplest and safest, and is the one therefore which is strongly recommended for use in this particular region of the body.

Another reason for employing it is because clinical experience has shown that for the deactivation of cervical MTrPs any neural stimulation other than a very lightly applied one is liable to give rise to much post-treatment soreness and, not infrequently, a temporary exacerbation of the pain. This would seem to be particularly so when deactivating TrPs in the sternocleidomastoid muscle for, as Simons et al (1999f) have pointed out, the strong stimulation provided by any deeply applied deactivating procedure gives rise to such a high incidence of post-treatment soreness that following the treatment the patient needs to rest in bed and to apply moist hot packs to the neck.

It is particularly important to employ SDN for the deactivation of cervical MTrPs in patients with a history of migraine, because they are in general strong responders (see Ch. 7) and therefore any neural stimulation other than a very lightly applied one is liable to bring on an attack.

Similarly, it has been found that when deactivating tender points and TrPs in the neck and other regions of patients with fibromyalgia, only very lightly applied SDN is required. Any neural stimulation stronger than this, such as is likely to be delivered by one of the more deeply applied techniques discussed in Chapter 7, tends to be counter-productive (Baldry 2000).

Deactivation of TrPs in the neck muscles should initially be carried out with the patient lying down rather than seated because in the latter position there is a greater risk of vasovagal attack occurring. This is especially likely to happen when deactivating TrPs in either the sternocleidomastoid or trapezius muscle because the spinal accessory nerve that innervates both of these has vagal components (Dworkin et al 1990). However, in patients who are not prone to developing vasovagal attacks the deactivation of cervical TrPs is far more easily carried out with them sitting down.

Muscle stretching exercises

Following deactivation of cervical MTrPs, the neck muscles should be stretched and the patient taught how to carry out muscle stretching exercises on a daily basis.

Prevention of myofascial trigger point reactivation

After the deactivation of TrPs in the neck in order to prevent activity in them recurring, the following are some of the measures that may have to be taken.

Pursuits which involve persistent hyperextension or hyperflexion of the neck should be avoided. This includes not sitting bent over a desk or workbench for any length of time without periodically standing up and stretching the muscles. Furthermore, anyone who has to use a computer should check that the position of the screen and keyboard is such as not to cause the shoulders to be kept in a persistently elevated position. The height of the desk or chair should be adjusted accordingly.

Also to be avoided is the neck becoming kinked during sleep as a result of resting the head on too many or too few pillows (Fig. 8.1).

Any leg length inequality should be corrected, for the scoliosis produced by this is liable to cause sagging of a shoulder with, as a consequence, overloading of the neck muscles on that side (p. 122).

It is necessary to provide adequate support for the elbows in someone whose upper arms are abnormally short. This is because this anomaly, by preventing the elbows from reaching the arm rests of a chair, is liable to cause a strain to be imposed upon the muscles of the neck. Therefore a person with this deformity should either be careful to sit in a chair with arm rests of sufficient height or have these raised by one means or another (Fig. 8.15).

CERVICAL WHIPLASH INJURIES
Terminological confusion

There are many ways in which a cervical whiplash injury may be brought about. Some of the more frequently occurring ones include diving into shallow water, falling from a horse, tripping when descending stairs and involvement in a vehicular collision. Although this type of injury is extremely common there continues to be a regrettable failure to recognise that often much of the pain produced by it emanates from MTrPs. For this reason its pathogenesis, clinical manifestations and management will be considered at some length.

The term 'whiplash' was first introduced by Crowe in 1928, at a meeting of the Western Orthopedic Association in San Francisco, at a time when he was discussing eight cases of head injury brought about by traffic accidents. However, he later admitted that he had come to regret ever having employed what he eventually called 'this unfortunate term' for as he explained (Crowe 1964), 'this expression was intended to be a description of motion but it has been accepted by physicians, patients and attorneys as a name of a disease'.

Davis (1945), for example, was not only guilty of this but he also committed the error of stating that the movement of the neck with this type of injury is one of 'hyperflexion followed by a spontaneous extension recoil'.

It has since been realised that this particular sequence of movements only takes place with certain types of neck injury such as, for example, when a stationary car is hit from the front end. The term whiplash injury should only be used in those cases where the movements of the neck brought about by it are the same as those taken by a whip during the course of it being cracked, i.e. acute hyperextension followed by forceful flexion. A sequence of movements which Severy et al (1955), from the carrying out

of controlled car collisions with the help of high speed photography, have shown only

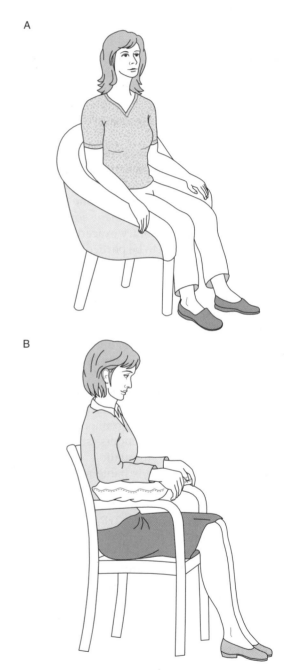

Figure 8.15 A person with abnormally short upper arms should sit in a chair with arm rests of sufficient height to allow the elbows to reach them (A) or have the arm rests raised by one means or another (B).

occurs when a stationary car is hit from the rear (Fig. 8.16).

Porter (1989) has therefore argued that, because the term whiplash injury is often inappropriately employed, it should be abandoned and replaced by that of acute neck sprain.

This has much to commend it for in the vast majority of cases the damage is confined to the soft tissues of the neck with stretching and bruising of the muscles and ligaments (Jeffreys 1980, Norris & Watt 1983). However, when the trauma is particularly severe discs (Barnsley et al 1994a) and facet joints (Aprill & Bogduk 1992, Bogduk & Marsland 1988) may become damaged. Vertebrae also may be fractured (Clark et al 1988).

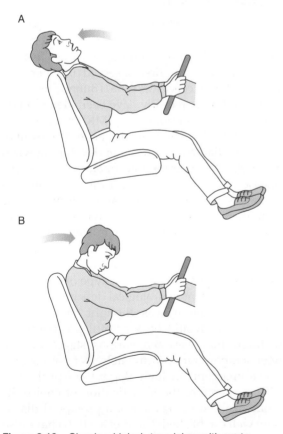

Figure 8.16 Classic whiplash-type injury with acute hyperextension of neck (A) followed by forceful flexion of it (B) brought about as a result of vehicle being hit from the rear.

Myofascial trigger point pain

Muscles subjected to a whiplash injury are liable to become bruised, and at times partially or completely torn with, as a consequence, bleeding into the tissues. Despite damage of this type usually healing within a matter of weeks, pain is liable to persist for months or even years. One common reason for this is the development of trauma-induced MTrP nociceptor activity (Evans 1992, Fricton 1993) with the MTrP pain tending to continue for an appreciable period of time because of the setting up of self-perpetuating MTrP nociceptor-activating circuits and the development of dorsal horn neuronal plasticity (Ch. 4).

Gerwin (1999) has observed that whilst some of his patients with whiplash injuries have discogenic pain and/or facet joint pain, all of them have MTrP pain. It therefore follows that the physical examination of a patient with an acute neck sprain should always include a search for MTrPs. The muscles in which these are liable to be found include the sternocleidomastoid (p. 129), the levator scapulae (p. 126), the posterior cervical muscles (p. 125), the trapezius (p. 128), the rhomboids (Ch. 14), the supraspinatus (Ch. 9) and the infraspinatus (Ch. 9); also, the scalenus anterior (p. 130) and the pectoralis minor (Ch. 14), with TrP activity in either of these two being responsible for the development of the thoracic outlet syndrome.

The thoracic outlet syndrome

There are many reasons for the development of the thoracic outlet syndrome. One of the commoner is a whiplash injury.

Roos & Owens (1966) reported that out of 138 cases of this syndrome one-third occurred as a result of injuries to the neck, a finding which led them to conclude that 'any injury causing a severe jerk of the shoulder or neck may precipitate the syndrome including the so-called "whiplash" auto injury'.

In the last few years it has become increasingly apparent that the thoracic outlet syndrome when it arises as a complication of a whiplash injury does so because of neurovascular compression brought about by MTrP-induced shortening and abnormal tautness of two muscles – the scalenus anterior and the pectoralis minor. A search for MTrPs in these two muscles in all such cases is therefore mandatory.

Scalenus anterior muscle

MTrP-induced tautness and shortening of the scalenus anterior by elevating the first rib causes pressure to be exerted on the lower trunk of the brachial plexus with, as a result, the development of pain extending down the inner side of the arm to the medial side of the hand with numbness and paraesthesiae in the fourth and fifth fingers. Occasionally pressure is also exerted on the subclavian vein with as a consequence distension of the veins in the arms and the development of oedema of the hand.

The pectoralis minor muscle

Hong & Simons (1993) have also found that whiplash injury victims are liable to develop TrP activity in the pectoralis minor and that when this happens, the TrP-induced tautness and shortening of the muscle causes pressure to be exerted on the lower trunk of the brachial plexus with, as a result, the referral of pain to the anterior chest wall, the shoulders, the medial aspect of the arm, the ulnar aspect of the forearm and hand. And in addition, paraesthesiae in the ring and little fingers.

The neurovascular entrapment symptoms produced by MTrP-induced shortening of the scalenus anterior and pectoralis minor are therefore so similar as to be virtually indistinguishable. And it is essential to remember that with a whiplash injury, MTrP activity not infrequently develops in these two muscles concomitantly.

Ulnar nerve conduction test

In the diagnosis of the thoracic outlet syndrome the ulnar nerve motor conduction velocity test (Caldwell Crane & Krusen 1971, Capistrant 1977) is of considerable help as there is invariably a significant decrease in the conduction velocity across the thoracic outlet. This test has proved to be of particular help in cases where litigation is pending as it helps to provide objective evidence that the symptoms complained of by the litigant have an organic basis.

Treatment of thoracic outlet syndrome

The deactivation of any MTrPs found to be present in these two muscles is clearly essential. It is often necessary to repeat this procedure at weekly intervals for a time. And in those cases where this fails to give any long-lasting relief, the first rib may have to be resected (Urschell & Razzuk 1972).

Discogenic pain

A whiplash injury to the neck may cause pain to develop if there is a tear in the richly innervated outer third of a disc's annulus fibrosus. Tears in this structure were first observed in cineradiograms of the cervical spine (Buonocore et al 1966), and more recently have been identified on magnetic resonance imaging (MRI) scans (Davis et al 1991). Disc pain may also arise as a result of a sterile inflammatory reaction developing when an endplate compression fracture causes the release of destructive enzymes into the nucleus pulposus. Another cause is avulsion of the disc from the vertebral endplate (Davis et al 1991). In addition, herniation of the nucleus pulposus through a ruptured annulus fibrosus may give rise to a radiculopathy or myelopathy with the development of a neuropathic type of pain and a clinically evident neurological deficit.

At one time it was thought that cervical discography would be a helpful procedure for distinguishing between various stages of disc degeneration but unfortunately its false-positive rate is unacceptably high (Bogduk & Aprill 1993). MRI is therefore the investigation of choice. Its value in the investigation of a prolapsed disc is now well established. Davis et al (1991) have also drawn attention to its usefulness in identifying other pain-producing lesions such as vertebral endplate avulsions and annular tears.

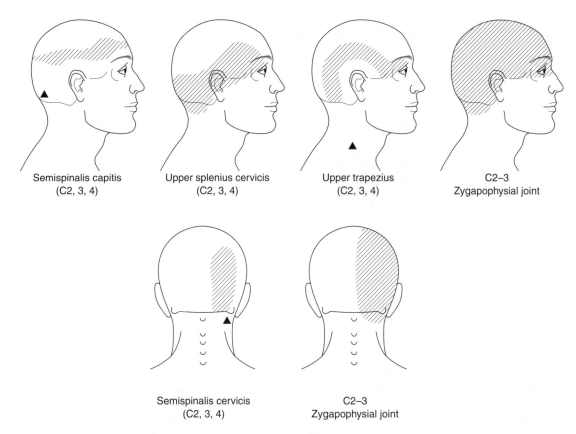

Figure 8.17 Sketches of the pain patterns of trigger points in various upper, posterior neck muscles and the pain pattern of the C2–C3 zygapophysial joint. The innervation of each muscle (depicted in parentheses) is concordant with that of the joint. (Reprinted from: Bogduk N, Simons D 1993 Neck pain: joint pain or trigger points? In: Voeroy H, Merskey H (eds) Progress in fibromyalgia and myofascial pain (Ch. 20), with permission of Elsevier Science and Dr David Simons.)

Median nerve entrapment pain (carpal tunnel syndrome)

Entrapment of the median nerve in the carpal tunnel may develop in patients with a whiplash injury because of the development of perineural oedema. This may arise as a result of subclavian vein compression or because of a hyperextension injury to the wrist caused by excessive gripping of the steering wheel or bracing the hands on the dashboard during the collision (Evans 1992).

Pain from this disorder usually comes on at night. It extends from the wrist up the arm often as far as the shoulder. It is characteristically relieved by hanging the affected limb out of bed. On waking the hand feels stiff, clumsy and subject-ively swollen. In addition, paraesthesiae develop in either all of the fingers or the outer three.

Paraesthesiae in the fingers following a whiplash injury may therefore arise because of the development of either the thoracic outlet syndrome, a cervical radiculopathy or the carpal tunnel syndrome.

Confirmation of the diagnosis of this latter syndrome may be obtained with electrical conduction studies. Treatment, as for other causes of it, is principally by surgical decompression.

Facet joint pain

Trauma to the neck from a whiplash injury may at times be responsible for the development

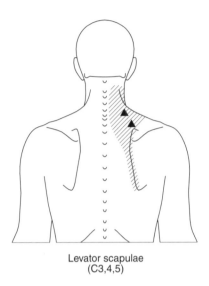 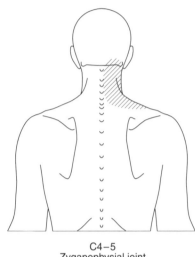

Levator scapulae
(C3,4,5)

C4–5
Zygapophysial joint

Figure 8.18 Sketches of the pain patterns from trigger points in the levator scapulae (innervation in parenthesis) and for the C4–C5 zygapophysial joint. (Reproduced from: Bogduk N, Simons D 1993 Neck pain: joint pain or trigger points? In: Voeroy H, Merskey H (eds) Progress in fibromyalgia and myofascial pain (Ch 20), with permission of Elsevier Science and Dr David Simons.)

of facet joint pain. Possible causes for this developing include occult fractures, capsular ruptures and intra-articular haemorrhages (Jónsson et al 1991).

Experimental studies have shown that each of the facet joints in the neck has its own specific pattern of pain referral (Aprill et al 1990, Dwyer et al 1990). Furthermore, Bogduk & Simons (1993) have pointed out that a facet joint and the muscles around it share the same nerve supply and that, because of this, the pattern of pain referral from TrPs in these muscles and from the joint is the same. Thus, for example, they have shown that the referral of pain both from a C2–C3 facet (zygapophysial) joint and from TrPs in posterior cervical muscles high up in the neck (semispinalis capitis, the upper part of the trapezius and the upper part of the splenius cervicis) is along the outer side of the head to the temporal region and the eye (Fig. 8.17). And the referral of pain both from a C4–C5 facet joint and from MTrPs in the levator scapulae muscle is along the side of the neck (Fig. 8.18).

As therefore the distribution of pain either from TrPs in muscles or from an adjacent damaged facet joint may be similar, the correct procedure is firstly to deactivate any MTrPs that

may be present. If this relieves the pain then clearly nothing further needs to be done. If, however, this is not so and particularly if the pain is reproduced by moving a facet joint, the possibility that it may be arising from that joint has to be taken into consideration and a diagnostic block of the nerves supplying it should be carried out (Bogduk & Marsland 1988).

Barnsley et al (1995) were the first to carry out a double-blind trial to study the reliability of diagnosing whiplash-injury-induced facet joint pain on clinical grounds alone. Fifty consecutive patients with whiplash-injury-induced chronic neck pain suspected clinically to be emanating from a facet joint, were entered into the trial. Twelve patients for a variety of reasons did not complete the study. Each of the remaining 8 cases received two nerve blocks of a possible painful facet joint. The first with short-acting lignocaine (Lidocaine) (2%) and the second with longer-acting bupivacaine (0.5%). Of the 38 patients who completed the investigation 27 (54%) met predetermined criteria for certain facet joint pain, i.e. they obtained complete relief with each of the two anaesthetic agents and it was longer-lasting with bupivacaine.

Headaches

Headache is a frequent complaint following a whiplash injury (Maimaris et al 1988). Possible causes for this immediately following such an injury include haemorrhage into the brain and concussion.

At a later stage persistent headache mainly occurs as a result of it being referred from TrPs either in the posterior cervical muscles (p. 124), in the upper part of the trapezius muscle (p. 127), or in the sternocleidomastoid muscle (p. 128).

Headache may also arise as a result of it being referred from a damaged C2–C3 facet joint.

Cognitive impairment

Psychometric assessment of patients with whiplash injuries have provided objective evidence of various cognitive disorders such as impaired attention, concentration and memory (Kischka et al 1991, Radanov et al 1991).

It seems unlikely that brain damage makes any appreciable contribution to these disorders for although an electroencephalographic study carried out many years ago by Torres & Shapiro (1961) in a group of patients with whiplash injuries and a control group showed abnormalities in 40–50% of the patients and in 1% of the control group, a more recent study has demonstrated no more than minimal changes in a minority of whiplash injury victims (Jacome 1987). Moreover, studies using computed tomographic (CT) scans and MRI in such patients have only shown non-specific abnormalities in a very small number of them (Ettlin et al 1992, Yarnell & Rossie 1988).

Other more probable reasons for cognitive disorders arising include the distracting influence of persistent intense neck and head pain, the anxiety and depression which develops as a result of such pain and the effects of drugs employed to combat these symptoms (Merskey 1993, Radanov et al 1992, Shapiro et al 1993).

Visual defects

Whiplash injuries frequently lead to the development of visual defects. A carefully conducted controlled study by Hildingsson et al (1989) showed objective evidence of oculomotor dysfunction in patients with long-standing cervical spine injuries. The reason for this is not clear but it may possibly have been due to damage to the midbrain occurring as a result of this structure becoming impacted against Blumenbach's clivus – the bony surface which slopes down from the pituitary fossa.

In addition, blurring of vision and difficulty in focusing sometimes develops. The reason for this too is not known for certain but it may be due to accommodation difficulties brought about by increased sympathetic efferent activity (Barnsley et al 1994a).

Spatial disorientation

The spatial disorientation that is liable to arise as a result of a whiplash injury may take the form of a true vertigo with rotation either of the person concerned or his or her surroundings together with spontaneous or latent nystagmus and abnormal vestibular tests (Toglia 1976). Alternatively, it may take the form of dizziness and light-headedness that causes a sudden loss of balance and a tendency to veer to one side when walking.

The two main causes of the development of this spatial disorientation are vertebrobasilar artery insufficiency and disordered proprioception in the neck.

Vertebrobasilar artery insufficiency is liable to develop either as a result of trauma-induced thrombosis of a vertebral artery (Carpenter 1961, Schneider & Schemm 1961) or because of the vertebral artery becoming compressed against the transverse process of the seventh cervical vertebra by a contracted deep cervical fascia (Compere 1968).

Spatial disorientation occurring as a result of disordered proprioception in the neck has been extensively investigated by Cohen (1959, 1961) in experiments carried out on monkeys. From these he was able to show that although information concerning the position of the head is provided by the labyrinths, information concerning the position of the head in relationship to the body comes from a proprioceptive mechanism in the neck so that unsteadiness and loss of balance may be produced by cutting the sensory anterior primary rami of the second and third cervical nerves.

In view of Cohen's observation just described it is interesting to note that in humans the sternocleidomastoid muscle is supplied by branches from the anterior primary rami of the second and third cervical nerves. And that following a whiplash injury, it is not uncommon for unsteadiness and loss of balance with a tendency to veer to one side on walking to come on, when movements of the body or head cause a change in tension to take place in the clavicular part of a sternocleidomastoid muscle that has become shortened as a result of trauma-induced MTrP activity in it (Travell 1967, Weeks & Travell 1955).

Such symptoms are all too frequently allowed to persist for an unnecessarily long period of time because of it erroneously being assumed that their development is due to a neurosis brought on by the shock of the accident. However, they disappear relatively quickly once the MTrPs have been deactivated about two to three times at weekly intervals.

Emotional disturbances

Anxiety and depression

Most people who suffer from a whiplash injury recover from it within 3–6 months. In a small number of cases, however, the pain persists with the development of what has become known as the late whiplash syndrome. The development of this syndrome has traditionally been attributed to neuroticism and a subconscious or even conscious desire for compensation (Balla 1980, Farbman 1973, Gay & Abbott 1953, Pearce 1989). However, it is becoming increasingly well recognised that emotional instability is not the cause of the pain persisting but, conversely it is severe unremitting pain that causes anxiety and depression to develop (Merskey 1993). And furthermore it is the job insecurity, marital disharmony and social disruption brought about by the persistent pain that makes these emotional disorders worse. This notwithstanding it has to be admitted that the pain is liable to be made worse by any

anxiety-arousing experience such as the legal proceedings associated with a compensation claim.

Phobias and the post-traumatic stress disorder

It has been estimated that as many as 70% of people who suffer from a whiplash injury as a result of a motor vehicle accident develop trauma-induced phobias. A common one is for such a person to have a feeling of insecurity when travelling in a vehicle and to become particularly apprehensive when for some reason it suddenly has to be brought to a halt.

An even more disabling condition is the post-traumatic stress disorder. With this there is a feeling of acute anxiety in returning to the site of the accident; also, the person concerned has vivid dreams about it at night and disturbing memories about it during the day. People most likely to experience this would seem to be those who feel victimised by the pain and disability and resentful towards the driver responsible for the accident. And in particular, those who in addition to this, have cause to be aggrieved when relatives, doctors or lawyers unjustly attribute the persistence of pain to psychological problems or even frank malingering (Shapiro & Roth 1993).

Erroneously diagnosed conversion hysteria

As already discussed in Chapter 2, regional pain arising as a result of trauma-induced MTrP nociceptor activity does not follow a strictly dermatomal pattern or nerve root distribution. Clinicians who are neither aware of this nor familiar with the specific patterns of regional pain referral from TrPs in individual muscles of the body tend not to recognise that the MTrP pain which occurs as a result of a whiplash injury is of organic origin and instead mistakenly consider it to be a manifestation of a conversion hysteria (Walters 1961, Weintraub 1988). As Merskey (1988) has correctly and categorically stated, 'regional pain is rarely hysterical'.

Blurring of vision and dizziness are two other complaints that are liable to be assumed to be hysterical despite both of them usually having a physical cause (see p. 139).

Late whiplash syndrome

From various prospective follow-up studies (Miles et al 1988, Norris & Watt 1983, Pennie & Agambar 1990) and retrospective ones (Deans et al 1987, Gargan & Bannister 1990, Maimaris et al 1988, Watkinson et al 1991) it has been deduced that between 14 and 42% of patients with whiplash injuries develop chronic pain and that approximately 10% of these have constant severe pain indefinitely (Barnsley et al 1994a).

In general terms therefore approximately 75% of patients with whiplash injuries recover within 3–6 months and about 25% develop what is known as the late whiplash syndrome – a condition in which symptoms persist for more than 6 months.

As stated previously, present evidence is against attributing the persistence of symptoms following a whiplash injury to either neuroticism or compensation-seeking avarice.

Factors which Radanov et al (1991), in a study primarily concerned with psychosocial influences, have identified as being predictive of symptoms lasting for more than 6 months include: severe initial neck pain; cognitive disturbances such as impaired attention, concentration and memory; and increasing age.

With respect to the pain it should be noted that the timing of its onset and its severity are related to the intensity of the trauma causing the injury. With mild to moderate amounts of injury the pain is delayed for 24–48 hours and when it eventually does come on it is usually no more than a widespread persistent dull ache. It is only when the trauma is considerable that the pain is both severe and present from the beginning.

Cognitive disturbances too relate to the severity of the pain because, as previously discussed, reasons for them developing include the distracting influence of severe pain, the anxiety it causes, and the effects of drugs used to combat it.

The presence of cervical spondylosis has also been said to be indicative of a poor prognosis (Maimaris et al 1988, Miles et al 1988, Norris & Watt 1983, Watkinson et al 1991). However, radiographically demonstrable cervical spondylosis is known to become commoner and more extensive with advancing years (see p. 145) so this finding may simply confirm Radanov et al's (1991) observation that the prognosis for whiplash injury is age related.

It would certainly seem from all this that one of the main reasons for the persistence of symptoms is severe trauma but this cannot be the only one for not infrequently the late whiplash syndrome develops in those who have been subjected to no more than mild or moderate injury. Some other possible reasons for its development therefore have to be considered. These include undiagnosed and therefore untreated MTrP nociceptor activity, facet joint injury and intervertebral disc damage; and also, the neuroplastic changes in dorsal horn transmission neurons that develop as a result of the sensory afferent barrage produced by persistently activated and sensitised nociceptors in these structures (see Chs 2 and 4). So far as MTrP pain in particular is concerned, other possible factors are the self-perpetuating pain-producing circuits which are believed to develop as a result of biochemical changes taking place locally at MTrP sites and as a result of the setting up of motor and sympathetic efferent activity (see Ch. 4).

Post-whiplash injury fibromyalgia

That the fibromyalgia syndrome (FS) may develop as a late complication of a whiplash injury is shown by the results of a survey carried out by Buskila et al (1997).

In this study there was a group of 102 patients with neck injury trauma and of these 90% had been subjected to a classic whiplash type of injury with sudden hyperflexion followed by hypertension of the neck in a rear impact-type vehicle collision. In addition there was a control group made up of 59 patients with leg fractures.

Clinical examination showed that the American College of Rheumatology criteria for the diagnosis of FS (Wolfe et al 1990) were present in 21.6% of the 102 patients with neck injuries and that this syndrome had developed on average 3.2 months after the trauma. In the control group only 1.7% were found to have developed FS.

From these results Buskila et al (1997) concluded that FS develops 13 times more frequently following trauma to the neck than it does following a lower extremity injury.

Whiplash compensation claims

There is a widespread feeling among many doctors and lawyers that a whiplash injury is no more than a muscle sprain from which the patient should recover in a relatively short period and that any persistence of pain and disability long after the injury is caused by neuroticism and/or a subconscious or even conscious desire to obtain financial compensation.

As stated in Chapter 3, Miller (1961, 1966) did much to encourage this concept by what he had to say concerning accident compensation claimants in a series of lectures delivered in the early 1960s. Regrettably his belief that the prolongation of symptoms by accident victims is fostered by the quest for compensation and that symptoms quickly resolve once this has been achieved was based on findings obtained from a follow-up of a small subset of 50 head injury patients especially selected because of their 'gross neurotic symptoms' from a total of 4000 patients. As Barnsley et al (1994a) in their comprehensive review of whiplash injury have commented, it is impossible to draw any valid conclusions from such biased sampling. Nevertheless, it was because Miller was a leading British neurologist that his opinion has done so much over the years to cause doctors and lawyers to adopt a hostile attitude towards accident compensation seekers. And it is whiplash injury claimants who are amongst those who suffer most from this.

During the 1970s and 1980s the view that symptoms which persist following whiplash injuries tend to be exaggerated and clear up once compensation has been awarded was repeatedly reiterated (Balla 1980, Gorman 1974, Hodge 1971, Mills & Horne 1986, Pearce 1989). Pearce even went so far as to say that most victims of whiplash injury have 'sustained no more than a minor sprain to the soft tissues and unusu-

ally severe or protracted complaints may demand explanations which lie outside the fields of organic and psychiatric illness'.

The climate of opinion, however, is now gradually changing, particularly since three large well-conducted prospective studies (Maimaris et al 1988, Norris & Watt 1983, Pennie & Agambar 1990) have shown that there are many reasons for symptoms persisting following whiplash injuries and that the desire for compensation is not one of them. It is evident from these studies that although admittedly some patients improve or recover once compensation has been paid, an equal number do not, so that there is no direct relationship between financial settlement and the length of time for which symptoms persist.

A similar conclusion was reached by Mendelson (1992) after studying the fate of a large number of people seeking compensation for a variety of different injuries in Australia. With respect to whiplash injuries in particular, Mendelson followed up 42 patients with car-accident-induced cervical sprains and found that of these 25 (60%) had resumed work before compensation had been awarded and that of the remaining 17 only 2 were able to return to work following settlement of their claims. A finding which together with similar ones from other types of accidents led him pithily to state that 'compensation claimants are not cured by a verdict' (Mendelson 1982).

Admittedly the possibility of secondary gain, exaggeration and malingering have to be taken into account when assessing any claimant for as Newman (1990) has said, 'conscious or unconscious fabrication of symptoms undoubtedly occurs ... but experience shows that it is usually the persistence of symptoms that leads a patient to litigation and not vice versa. After settlement of a claim many patients remain symptomatic and the chronic pain syndrome is seen in patients not involved in litigation'.

The balance of evidence therefore is that patients with whiplash injuries who exaggerate their symptoms or resort to malingering are only a small minority (Barnsley et al 1994a, Evans 1992).

The effects of litigation on recovery from whiplash injuries

There is no doubt that the adversarial nature of the litigation process in many countries has a profoundly harmful effect on whiplash injury victims with, in particular, a significant increase in the intensity of pain.

Support for this view is provided by the results of a study that was carried out by Teasell et al (1993). In that study 62 patients with whiplash injuries were divided into two groups. One group included 41 patients involved in ongoing litigation and the other was made up of 21 patients who had obtained compensation. From a comparison of these two groups it was evident that the group currently engaged in the litigation process had more intensive and widespread pain, more marked impairment of movements and a significantly greater intake of analgesics.

One of the main reasons for this increase in the intensity of the pain during the course of litigation is the emotional turmoil this protracted process engenders (Farbman 1973). The hostility shown towards litigants by doctors and lawyers acting for insurance companies and the scepticism shown by these professionals as to the veracity of their claims are two other important contributory factors (see Ch. 3).

Management of whiplash injuries

Orthopaedic collar support versus mobilisation

There is considerable controversy as to whether immediately following a whiplash injury the neck should either be supported by a collar or mobilised.

It is traditional to place the neck in a collar but Mealy et al (1986), in a study of 61 patients followed up for 8 weeks, compared the effect of early mobilisation of the neck employing Maitland-type exercises with that of keeping the neck in a collar for 2 weeks and then giving graduated exercises. They found that the group treated by early mobilisation did better with a significantly greater reduction in pain and stiffness.

Pennie & Agambar (1990) in a study of 135 patients seen over a 20-week period at two accident units came to a different conclusion. In their study the patients were divided into two groups. One group (74 patients) had their necks immobilised in a collar for the first 2 weeks and following this were taught a programme of active exercises. A second group (61 patients) were given intermittent neck traction (5.4 kg applied for 30 seconds with 30-second rest periods for 10 minutes) twice a week. In addition to this, they were encouraged to perform simple neck and shoulder exercises in their homes. The results with these two types of treatment were similar but as traction in a physiotherapy department is more expensive they decided to recommend the use of a collar. Furthermore, they found that an individually moulded thermoplastic polyethylene foam type of collar which keeps the neck slightly flexed gives more pain relief than the standard type which tends to splint the neck in slight extension.

The use of an orthopaedic collar continues to be popular but, as stated, when discussing the management of the primary cervical MTrP pain syndrome, it should never be worn continuously for more than 2 weeks. The patient should then be gradually weaned off it over the following week and during that time a neck exercise programme should be instituted (Teasell et al 1993).

Neck muscle stretching exercises

Exercises designed to strengthen the muscles of the neck should be avoided as they cause already damaged muscles to become overloaded and as a consequence are liable to increase the pain. Exercises to stretch muscles that have become shortened as a result of MTrP activity have, however, much to recommend them as, by assisting with the MTrP nociceptor deactivating process, they help to alleviate the pain. Initially they should be carried out under the supervision of a physiotherapist and then patients should continue with them on a regular daily basis on their own.

Traction

Mechanically applied traction has for long been employed (MacNab 1964, 1971). Newman (1990), however, considers its use to be illogical. Teasell et al (1993) have found that because it is liable to damage the tissues, it often makes the pain worse and that it is no substitute for muscle stretching exercises.

Manipulation

As previously stated when considering the use of manipulation in the treatment of the primary cervical MTrP pain syndrome (p. 132), a recent whiplash injury to the neck is a contraindication to its employment (Wells 1994).

Heat and cold

Heat provided by ultrasound or interferential stimulation is often employed but it cannot be expected to give more than some non-specific short-term pain relief.

The application of ice packs may also afford some temporary comfort.

Analgesics

The administration of an analgesic during the first few weeks following a whiplash injury is essential.

There is little to be gained from the use of a non-steroidal anti-inflammatory drug as any effect it may have on pain of this type is likely to be due more to its non-specific analgesic action than to any specific anti-inflammatory properties it may possess.

It is therefore better to prescribe non-narcotic analgesics (e.g. aspirin and paracetamol) and low-efficacy narcotics (e.g. codeine, dihydrocodeine and dextropropoxyphene) either individually or in various combinations. During the first few days the administration of a high-efficacy opioid such as morphine may prove necessary should the pain be particularly severe. And at a later stage the pain-relieving effect of the tricyclic antidepressant amitryptyline in a dose of 10–30 mg nocte may be of value.

Cervical epidural steroid injection

In experienced hands this is a safe procedure (Cicala et al 1989). Nevertheless, although commonly carried out its benefit is questionable because the soft tissues which are damaged in this type of injury lie outside the epidural space (Teasell et al 1993).

Deactivation of MTrPs

As invariably with a whiplash injury the muscles of the neck are sprained, with as a consequence, the development of activity in MTrPs, clearly their deactivation by one or other method is essential.

The only controlled trials that have been carried out are those by Byrn and his colleagues in Scandinavia. In their first one they showed that it is possible to relieve the myofascial pain of a whiplash injury by injecting water into the skin overlying MTrPs (Byrn et al 1991). As an injection of this type is extremely painful they next decided to compare the relative effectiveness of subcutaneous injections of water and subcutaneous injections of saline at MTrP sites. This showed that although water injected under the subcutaneous tissues gives rise to a brief but intense burning sensation its MTrP pain-relieving effect is significantly better than that of saline (Byrn et al 1993).

This notwithstanding there remains an urgent need for controlled blinded trials to evaluate objectively the comparative safety, simplicity, patient acceptability and the pain-relieving efficacy of all the currently available procedures discussed in Chapter 7. In the meantime, for reasons stated both in this chapter and elsewhere, superficial dry needling at MTrP sites remains my personal choice for the alleviation of myofascial pain in patients with whiplash injuries.

Deactivation of all the MTrPs present should be carried out as soon as possible and repeated every 3 days for the first 2–3 weeks. Following this it should be done once a week for a few weeks and then at increasingly long intervals. Eventually the pain may disappear altogether but in some cases this is not so and treatment has to be repeated every 4–6 weeks on a long-term basis. This is the usual outcome when for one reason or another MTrP pain is allowed to persist for some time before MTrP deactivation is commenced. In fairness, however, it has to be said that it may also happen despite this being started at an early stage. Clinical trials are therefore required to show whether MTrP deactivation is simply a palliative procedure or one which if started early enough is capable of significantly influencing the natural history of the pain and preventing it from becoming chronic.

Treatment of facet joint pain

Whenever pain is thought to have arisen as a result of a damaged facet joint a local anaesthetic block of the nerves supplying it should be carried out (Barnsley et al 1995, Bogduk & Marsland 1988). Such a procedure requires both skill and the availability of radiographic facilities. The best means of providing long-term relief from the pain has, however, still to be decided. There have been some encouraging reports of the use of intra-articular corticosteroids (Hove & Gyldensted 1990, Roy et al 1988). A recent study, however, has disputed the efficacy of this form of treatment (Barnsley et al 1994b).

Percutaneous radiofrequency facet joint denervation also has its advocates (Hildebrandt & Argyrakis 1986, Schaerer 1988) but as yet this method of treatment has not been subjected to a clinical trial.

Treatment of disc prolapse

Whenever following a whiplash injury pain in the neck and arm is accompanied by physical signs of nerve root entrapment, and magnetic resonance imaging confirms the presence of a prolapsed disc at the same segmental level, then clearly if the pain does not resolve with conservative methods a laminectomy may prove necessary.

CERVICAL SPONDYLOSIS

Because of widespread confusion concerning the part played by cervical spondylosis in the production of persistent neck pain, the pathology

and clinical manifestations of this disorder will be discussed in some detail.

Spondylosis, a disorder which is liable to affect the cervical and lumbar regions of the spine, is one in which degenerative changes take place in the intervertebral discs and facet joints.

Vernon-Roberts & Pirie (1977), from a dissection of over 100 lumbar spines, showed that degenerative changes firstly take place in the discs and at a later stage in the facet joints.

Confirmation of this sequence of events has recently been provided by Butler et al (1990) who, from a study in which they employed MRI to detect lumbar intervertebral disc degeneration and CT to detect lumbar facet joint arthritis, showed that disc degeneration is frequently present on its own but facet joint arthritis only develops once disc degeneration has taken place.

There is every reason to believe that this also applies to cervical discs for the degenerative changes cause them to lose height (Uttley & Monroe 1989), and when this happens an abnormal load is placed on the nearby facet joints so that degenerative changes then start to take place in them also (Dunlop et al 1984).

Cervical discs gradually undergo this degenerative process as part of normal ageing but the speed with which this happens is liable to be accelerated should the spine be subjected to injury (Irvine et al 1965).

The degenerative process in the discs leads to the formation of osteophytes on their anterolateral and posterior borders. Osteophytes also develop on the anterior and posterior aspects of degenerative facet joints. However, with both the discs and facet joints it is only the posteriorly situated osteophytes that are of any clinical significance for it is these together with hypertrophied ligaments that are responsible for compressing nerve roots.

Asymptomatic spondylosis

The incidence of cervical spondylosis increases with advancing years so that whereas between the ages of 20 and 29 only 13% of men and 5% of women have the characteristic appearances of it on plain X-rays of the neck, from the age of 70 upwards, 100% of men and 96% of women have radiographic evidence of it (Irvine et al 1965).

However, although the radiographic appearances tend to become more marked with increasing age there is no correlation between this and the development of pain for it is not uncommon to find advanced degenerative changes in neck X-rays of asymptomatic elderly people (Friedenberg & Miller 1963, Heller et al 1983, Pallis et al 1954).

Heller et al (1983) compared the neck radiographs of a group of patients over the age of 60 who had been specifically referred to their department of radiology during the course of one particular year for X-ray examination of the neck with those of a group of patients, also over the age of 60, who had been referred during the same year, for barium studies of the gastrointestinal tract. This survey not only showed that the incidence of cervical spondylosis in the two groups was similar but also that there was no consistent relationship between symptoms and the changes observed radiographically.

It therefore follows that finding evidence of cervical spondylosis on the radiographs of a patient suffering from pain in the neck and arm does not necessarily imply that the pain is due to that disorder. Frequently examination of the neck of such a person reveals the presence of MTrPs and should the pain disappear once these have been deactivated it is reasonable to conclude that the abnormal radiographic appearances were no more than a chance investigatory finding of no clinical significance.

Spondylotic nerve root entrapment

Pain in the neck and arm can only safely be attributed to cervical spondylosis when, in addition to the characteristic radiographic appearances of this degenerative process, there are objective neurological signs of nerve root entrapment such as, for example, muscle wasting, sensory loss and depression of a tendon jerk. Usually in such cases lateral radiographs show the presence of posteriorly situated osteophytes. This nerve root entrapment is due to degenerative disc material, osteophytes and hypertrophied ligaments narrowing the intervertebral foramina through which the spinal roots pass. The sudden involvement of one spinal nerve root may lead to symptoms and signs resembling those of an acute disc prolapse (see p. 147) but it is commoner for more than one root to be involved. Usually it is the sixth and seventh cervical ones that are affected.

Compression of the sixth root causes pain to be referred to the shoulder and upper arm. In addition, it may give rise to tingling and numbness in the index finger and thumb. The biceps and brachioradialis tendon reflexes are depressed. Weakness and wasting of these muscles may also be observed.

Compression of the seventh root causes pain to be referred down the arm and forearm, and also sometimes around the chest wall. Paraesthesiae may be experienced in the middle finger. The triceps reflex is depressed and in severe cases weakness of this muscle is observed.

Clinical examination may also reveal some sensory loss with diminished appreciation of light touch, tactile discrimination and pin prick. The distribution of these sensory changes is dependent on which nerve root or roots are involved.

As pointed out by Hopkins (1993), it is not known why pain suddenly arises from a root or roots that must undoubtedly have been compressed by osteophytes for some considerable time or why, eventually, as is usually the case, it spontaneously disappears. One possible explanation is that trauma to the nerve leads to the development of inflammatory oedema of the tissues around the root or roots and that, over the course of time this gradually subsides.

Superimposed myofascial trigger point pain

When a cervical nerve root becomes entrapped, whether this be due to spondylosis, disc prolapse (p. 147) or some other cause, there may be not only nociceptive nerve pain (syn: nerve trunk pain; see Ch. 5) but in some cases superimposed MTrP pain due to the development of TrP activity in muscles supplied by the damaged nerve root.

Electromyographic studies carried out by Chu (1995) on patients with lumbar radiculopathy provide grounds for believing that a likely reason for this MTrP pain developing is the effect motor nerve compression has on motor endplates at MTrP sites (see Ch. 4).

Treatment

It might be thought that when nerve root entrapment occurs as a result of cervical spondylosis, surgical decompression of the root in its exit canal would need to be carried out as soon as possible. This, however, is not so because, as already stated, the pain usually spontaneously disappears after a few months and it is only in the exceptional case that persisting pain and weakness necessitates surgical intervention.

As initially cervical spondylotic nerve root entrapment pain is very severe the use of analgesics on a regular basis is essential.

It is also customary to attempt to restrict the movements of the neck by the wearing of an orthopaedic collar. The value of this, however, is doubtful for trials have shown that the effect of a collar on neck movements is minimal (Colachis et al 1973) and that any pain relief it may afford is no more than a placebo effect (British Association of Physical Medicine 1966). Moreover, as Huston (1988) has pointed out, its potential disadvantages still need to be further studied. Despite all this most patients appear to derive some comfort from wearing a collar but for reasons already discussed it should not be worn on a continuous basis for more than 2 weeks.

Various forms of heat treatment such as short wave diathermy and ultrasound are commonly employed but their pain-relieving effect is very limited (Koes et al 1992). Manipulation has its advocates but in an elderly person is not without its risks.

Manual traction applied by a physiotherapist may sometimes alleviate the pain for a short time but gives no lasting relief (Steinberg & Mason 1959).

When active MTrPs are found to be present their deactivation at regular intervals helps to decrease the intensity of the pain.

Chu (1997) has shown that deep needling of the MTrPs with the evocation of twitch responses, a technique called by her twitch-obtaining intramuscular stimulation (see Ch. 7), effectively alleviates MTrP pain that arises secondary to the development of a cervical radiculopathy.

CERVICAL DISC PROLAPSE

A patient with prolapse of a cervical intervertebral disc often has recurrent brief attacks of pain in the neck before it eventually becomes suddenly much more severe and radiates down the arm. The movements of the neck on the affected side then become markedly limited, partly because of the pain but also because of considerable muscle spasm. The pain and muscle spasm is due to entrapment of a nerve root, usually the seventh with, as a consequence, weakness of the triceps muscle and loss of the triceps jerk, and the development of slight sensory changes and paraesthesiae in one or more fingers (Matthews 1975). In addition, TrP nociceptors in the neck muscles are liable to become activated with, as a result, the development of MTrP pain.

Investigations

Plain X-rays of the cervical spine show no abnormality. Myelography was for long one of the best means of visualising disc prolapse-induced nerve root entrapment but in recent years MRI has become increasingly more widely used for this purpose.

It has to be remembered, however, that not uncommonly bulging of a disc may be apparent on an MRI of an otherwise fit person and that such a finding therefore is only of significance when, in addition to this, there are symptoms and physical signs of nerve root entrapment at the same segmental level.

Treatment

The pain is usually so severe that initially bed rest and the prescribing of analgesics are essential. Immobilisation of the neck with sand bags or a collar and the application of intermittent neck traction during the initial stage may afford some symptomatic relief.

The deactivation of secondarily activated MTrPs provides a certain amount of pain relief but as this is liable to be short lasting it needs to be repeated at regular intervals.

The use of one or other form of heat or altern-

atively the application of ice packs helps to reduce the muscle spasm.

An episode of disc prolapse is usually self-limiting with a significant reduction in the severity of the pain after 2–3 weeks and its disappearance after about 6–8 weeks. Occasionally, however, either because of the persistence of pain or because of its recurrence surgical removal of the herniated disc becomes necessary.

REFERENCES

Aprill C, Bogduk N 1992 The prevalence of cervical zygapophysial joint pain: a first approximation. Spine 17:744–747

Aprill C, Dwyer A, Bogduk N 1990 Cervical zygapophysial joint pain patterns II. A clinical evaluation. Spine 15:458–461

Baldry P E 2000 Superficial dry needling. In: Chaitow L (ed) Fibromyalgia syndrome: a practitioner's guide to treatment. Churchill Livingstone, Edinburgh, pp 77–90

Balla J I 1980 The late whiplash syndrome. Australian and New Zealand Journal of Surgery 50:610–614

Barnsley L, Lord S M, Bogduk N 1994a Whiplash injury. Pain 58:283–307

Barnsley L, Lord S M, Wallis B J, Bogduk N 1994b Level of effect of intra-articular corticosteroids for chronic pain in the cervical zygapophysial joints. New England Journal of Medicine 330:1047–1050

Barnsley L, Lord S M, Wallis B J, Bogduk N 1995 The prevalence of chronic cervical zygapophysial joint pain after whiplash. Spine 20(1):20–26

Bogduk N, Aprill C 1993 On the nature of neck pain, discography and cervical zygapophysial joint blocks. Pain 54:213–217

Bogduk N, Marsland A 1988 The cervical zygapophysial joints as a source of neck pain. Spine 13:610–617

Bogduk N, Simons D G 1993 Neck pain: joint pain or trigger points? In: Voeroy H, Merskey H (eds) Progress in fibromyalgia and myofascial pain. Elsevier, Amsterdam, pp 267–273

British Association of Physical Medicine (1966) Pain in the neck and arm. A multicentre trial of the effects of physiotherapy. British Medical Journal i:253–258

Buonocore E, Hartman J T, Nelso C L 1966 Cineradiograms of cervical spine in diagnosis of soft-tissue injuries. Journal of American Medical Association 198:143–147

Buskila D, Neumann L, Vaisberg G, Alkalay D, Wolfe F 1997 Increased rates of fibromyalgia following cervical spine injury. A controlled study of 161 cases of traumatic injury. Arthritis and Rheumatism 40(3):446–452

Butler D, Trafimow J H, Andersson J, McNeill T W, Huckman M S 1990 Discs degenerate before facets. Spine 15(2):111–113

Byrn C, Borenstein P, Linder L E 1991 Treatment of neck and shoulder pain in whiplash syndrome patients with intracutaneous sterile water injections. Acta Anaesthesiologica Scandinavica 35:52–53

Byrn C, Olsson I, Falkheden L et al 1993 Subcutaneous sterile water injections for chronic neck and shoulder pain following whiplash injuries. Lancet 341:449–452

Caldwell J W, Crane C R, Krusen U L 1971 Nerve conduction studies: an aid in the diagnosis of thoracic outlet syndrome. Southern Medical Journal 64:210–212

Capistrant T D 1977 Thoracic outlet syndrome in whiplash injury. Annals of Surgery 185:175–178

Carpenter S 1961 Injury of neck as cause of vertebral artery thrombosis. Journal of Neurosurgery 18:849–853

Chu J 1995 Dry needling (intramuscular stimulation) in myofascial pain related to lumbosacral radiculopathy. European Journal of Physical Medicine and Rehabilitation 5(4):106–121

Chu J 1997 Twitch-obtaining intramuscular stimulation (TOIMS): effectiveness for long-term treatment of myofascial pain related to cervical radiculopathy. Archives of Physical Medicine and Rehabilitation 78:1042

Cicala R S, Westbrook L, Angel J J 1989 Side effects and complications of cervical epidural steroid injections. Journal of Pain Symptom Management 4:64–66

Clark C R, Ingram C M, el Khoury G Y, Ehara S 1988 Radiographic evaluation of cervical spine injuries. Spine 13:742–747

Cohen L A 1959 Body orientation and motor co-ordination in animals with impaired neck sensation. Federation Proceedings 18:26

Cohen L A 1961 Role of neck and eye proprioceptive mechanisms in body orientation and motor co-ordination. Journal of Neurophysiology 24:1–11

Colachis S C, Strohm B R, Ganter E L 1973 Cervical spine motion in normal women. Radiographic study of the effect of cervical collars. Archives of Physical Medicine and Rehabilitation 54:161–169

Compere W E 1968 Electronystagmographic findings in patients with whiplash injuries. Laryngoscope 78:1226–1233

Crowe H 1964 A new diagnostic sign in neck injuries. Californian Medicine 100:12–13

Davis A G 1945 Injuries of the cervical spine. Journal of the American Medical Association 127:149–156

Davis S J, Teresi L M, Bradley W G J, Ziemba M A, Bloze A C 1991 Cervical spine hyperextension injuries. M R findings. Radiology 180:245–251

Deans G T, Magalliard J N, Kerr M, Rutherford W H 1987 Neck pain – a major cause of disability following car accidents. Injury 18:10–12

Dunlop R B, Adams M A, Hutton W C 1984 Disc space narrowing and the lumbar facet joints. Journal of Bone and Joint Surgery 66B:706–710

Dworkin S P, Truelove E L, Bonica J J, Sola A 1990 Facial and head pain caused by myofascial and temporomandibular disorders. In: Bonica J J (ed) The management of pain, 2nd edn. Lea & Febiger, Philadelphia, p 743

Dwyer A, Aprill C, Bogduk N 1990 Cervical zygapophysial pain patterns I: a study in normal volunteers. Spine 15:453–457

Easton J D, Sherman D G 1986 Cervical manipulation and stroke. Stroke 8:594–597

Ettlin T M, Kischka V, Reichman S et al 1992 Cerebral symptoms after whiplash injury of the neck: a prospective clinical and neurophysiological study of whiplash injury. Journal of Neurology, Neurosurgery and Psychiatry 55:943–948

Evans R W 1992 Some observations on whiplash injuries. Neurologic Clinics 10(4):975–997

Farbman A A 1973 Neck sprain: associated factors. Journal of the American Medical Association 223:1010–1015

Fast A, Zincola D V, Marin E L 1987 Vertebral artery damage complicating cervical manipulation. Spine 12:840–842

Fricton J R 1993 Myofascial pain and whiplash. Spine: State of the Art Reviews 7:403–422

Fricton J R, Kroening R, Haley D, Siegert R 1985 Myofascial pain syndrome of the head and neck: a review of clinical characteristics of 164 patients. Oral Surgery, Oral Medicine, Oral Pathology 60:615–623

Friedenberg Z B, Miller W T 1963 Degenerative disc disease of the cervical spine. A comparative study of asymptomatic and symptomatic patients. Journal of Bone and Joint Surgery 45A:1171–1178

Gargan M F, Bannister G C 1990 Long term prognosis of soft-tissue injuries of the neck. Journal of Bone and Joint Surgery (Br) 72:901–903

Gay J R, Abbott K H 1953 Common whiplash injuries of the neck. Journal of the American Medical Association 152:1698–1704

Gerwin R 1995 Myofascial back and neck pain. Spine: State of the Art Reviews 9(3):1–15

Gerwin R 1999 Differential diagnosis of myofascial pain syndrome and fibromyalgia. Journal of Musculoskeletal Pain 7(1/2):209–215

Gorman W 1974 The alleged whiplash injury. Arizona Medicine 31:411–413

Grieve G 1986 Modern manual therapy of the vertebral column. Churchill Livingstone, Edinburgh

Grosshandler S L, Stratas N E, Toomey T C, Gray W F 1985 Chronic neck and shoulder pain, focusing on myofascial origins. Postgraduate Medicine 77(3):149–158

Heller C A, Stanley P, Lewis-Jones B, Heller R F 1983 Value of X-ray examinations of the cervical spine. British Medical Journal 287:1276–1278

Hildebrandt J, Argyrakis A 1986 Percutaneous nerve block of the cervical facet – a relatively new method in the treatment of chronic headache and neck pain. Manual Medicine 2:48–52

Hildingsson C, Wenngren B J, Bring G, Toolanen G 1989 Oculomotor problems after cervical spine injury. Acta Orthopaedica Scandinavica 60:513–516

Hodge J R 1971 The whiplash neurosis. Psychosomatics 12:245–249

Hong C-Z, Simons D G 1993 Response to treatment for pectoralis minor myofascial pain syndrome after whiplash. Journal of Musculoskeletal Pain 1(1):89–131

Hopkins A 1993 Clinical neurology. University Press, Oxford, p 336

Hove B, Gyldensted C 1990 Cervical analgesic facet joint arthrography. Neuroradiology 32:456–459

Huston G J 1988 Collars and corsets. British Medical Journal 296:276

Irvine D H, Fisher J B, Newell D J et al 1965 Prevalence of cervical spondylosis in a general practice. Lancet i:1089–1092

Jacome D E 1987 EEG in whiplash: a reappraisal. Clinical Electroencephalography 18:41–45

Jeffreys E 1980 Soft tissue injuries of the cervical spine. Disorders of the cervical spine. Butterworth, Oxford, pp 81–89

Jónsson H J R, Bring G, Rauschning W, Sahlstedt B 1991 Hidden cervical spine injuries in traffic accident victims with skull fractures. Journal of Spinal Disorders 4:251–263

Kischka V, Ettlin T, Heim S, Schmid G 1991 Cerebral symptoms following whiplash injury. European Neurology 31:136–140

Kleynhans A M 1980 Complications and contraindications to spinal manipulative therapy. In: Haldeman S (ed) Modern developments in the principles and practice of chiropractice. Appleton-Century-Crofts, Norwalk, CT, pp 359–384

Koes B W, Bouter L M, van Maineren H et al 1992 Randomized clinical trial of manipulative therapy and physiotherapy for persistent back and neck complaints: result of one year follow-up. British Medical Journal 304:601–605

Long C 1956 Myofascial pain syndromes Part 2 – syndromes of the head, neck and shoulder girdle. Henry Ford Hospital Medical Bulletin 4:22–28

MacNab I 1964 Acceleration injuries of the cervical spine. Journal of Bone and Joint Surgery (Am) 46:1797–1799

MacNab I 1971 The whiplash syndrome. Clinical Neurosurgery 20:232–241

Maimaris C, Barnes M R, Allen M J 1988 Whiplash injuries of the neck: a retrospective study. Injury 19:393–396

Matthews W B 1975 Practical neurology, 3rd edn. Blackwell Scientific Publications, Oxford, p 125

Mealy K, Brennan H, Fenelon G E 1986 Early mobilization of acute whiplash injuries. British Medical Journal 292:656–657

Mendelson G 1982 Not 'cured by a verdict': effects of legal settlement on compensation claims. Medical Journal of Australia 2:132–134

Mendelson G 1992 Compensation and chronic pain. Pain 48:121–123

Merskey H 1988 Regional pain is rarely hysterical. Archives of Neurology 45:915–918

Merskey H 1993 Psychological consequences of whiplash. Spine: State of the Art Reviews 7:471–480

Michele A A, Eisenberg J 1968 Scapulocostal syndrome. Archives of Physical Medicine and Rehabilitation 49:383–387

Michele A A, Davies J J, Kreuger F J, Lichtor J M 1950 Scapulocostal syndrome (fatigue-postural paradox). New York State Journal of Medicine 50:1353–1356

Miles K A, Maimaris C, Finlay D et al 1988 The incidence and prognostic significance of radiological abnormalities in soft tissue injuries in the cervical spine. Skeletal Radiology 17:493–496

Miller H 1961 Accident neurosis. British Medical Journal i:919–925

Miller H 1966 Accident neurosis. Proceedings of the Medico-Legal Society, Victoria 10:71–82

Mills H, Horne G 1986 Whiplash – man made disease? New Zealand Medical Journal 99:373–374

Newman P K 1990 Whiplash injury. British Medical Journal 301:395–396

Norris S H, Watt I 1983 The prognosis of neck injuries resulting from rear-end vehicle collisions. Journal of Bone and Joint Surgery (Br) 65:608–611

Ochsner A, Gage M, DeBakey M 1935 Scalenus anticus (Naffziger) syndrome. American Journal of Surgery 28:669–695

Pallis C, Jones A M, Spillane J D 1954 Cervical spondylosis. Incidence and implications. Brain 77:274–289

Pearce J M 1989 Whiplash injury: a reappraisal. Journal of Neurology, Neurosurgery and Psychiatry 52:1329–1331

Pennie B, Agambar L J 1990 Patterns of injury and recovery in whiplash. Injury 22:57–59

Porter K M 1989 Neck sprains after car accidents. British Medical Journal 298:973–974

Radanov B P, Stefano G, Schnidrig A, Ballinari P 1991 Role of psychosocial stress in recovery from common whiplash. Lancet 338:712–715

Radanov B P, Schnidrig A, Stefano G, Sturzenegger M 1992 Illness behaviour after common whiplash. Lancet 339:749–750

Roos D B, Owens J C 1966 Thoracic outlet syndrome. Archives of Surgery 93:71–75

Roy D F, Fleury J, Fontaine S B, Dussault R G 1988 Clinical evaluation of cervical facet joint infiltration. Journal of the Canadian Association of Radiologists 39:118–120

Russek A S 1952 Diagnosis and treatment of scapulocostal syndrome. Journal of the American Medical Association 150:25–27

Schaerer J P 1988 Treatment of prolonged neck pain by radiofrequency facet rhizotomy. Journal of Neurological and Orthopaedic Medicine and Surgery 9:74–76

Schneider R C, Schemm G W 1961 Vertebral artery insufficiency in acute and chronic spinal trauma. Journal of Neurosurgery 18:348–360

Severy D M, Mathewson J H, Bechtol C O 1955 Controlled automobile rear-end collisions, an investigation of related engineering and medical phenomena. Canadian Services Medical Journal 11:727–759

Shapiro A P, Roth R S 1993 The effect of litigation on recovery from whiplash. Spine: State of the Art Reviews 7(3):531–556

Shapiro A P, Teasell R W, Steenhuis R 1993 Mild traumatic brain injury following whiplash. Spine: State of the Art Reviews 7:455–470

Simons D G, Travell J G, Simons L S 1999a–f Travell & Simons myofascial pain and dysfunction. The trigger point manual, 2nd edn. Williams & Wilkins, Baltimore, vol 1, pp 237–277 (a), p 436 (b), p 310 (c), p 514 (d), p 510 (e), p 324 (f)

Sola A E, Kuitert J H 1955 Myofascial trigger point pain in the neck and shoulder girdle. Northwest Medicine 54:980–984

Sola A E, Williams R L 1956 Myofascial pain syndromes. Neurology (Minneapolis) 6:91–95

Steinberg V, Mason R 1959 Cervical spondylosis. Pilot therapeutic trial. Annals of Physical Medicine 5:37

Teasell R W, Shapiro A P, Mailis A 1993 Medical management of whiplash injuries: an overview. Spine: State of the Art Reviews 7(3):481–499

Toglia J U 1976 Acute flexion–extension injury of the neck. Electronystagmographic study of 309 patients. Neurology 26:808–814

Torres F, Shapiro S K 1961 Electroencephalograms in whiplash injury. Archives of Neurology 5:28–35

Travell J 1955 Sternomastoid syndrome of headache and dizziness. New York State Journal of Medicine 55:331–339

Travell J 1960 Temporomandibular joint pain referred from muscles of the head and neck. Journal of Prosthetic Dentistry 10:745–763

Travell J 1967 Mechanical headache. Headache 7:23–29

Urschell H C, Razzuk M A 1972 Management of the thoracic outlet syndrome. New England Journal of Medicine 286(21):1140–1143

Uttley D, Monro P 1989 Neurosurgery for cervical spondylosis. British Journal of Hospital Medicine 42:62–70

Vernon-Roberts B, Pirie C J 1977 Degenerative changes in the intervertebral discs of the lumbar spine and their sequelae. Rheumatology and Rehabilitation 16:13–21

Walters W 1961 Psychogenic regional pain alias hysterical pain. Brain 84:1–18

Watkinson A, Gargan M F, Bannister G E 1991 Prognostic factors in soft tissue injuries of the cervical spine. Injury 22:307–309

Weeks V D, Travell J 1955 Postural vertigo due to trigger areas in the sternocleidomastoid muscle. Journal of Pediatrics 47:315–327

Weinberger L M 1976 Trauma or treatment? The role of intermittent traction in the treatment of cervical soft tissue injuries. Journal of Trauma 15:377–382

Weintraub M I 1988 Regional pain is usually hysterical. Archives of Neurology 45:913–914

Wells P E 1994 Manipulative procedures. In: Wells P E, Frampton V, Bowser D (eds) Pain management by physiotherapy, 2nd edn. Butterworth-Heinemann, Oxford, ch 17

Wolfe F, Smythe H A, Yunus M B, Bennett R M et al 1990 The American College of Rheumatology 1990 Criteria for the Classification of Fibromyalgia: report of the multicenter criteria committee. Arthritis and Rheumatism 33:160–172

Yarnell P R, Rossie G V 1988 Minor whiplash head injury with major debilitation. Brain Injury 2:255–258

9

The shoulder

INTRODUCTION

When investigating the cause of pain in the shoulder region disorders such as rheumatoid arthritis, other inflammatory arthritides, crystal arthropathy and haemarthrosis of the glenohumeral joint, osteoarthritis of the acromioclavicular joint and occasionally of the glenohumeral joint, diseases of the bone, diseases of the lung, and myocardial infarction all have to be included in the differential diagnosis. The possibility that the pain may have been referred to the shoulder from a disorder in the vicinity of the diaphragm stimulating the phrenic nerve also has to be considered.

This chapter, however, will mainly be concerned with the primary referral of pain to the shoulder region from myofascial trigger points (MTrPs) in the neck, shoulder girdle, chest wall and upper arm. The secondary development of MTrP pain in rotator cuff tendinitis and adhesive capsulitis will also be discussed.

PRIMARY REFERRAL OF MTrP PAIN TO THE SHOULDER REGION

That MTrP pain may be referred to the shoulder region when one or more of a number of different muscles in the neck, shoulder girdle, chest wall and upper arm become acutely strained or chronically overloaded is still not well recognised despite attention having first been drawn to it as long ago as the early 1940s by Kelly (1942) whilst he was serving in the Australian Army Medical Corps and by Travell and her co-workers in America (Travell et al 1942). Unfortunately their reports, when first published, seem to have been largely ignored but as in recent years the importance of this particular cause of shoulder pain has once again been stressed (Simons & Travell 1984, Sola 1994), it is to be hoped that it will now begin to receive the attention it merits.

The muscles from which TrP pain may be referred to the shoulder region include the supraspinatus, infraspinatus, teres minor, deltoid, biceps brachii, long head of the triceps (Ch. 10), clavicular section of pectoralis major (Ch. 14), coracobrachialis, latissimus dorsi (Ch. 14), teres major and subscapularis.

Supraspinatus muscle (Fig. 9.1)

Anatomical attachments

This muscle occupies the whole of the supraspinous fossa. From there its fibres pass under the acromion to form a tendon which adheres to the capsule of the shoulder joint before being inserted into the greater tuberosity of the humerus.

Factors responsible for development of trigger point activity

TrP activity may develop in this muscle when it is subjected to strain as, for example, by carrying a heavy load such as a suitcase with the arm hanging by the side, by lifting a heavy object up to, or above, the shoulder level with the arm outstretched, or by the carrying out of any task that requires repeated or prolonged elevation of the arm.

Trigger point examination

When searching for TrPs in this muscle the patient should sit comfortably, or lie with the affected side uppermost. As the TrPs have to be palpated through the trapezius muscle they are often located more readily if the muscle is put on

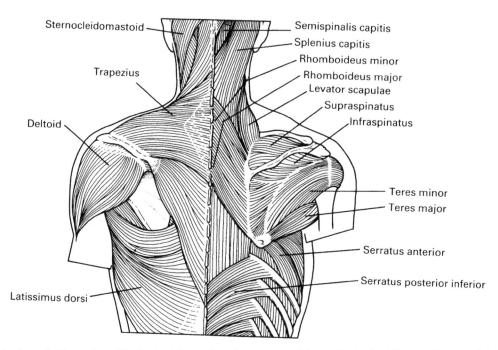

Figure 9.1 Superficial muscles of the back of the neck and upper part of the trunk. On the left, the skin, superficial and deep fasciae have been removed. On the right, the sternocleidomastoid, trapezius, latissimus dorsi and deltoid have been dissected away.

the stretch by placing the forearm of the patient behind the back at waist level.

Trigger point sites

TrP sites are usually located either at the medial or lateral parts of the muscle, or in both places (Fig. 9.2). In addition, a TrP may develop in the tendon of the muscle near to its insertion (Fig. 9.3).

Associated trigger points

TrP activity may develop in the supraspinatus muscle alone, but more often it develops in the infraspinatus at the same time, and also quite often in trapezius, levator scapulae and deltoid muscles.

Specific pattern of pain referral

Pain from TrPs in the belly of this muscle is referred to the region of the deltoid muscle. From there it frequently extends down the arm and forearm and, as stated by Simons et al (1999a), is often felt particularly strongly over the lateral epicondyle (Fig. 9.2).

Pain from TrPs in its tendon is felt locally at that site (Fig. 9.3).

Referred pain from TrPs in this muscle is similar in distribution to that of the pain of a C5–C7 radiculopathy (Reynolds 1981). Unlike with the latter, however, there is no neurological deficit or electromyographic abnormality.

Movements aggravating the pain

Referred pain from this muscle is made worse by abducting the arm, and by passively stretching

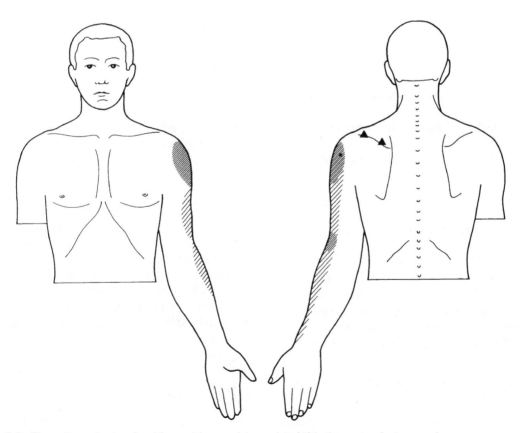

Figure 9.2 The pattern of pain referral from a trigger point or points (▲) in the supraspinatus muscle.

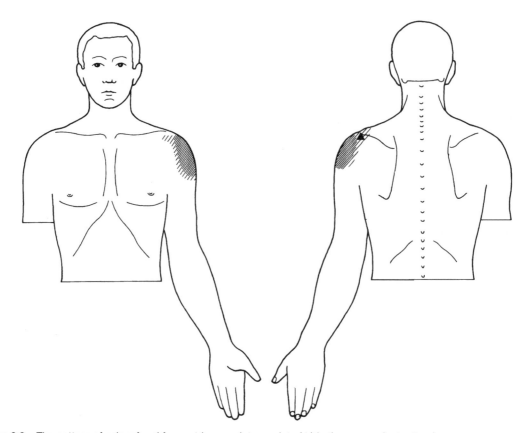

Figure 9.3 The pattern of pain referral from a trigger point or points (▲) in the supraspinatus tendon.

the muscle by adducting the arm behind the back. Some of the commoner types of movements likely to aggravate the pain include reaching upwards either to brush the hair, to shave, or to clean the teeth.

Infraspinatus muscle (Fig. 9.1)

Anatomical attachments

This thick triangular muscle occupies most of the infraspinous fossa. Its fibres converge to form a tendon which, after passing across the posterior part of the capsule of the shoulder joint, is inserted into the greater tuberosity of the humerus.

Factors responsible for development of trigger point activity

This is usually brought about by the muscle being subjected to some sudden strain such as,

for example, when reaching backwards either for support when falling, or to pick up objects from the back of a car when sitting in the front of it.

Trigger point sites

When searching for TrPs the patient should be seated with the muscle put on the stretch by bringing the hand and arm across the front of the chest to grasp the contralateral arm rest of the chair. Flat palpation of the infraspinatus fossa should then be carried out systematically. One or more TrPs are likely to be found somewhere along a line immediately beneath the spine of the scapula.

Specific pattern of pain referral

Referred pain from TrP activity in this muscle is experienced deep inside the front of the shoulder

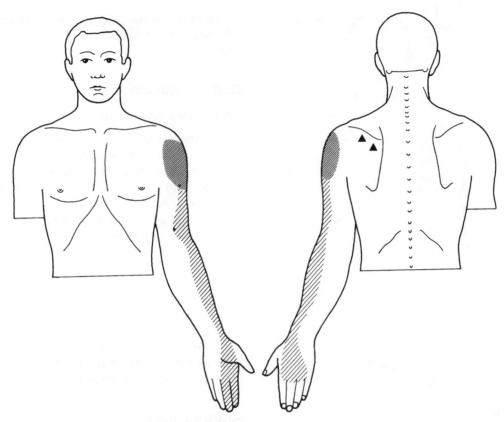

Figure 9.4   The pattern of pain referral from a trigger point or points (▲) in the infraspinatus muscle.

and for this reason is sometimes erroneously thought to be due to an arthritis of the gleno-humeral joint. It may also radiate down the anterolateral aspect of the arm and forearm to the radial aspect of the hand, sometimes reaching the thumb and first two fingers (Fig. 9.4) (Pace 1975, Rubin 1981, Sola & Williams 1956, Travell et al 1942, Travell 1952). This particular type of shoulder pain is particularly disturbing at night because it not only prevents the patient from lying on the affected side but it is also trouble-some when lying on the unaffected side.

Referred pain to the shoulder from TrP activity in the infraspinatus muscle may closely simulate that arising from glenohumeral joint disease. And as it causes pain to radiate down the arm in a similar distribution to that occurring with irri-tation of the 5th, 6th and 7th cervical nerve roots, a full neurological examination is essential and, at times, an EMG may be necessary to distin-guish between them. Confusion is particularly likely to occur in patients who also have neck pain (see Ch. 8).

The particular pattern of pain referral in what Long (1956) called the scapulo-humeral syn-drome is liable to include referral from TrPs in the infraspinatus and also from TrPs in the pec-toralis muscles and the long head of the biceps brachii (Simons et al 1999b).

Characteristic disorder of movements

There is an inability to internally rotate and adduct the arm at the shoulder. As a con-sequence, it is not possible to reach the spine of the contralateral scapula with the finger tips when placing the arm behind the back (Fig. 9.5), a restriction of movement that makes it difficult to do up buttons or manipulate a zip fastener on the back of clothing.

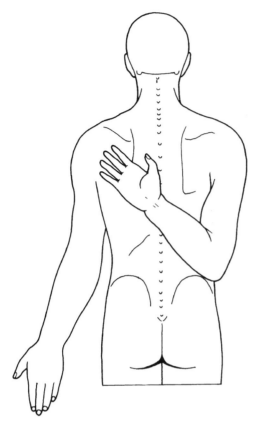

Figure 9.5 To illustrate how a normal person, on placing an arm behind the back, is able to reach the spine of the contralateral scapula with the finger tips. With trigger point activity in either the supraspinatus or infraspinatus or both, this is not possible.

Teres minor (Fig. 9.1)

This muscle with its attachments immediately adjacent to and just below those of the infraspinatus and having actions which are almost identical to the latter, has TrP activation brought about by exactly similar stresses, i.e. stretching and reaching behind the shoulder. However, unlike the infraspinatus, it is one of the less commonly involved muscles. Sola & Kuitert (1955) found only about 7% of their patients with shoulder pain had TrPs in this muscle. Teres minor is rarely involved without simultaneous involvement of the infraspinatus, and usually notice is drawn to it by the patient continuing to complain of the pain in the posterior part of the shoulder, once pain deep in

the front of the shoulder has been satisfactorily alleviated by deactivating TrPs in the infraspinatus.

Deltoid muscle (Fig. 9.1)

Anatomical attachments

The deltoid muscle is so-called because being triangular in shape it resembles the Greek letter Δ (delta). It arises from the lateral one-third of the clavicle, from the acromion and from the spine of the scapula. After covering the shoulder joint its fibres converge to form a thick tendon which is inserted into a tuberosity on the outer side of the shaft of the humerus.

The muscle is made up of three parts – anterior, middle and posterior.

TrP activity may develop either in its anterior part, its posterior part or both together. It often occurs as a secondary event in both the anterior and posterior parts simultaneously, when pain is referred to that area from TrPs in the supraspinatus and infraspinatus muscles.

Anterior part

Factors responsible for development of trigger point activity

Primary TrP activity in the anterior part of this muscle may be brought about by direct trauma to the upper part of the arm such as may occur with a fall, or when it is damaged by the impact of a ball, or the recoil of a gun. Also when it is suddenly overloaded, such as when grasping a rail to break a fall, or is recurrently overloaded such as may occur when some heavy object such as a tool or instrument is repeatedly held at shoulder level.

Trigger point pain referral

The patient complains of pain at rest over the anterior part of the deltoid muscle (Fig. 9.6). It is made worse by movement, and in particular there is difficulty in raising the arm to the horizontal so that drinking becomes troublesome.

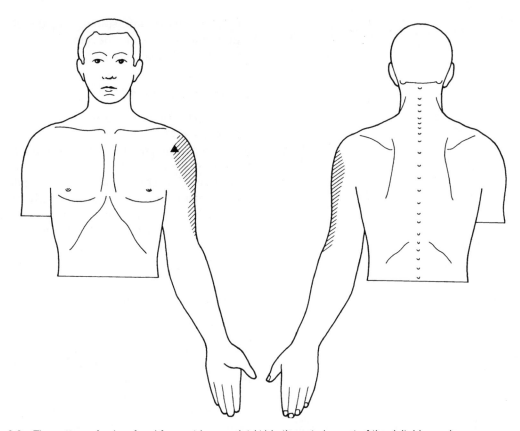

Figure 9.6 The pattern of pain referral from a trigger point (▲) in the anterior part of the deltoid muscle.

It is aggravated by asking the patient to abduct the arm with the elbow straight and the palm to the front. In addition, the patient has difficulty in passing the hand across the small of the back. Normally it is possible to rest the hand on the back of the opposite arm. With anterior deltoid TrP activity, it may only be possible to reach the midline (Fig. 9.7).

Posterior part

Factors responsible for development of trigger point activity

Primary TrP activation may occur as a result of injecting some irritant substance such as an antibiotic, vitamin or vaccine into this part of the muscle, or when it is subjected to excessive strain during sporting activities.

Trigger point pain referral

Pain from TrPs in this part of the muscle is referred to the back of the shoulder (Fig. 9.8). Movement of the shoulder joint makes it worse. In addition, because of the pain external rotation of the joint is limited so that whilst the hand can be brought up to the head it cannot be wrapped around the back of it. The pain is also aggravated by asking the patient to abduct the arm with the elbow straight and the palm facing backwards.

Trigger point examination

When searching for TrPs in both the anterior and posterior part of this muscle it should be put

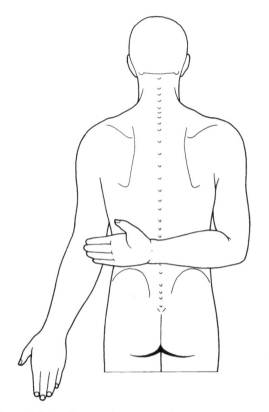

Figure 9.7 To illustrate how a normal person on putting the arm behind the back can reach across to rest the back of the hand on the opposite arm. With trigger points in either the anterior deltoid or coracobrachialis muscle it is usually not possible to reach past the midline.

under moderate tension by slightly abducting the arm.

TrPs in the anterior part of the muscle are usually found high up in the muscle in contrast to TrPs in the posterior part, which are usually found in the lower part of the muscle (Fig. 9.9).

Associated trigger points

TrP activity is rarely confined to the deltoid muscle alone. TrP activity in the anterior part of this muscle is often accompanied by similar activity in TrPs present in the clavicular section of the pectoralis major and biceps brachii. TrP activity in the posterior part of this muscle, the long head of the triceps, the latissimus dorsi and teres major not infrequently develops concurrently. In addition, referral of pain from TrPs in the

supraspinatus or infraspinatus to the shoulder region may lead to the development of satellite TrP activity in this muscle.

Differential diagnosis

Deltoid TrP pain in the shoulder region has to be distinguished from the pain of various other disorders including rotator cuff tendinitis, bicipital tendinitis, glenohumeral joint arthritis, acromioclavicular joint sprain and a C5 radiculopathy. Such a distinction can usually readily be made provided the physical examination includes a search for TrPs. Occasionally, however, deltoid TrP activity and one or other of these disorders develop concurrently.

Biceps brachii muscle (Fig. 9.10)

Anatomical attachments

This long muscle, which is situated on the front of the upper part of the arm, is so called because it has two heads. A short head arises by a thick tendon from the coracoid process. And a long head arises within the capsule of the shoulder joint from a tubercle at the apex of the glenoid cavity. Distally the muscle is attached by means of a tendon to the tuberosity of the radius.

Factors responsible for development of trigger point activity

TrP activity may develop in the lower part of the muscle should it become strained by the lifting of a heavy object with the arm outstretched, or the carrying out of some task with the elbow flexed for a long time as, for example, when cutting a hedge. It may also develop as a result of repeated supination of the arm against resistance, such as when using a screwdriver. Another possible factor, as with the infraspinatus muscle, is sudden stretching as when reaching backwards for support to prevent a fall.

Trigger point examination

When searching for TrPs in this muscle the patient is seated with the elbow resting on a

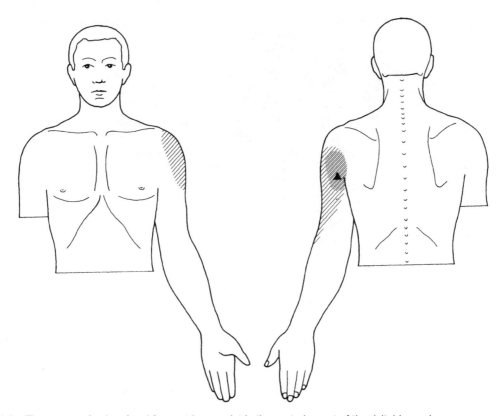

Figure 9.8   The pattern of pain referral from a trigger point in the posterior part of the deltoid muscle.

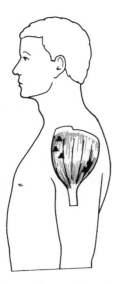

Figure 9.9   To illustrate the usual location of trigger points in the upper anterior part and lower posterior part of the deltoid muscle.

table. With the hand supinated, the elbow is slightly flexed to slacken the biceps muscle.

Trigger point sites

TrPs in elongated tense bands are usually found in the distal part of the muscle (Winter 1944) just above the elbow (Fig. 9.11).

Trigger point pain referral

Pain from these TrPs is referred upwards to the anterior surface of the shoulder joint, and sometimes to a lesser extent to the suprascapular region (Fig. 9.12). There is no restriction of movement at the shoulder joint but pain is aggravated by raising the hand above the head.

Bicipital tendinitis

This, together with rotator cuff tendinitis, will be discussed later in the chapter.

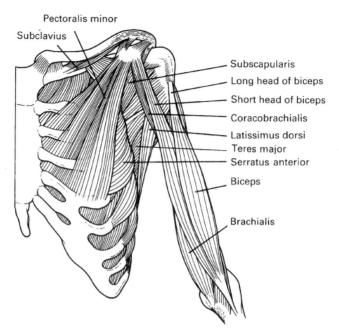

Figure 9.10   The deep muscles of the front of the chest and arm. Left side.

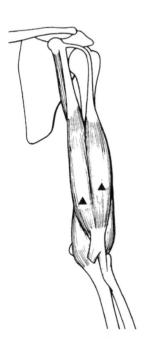

Figure 9.11   To show the usual location of trigger points in the lower part of the biceps muscle just above the elbow.

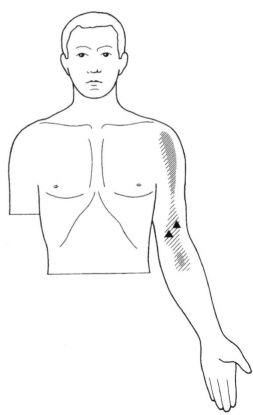

Figure 9.12   The pattern of pain referral from trigger points (▲) in the lower part of the biceps muscle.

Triceps (long head)

A detailed account of various parts of the triceps muscle and the effects of TrP activation in them will be given when discussing pain around the elbow joint in Chapter 10, but reference must be made here to the long head of this muscle because when TrP activity develops in the posterior part of the deltoid it may also arise in the latissimus dorsi, the teres major and this part of the muscle. TrPs in the long head cause pain to be referred upwards over the back of the arm to the posterior part of the shoulder and sometimes downwards along the back of the forearm (see Fig. 10.2).

A person suffering from this, when instructed to raise both arms above the head with the elbows straight and the palms to the front, finds it impossible to hold the affected arm tight against the side of the head (see Fig. 10.3).

Clavicular section of the pectoralis major muscle (see Fig. 14.3)

TrPs in the clavicular section of this muscle refer pain to the front of the shoulder, and may also cause abduction of the arm at the shoulder joint to be restricted. A detailed discussion of this muscle and its TrP pain referral patterns will be given in Chapter 14.

Coracobrachialis (Fig. 9.10)

Anatomical attachments

This muscle, together with the pectoralis minor and the short head of the biceps, is attached at its upper end to the coracoid process, and at its lower end to the middle of the humerus.

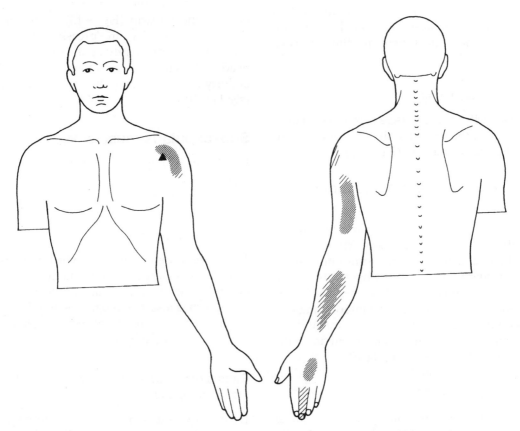

Figure 9.13   the pattern of pain referral from a trigger point or points (▲) in the coracobrachialis muscle.

Factors responsible for development of trigger point activity

TrP activity in this muscle develops as a secondary event following the primary activation of TrP nociceptors in muscles with which it acts synergistically, such as the anterior deltoid, short head of the biceps and pectoralis major, and also following the development of TrP activity in its antagonists. These include the posterior deltoid, latissimus dorsi, teres major and long head of the triceps.

With regard to this Simons et al (1999c) have stated, 'Involvement of the coracobrachialis is usually discovered when the patient returns following successful inactivation of multiple TrPs in other shoulder muscles, especially the anterior deltoid'.

Trigger point sites

Sites where TrPs are likely to be found in this muscle include the mid-part of its belly and close to its proximal attachment to the coracoid process.

Trigger point pain referral

Pain from TrPs in this muscle is referred mainly to the front of the shoulder and to a lesser extent down the back of the arm (Fig. 9.13).

Latissimus dorsi and teres major
(Fig. 9.1)

These muscles, which together form the posterior axillary fold, often develop TrP activity in them at the same time. The latissimus dorsi muscle is considered in detail in Chapter 14 as TrP activity in this muscle mainly causes pain to be felt in the chest wall around the inferior angle of the scapula but in addition it may also be referred to the back of the shoulder and down the inner side of the arm (see Fig. 14.10).

Teres major (Fig. 9.1)

This muscle is attached medially to the lower part of the scapula; and laterally converges with the latissimus dorsi muscle to form the posterior axillary fold before being inserted into the tuberosity close to the latissimus dorsi in the bicipital groove.

Trigger point sites and patterns of pain referral

TrPs may occur at both the inner and outer ends of the muscle (Fig. 9.14). TrPs occurring medially at the insertion of the muscle into the lower lateral border of the scapula may be located by applying pressure against the underlying scapula. TrPs occurring laterally in the posterior axillary fold may be located by gripping the fold between the thumb and fingers. This may be done with the patient sitting but it is probably easier to do it with the patient lying supine and the arm abducted to 90°.

Pain from these TrPs is felt in the posterior part of the shoulder when reaching forwards and upwards and occasionally along the back of the forearm (Fig. 9.15). A person with this has difficulty in pressing the raised outstretched arm tightly against the side of the head in the same way as someone does with TrP activity in the long head of the triceps (see Fig. 10.3).

Subscapularis muscle (Fig. 9.16)

Finally, it is important not to overlook TrPs hidden away in the subscapularis muscle as a cause of persistent pain in the shoulder.

Anatomical attachments

This large triangular muscle, which fills the subscapular fossa, arises from its medial two-thirds. From there its fibres pass laterally to end in a tendon which is inserted into the lesser tuberosity of the humerus and the front of the capsular ligament of the shoulder joint.

Factors responsible for the development of trigger point activity

TrP activity in this muscle is liable to develop as a result of one or other of the following: repeated

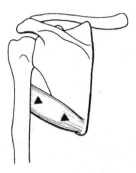

Figure 9.14 To show sites at which trigger points are liable to become activated in the teres major muscle.

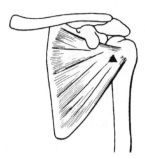

Figure 9.16 The subscapularis muscle with a trigger point (▲) near to the insertion of this muscle into the humerus.

Myofascial trigger point sites and pattern of pain referral

TrPs are usually located along the axillary border of the subscapular fossa but they are difficult to palpate unless the arm is well abducted with traction applied to the arm to abduct the scapula.

The pain from TrPs in this muscle is very severe even at rest and made worse by movement. It is predominantly felt over the back of the shoulder but also extends up towards the scapula, down the back of the arm to the elbow and occasionally as far as the back of the wrist (Fig. 9.17). Because of pain and TrP-induced shortening of the muscle there is liable to be restriction of abduction and external rotation of the shoulder joint.

Associated trigger points

TrP activity in this muscle is liable to be associated with similar activity in the pectoralis major, latissimus dorsi, teres major, long head of the triceps, and the anterior and posterior part of the deltoid muscles.

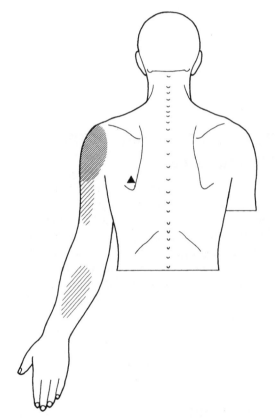

Figure 9.15 The pattern of pain referral from a trigger point at the inner end of the teres major muscle.

Deactivation of shoulder-pain-referring MTrPs

When deactivating MTrPs that refer pain to the shoulder region any of the deeply applied techniques which involve inserting a needle into the MTrP itself runs the risk, as elsewhere in the body, of damaging neighbouring structures.

For example, when inserting a needle into TrPs in the lower part of the biceps, care has to be taken not to damage the median and radial

movements involving a considerable amount of internal rotation; direct trauma to the shoulder; and immobilisation of the shoulder joint for a protracted period in the adducted and internally rotated position.

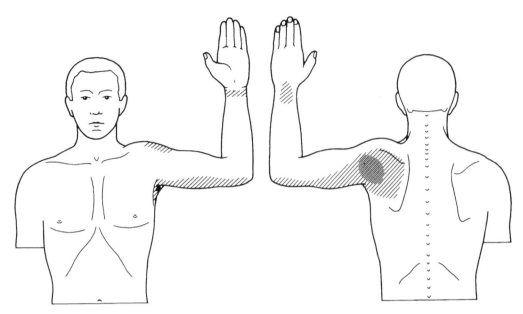

Figure 9.17   The pattern of pain referral from a trigger point or points (▲) in the axillary part of the subscapularis muscle.

nerves which run respectively along the inner and outer borders of the distal part of this muscle. Similarly, with TrPs in the coracobrachialis muscle it is necessary to avoid damaging the brachial artery. And with TrPs in muscles such as the pectoralis major, subscapularis and infraspinatus it is essential to avoid penetrating the pleura.

Superficial dry needling is therefore recommended for it is not only far easier to carry out but seemingly just as effective and has the added merit of avoiding these hazards. However, even with this, when deactivating TrPs in muscles in the vicinity of the chest wall the needle must be inserted at an oblique angle in order to avoid any possibility of inducing a pneumothorax.

Furthermore, as elsewhere in the body, superficial dry needling may be employed not only for deactivating TrPs in muscles that lie just below the surface, but also for deactivating deeply situated ones such as the supraspinatus, which is covered by the trapezius muscle.

SECONDARY DEVELOPMENT OF MTrP PAIN

MTrP pain in the shoulder region may develop as a secondary event in rotator cuff tendinitis and associated disorders and in adhesive capsulitis.

ROTATOR CUFF TENDINITIS
The rotator cuff

The musculotendinous rotator cuff comprises the conjoined tendon of the supraspinatus, infraspinatus and teres minor muscles which inserts into the greater tuberosity of the humerus, and also the subscapularis tendon which inserts into the lesser tuberosity. This rotator cuff of muscles together with the tendon of the long head of the biceps muscle serves to stabilise the humeral head in the glenoid fossa and prevents the deltoid muscle from pulling the head upwards towards the acromion during the initiation of either shoulder abduction or elevation.

Pathogenesis

In young adults rotator cuff tendinitis develops acutely as a result of reversible oedematous and haemorrhagic changes taking place in the cuff muscles. People with glenohumeral instability are particularly liable to develop it. It commonly occurs when the rotator cuff muscles are suddenly overloaded with the arm in the elevated position such as may happen when throwing a ball.

In older people the disorder has a more insidious onset and develops as a result of slowly progressive degenerative and ischaemic changes taking place in the cuff. Eventually these cause the cuff to become so weakened as to allow the humeral head to move upwards during abduction and elevation of the upper arm, with the result that the supraspinatus tendon becomes compressed between the humeral head and the overlying acromion and coracoacromial ligament. In addition to impingement taking place in this way, it also occurs as a result of bony changes developing in the acromion and humeral head. Attrition of the cuff may eventually cause it to rupture.

Clinical manifestations

In the young adult there is usually a sudden onset of severe pain in the deltoid region that develops when overloading of the cuff muscles causes their tendinous insertion to become acutely inflamed. This is particularly liable to happen during the course of some athletic pursuit such as swimming or one that involves throwing of a ball.

In a middle-aged person the pain tends to develop more gradually and to come on as a result of repeated strenuous use of the upper arm, particularly when this involves much sustained overhead activity.

In the elderly the onset may be even more insidious for in this age group there is often no history of trauma with the disorder frequently arising spontaneously as a result of the rotator cuff undergoing slowly progressive ischaemia-induced degenerative changes.

Initially the abduction of the arm is full but pain is experienced as it is moved through a range of 70–120°. And then when lowering the arm from full abduction, pain is again felt in this mid-part of the movement. There is often difficulty in reaching up behind the back when dressing. Also, a patient with this disorder is often awakened from sleep by pain when turning on to the affected side. Passive movements of the upper arm remain full but active movements become increasingly more restricted.

The pain is increased when various movements are carried out against resistance. Pain from inflammation of the supraspinatus part of the cuff is made worse by resisted abduction. Pain from inflammation of the infraspinatus part of the tendon is aggravated by resisted external rotation. And pain from inflammation of the subscapularis part is increased by resisted internal rotation.

MTrP activity

The examination of a patient with rotator cuff tendinitis should include a search for TrPs in the rotator cuff itself, and also in the muscles of the neck, the shoulder girdle, the upper arm and the anterior chest wall.

In most accounts of this disorder attention is drawn to a point of exquisite tenderness at the site where the supraspinatus tendon inserts into the greater tuberosity and another where the subscapularis tendon inserts into the lesser tuberosity. What, however, is not sufficiently well recognised is that these points of maximum tenderness are MTrPs (Simons et al 1999a). TrP activity in this disorder may be either a primary or secondary event.

The trauma responsible for the tendinitis initially developing may also lead to the development of primary TrP activity in nearby muscles. In addition, the pain that arises as a result of the tendinitis may cause muscles in the immediate vicinity of the shoulder joint to go into spasm with, as a consequence, the development of secondary MTrP activity. In addition, the latter may also develop in shoulder girdle, neck and chest wall muscles as a result of the tendinitis pain causing the patient to hold these in a persistently contracted state.

Deposition of calcium

Calcium crystals may become deposited in the rotator cuff tendon. This may be symptomless and only found on radiographic examination. It may, however, be a cause of chronic aching in the shoulder aggravated by movements of the upper arm. And sometimes when large amounts of calcium are deposited over a short period of time there is a sudden onset of excruciating pain in the shoulder with considerable limitation of its movements.

Radiographic changes

In addition to calcific deposits at times being observed on a plain radiograph other abnormalities that may be seen, particularly in long-standing cases, are cystic and sclerotic changes in the region of the cuff's insertion into the greater tuberosity; also, osteophytes in the acromion.

Management

The treatment of this disorder is far from easy as there is no evidence to suggest that any form of therapy influences its natural history. Therefore all that can be done is to encourage shoulder movements during the weeks or months it takes for the lesion to undergo spontaneous resolution whilst, at the same time, relieving the pain by the use of anti-inflammatory physical modalities and drugs, and by deactivating MTrPs.

Exercises

The arm should initially be rested for several days. Following this gentle pendular exercises carried out with the arm dangling, as first described by Codman (1934), should be started and then over the weeks these should be supplemented by more active exercises. The only movement that should be avoided is abduction as this tends to cause the greater tuberosity to impinge upon the acromion with, as a consequence, a worsening of the inflammation and an increase in the damage to the cuff.

Anti-inflammatory physical modalities

These traditionally include various forms of heat such as ultrasound. Cailliet (1991), however, believes that during the acute phase this may possibly increase the swelling of an inflamed cuff and, as a consequence do more harm than good by causing greater encroachment within an already narrowed suprahumeral space. For this reason he is of the opinion that for the first few days it is better to apply ice packs for 20 minutes several times a day.

Anti-inflammatory drug therapy

Petri et al (1987) were the first to carry out a double-blind placebo-controlled trial to compare the effects of an orally administered non-steroidal anti-inflammatory drug (NSAID; naproxen), a subacromial injection of a steroid (triamcinolone) and a placebo in the treatment of the painful shoulder. They concluded that both naproxen and triamcinolone were more effective than a placebo and that the pain relief obtained with a triamcinolone injection into the subacromial bursa was better than that provided by naproxen. Also, that there was no advantage in using a combination of naproxen and triamcinolone.

It should be noted that in this trial the steroid was injected into the subacromial bursa rather than into the region of the supraspinatus tendon. This was because it is a more easily taught technique, reduces the risk of tendon rupture (Fearnley & Vadasz 1969, Simkin 1983), and has the advantage of providing a repository of corticosteroid that can spread diffusely to the adjacent tendons. The injection in this trial consisted of a triamcinolone/lignocaine (lidocaine) mixture, the purpose of the local anaesthetic being to prevent the development of post-injection pain.

Currently the most widely adopted regime (Barry & Jenner 1996, Dalton 1995) is firstly to prescribe an orally administered NSAID. And in those cases where this does not prove sufficient to inject a corticosteroid/local anaesthetic mixture into the subacromial bursa. The pain-relieving effect of a steroid injection is not long-lasting and may have to be repeated at intervals. With respect to this, Barry and Jenner (1996) point out that 'long acting deep preparations of corticosteroids such as methylprednisolone should be used with caution because of the possibility of atrophy of soft tissue or rupture of the tendon if this is injected inadvertently'. There is therefore a case for employing the shorter-acting hydrocortisone acetate (Hazelman 1990).

Deactivation of myofascial trigger points

Pain-producing TrPs both in the rotator cuff itself and in the surrounding muscles should be deactivated.

Surgery

When symptoms persist for more than 12 months subacromial decompression by means of an acromioplasty and resection of the coracoacromial ligament should be carried out arthroscopically (Dalton 1995).

Rotator cuff tears

A rotator cuff tear may be partial or complete. A partial tear may occur at any age but a complete one is rarely seen under the age of 40. Probably the most frequent reason for the tearing of a cuff is its subjection to trauma when already weakened by a long-standing degenerative process.

Some common forms of trauma include falling on the outstretched arm, falling on the side of the shoulder, and hyperabduction of the arm with impingement of the cuff against the acromion and coracoacromial ligament. In addition, with patients over the age of 40 there is a close association between the tearing of a cuff and dislocation of the shoulder (Hawkins et al 1986).

Clinical manifestations

The patient complains of pain on abduction of the shoulder joint and an inability to hold the arm in this position for more than a short time before it falls to the side. Flexion and external rotation may also be weak depending on which part of the cuff has ruptured. Failure to be able to externally rotate the arm against resistance is also indicative of a torn cuff. The bellies of the infraspinatus and supraspinatus muscles may show evidence of wasting.

Investigations

A plain radiograph is likely to show evidence of chronic degeneration with sclerosis and cystic changes in the greater tuberosity. Osteophytes may also be seen in the acromion. Narrowing of the subacromial space as a result of the migration of the humeral head upwards may also be evident. A contrast arthrogram is of considerable value in demonstrating the presence of a full thickness tear. Magnetic resonance imaging may also be used for this purpose. Arthroscopy is a particularly helpful investigation as it permits visualisation of the rotator cuff, the subacromial bursa and the intra-articular part of the biceps tendon, and allows the size of the cuff tear to be estimated.

Management

A partial cuff tear should be managed conservatively using the methods employed for the treatment of a rotator cuff tendinitis except that the injection of a steroid should be avoided during the first 4–6 weeks. A sudden complete tear in an active young person should be repaired immediately. In older people, however, it should initially be treated conservatively and only if there is no significant improvement within 3 weeks should a subacromial decompression and repair be carried out (Hawkins et al 1985).

ASSOCIATED DISORDERS

Two disorders which may occur either alone or in association with rotator cuff tendinitis are acromioclavicular joint osteoarthritis and bicipital tendinitis.

Osteoarthritis of the acromioclavicular joint

Pathogenesis

Degenerative changes may take place in the acromioclavicular joint as part of a widespread osteoarthritis. Alternatively they may affect this joint alone, particularly when at some time in the past it has been subjected to trauma. In such cases rotator cuff tendinitis often develops concomitantly. When this happens osteophytes on the inferior aspect of the acromioclavicular joint may contribute to the development of a rotator cuff tear.

Clinical manifestations

In this disorder pain, made worse by abduction of the arm, is confined to the joint. On examination, the joint is found to be tender and often enlarged as a result of osteophyte formation. Crepitus is frequently elicited.

Investigations

The degenerative changes in this joint are evident on a plain radiograph.

Management

The pain may be alleviated by the use of analgesics and NSAIDs. In addition, exercises designed to restore normal scapulohumeral rhythm and glenohumeral movements should be instituted. Should symptoms persist despite conservative treatment it may be necessary to carry out an excision arthroplasty. Care has to be taken to exclude the presence of a rotator cuff tear for if present it may need to be repaired.

Bicipital tendinitis

Pathogenesis

Acute inflammation of the tendon of the long head of the biceps muscle may develop as a result of an overuse injury incurred during some sporting activity. Chronic inflammation may result from the prolonged and repeated carrying of a heavy load.

The inflammation may develop alone but more often it does so in association with rotator cuff tendinitis. This is because the biceps tendon and the rotator cuff stabilise the humeral head and, therefore, both rotator cuff tendinitis and bicipital tendinitis are prone to develop whenever there is glenohumeral instability.

Rupture of the tendon is comparatively rare. However, in a younger person this is liable to happen suddenly should the tendon be subjected to excessive overloading, and in an older person should it become thin and attenuated.

Clinical manifestations

The pain in this disorder is felt over the anterior aspect of the shoulder and down into the belly of the biceps muscle. It is exacerbated by overhead movements, shoulder extension and elbow flexion. It may be reproduced either by resisted elbow flexion or supination. On palpating the bicipital groove the tendon is found to be tender. Comparison with the non-affected side, however, is essential as a normal tendon may be slightly tender. Rupture of the tendon gives rise to a characteristic lump in the upper arm.

Management

Bicipital tendinitis should be treated by resting the arm and administering a NSAID. If symptoms persist despite this a corticosteroid should be injected into the tissues around the tendon, care being taken not to inject it into the tendon itself as this may cause it to rupture. Rupture of the tendon is usually treated conservatively.

ADHESIVE CAPSULITIS

Terminology

Over the years there has been considerable controversy as to the nature of this disorder with, as a consequence, much confusion concerning its terminology. Duplay (1896) first termed the condition 'de la periarthrite scapulo-humerale' and in line with this others have since called it periarthritis (Lee et al 1974, Lloyd-Roberts & French 1959). In 1945 Neviaser coined the term adhesive capsulitis. He did this because of the appearances he found during the course of operating on patients with this disorder. These included thickening and contraction of the capsule together with adhesions between the synovial surfaces. It was not, however, because of seeing adhesions that he described the capsulitis as being adhesive but rather because at operation the capsule separates from the head of the humerus in the same manner as adhesive strapping peels from the skin. Previous to this Codman (1934) had introduced the term frozen shoulder for this condition. Although this has had much popular appeal it has regrettably over the years tended to be used in an indiscriminate and imprecise manner for any disorder in which there is pain and severely restricted movements of the shoulder joint regardless of the underlying cause. Moreover, as Bunker (1985) has pointed out, the widespread acute inflammatory reaction and increased vascularity in the capsule and rotator cuff in this disorder make these structures abnormally warm so that the term frozen shoulder is somewhat of a misnomer and for this reason alone is better avoided.

Pathogenesis

Adhesive capsulitis is liable to develop whenever movements of the shoulder joint become restricted. Thus it may come on following an injury to the shoulder either in the form of repeated episodes of minor trauma or a single episode of severe trauma (Wright & Haq 1976). It also not infrequently develops as a complication of rotator cuff tendinitis. It may in addition occur when an arm becomes paralysed following a cerebrovascular accident, particularly if the arm is allowed to remain immobile and not put through a full range of movements every day (McLaughlin 1961). For the same reason it may arise as a complication of various chronic neurological disorders such as Parkinson's disease. In the past it not uncommonly developed when people suffering from disorders such as myocardial infarction and tuberculosis were confined to their beds for prolonged periods. It frequently arises in those engaged in sedentary work shortly after they have taken up what is for them some relatively strenuous physical activity such as golf, tennis or bowling. Capsulitis is particularly prevalent in diabetics and when it arises as a complication of this disease it not infrequently develops bilaterally (Satter & Luqman 1985). The reason for it developing in this disorder is not certain but it is thought it may be because of a

predilection to infection or because of a vasculitis (Nash & Hazelman 1989). Patients with hypothyroidism (Bowman et al 1988) and hyperthyroidism (Wohlgethan 1987) also appear to be particularly susceptible to developing it.

Clinical manifestations

The disorder is rare under the age of 40. Dalton (1995) has defined it as being, 'a condition of unknown etiology in which there is a painful global restriction of glenohumeral movements in all planes, both active and passive, in the absence of joint degeneration sufficient to explain this restriction'. The intense pain and severe limitation of movements cause difficulty in carrying out such everyday tasks as dressing and combing the hair. There is also difficulty in placing the hand in the back pocket of trousers and in reaching upwards behind the back. The natural history of the disorder is such that the course taken by it may conveniently be divided into three stages: the painful stage, the adhesive stage and the recovery stage.

The painful stage

This stage, which lasts for 3–8 months, is characterised by increasingly severe pain that is made worse by shoulder movements and is liable to waken the patient from sleep when pressure is exerted on the shoulder as a result of lying on the affected side. The pain is partly due to the capsulitis itself and partly due to the development of TrP activity in muscles in the vicinity of the shoulder joint.

TrP activity in these muscles has two causes. It is liable to be brought on by the trauma initially responsible for the development of the capsulitis. In may also arise secondarily to the onset of capsulitis pain-induced muscle spasm. In addition, TrPs in muscles in the neck and shoulder girdle may become active as a result of the capsulitis pain causing the patient to hold them in a persistently contracted state.

During this stage all movements of the glenohumeral joint, both active and passive, are severely restricted.

Adhesive stage

During this stage, which lasts for 4–6 months, there is a gradual reduction in the intensity of the pain but the movements of the shoulder become increasingly more restricted.

Recovery stage

Recovery is a slow process, often taking 1–3 years. During this stage the pain gradually disappears and the movements slowly increase in range although not infrequently there is some long-term reduction of them.

Hazelman (1972) in a retrospective survey of 130 patients found that 15% of them had a persistent disability. And Reeves (1976) in a prospective 5–10-year study of 49 patients found that 3 had a severe and 22 had a mild persistent disability. However, Binder et al (1984), in a prospective study of 40 patients followed up for between 40 and 48 months (mean 44), found that even when objective restriction of their movements persisted they were frequently unaware of this and had little or no functional disability.

Shoulder–hand syndrome

This severely disabling complication of the disorder (Bonica & Sola 1990) will be discussed at some length in Chapter 10.

Arthrography

The glenohumeral joint is normally capable of accommodating 10–15 ml of contrast fluid. With moderate capsulitis this is frequently reduced to 5–10 ml and with severe capsulitis it is often reduced to even less (Bruckner 1982). However, a significant number of patients diagnosed as having adhesive capsulitis have normal arthrographic findings (Binder et al 1984).

Management

Clinical trials in this disorder have shown that no forms of therapy influence its natural history but that certain types of treatment given during the initial phase are helpful. The consensus is that during the initial phase treatment should be aimed at providing symptomatic pain relief and encouraging movement of the joint.

Symptomatic pain relief

The pain is so severe that simple analgesics are of very limited value and NSAIDs have not been found to be particularly useful. For example, in a prospective clinical trial carried out by Bulgen et al (1984) half the patients prior to being admitted to this had been given a NSAID but only 3 out of 21 had found it to be helpful.

A number of trials have shown that a corticosteroid administered either orally or by local injection gives some worthwhile short-term symptomatic pain relief.

Cyriax & Trosier (1953) were among the first to treat what they termed 'freezing arthritis' with an intra-articular injection of hydrocortisone.

Roy and Oldham (1976) afforded considerable relief to 55 patients by injecting hydrocortisone both into the subacromial bursa and into the shoulder joint on two to three occasions at weekly intervals. Roy et al (1982) reported similarly good results and stressed the effectiveness of injecting it into both the subacromial bursa and joint rather than into the joint alone.

Bulgen et al (1984), in a prospective controlled study in which they evaluated three treatment regimes (intra-articular steroids, mobilisation and ice therapy), therefore employed the same technique in the group given a corticosteroid (0.5 ml of methyl prednisolone (20 mg) and 1% lignocaine (lidocaine) injected into each of the two sites weekly for 3 weeks). Their conclusion, like that reached earlier by Lee et al (1974) and Richardson (1975), was that 'steroid injections may benefit pain and range of movement in the early stages of the condition'.

Binder et al (1986) in a controlled study of oral prednisolone in frozen shoulders have shown that this too gives symptomatic short-term pain relief.

Mobilisation of the joint

It is generally agreed that patients should be taught to carry out pendular exercises for 2–3 minutes every hour (Bulgen et al 1984). In addition, there is evidence to show that mobilisation of the joint by a physiotherapist employing a technique such as that devised by Maitland (1983) is helpful. With respect to this, however, it should be noted that Dacre et al (1989) carried out an interesting study comparing the cost and efficacy of treating what they termed periarthritis of the shoulder either with a local steroid injected anteriorly around the shoulder joint, or with physiotherapy mainly in the form of mobilisation carried out for 6 weeks, or with a combination of both. Their results showed that a local steroid injection is as effective as physiotherapy alone or a combination of the two and is also the most cost effective. (In 1989 a steroid injection cost £2.10 as opposed to £48.50 for a 6-week course of physiotherapy.)

Deactivation of myofascial trigger points

Some of the pain in patients with capsulitis emanates from activated TrP nociceptors in nearby muscles and as long ago as 1942 Travell, Rinzler and Herman stressed the importance of deactivating these. More recently Sola (1994) has again drawn attention to the necessity for doing it in this disorder.

Manipulation under an anaesthetic

This is never carried out in the initial painful stage but can be of value in restoring movements during the adhesive phase (Lloyd-Roberts & French 1959, Lundberg 1969, Reeves 1976). As Dalton (1995), however, has pointed out, 'For many patients, once the painful phase of this condition has subsided the prospect of this painful procedure is not appealing'.

Recognition and management of depression

The treatment of capsulitis is far from satisfactory. A certain amount of pain relief can be obtained by injecting steroids into the subacromial bursa and shoulder joint and by deactivating MTrPs; but such procedures do nothing to curtail the natural history of this profoundly disabling disorder. It is hardly surprising therefore that patients with it often suffer from depression which when present needs to be recognised and treated.

REFERENCES

Barry M, Jenner J R 1996 Pain in the neck, shoulder and arm. In: Snaith M I (ed) ABC of rheumatology. BMA Publishing Group, London

Binder A, Bulgen D Y, Hazelman B L, Roberts S 1984 Frozen shoulder. A long-term prospective study. Annals of Rheumatic Diseases 43:361–364

Binder A, Hazelman B L, Parr G, Roberts S A 1986 Controlled study of oral prednisolone in frozen shoulder. British Journal of Rheumatology 25:288–292

Bonica J J, Sola A E 1990 Other painful disorders of the upper limb. In: Bonica J J (ed) The management of pain, 2nd edn. Lea & Febiger, Philadelphia, vol 1, p 955

Bowman C, Jeffcoate W, Patrick M, Doherty M 1988 Bilateral adhesive capsulitis, oligoarthritis, and proximal myopathy as a presentation of hypothyroidism. British Journal of Rheumatology 27:62–64

Bruckner F E 1982 Frozen shoulder (adhesive capsulitis). Journal of the Royal Society of Medicine 75:688–689

Bulgen D Y, Binder A, Hazelman B L, Dutton J, Roberts S 1984 Frozen shoulder: prospective clinical study with an evaluation of three treatment regimens. Annals of Rheumatic Diseases 43:353–360

Bunker T D 1985 Time for a new name for 'frozen shoulder'. British Medical Journal 290:1233–1234

Cailliet R 1991 Shoulder pain, 3rd edn. F A Davis, Philadelphia, p 73

Codman E A 1934 The shoulder. Thomas Todd, Boston

Cyriax J, Trosier O 1953 Hydrocortisone and soft tissue lesions. British Medical Journal 11:966–968

Dacre J E, Beeney N, Scott L 1989 Injections and physiotherapy for the painful stiff shoulder. Annals of the Rheumatic Diseases 48:322–325

Dalton S E 1995 The shoulder. In: Klippel J, Dieppe P (eds) Practical rheumatology. Mosby, London, ch 7

Duplay S 1896 De la periarthrite scapulo-humerale. L'Abeille Medicale 53:226

Fearnley M, Vadasz I 1969 Factors influencing the response of lesions of the rotator cuff of the shoulder to local steroid injection. Annals of Physical Medicine 10:53–63

Hawkins R J, Misamore G W, Hobeika P E 1985 Surgery for full-thickness rotator cuff tears. Journal of Bone and Joint Surgery 67A:1349–1355

Hawkins R J, Bell R H, Hawkins R A, Koppert G J 1986 Anterior dislocation of the shoulder in the older patient. Clinical Orthopaedics 206:192–198

Hazelman B L 1972 The painful stiff shoulder. Rheumatology and Rehabilitation 11:413–421

Hazelman B 1990 Musculoskeletal and connective tissue disease. In: Souhami R L, Moxham J (eds) Textbook of medicine. Churchill Livingstone, Edinburgh, p 1037

Kelly M 1942 New light on the painful shoulder. Medical Journal of Australia 1:488–493

Lee R N, Lee M, Haq A M, Longton E B, Wright V 1974 Periarthritis of the shoulder: trial of treatments investigated by multivariate analysis. Annals of Rheumatic Diseases 33:116–119

Lloyd-Roberts G C, French P R 1959 Periarthritis of the shoulder. British Medical Journal i:1569–1571

Long C 1956 Myofascial pain syndromes part II – syndromes of the head, neck and shoulder girdle. Henry Ford Hospital Medical Bulletin 4:22–28

Lundberg B J 1969 The frozen shoulder. Acta Orthopaedica Scandinavica 119(suppl):1–59

McLaughlin H L 1961 The 'frozen shoulder'. Clinical Orthopedics 20:126–131

Maitland G D 1983 Treatment of the glenohumeral joint with passive movements. Physiotherapy 69:3–6

Nash P, Hazelman B L 1989 Frozen shoulder. In: Hazelman B L, Dieppe P A (eds) The shoulder joint. Baillière's Clinical Rheumatology, London, pp 551–566

Neviaser J S 1945 Adhesive capsulitis of the shoulder. Journal of Bone and Joint Surgery 27:211–222

Pace J B 1975 Commonly overlooked pain syndromes responsive to simple therapy. Postgraduate Medicine 59:107–113

Petri M, Dobrow R, Neiman R, Whiting-O'Keefe Q, Scaman W E 1987 Randomized, double-blind, placebo-controlled study of the treatment of the painful shoulder. Arthritis and Rheumatism 30(9):1040–1045

Reeves B 1976 The natural history of the frozen shoulder syndrome. Scandinavian Journal of Rheumatology 4:193–196

Reynolds M D 1981 Myofascial trigger point syndromes in the practise of rheumatology. Archives of Physical Medicine and Rehabilitation 62:111–114

Richardson A T 1975 The painful shoulder. Proceedings of the Royal Society of Medicine 8:731–736

Roy S, Oldham R 1976 Management of the painful shoulder. Lancet i:1322–1324

Roy S, Oldham R, Nichol F E 1982 Frozen shoulder: adhesive capsulitis. British Medical Journal 284:117–118

Rubin D 1981 An approach to management of myofascial trigger point syndromes. Archives of Physical Medicine and Rehabilitation 62:107–110

Satter M A, Luqman W A 1985 Periarthritis: another duration-related complication of diabetes mellitus. Diabetes Care 8:507–510

Simkin P 1983 Tendinitis and bursitis of the shoulder, anatomy and therapy. Postgraduate Medicine 73:177–190

Simons D G, Travell J G 1984 Myofascial pain syndromes. In: Wall P D, Melzack R (eds) Textbook of pain. Churchill Livingstone, Edinburgh, p 267

Simons D G, Travell J G, Simons L S 1999a–c Travell & Simons Myofascial pain and dysfunction. The trigger point manual. Vol 1 Upper half of the body, 2nd edn. Williams & Wilkins, Baltimore, p 538 (a), p 558 (b), p 641 (c)

Sola A E 1994 Upper extremity pain. In: Wall PD, Melzack R (eds) Textbook of pain, 3rd edn. Churchill Livingstone, Edinburgh, ch 25

Sola A E, Kuitert J H 1955 Myofascial trigger point pain in the neck and shoulder girdle. Northwest Medicine 54:980–984

Sola A E, Williams R L 1956 Myofascial pain syndromes. Neurology 6:91–95

Travell J 1952 Pain mechanisms in connective tissues. In: Ragan C (ed) Connective tissues, transactions of the second conference 1951. Josiah Macy Jr Foundation, New York

Travell J, Rinzler S, Herman M 1942 Pain and disability of the shoulder and arm: treatment by muscular infiltration with procaine hydrochloride. Journal of the American Medical Association 120:417–422

Winter S P 1944 Referred pain in fibrositis. Medical Record 157:34–37

Wohlgethan J R 1987 Frozen shoulder in hyperthyroidism. Arthritis and Rheumatism 30:936–939

Wright V, Haq A M M 1976 Periarthritis of the shoulder. 1. Aetiological considerations with particular reference to personality factors. Annals of Rheumatic Diseases 35:126–131

10

The arm

INTRODUCTION

When investigating the cause of pain in the arm
it is essential to exclude the possibility that it is
arising from myofascial trigger points (MTrPs).
And in order to do this it is essential to carry out
a systematic search for these not only in the muscles of the arm itself but also in the neck, shoulder girdle and chest wall. And when considering
possible reasons for MTrP activity developing in
these muscles it has to be remembered that it

may be due not only to local causes but also to distant ones including structural and mechanical disorders as far away as in the leg and foot (Gerwin 1997).

In this chapter various brachial MTrP pain syndromes will be considered together with other disorders from which these have to be distinguished including cervical radiculopathy, epicondylar enthesopathy and the carpal and cubital tunnel syndromes.

The highly controversial brachial pain disorder that has been accorded a multiplicity of names, including repetitive strain injury, will also be discussed. In addition, reasons will be given as to why brachial MTrP pain and sympathetically mediated pain may develop concomitantly. And finally attention will be drawn to the clinical manifestations and treatment of the shoulder–hand syndrome.

CERVICAL RADICULOPATHIC AND MTrP BRACHIAL PAIN – DIFFERENTIAL DIAGNOSIS

Much diagnostic confusion tends to arise because pain that radiates down the arm from TrPs in either the supraspinatus (see Fig. 9.2), infraspinatus (see Fig. 9.4) or scalenus anterior muscle (see Fig. 8.13) has the same distribution as that of the pain of a C5–C7 radiculopathy (Reynolds 1981). However, it cannot be too strongly emphasised that pain down the arm should not be attributed to nerve root entrapment without clinical evidence of a neurological deficit and preferably without electromyographic evidence of muscle denervation. This dictum applies even when magnetic resonance imaging of the spine shows evidence of a structural disorder that is potentially capable of entrapping a nerve.

Errors of diagnosis and the employment of inappropriate treatment, however, are mainly due to a failure to search routinely for MTrPs when investigating the cause of pain radiating down an arm from the neck (Aronson et al 1971). This notwithstanding, it has to be said that the presence of MTrPs does not of itself exclude the possibility of there being an underlying radicu-

lopathy. This is because TrP activity is liable to develop as a secondary event in muscles innervated by an entrapped nerve root due to the effect motor nerve compression has on a TrP's motor endplates.

It also has to be remembered that TrP activity in a muscle is liable to cause it to become shortened and as a consequence to exert pressure on adjacent nerves. An example of this is pain in the arm brought about as a result of TrP-induced shortening of either a scalene muscle or the pectoralis minor muscle giving rise to compression of the brachial plexus.

BRACHIAL PAIN FROM TrPs IN NECK, SHOULDER GIRDLE AND CHEST WALL MUSCLES

When investigating the cause of pain in the arm it is essential for the clinical examination to include a systematic search for TrPs not only in muscles in the arm itself but also in muscles situated in the neck, shoulder girdle and chest wall.

Neck

The muscles in the neck that have to be examined for TrP activity include the levator scapulae (Ch. 8) and the scalenus anterior (Ch. 8).

Shoulder girdle

The muscles in the shoulder girdle that have to be examined include the supraspinatus (Ch. 9), the infraspinatus (Ch. 9) and the subscapularis (Ch. 9).

Chest wall

The muscles in the chest wall that have to be examined include anteriorly, the clavicular section of the pectoralis major (Chs 9 and 14), pectoralis minor (Ch. 14) and coracobrachialis (Ch. 9). And, posteriorly, the latissimus dorsi (Chs 9 and 14), teres major (Ch. 9) and teres minor (Ch. 9).

PAIN FROM TrPs IN THE UPPER ARM MUSCLES

The muscles in the upper arm that have to be examined for TrP activity include the deltoid, biceps brachii, triceps brachii and brachialis. As pain from TrPs in the deltoid and biceps brachii is referred to the shoulder region, these two muscles were considered in Chapter 9. It therefore only leaves the triceps and brachialis muscles to be discussed.

Triceps brachii muscle (Fig. 10.1)

Anatomical attachments

This muscle, as its name implies, arises from three heads, the long, lateral and medial.

Proximally, the long head attaches to the scapula. And distally, it ends in a common tendon which, beginning above the middle of the muscle, is inserted into the olecranon process of the ulna.

The lateral and medial heads are attached proximally to the humerus and distally by the common tendon to the olecranon process.

Factors responsible for the development of TrP activity

TrP activity in this muscle is liable to develop when it is overloaded, such as during the course of sporting activities. It may also be caused by sitting for long periods with the unsupported elbow held forwards in front of the body, such as may occur, for example, when driving a car or sitting in a chair doing needlework.

MTrP sites and patterns of pain referral

Long head   A common site for TrP activity to develop in the long head of the muscle is

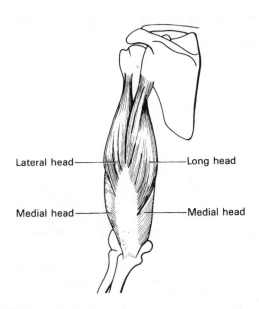

Figure 10.1   The medial, lateral and long heads of the triceps muscle. It should be noted that the lower part of the medial head just above the elbow extends from one side of the arm to the other beneath the muscle's comon tendon of attachment to the olecranon process of the ulna

Lateral head

Long head

Medial head

Medial head

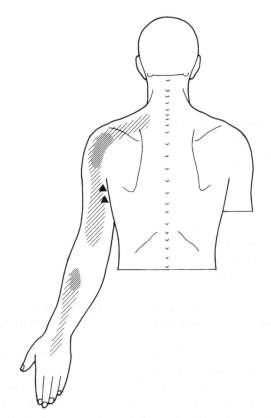

Figure 10.2   The pattern of pain referral from a trigger point or points (▲) in the long head of the triceps muscle.

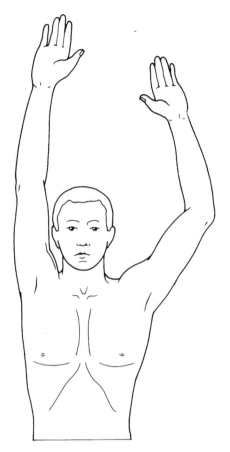

Figure 10.3   To illustrate the difficulty experienced in bringing the ipsilateral arm up against the ear when there is trigger point activity in either the long head of the triceps or the teres major muscle.

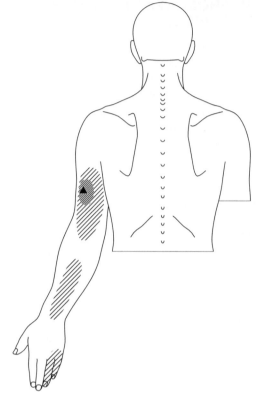

Figure 10.4   The pattern of pain referral from a trigger point (▲) in the lateral border of the lateral head of the triceps muscle.

on its medial side just below the posterior axillary fold. The TrP lies deep in the belly of the muscle and requires very firm palpation in order to locate it. Pain from a TrP at this site is referred both around it and upwards to the back of the shoulder. Occasionally it is also referred up the back or the neck, and down the back of the forearm (Fig. 10.2).

A person with pain from a TrP in the long head, when instructed to raise both arms above the head with the elbows straight and the palms to the front, finds it impossible to hold the arm on the affected side tight against the side of the head (Fig. 10.3).

Lateral head A TrP is liable to be found midway down the arm in the lateral head of this posteriorly situated muscle. From this, pain is referred locally around that site and occasionally down the forearm (Fig. 10.4).

Medial head TrP activity in this head is liable to develop either in its lateral or medial border just above the elbow where it extends across the upper arm beneath this muscle's tendon (Fig. 10.1).

A TrP in its lateral border just above the lateral epicondyle refers pain to this region of the elbow (Fig. 10.5A and B).

A TrP in its medial border just above the medial epicondyle refers pain both to this and down the inner side of the anterior forearm to the ring and little fingers (Fig. 10.6).

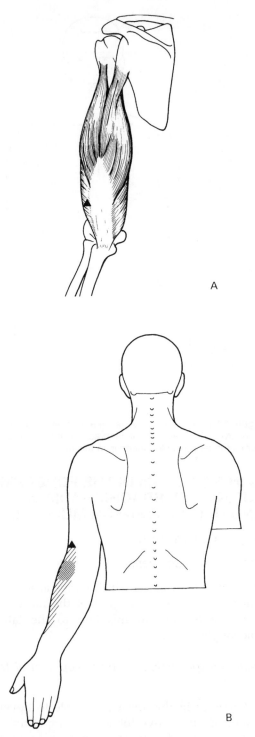

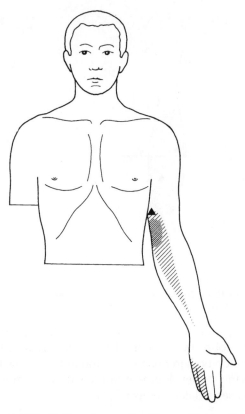

Figure 10.6 Pattern of pain referral from a trigger point in the medial border of the medial head of the triceps muscle.

Brachialis muscle (Fig. 10.7)

Anatomical attachments

This muscle, which covers the lower half of the humerus and front of the elbow, is attached above to the lower half of the anterior aspect of the humerus and below is inserted into the ulnar tuberosity by means of a thick tendon.

It lies in front of the humerus immediately behind the biceps muscle. Its main action is to flex the elbow joint.

Factors responsible for the development of TrP activity

TrPs are liable to become active in this muscle should it become overloaded whilst flexing the forearm during the course of heavy lifting; also, when the elbow is kept in the flexed position for

Figure 10.5 A: Trigger point in the lateral border of the medial head of the triceps muscle. B: Pattern of pain referral from this trigger point.

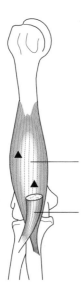

Figure 10.7 The brachialis muscle with trigger points (▲) situated deep to the biceps muscle.

a long time such as, for example, when playing the violin. In addition, TrP activity is liable to develop both in this muscle and in the biceps following its development in the supinator muscle in cases of lateral epicondylitis.

MTrP sites and patterns of pain referral

In order to locate TrPs in this muscle and to deactivate them by one means or another the elbow should be partially flexed, the forearm supinated and the biceps pushed medially out of the way. They are usually to be found in the lower part of this muscle just above the elbow.

Pain from these TrPs is referred mainly to the thumb but also at times to the front of the elbow.

They may also be found high up the arm where the muscle lies beneath the biceps muscle. Pain from these is referred up the arm in a similar manner to that from TrPs in the biceps muscle (Fig. 10.8).

Nerve entrapment

Should the muscle become shortened as a result of TrP activity the radial nerve which runs along its lateral border is liable to become entrapped. When this happens numbness around the dorsum of the thumb develops.

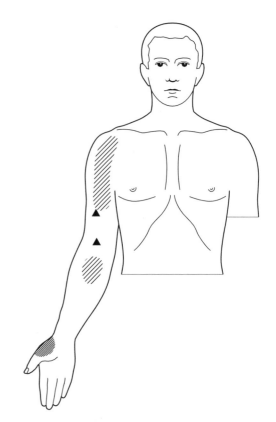

Figure 10.8 The pattern of pain referral from a trigger point (▲) in the lower part of the brachialis muscle and from a trigger point (▲) higher up in this muscle.

PAIN FROM TrPs IN THE FOREARM'S SUPINATOR, BRACHIORADIALIS AND HAND EXTENSOR MUSCLES

Supinator muscle

Anatomical attachments

This small flat muscle which wraps around the outer side of the upper part of the radius has attachments both to this and to the lateral epicondyle.

Factors responsible for the development of TrP activity

TrP activity in this muscle is liable to develop whenever it is overloaded by repetitive or sustained forceful twisting movement at the elbow, particularly when this is carried out with the forearm in the extended position. There are

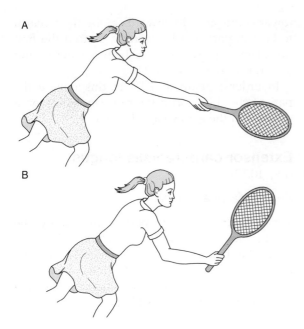

A

B

Figure 10.9   A: Overloading the supinator muscle as a result of incorrect holding of a tennis racquet. B: Avoidance of this by holding the racquet with elbow slightly bent and wrist cocked.

many activities when this may happen. Examples include playing tennis, turning a stiff door knob and unscrewing a tight lid. Overloading whilst playing tennis is particularly liable to happen when a tennis ball is hit with the racquet held by an arm that is kept straight at the elbow and the wrist dropped rather than as it should be with the elbow slightly bent and the wrist cocked (Fig. 10.9).

MTrP sites and pattern of pain referral

In order to examine this muscle for TrP activity the forearm should be fully supinated and the elbow slightly flexed as this relaxes the brachioradialis muscle and allows it to be pushed out of the way. A common site for a TrP to be found in this muscle is on the anterior surface of the forearm just lateral to the biceps tendon.

Pain from this TrP is referred locally to the lateral epicondylar region. And also, as pointed out many years ago by Travell & Rinzler (1952), to the back of the thumb (Fig. 10.10). Two other muscles

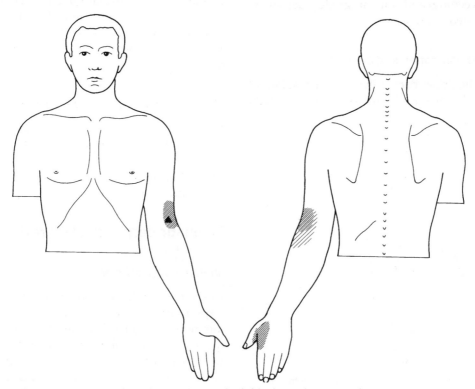

Figure 10.10   The pattern of pain referral from a trigger point (▲) in the supinator muscle.

with a similar TrP pain referral pattern are the brachoradialis and exterior carpi radialis longus.

Brachioradialis (see Fig. 10.18)

Anatomical attachments

This is the most superficial muscle on the radial side of the forearm. Its upper attachment is to the lateral supracondylar ridge of the humerus. And its fibres end in the middle of the forearm in a flat tendon that is inserted into the outer lower end of the radius.

Factors responsible for the development of TrP activity

TrPs in this muscle, like those in the exterior carpi radialis longus and brevis, develop activity as a result of repetitive twisting movements combined with forceful gripping of the hand. Examples include hitting a tennis ball with the arm held in the same faulty position as that which overloads the supinator muscle; prolonged weeding and similar garden activities; also, repeated hand-shaking.

MTrP sites and patterns of pain referral

A TrP in the upper part of this muscle just below the lateral epicondyle refers pain upwards

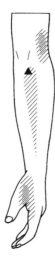

Figure 10.11 The pattern of pain referral from a trigger point (▲) in the brachioradialis muscle.

towards this and downwards along the forearm to be felt, particularly strongly, around the first dorsal interosseous muscle between the thumb and index finger (Fig. 10.11).

In order to palpate TrPs in this muscle the patient should sit with the forearm resting on a pillow and the elbow slightly bent.

Extensor carpi radialis longus
(Fig. 10.12)

Anatomical attachments

This muscle, which is partly covered by the brachioradialis, like the latter also mainly arises from the lateral supracondylar ridge of the humerus. And distally its tendon which runs along the lateral border of the radius is inserted into the second metacarpal bone.

Factors responsible for the development of TrP activity

The factors responsible for the development of TrP activity in this muscle, the extensor carpi radialis brevis and ulnaris are the same as those responsible for this in the brachioradialis.

MTrP sites and patterns of pain referral

TrPs in this muscle, like those in the brachioradialis, tend to be found just below the lateral epicondyle. Pain from them is referred to the lateral epicondyle and down the forearm to the base of the thumb (Fig. 10.13).

Extensor carpi radialis brevis
(Fig. 10.12)

Anatomical attachments

This muscle, which is covered by the extensor carpi radialis longus, mainly arises from the common extensor tendon attached to the lateral epicondyle. And, about the middle of the forearm, its fibres converge to a flat tendon which, distally, attaches to the second and third metacarpal bones.

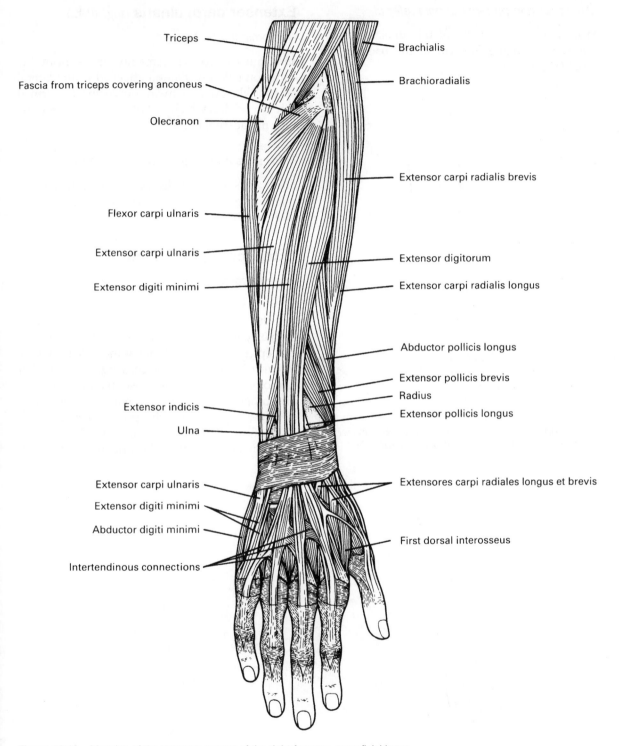

Figure 10.12   Muscles of the extensor aspect of the right forearm, superficial layer.

MTrP sites and patterns of pain referral

From a TrP in the belly of this muscle pain is referred down the forearm to the back of the wrist (Fig. 10.14).

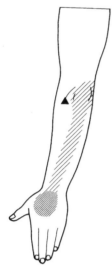

Figure 10.13 The pattern of pain referral from a trigger point (▲) in the extensor carpi radialis longus muscle.

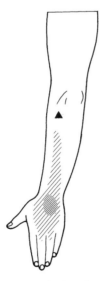

Figure 10.14 The pattern of pain referral from a trigger point (▲) in the extensor carpi radialis brevis muscle.

Extensor carpi ulnaris (Fig. 10.12)

Anatomical attachments

This muscle, likewise, mainly arises from the common extensor tendon attached to the lateral epicondyle. And, halfway down the forearm it forms a tendon which distally is inserted into the fifth metacarpal bone.

MTrP sites and patterns of pain referral

From TrPs in the belly of this muscle pain is referred to the posteromedial aspect of the wrist (Fig. 10.15).

Extensor digitorum muscle (Fig. 10.12)

Anatomical attachments

This muscle, the extensor carpi radialis brevis and the extensor carpi ulnaris arise from a common extensor tendon which is attached to the lateral epicondyle. Two-thirds of the way down the forearm its muscle fibres converge to form four tendons with each of these having complex attachments to a metacarpophalangeal joint so as to allow it to extend the proximal phalanx of an individual finger. This muscle also has the function of separating the fingers at the same

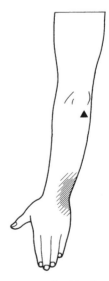

Figure 10.15 The pattern of pain referral from a trigger point (▲) in the extensor carpi ulnaris muscle.

time as it extends them. In addition, it can assist with extending the wrist.

Factors responsible for the development of TrP activity

Forceful repetitive movements of the fingers such as those carried out by craftsmen and musicians are liable to cause TrP activity to develop in this muscle.

MTrP sites and patterns of pain referral

The middle finger extensor is the one in which TrP activity most often develops. Because a TrP in the fibres of the muscle which supplies this finger tends to be near the surface there is no difficulty in locating it. Also its associated taut band is easily felt and a local twitch response readily evoked.

Pain from the TrP is referred down the back of the forearm, wrist and hand as far as the proximal interphalangeal joint of this finger (Fig. 10.16).

Because TrPs in the fibres of the muscle which supplies the ring and little fingers lie at a deep level they are more difficult to locate.

Pain from them is not only referred downwards to the respective fingers but also upwards to the lateral epicondylar region (Fig. 10.17).

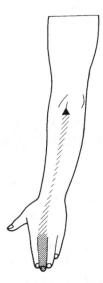

Figure 10.16   The pattern of pain referral from a trigger point (▲) in the extensor digitorum muscle (middle finger extensor).

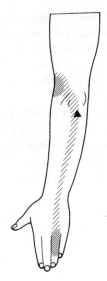

Figure 10.17   The pattern of pain referral from a trigger point (▲) in the extensor digitorum muscle (ring finger extensor).

TrP activity in this muscle is also responsible for a loss of power when attempting to grip with the hand and any attempt to grip firmly, such as when shaking hands, markedly exacerbates the pain.

LATERAL EPICONDYLITIS (SYN: TENNIS ELBOW)

Pathogenesis

Lateral epicondylitis or 'tennis elbow' is an extremely common disability but both terms are misnomers as there is neither inflammation of the epicondyle itself nor is it only tennis players who suffer from it. Although admittedly 40–50% of middle-aged tennis players are liable to develop it, of the total number of people affected, tennis is an aetiological factor in less than 5% (Coonrad & Hooper 1973). And surprisingly, despite repeated microtrauma contributing to its development, the majority affected are neither athletes nor manual workers (Binder & Hazelman 1983).

It is now generally agreed that the basic lesion is an enthesopathy (Neipal & Sitaj 1979) with the initial pathological change being an inflammatory reaction at the common extensor tendon's attachment to the lateral epicondyle.

Infrared thermographs of the affected elbow show a well-demarcated area of increased heat near the lateral epicondyle in 98% of cases (Binder et al 1983).

Chard & Hazelman (1989) have found that biopsies taken prior to surgery being carried out at a relatively late stage of the disorder show that over the course of time the initial inflammatory changes have been supplanted by degenerative ones.

The disorder rarely arises before the age of 30 and mainly affects middle-aged people who, for one reason or another, have subjected the epicondylar–tenoperiosteal junction (enthesis) to repeated overloading.

The pain, which initially is localised to the lateral epicondyle and later spreads up and down the arm, is largely due to the enthesopathy but as Simons et al (1999a) have stated, clinical examination shows that it also often emanates from TrPs in various muscles around the elbow, including the supinator, brachioradialis, extensor carpi radialis longus and brevis, the extensor digitorum and the lower end of the lateral margin of the medial head of the triceps.

Resisted dorsiflexion of the wrist with the elbow in extension aggravates the pain.

Differential diagnosis

Other causes of lateral epicondylar pain include arthritis of the elbow, referral to that region as a result of cervical nerve entrapment and from TrPs in the supraspinatus muscle.

Treatment

The standard treatment is to counteract the inflammatory changes present in and around the common extensor tendon by injecting a corticosteroid into the tissues immediately distal to the lateral epicondyle.

One well-recognised method of doing this is as follows. With the elbow supported by resting the arm on a pillow, and the forearm extended and

fully supinated, the tissues around the lateral epicondyle are palpated to find a point of maximum tenderness. This is usually just below the epicondyle. A needle is then inserted deep into the tissues at this site until it reaches the tenoperiosteal junction and 2–5 ml of either hydrocortisone (10–25 mg), triamcinolone (5–10 mg) or methylprednisolone (10–20 mg), mixed with 1% lignocine (Lidocaine), is injected through it (Chard 1995).

Assendelft et al (1996), from a review of 12 clinical trials, have concluded that the pain relief obtained with a corticosteroid injection carried out in this manner is relatively short-lasting and frequently has to be repeated after 4–6 weeks. It is generally agreed that if there is no response to two injections further ones are unlikely to be effective (Calvert et al 1985).

There are grounds for believing that the treatment of this disorder is considerably more effective when it includes the deactivation of MTrPs in the vicinity of the lateral epicondyle. However, it has to be admitted that objective proof of this is lacking and there is an urgent need for clinical trials to be carried out to compare the relative effectiveness of a steroid injection, TrP deactivation, and a combination of both of these.

Finally, it has to be said that when conservative treatment provides no more than temporary relief, surgical release of the common extensor tendon at the epicondyle may have to be carried out (Bosworth 1965, Rosen et al 1980).

PAIN FROM TrPs IN THE FOREARM'S HAND AND FINGER FLEXOR MUSCLES

The forearm flexor muscles in which TrP activity is liable to cause pain to be referred to the front of the wrist and hand include the flexor carpi radialis, the flexor carpi ulnaris, and the flexor digitorum (superficialis and profundus), all of which are attached proximally to the medial epicondyle by means of a common tendon, and the flexor pollicis longus, which is attached proximally to the radius. Distally these muscles have tendinous attachments to the phalanges.

Anatomical relationships of these muscles

In order to be able to identify in which of these various muscles a particular TrP is located, it is helpful to remember that they are arranged in three layers with the superficial layer consisting of the flexor carpi radialis and the flexor carpi ulnaris, separated by the palmaris longus; the intermediate layer consisting of the flexor digitorum superficialis; and the deep layer consisting of the flexor digitorum profundus and the flexor pollicis longus.

Factors responsible for the development of TrP activity in the forearm flexor muscles

TrPs in these muscles are liable to develop activity as a result of prolonged gripping. It commonly occurs, for example, when the steering wheel of a car is held tightly during a long journey, particularly when the hands are placed on top of the steering wheel in the flexed position. In addition to this TrPs in the flexor pollicis longus are liable to become active as a result of gripping tightly with the thumb whilst carrying out any continued twisting and pulling movement such as may occur when weeding.

Flexor carpi radialis and flexor carpi ulnaris (Fig. 10.18)

MTrP sites and patterns of pain referral

TrPs in both of these muscles are liable to be found high up the forearm just below where each of them is attached to the medial epicondyle. As both muscles are in the superficial layer, TrPs in them are easily recognised by their exquisite tenderness to light touch. Also, by sustained pressure evoking a readily visible local twitch response, and their specific pattern of pain referral.

Pain from these TrPs is referred either to the radial aspect or the ulnar aspect of the palmar surface of the wrist according to which one is involved (Fig. 10.20A and B).

Flexor digitorum superficialis and profundus (Figs 10.18 and 10.19)

MTrP sites and patterns of pain referral

TrPs in these two muscles tend to be found in the same part of the forearm as those in the flexor carpi radialis and ulnaris. However, as they lie at a deeper level locating them requires the application of very firm pressure and even with this, local twitch responses cannot be obtained.

TrPs in these two muscles refer pain to individual fingers (Fig. 10.21).

Flexor pollicis longus (Fig. 10.19)

MTrP sites and patterns of pain referral

As this muscle is also deeply placed, firm pressure is required to elicit any TrP activity in it. The site at which a TrP is usually found is on the radial side of the forearm about one-quarter of the way up from the wrist crease.

Pain from the TrP is referred to the thumb (Fig. 10.22).

PAIN FROM TrPs IN THE PALMARIS LONGUS AND PRONATOR TERES MUSCLES

TrP activity in these two forearm muscles may also cause pain to be referred to the hand.

Palmaris longus (Fig. 10.18)

This vestigial muscle, which is situated in the superficial layer of the flexor forearm muscles between the flexor carpi ulnaris and the flexor carpi radialis, is not always present but when it is, it also is attached proximally to the medial epicondyle and distally to the palmar fascia and has, as its main action, the cupping of the hand. It also assists flexion of the hand at the wrist.

Factors responsible for the development of TrP activity

TrPs in this muscle are liable to become activated should it be subject to direct trauma or following the repeated, excessively tight gripping of some object such as a tennis racquet or tool. They may also develop activity as a secondary event whenever pain is referred to the upper part of the forearm from TrPs just above the medial epicondyle in the medial head of the triceps muscle. In addition, Simons et al (1999b) have found that patients with Dupuytren's contracture invariably have one or more active TrPs in this forearm muscle.

MTrP sites and pattern of pain referral

TrPs in this muscle are liable to be found high up in the forearm just below the medial epicondyle.

Activity in them causes a persistent unpleasant tingling sensation to be felt in the palm of the hand (Fig. 10.23) and the patient complains of discomfort on applying pressure to any object held in the palm. This therefore makes the handling of tools difficult.

Deactivation of trigger points

Deactivation of these TrPs just below the elbow is carried out with the forearm extended and well supported.

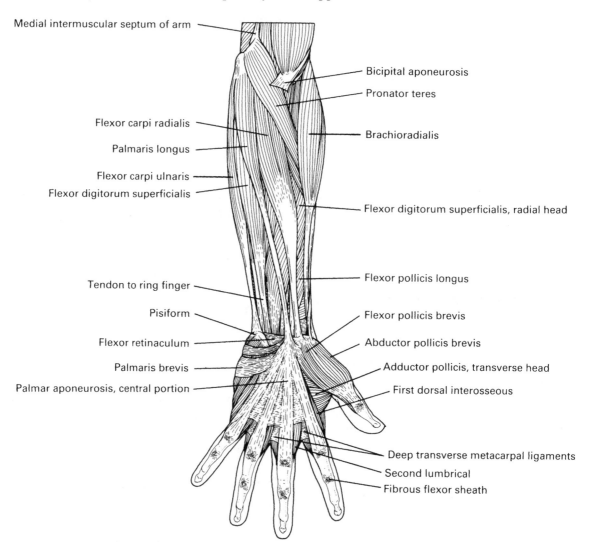

Figure 10.18 The superficial flexor muscles of the left forearm, the palmar aponeurosis and the digital fibrous flexor sheaths.

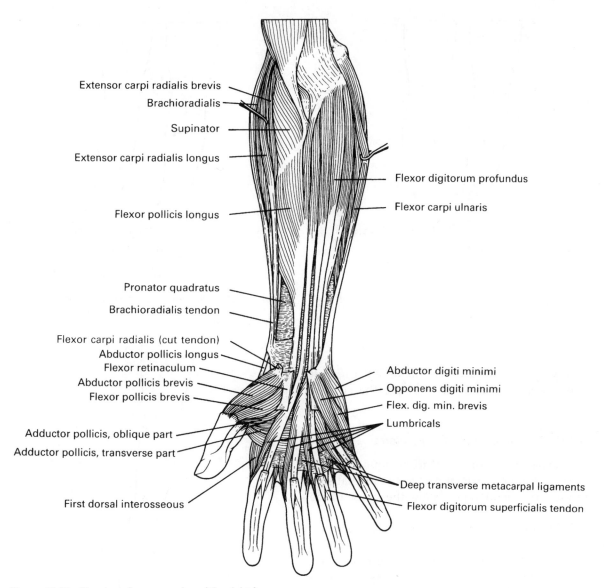

Extensor carpi radialis brevis
Brachioradialis
Supinator
Extensor carpi radialis longus

Flexor pollicis longus

Pronator quadratus
Brachioradialis tendon

Flexor carpi radialis (cut tendon)
Abductor pollicis longus
Flexor retinaculum
Abductor pollicis brevis
Flexor pollicis brevis

Adductor pollicis, oblique part
Adductor pollicis, transverse part

First dorsal interosseous

Flexor digitorum profundus
Flexor carpi ulnaris

Abductor digiti minimi
Opponens digiti minimi
Flex. dig. min. brevis
Lumbricals

Deep transverse metacarpal ligaments
Flexor digitorum superficialis tendon

Figure 10.19 The deep flexor muscles of the right forearm.

Pronator teres (Fig. 10.18)

This forearm muscle, which has a close anatomical relationship to the flexor forearm muscles, is attached above by two heads, its humeral head arising from the medial epicondyle, and its ulnar head from the coronoid process of the ulna. The median nerve enters the forearm between these

two heads. Distally it is attached to the lateral surface of the radius.

Factors responsible for the development of TrP activity

TrP activity in this muscle is particularly liable to develop following a fracture at the wrist or

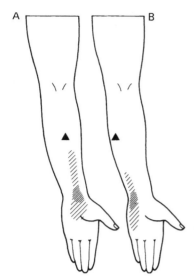

Figure 10.20 The patterns of pain referral from trigger points (▲) in (A) the flexor carpi radialis muscle and (B) the flexor carpi ulnaris muscle.

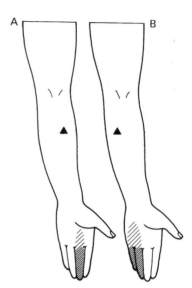

Figure 10.21 The patterns of pain referral from trigger points (▲) in the flexor digitorum superficialis (A) radial head (B) humeral head.

elbow. This TrP activity makes it difficult and extremely painful to supinate the cupped hand.

MTrP sites and pattern of pain referral

The usual place for a TrP to be found in this muscle is in its proximal part to the medial side of the biceps tendon just below the crease of the elbow.

Pain from this is referred down the outer side of the anterior surface of the forearm and is particularly pronounced around the radial side of the wrist, in much the same area as pain from TrP activity in the flexor carpi radialis (Fig. 10.24).

A patient with an active TrP in this muscle finds it difficult to turn the hand into the fully supinated position and is usually not able to turn it beyond the mid position.

MEDIAL EPICONDYLITIS

This enthesopathy, which is far less common than lateral epicondylitis, is brought about as a

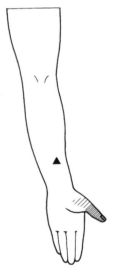

Figure 10.22 The pattern of pain referral from a trigger point (▲) in the flexor pollicis longus muscle.

result of the overloading of the forearm's hand and finger flexor muscles. Much of its pain is due to inflammatory and ultimately degenerative changes taking place in the common flexor tendon at its attachment to the medial epicondyle. Also to the development of TrP activity in forearm flexor muscles in the vicinity of their upper tendinous attachment and in the medial border

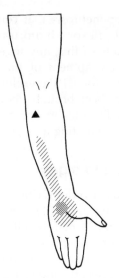

Figure 10.23   The pattern of pain referral from a trigger point (▲) in the palmaris longus muscle.

of the medial head of the triceps just above the elbow (p. 176).

It is characteristic of this disorder that resisted flexion of the wrist, when the elbow is extended, aggravates the pain.

The advantages and disadvantages of a local corticosteroid injection are similar to those when it is used in the treatment of lateral epicondylitis.

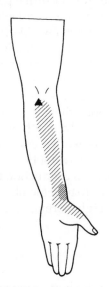

Figure 10.24   The pattern of pain referral from a trigger point (▲) in the pronator teres muscle.

And, as with the latter, deactivation of TrPs is often helpful in relieving the pain.

CUBITAL TUNNEL SYNDROME

The ulnar nerve at the elbow is held in a groove behind the medial epicondyle by a fibrous expansion of the common flexor tendon. From there it enters the forearm beneath an arch formed by the humeral and ulnar heads of the flexor carpi ulnaris muscle to occupy a space that is bounded by the flexor carpi ulnaris superficially and medially, the flexor digitorum superficialis above it and the flexor digitorum profundus behind it. Compression of the ulnar nerve at the elbow gives rise to what is known as the cubital tunnel syndrome.

Pathogenesis

The ulnar nerve is at risk of being damaged in the elbow region by external pressure applied to it where it lies behind the medial epicondyle. In addition, it may be compressed in the cubital tunnel by arthritic or other structural changes affecting the elbow or as a result of TrP-induced shortening of muscles in that region, particularly the flexor carpi ulnaris (Simons et al 1999c). Not infrequently, however, the syndrome arises in the absence of any obvious predisposing cause.

Symptoms and signs

The syndrome manifests itself by the gradual onset of numbness on the dorsum of the hand, tingling affecting the fifth finger and the ulnar half of the ring finger and, at a later stage, by weakness and wasting of the small muscles of the hand. There may, in addition, be pain along the ulnar border of the forearm and hand.

The clinical manifestations of the cubital tunnel syndrome have to be distinguished from those arising as a result of cervical nerve root (C8T1) entrapment; TrP activity in the levator scapulae (Ch. 8); TrP activity in the medial border of the medial head of the triceps (p. 176); and from those caused by the lower trunk of the brachial plexus becoming stretched as a result of it passing over a first rib or occasionally a cervical rib that has become elevated because of MTrP-induced shortening of the scalenus anterior or medius (thoracic outlet syndrome).

The diagnosis may be confirmed by demonstrating the presence of a delayed nerve conduction velocity at the point of entrapment.

Treatment

In those cases where the syndrome is caused by the activation of TrPs in the vicinity of the medial epicondyle the deactivation of these by relaxing the muscles containing them may prove sufficient to relieve the pressure on the nerve. When, however, the nerve has been damaged by external pressure applied to it or is bound down by fibrous tissue, a surgical operation to release it from the groove and transpose it to the front of the elbow is necessary.

CARPAL TUNNEL SYNDROME

Although compression of the median nerve in the carpal tunnel became recognised as a clinical entity soon after the Second World War (Brain et al 1947), and there are now good descriptions of the syndrome in standard textbooks, a brief account of it will be given here as one not sufficiently well-recognised possibility is that the disorder may occasionally develop as a result of compression of the nerve by taut bands at TrP sites either in the pronator teres or in the flexor digitorum superficialis.

Pathogenesis

This syndrome principally affects middle-aged women, but may arise in younger women and is occasionally seen in men.

It is in the main an idiopathic disorder but may at times be due to either a tenosynovitis in rheumatoid arthritis, fluid retention during pregnancy, or swelling of the soft tissue in either myxoedema or acromegaly. In addition, as Simons et al (1999d) have pointed out, the median nerve in the forearm passes behind the humeral and ulnar heads of the pronator teres (p. 187) and then

beneath the aponeurosis that connects the two heads of the flexor digitorum superficialis (p. 156). In view of this, any investigation as to the cause of entrapment of this nerve should include a search for TrPs to exclude the possibility that this has been brought about as a result of taut bands at TrP sites in one or other of these two muscles constricting it.

Symptoms and signs

The pain in this disorder is characteristically nocturnal, awakening the patient in the early hours of the morning. It is mainly felt at the wrist, but often ascends up the arm, at times as high as the shoulder. In addition, there are paraesthesiae which usually affect the index, middle and radial side of the ring finger, but surprisingly on occasions may also involve the little finger.

These nocturnal symptoms are often relieved by hanging the arm over the side of the bed. On waking in the morning, the hand frequently feels stiff and swollen.

During the day, there is little or no pain but the paraesthesiae persist and are made worse by any activity such as knitting or holding a book.

The condition, as might be expected, most often affects the dominant side but eventually it may become bilateral. The nocturnal pain and the nocturnal and diurnal paraesthesiae may persist for many months without any objective neurological signs developing, but eventually weakness and wasting of two of the thenar muscles (abductor pollicis brevis and opponens pollicis) cause flattening of the outer half of the thenar eminence.

On examination, the pain and tingling can often be provoked by applying pressure to a point of exquisite tenderness over the anterior carpal ligament. If any doubt as to the diagnosis remains, an electrical conduction test may be carried out but it has to be remembered that this test may be misleadingly normal in cases with a short history.

Treatment

When the history is short, conservative measures are justifiable. The avoidance of activities which aggravate the symptoms is advisable, and the wearing of a splint at night is beneficial. In addition, the local injection of a corticosteroid may prove helpful. Care has to be taken, however, not to inject the material into the median nerve, or into the tendon of the palmaris longus.

In those cases where clinical examination reveals the presence of TrPs in the pronator teres or flexor digitorum superficialis, then clearly deactivation of these by one or other of the methods discussed in Chapter 7 should be carried out.

When symptoms are long-standing and particularly where there is evidence of muscle wasting, decompression of the median nerve by division of the flexor retinaculum is essential.

TENOSYNOVITIS OF THE WRIST

Inflammation of the synovial sheaths surrounding the tendons around the wrist joint is liable to occur whenever the forearm muscles are used excessively or the fingers are worked both hard and rapidly such as, for example, during the course of some athletic or occupational pursuit.

The pain, which can be quite severe, is felt along the line of one or more of the tendons at the wrist. It is usually associated with swelling around an affected tendon and characteristically crepitus will be felt on the movement of it.

The disorder known as de Quervain's tenosynovitis is one which affects the conjoined tendons of the extensor pollicis brevis and extensor pollicis longus as they pass over the styloid process of the radius. It is liable to occur as a result of any activity associated with strenuous repetitive movement of the thumb and leads to the development of pain and tenderness over the styloid process with crepitus on extending the thumb. Athletes, manual workers and patients with rheumatoid arthritis, psoriatic arthritis and other inflammatory synovitides are prone to developing it.

Treatment

Treatment includes resting the affected part on a splint or in a plaster cast. Cases which do not respond to this should have an injection of a corticosteroid into an affected tendon sheath.

Extreme care, however, has to be taken not to inject the material into the tendon itself as this may cause it to rupture.

PAIN FROM MTrPs AROUND THE THUMB

The muscles around the thumb include the adductor pollicis and a group of muscles made up of the opponens pollicis covered by the abductor and flexor pollicis brevis. Of these, it is the adductor pollicis and opponens pollicis which most commonly develop TrP activity. This is because their function is to assist with gripping objects between the thumb and fingers.

The action of the adductor pollicis is to bring the thumb into contact with the palm of the hand. The action of the opponens pollicis is to bring the palmar surface of the thumb into contact with the palmar surface of the top of any of the fingers. TrP activity is therefore liable to develop in either of these two muscles should it become overloaded as a result of forceful gripping. Examples of when this is liable to happen include prolonged sewing, writing and pulling up firmly embedded roots.

The anatomical location of these two thumb muscles is shown in Figure 10.25 and their patterns of MTrP pain referral are depicted in Figures 10.26 and 10.27.

In order to locate and deactivate a TrP in the adductor pollicis, the pronated hand should be placed on a pillow. Palpation is carried out with the first dorsal interosseous muscle pushed to one side.

In order to locate and deactivate a TrP in the opponens pollicis the supinated hand should be place on a pillow and palpation carried out over the thenar eminence.

TrP activity in either of these two muscles is usually accompanied by TrP activity in the first dorsal interosseous muscle.

FIRST CARPOMETACARPAL JOINT OSTEOARTHRITIS

MTrP pain around the base of the thumb has to be distinguished from osteoarthritis involving the first carpometacarpal joint.

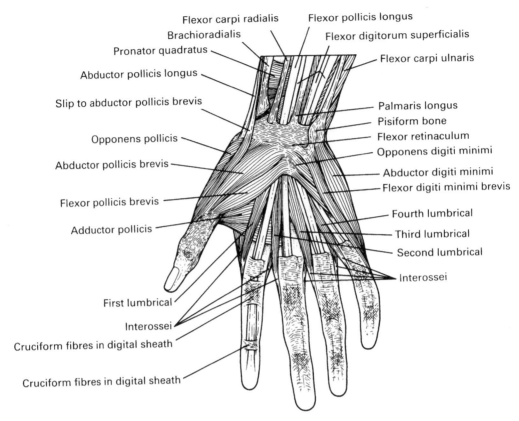

Figure 10.25   Superficial dissection of muscles of the palm of the right hand.

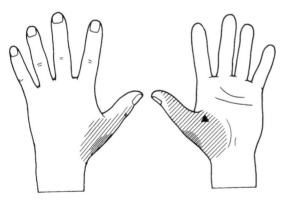

Figure 10.26   The pattern of pain referral from a trigger point (▲) in the adductor pollicis muscle.

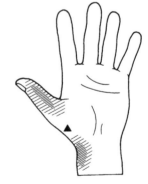

Figure 10.27 The pattern of pain referral from a trigger point (▲) in the opponens pollicis muscle.

Palpation of the joint reveals the presence of one or more periarticular tender points. And superficial dry needling of A-delta fibres in the skin and subcutaneous tissues at these points is often helpful in relieving the pain.

MTrP PAIN IN THE FINGERS

As stated earlier, pain may be referred to the fingers from TrPs in the flexor digitorum superficialis and profundus (p. 188) and the extensor digitorum (p. 183).

Pain in the fingers with stiffness of their movements may also occur because of TrP activity developing in an interosseous muscle (Fig. 10.22) when it becomes overloaded as a result of two fingers being closely approximated for the purpose of obtaining a sustained or repetitive pincer grasp.

TrPs in these muscles are difficult to palpate but it is important to be able to distinguish between pain emanating from them, pain referred to the fingers from forearm muscle TrPs and pain developing in them as a result of various other disorders such as cervical radiculopathy (Ch. 8), ulnar nerve compression (p. 189) and brachial plexus entrapment (Ch. 9).

OSTEOARTHRITIC SMALL JOINTS OF THE HAND

When osteoarthritic changes take place in a small joint of the hand palpation around it reveals the presence of periarticular tender points. And superficial dry needling of A-delta fibres in the skin and subcutaneous tissues at these points is often helpful in relieving the pain.

MANAGEMENT OF THE BRACHIAL MTrP PAIN SYNDROME

It is not only necessary to locate and deactivate all of the MTrPs in the neck, shoulder girdle, chest wall and arm from which pain in the arm may be emanating but also to identify what caused the MTrP activity to develop so that whenever possible measures may be taken to prevent it from recurring. And as discussed in the introduction to this chapter, these must perforce include a detailed examination of the musculoskeletal system from the feet upwards.

TrPs in both the superficial and deep muscles of the arm are usually readily deactivated by any of the methods described in Chapter 7 including superficial dry needling. And a particular advantage of this latter method is that with it there is less risk of damaging blood vessels and nerves. Thus, for example, when it

is used for deactivating TrPs in the deeply lying brachialis muscle the chance of injuring the radial or median nerve which lie respectively on the outer and inner borders of the muscle is minimal.

As elsewhere in the body it is essential for the deactivation of TrPs in the arm to be followed by muscle stretching exercises.

REPETITIVE STRAIN INJURY
A multiplicity of terms

When keyboard operators in Australia first began to complain of work-related pain in the arm during the early 1980s it was called repetitive strain injury (RSI).

Unfortunately, this term quickly acquired emotive connotations and partly because of this, and partly because of fallacious popular concepts concerning the nature of the disorder, its incidence rapidly increased. An epidemic of it was only brought under control once steps were taken to defuse this emotionally charged situation (Littlejohn 1986). Included amongst these was the Australian College of Physicians' advice in the mid 1980s to abandon the pejorative term RSI and to call it instead regional pain syndrome (Quintner 1991).

This term has since been widely adopted (Littlejohn 1996) but in an attempt to improve upon it, a plethora of other names have been introduced. These have included occupational cervicobrachial disorder (Aoyama 1985), occupational overuse syndrome (Ellis 1988), chronic upper limb pain syndrome (Miller & Topliss 1988), refractory cervicobrachial syndrome (Cohen et al 1992), localised fibromyalgia (Littlejohn 1995) and cumulative trauma disorder (Headley 1997).

Because none of these terms has any particular advantage over any of the others and because RSI is the one that is still most widely used, it will continue to be employed during the course of this discussion. Nevertheless, it has to be said that it is far from satisfactory, for in this context 'strain' is not used in its true mechanical sense and 'injury' implies culpability on the part of an employer that may or may not be justified (Barton et al 1992).

Epidemic in Britain

The 1990s saw a dramatic rise in the incidence of work-related upper limb pain in the United Kingdom, with the overall pattern of the epidemic being very similar to the one which prevailed in Australia during the 1970s and 1980s (Reilly 1995). Keyboard operators employed in large organisations such as the Inland Revenue, British Broadcasting Corporation, the Post Office, clearing banks and the newspaper industry have been amongst those especially affected by it.

The following are some of the more important contributory factors: the failure of doctors and employers to learn from the experience gained by their Australian counterparts; ignorance amongst doctors concerning the optimum management of the disorder; trade union intransigence and combativeness; dissemination of emotive and misleading information by both government-sponsored health authorities and patient-oriented support groups; media sensationalism; and protracted confrontational medicolegal proceedings.

The situation, however, would seem to be gradually improving due to an increasingly enlightened approach to the disorder by both doctors and employers with, above all, the provision of rehabilitation programmes that have as their aim a graduated return to normal work. Also, by an increasing reluctance of employees to become subjected to the stresses imposed upon them by the adversarial British legal system.

Aetiology

Repetitive muscular overactivity

The main aetiological factor is prolonged repetitive muscular movements carried out during the course of some occupational or recreational activity.

People liable to be affected

Women are affected about six times more often than men (Huskisson 1992).

A wide range of workers are particularly at risk of developing this disorder. These include keyboard operators, electronic assemblers, machine operatives, seamstresses, ceramic manufacturers, poultry pluckers, process workers and musicians. The disorder may also affect people who play computer games.

Emotional factors

It is widely believed that RSI is common among those of an anxious temperament. It has to be said, however, that much of the anxiety in people with this disorder is a secondary event that is brought on by the suffering caused by persistent pain and the worry this engenders concerning job security.

Biomechanical factors

The adoption of a faulty posture commonly causes this disorder to develop. For example, the incorrect height of a chair or desk may lead to a computer operator developing pain as a result of a wrist being held in a persistently hyperextended position.

Pathophysiology and clinical manifestations

In our present state of knowledge it is only possible to hypothesise about the pathophysiology of RSI (Cohen et al 1992). The pain in this disorder initially takes the form of an aching sensation localised to either the wrist, elbow or shoulder and is brought on by the carrying out of a task involving prolonged repetitive hand movements. At this early stage it is relieved by resting but if such type of work is continued with, the pain increases in intensity until eventually it becomes unremitting and extremely severe. Paraesthesiae in the hands and cramps may then also be experienced. The persistent pain is then liable to keep the patient awake and the loss of sleep may not only exacerbate the pain but may also lead to the development of early morning stiffness of the affected muscles.

Clinical examination shows that much, if not all, of the pain in this disorder emanates initially from MTrPs (Headley 1997, Lin et al 1997) and fibromyalgia-like tender points (Grange & Littlejohn 1993). The intense sensory afferent barrage set up by the nociceptor activity at these two types of points then leads to the rapid development of neuroplastic changes in dorsal horn nociceptive neurons – the phenomenon known as central sensitisation (Ch. 2).

One of the effects of this central sensitisation is to induce long-term changes in these dorsal horn neurons' synaptic processes with, as a consequence, an increase in the number of them that respond to the sensory afferent barrage from the peripheral nociceptive source (Mense 1997). And it may be this that accounts for the rapid spread of pain in this disorder.

Another of its effects is the development of widespread hyperalgesia due to A-beta-mediated pain arising as a result of these sensitised dorsal horn neurons responding to light touch-induced stimulation of mechanoreceptors in the skin (Ch. 2). In addition, the sensory afferent input to the dorsal horn has a stimulating effect on sympathetic preganglionic neurons there with, as a result, the development of sympathetic efferent activity (Livingston 1943). The latter, as Roberts (1986) has postulated, may activate A-beta mechanoreceptors in the skin in a similar manner to that normally brought about by cutaneous stimulation. The effect of this would then be to stimulate sensitised dorsal horn nociceptive neurons with, as a consequence, the development of sympathetically maintained pain. It is presumably because of the development of this sympathetically mediated activity that the pain in this disorder may over the course of time develop a burning character and why allodynia, coldness of the limb and tissue swelling may also be prominent features.

Management

Pain

Those physicians who have come to realise that myofascial trigger points and tender points are important sources of pain in this disorder

(Simons et al 1999e) deactivate them by one means or another. However, clinical trials need to be carried out to show whether this alone is sufficient to control the pain or whether it needs to be combined with other currently employed forms of treatment. Also, to see whether deactivating TrPs immediately the disorder develops helps to reduce the incidence of dorsal horn neuroplasticity and the adverse clinical effects produced by it.

All this notwithstanding Littlejohn (1995) has found that when treatment is started at a very early stage a simple analgesic is often all that is required to control the pain.

Sleep disturbance

Patients with RSI, like those with fibromyalgia, are liable to have non-restorative sleep. In such cases a tricyclic antidepressant such as amitriptyline (10–20 mg at night) often improves the sleep pattern and ameliorates the early morning muscle aching and stiffness.

Stress

The use of some simple stress-relieving technique such as hypnotherapy is often helpful in the same way as it is for patients with fibromyalgia (Haanen et al 1991). Alternatively, the somewhat more complex cognitive-behavioural therapy employed by psychotherapists has been shown to be effective (Spence 1989).

Adjustments to working conditions

It is generally agreed that the aim should be to get a person affected by the disorder back to work as soon as possible, for the longer this is delayed the more difficult it becomes. At the same time it is essential that any necessary adjustments to working conditions are made as otherwise a recurrence of symptoms is inevitable. However, it has to be admitted that in a severe case a change of occupation may prove unavoidable (Huskisson 1992).

Avoidance of RSI

Avoidance of this disorder is largely the responsibility of employers and supervisors. They should insist that work which entails the use of rapid hand movements should only be carried out for 1–2 hours at a time, followed by breaks of about 15 minutes. And that tasks liable to bring on the syndrome should be interspersed with others which do not carry this risk. They should also ensure that working conditions are such that faulty postures may be avoided; that employees work as far as possible in a stress-free environment; that they receive adequate training; and that they are not coerced into working excessively long hours by bonus and overtime incentives. In addition, employers are legally obligated to warn workers of any particular occupational risks, to heed employees' complaints and, once symptoms of the disorder appear, to withdraw the employee immediately from the type of work responsible for its development.

Differential diagnosis

RSI has to be distinguished from a number of other disorders that are liable to be brought on by repetitive movements carried out during the course of occupational or sporting activities. These include the rotator cuff syndrome, lateral epicondylitis, carpal tunnel syndrome, tenosynovitis and writer's cramp.

Rotator cuff tendinitis

This disorder (Ch. 9) is prone to affect athletes such as swimmers who use high overhead actions (Hawkins & Kennedy 1980). It may also develop in professional musicians, particularly string and wind players (Sola 1994).

Lateral epicondylitis (syn: tennis elbow)

Although this disorder (p. 183) is liable to be brought on by overuse of the extensors and supinators of the wrist there is no clear evidence that it is occupationally related (Barton et al 1992). Thus although Luopajarvi et al (1979) found it to

be commoner in assembly line workers than in shop assistants, Dimberg (1987) conversely, in a survey of staff at the Volvo aircraft engine division, found that its incidence among white collar and manual workers was the same.

Carpal tunnel syndrome

Differentiating clinically between RSI and the carpal tunnel syndrome is not always easy as in some cases the symptoms are similar. However, with RSI, electrical testing is normal and injecting the carpal tunnel with a steroid or surgically decompressing it is not helpful (Huskisson 1992).

To add to the difficulty there is reason to believe that certain occupational tasks may contribute to the carpal tunnel syndrome's development. Feldman et al (1987) found this syndrome to be common amongst those workers in an electronic factory who had to carry out repetitive hand movements. Birkbeck & Beer (1975) found a significant incidence of it in those who performed similar movements during the course of making boots and shoes. And both Lockwood (1989) and Sola (1994) have found that professional musicians, particularly pianists, clarinettists and oboists, are liable to develop it.

This notwithstanding, Nathan et al (1988), from the carrying out of nerve conduction studies on 471 employees doing 27 different types of work in 4 factories, concluded that there is no correlation between occupationally-related hand movements and the prevalence and severity of impaired median nerve conduction. And in support of this Hadler (1985) and Barton et al (1992) have failed to find evidence that occupationally related hand movements are responsible primarily for the syndrome developing, Barton et al (1992) only being willing to concede that 'if the disorder is already present certain tasks may exacerbate it'.

Tenosynovitis

As stated on p. 191, tenosynovitis is well recognised to be brought on by unaccustomed repetitive movements carried out during the course of some athletic or occupational pursuit and, with respect to the latter, Thompson et al (1951) found that movements of this type were the cause of it developing in 544 workers at the Vauxhall car factory. And Hochberg et al (1983) have reported a high incidence in professional musicians, particularly keyboard instrumentalists.

In addition, de Quervain's stenosing tenosynovitis, a disorder which affects the conjoined tendons of the extensor pollicis brevis and abductor pollicis longus (see p. 191), is liable to affect workers such as cooks and dressmakers who have to carry out tasks that involve pinching repetitive movements with the thumb whilst moving the wrist from side to side (Leao 1958).

Writer's cramp

Cramp in the hand brought on by prolonged periods of writing is a long-recognised entity. During the last century it was known as scriveners' palsy, the term scrivener being derived from the old French escrivain (a clerk) and the Latin scriba (a scribe). Samuel Solly, a physician at St Thomas' Hospital, wrote about it in 1864, describing how men whose employment caused them to write incessantly developed incapacitating pain of a burning or aching character together with cramp in the hand. Sir John Reynolds, in his textbook published in 1872, observed that it could also affect musicians (Huskisson 1992).

The disorder is now recognised to be a focal dystonia with tonic spasm causing a pen to be gripped too tightly. However, somewhat surprisingly, as Hopkins (1993) has pointed out, a person affected by it can use a word processor without any difficulty.

Lockwood (1989), during the course of discussing the medical problems of musicians, states that those with a focal dystonia report, 'incoordination while playing, frequently accompanied by involuntary curling or extension of fingers during passages of music that require rapid forceful finger movements'.

One difference, however, between focal dystonia in writers and musicians is that the incoordinated movements in the latter may, in some cases, be painless (Newmark & Hochberg 1987).

SYMPATHETICALLY MEDIATED BRACHIAL PAIN
Concomitant complex regional and MTrP pain syndromes

As discussed in Chapter 6, the complex regional pain syndrome type 1 (RSD) and the MTrP pain syndrome may develop in the arm concomitantly due to the main aetiological factor responsible for the development of this being trauma. In addition, they may develop occasionally following either a myocardial infarction or a cerebrovascular accident (see Chs 5 and 14).

Shoulder–hand syndrome

The sympathetically mediated brachial pain disorder now known as the shoulder–hand syndrome (Steinbrocker 1947) is a long-recognised one for as Bonica & Sola (1990) have pointed out, Mitchell first observed it in patients with coronary heart disease in 1874, Osler referred to it in his lectures on angina pectoris published in 1897 and Chevallier described its occurrence in hemiplegic limbs in 1867.

The disorder (see Ch. 9) develops as a complication of a frozen shoulder (adhesive capsulitis) that has arisen either spontaneously, or following a rotator cuff tendinitis, or as a result of the shoulder joint having been kept immobile for a long period following, for example, a myocardial infarction or stroke. Hazelman (1990) has pointed out that patients even with minor degrees of frozen shoulder are liable to develop it.

The syndrome has an insidious onset with its initial manifestations being a burning pain in the shoulder and vasomotor changes in the hand. And then, after a period of time, the shoulder pain tends to ease but progressively worsening trophic changes take place in the hand, including thickening of the palmar fascia and atrophy of the muscles and nails.

The treatment of this disorder is far from easy. The pain, which is liable to be intense, may require narcotics for its relief. In addition, sympathetic blocks and the deactivation of MTrPs may prove helpful. Exercises to maintain function should also be carried out (Sola 1994).

REFERENCES

Aoyama H 1985 Occupational cervicobrachial disorder. In: International labour office encyclopaedia of occupational health and safety. ILO, Geneva, vol 1, pp 440–442

Aronson P R, Murray D G, Fitzsimmons R M 1971 Myofascitis: a frequently overlooked cause of pain in cervical root distribution. North Carolina Medical Journal 32:463–465

Assendelft W J, Hay E M, Adshead R et al 1996 Corticosteroid injections for lateral epicondylitis: a systematic overview. British Journal of General Practice 46(405):209–216

Barton N J, Hooper G, Noble J, Steel W M 1992 Occupational causes of disorders in the upper limb. British Medical Journal 304:309–311

Binder A I, Hazelman B L 1983 Lateral humeral epicondylitis – a study of natural history and the effect of conservative therapy. British Journal of Rheumatology 22:73–76

Binder A, Parr G, Page T P, Hazelman B 1983 A clinical and thermographic study of lateral epicondylitis. British Journal of Rheumatology 22:77–81

Birkbeck M Q, Beer T C 1975 Occupation in relation to the carpal tunnel syndrome. Rheumatology & Rehabilitation 14:218–221

Bonica J J, Sola A E 1990 Other painful disorders of the upper limb. In: Bonica J J (ed) The management of pain, 2nd edn. Lea & Febiger, Philadelphia, p 955

Bosworth D M 1965 Surgical treatment of tennis elbow. New York State Journal of Medicine 79:1363–1366

Brain W R, Wright A D, Wilkinson M 1947 Spontaneous compression of both median nerves in the carpal tunnel. Lancet i:277–282

Calvert P T, Macpherson I S, Allum R L, Bentley G 1985 Simple lateral release in treatment of tennis elbow. Journal of the Royal Society of Medicine 78:912–915

Chard M D 1995 Aspiration and injection of joints and periarticular tissues – the elbow region. In: Klippel J H, Dieppe P A (eds) Practical rheumatology. Times Mirror International Publishers, London, pp 115–116

Chard M D, Hazelman B L 1989 Tennis elbow – a reappraisal. British Journal of Rheumatology 28(3):186–189

Chatterjee D S 1987 Repetitive strain injury: a recent review. Journal of Society of Occupational Medicine 37:100–105

Cohen M L, Arroyo J T, Champion G D, Browne D 1992 Hypothesis. In search of the pathogenesis of refractory cervicobrachial pain syndrome. A deconstruction of the RSI phenomenon. The Medical Journal of Australia 156:432–436

Coonrad R W, Hooper W R 1973 Tennis elbow: course, natural history, conservative and surgical management. Journal of Bone and Joint Surgery (Am) 55:1177–1187

Dimberg L 1987 The prevalence and causation of tennis elbow (lateral humeral epicondylitis) in a population of workers in an engineering industry. Ergonomics 30:573

Ellis N 1988 Occupational overuse syndrome. Patient Management 12(June):133–143

Feldman R G, Travers P H, Charico-Post J, Keyserling W M 1987 Risk assessment in electronic assembly workers: carpal tunnel syndrome. Journal of Hand Surgery (Am) 12A:849–855

Gerwin R D 1997 Myofascial pain syndromes in the upper extremity. Journal of Hand Therapy 10:130–136

Grange G, Littlejohn G O 1993 Prevalence of myofascial pain syndrome in fibromyalgia syndrome and regional pain syndrome: a comparative study. Journal of Musculoskeletal Pain 1(2):19–35

Haanen H C M, Hoenderdos H T W, Van Romunde L K J et al 1991 Controlled trial of hypnotherapy in the treatment of refractory fibromyalgia. Journal of Rheumatology 18:72–75

Hadler N M 1985 Illness in the workplace. The challenge of musculoskeletal symptoms. Journal of Hand Surgery (Am) 10A:451–456

Hawkins R J, Kennedy J S 1980 The impingement syndrome in athletes. American Journal of Sports Medicine 8:57–62

Hazelman B 1990 Musculoskeletal and connective tissue disease. In: Souhami R L, Moxham J (eds) Textbook of medicine, Churchill Livingstone, p 1032

Headley B J 1997 Physiologic risk factors. In: Sanders M (ed) Management of cumulative trauma disorders. Butterworth-Heinemann, London, pp 107–127

Hochberg F H, Letfert R D, Heller M D, Merriman L 1983 Hand difficulties among musicians. Journal of the American Medical Association 249:1869–1872

Hopkins A 1993 Clinical neurology. A modern approach. University Press, Oxford, pp 225–226

Huskisson E 1992 Repetitive strain injury: the keyboard disease. Charterhouse Conference and Communications Company, London

International Association for the Study of Pain Subcommittee on Taxonomy 1979 Pain terms: a list with definitions and notes on usage. Pain 6:249–252

Leao L 1958 De Quervain's stenosing tenovaginitis. A clinical and anatomical study. Journal of Bone and Joint Surgery (Am) 40A:1063–1070

Lin T Y, Teixeira M J, Fischer A A et al 1997 Work-related musculoskeletal disorders. Physical Medicine and Rehabilitation Clinics of North America, Philadelphia, pp 113–117

Littlejohn G O 1986 Repetitive pain syndrome: an Australian experience. Journal of Rheumatology 13:1004–1006

Littlejohn G O 1995 Key issues in repetitive strain injury. Journal of Musculoskeletal Pain 3(2):25–33

Littlejohn G O 1996 Clinical update on other pain syndromes. Journal of Musculoskeletal Pain 4(1/2):163–179

Livingston W K 1943 Pain mechanisms. Macmillan, New York

Lockwood A H 1989 Medical problems of musicians. New England Journal of Medicine 320:221–227

Luopajarvi V, Kuorinka I, Virolainen A, Holmberg M 1979 Prevalence of tenosynovitis and other injuries of the upper extremities in repetitive work. Scandinavian Journal of Work and Environmental Health 5(suppl 3):48–55

Mense S 1997 Pathophysiologic basis of muscle pain syndromes. An update. Physical Medicine and Rehabilitation Clinics of North America 8(1):23–53

Miller M H, Topliss D J 1988 Chronic upper arm pain syndrome (repetitive strain injury) in the Australian workforce: a systematic cross-sectional rheumatologic study of 229 patients. Journal of Rheumatology 15:1705–1712

Nathan P A, Meadows K D, Doyle E 1988 Occupation as a risk factor for impaired sensory conduction of the median nerve at the carpal tunnel syndrome. Journal of Hand Surgery (Br) 13B:167–170

Neipal G A, Sitaj S 1979 Enthesopathy. Clinics in rheumatic diseases 5:857–872

Newmark J, Hochberg F H 1987 Isolated painless manual incoordination in 57 musicians. Journal of Neurology, Neurosurgery and Psychiatry 50:291–295

Quintner J 1991 The RSI syndrome in historical perspective. International Disability Studies 13:99–104

Reilly P A 1995 Approaches to RSI in the United Kingdom. Journal of Musculoskeletal Pain 3(2):123–125

Reynolds M D 1981 Myofascial trigger point syndromes in the practice of rheumatology. Archives of Physical Medicine and Rehabilitation 62:111–114

Roberts W B 1986 A hypothesis on the physiological basis for causalgia and related pain. Pain 24:297–311

Rosen M J, Duffy F B, Miller E H et al 1980 Tennis elbow syndrome: results of the lateral release procedure. Ohio State Medical Journal 76:103–109

Simons D G, Travell J G, Simons L S 1999a–e Travell & Simons' myofascial pain and dysfunction. The trigger point manual, 2nd edn. Williams & Wilkins, Baltimore, vol 1, pp 734–736 (a), p 746 (b), pp 704–705 (c), p 765 (d), p 41 (e)

Sola A E 1994 Upper extremity pain. In: Wall PD, Melzack R (eds) Textbook of pain, 3rd edn. Churchill Livingstone, Edinburgh, ch 25

Spence S H 1989 Cognitive-behaviour therapy in the management of chronic occupational pain in the upper limbs. Behaviour Research and Therapy 27:435–446

Steinbrocker O 1947 The shoulder–hand syndrome. American Journal of Medicine 3:402

Thompson A R, Plewes L W, Shaw E G 1951 Peritendinitis crepitans and simple tenosynovitis: a clinical study of 544 cases in industry. British Journal of Industrial Medicine 8:150–159

Travell J, Rinzler S H 1952 The myofascial genesis of pain. Postgraduate Medicine 11:425–434

11

The head and face

INTRODUCTION

In this chapter attention will be drawn to three causes of pain in the head: myofascial trigger point (MTrP) cephalalgia, migraine and tension-type headaches. Also, to temporo-facial MTrP pain, trigeminal neuralgia, atypical facial pain, migrainous neuralgia and various disorders in and around the temporomandibular joint including the temporomandibular MTrP pain syndrome.

MYOFASCIAL TRIGGER POINT CEPHALALGIA

Cephalalgia arising as a result of the activation and sensitisation of nociceptors at TrP sites in muscles of either the scalp or neck is not included in the classification system (Box 11.1) devised by the Headache Classification Committee of the International Headache Society (1988). However, those who include a search for MTrPs as part of their routine physical examination in all cases of persistent head pain have come to realise that it is an extremely common but poorly recognised disorder.

Cephalalgia of this type is liable to arise as a result of TrP activity developing in one or more of the following muscles: in the scalp, the occipitofrontalis and temporalis muscles; and in the neck, the upper part of the trapezius, the sternocleidomastoid and the posterior cervical group of muscles.

Box 11.1 IHS Headache Classification Committee

A – Primary Headache Disorders
Migraine:
1.1   Migraine without aura (formerly common
         migraine)
1.2   Migraine with aura (formerly classical migraine)
1.3–1.7 Migraine sub-types
2   Tension-type headache (formerly tension
         headache, muscle contraction headache,
         psychogenic headache)
3   Cluster headache
4   Miscellaneous headaches without structural
         lesion
B – Secondary Headache Disorders
5   Headache associated with head trauma
6–13   Other secondary headache disorders

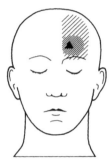

Figure 11.1 The pattern of pain referral from a trigger point in the frontalis belly of the occipitofrontalis muscle.

Occipitofrontalis muscle

Anatomical attachments

The occipitofrontalis scalp muscle consists of two occipital bellies and two frontalis bellies and an interconnecting epicranial aponeurosis (galea aponeurotica). The frontalis part of the muscle is attached anteriorly to the skin above the orbit. The occipitalis part is attached posteriorly to the occipital bone.

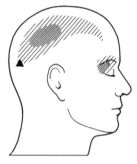

Figure 11.2 The pattern of pain referral from a trigger point in the occipitalis belly of the occipitofrontalis muscle.

Factors responsible for development of TrP activity

TrPs in the frontalis part of this muscle are liable to become active as a primary event in people who persistently have an anxiety-induced furrowed brow, and as a secondary event when pain is referred to the forehead from TrPs in the sternocleidomastoid muscle.

TrPs in its occipitalis part are liable to develop activity as a primary event when, because of anxiety or impaired visual acuity, the scalp muscles are held in a persistently contracted state. They may develop as a secondary event when pain is referred to the back of the head from TrPs in the posterior cervical muscles or the sternocleidomastoid muscle.

TrPs in the frontalis part are liable to be found near to its insertion immediately above the orbit. Pain from these TrPs is referred to the forehead (Fig. 11.1). TrPs in the occipital part are liable to

be found anywhere at the back of the head. Pain from these is referred forwards along the side of the head into the eye (Fig. 11.2).

Deactivation of myofascial trigger points

Because the frontalis part of this muscle is thin the carrying out of any of the deeply applied deactivating techniques discussed in Chapter 7 is technically difficult. Therefore superficial dry needling is recommended.

The occipitalis part of the muscle is thicker and therefore TrPs in it may readily be deactivated by any method.

Preventative measures

The patient must avoid persistently contracting the scalp. The teaching of a relaxation technique such as autohypnosis is often helpful. TrPs in other muscles liable to cause satellite TrP activity to develop in this muscle must be located and deactivated.

Temporalis muscle

TrP activity in this muscle may give rise to either cranial pain or craniofacial pain and develops principally as a result of masticatory dysfunction. Consideration of this muscle's TrP pain will therefore be deferred until masticatory disorders in general are discussed later in the chapter.

Upper part of the trapezius, sternocleidomastoid and posterior cervical group of muscles

As explained in Chapter 8, the concomitant development of TrP activity in several muscles of the neck is liable to give rise to restricted movements of the neck together with widespread pain in the head, neck and arm in the disorder known as the cervical MTrP pain syndrome. There are, however, in addition cases where TrP activity in one or more of the following muscles leads to the development of pain localised to the cranium.

Upper part of the trapezius muscle

Factors responsible for TrP-induced headaches

Circumstances liable to lead to the development of TrP activity in the upper part of the trapezius muscle with, as a consequence, the referral of pain along the side of the head to the temple (see Fig. 8.11) include sagging of the shoulder girdle as a result of the scoliosis of the spine that develops when one leg is shorter than the other; the setting up of a sustained pull on this muscle as a result of disproportionately short arms not allowing the elbows to reach the arm rests of the average chair; the overloading of this part of the muscle as a result of it having to provide support for the arm during, for example, the prolonged use of a telephone or computer; and as a result of it having to keep the shoulder girdle in a persistently elevated position such as, for example, when playing a violin. Also, the pressure of tight or heavy clothing.

Sternocleidomastoid muscle

Factors responsible for TrP-induced headaches

Reasons for TrPs becoming active in this muscle with, as a consequence, the referral of pain to the head (see Fig. 8.12A and B) include persistent hyperextension of the neck during the course of, for example, painting a ceiling or watching a play performed on a high stage; prolonged twisting of the neck, such as may happen when reading in bed by the aid of a light obtained from a lamp placed at the side of it (Fig. 11.3); overloading of the muscle as a result of sagging of the shoulder girdle when scoliosis of the spine develops in someone with one leg shorter than the other; and overloading of it as a result of sleeping with the neck in a kinked position.

In addition, because this muscle and its contralateral counterpart are accessory muscles of respiration they are liable to become overloaded during inspiration in chronic obstructive airways disease.

Posterior cervical group of muscles

Factors responsible for TrP-induced headaches

Reasons for TrPs becoming active in this group of muscles with, as a consequence, the referral of

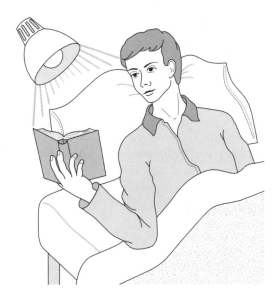

Figure 11.3 Overloading of the right sternocleidomastoid muscle as a result of prolonged kinking of the neck.

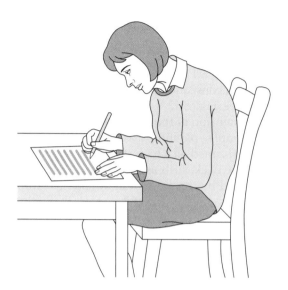

Figure 11.4   Overloading of the posterior cervical group of muscles as a result of sitting crouched over a desk.

pain to the head (see Figs 8.4 and 8.5) include the overloading of one or more of these muscles as a result of the adoption of a poor posture crouched over a desk or workbench (Fig. 11.4). And their overloading as a result of sleeping in the supine position with the neck hyperextended.

MIGRAINE

Classification

The Headache Classification Committee of the International Headache Society (1988) has divided migraine into no less than seven types (Box 11.1). The two main ones, however, are migraine without aura (formerly known as common migraine) and migraine with aura (formerly known as classical migraine).

Pathogenesis

The factors responsible for migraine developing are vascular, myofascial and emotional. These will be considered in turn as the long-term control of this disorder depends on directing treatment at any or all of them according to the needs of each individual patient.

Vascular nociceptive component

Vessels in the brain, meninges and venous sinuses have plexuses of unmyelinated C fibres in their walls. And, as a result of the activation of nociceptors in the peripheral terminals of these sensory afferents, noxiously generated information is conveyed to that part of the trigeminal brainstem's sensory nuclear complex known as the subnucleus caudalis which, because of its morphological and physiological similarities to spinal dorsal horns, is also known as the medullary dorsal horn. As will be discussed later, in addition to this vascular nociceptive input to the subnucleus caudalis there are also myofascial and supraspinal (emotional) ones and, following their integration in that structure, migraine-evoking activity is transmitted up the quinto-thalamic tract to the cerebral cortex (Fig. 11.5).

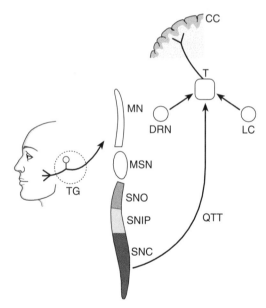

Figure 11.5   Diagram to show neuroanatomy of the trigeminal system with particular reference to the subnucleus caudalis (SNC) in which migraine-evoking activity is integrated before being transmitted up the quintothalamic tract (QTT) to the cerebral cortex (CC) via the thalamus (T). The thalamic processing of this information is influenced by a serotonergic input from the midbrain's dorsal raphe nucleus (DRN) and by a catecholaminergic input from the pontine locus coeruleus (LC). TG, Trigeminal ganglion; MN, mesencephalic nucleus; MSN, main sensory nucleus; SNO, subnucleus oralis; SNIP, subnucleus interpolaris.

Neurogenic inflammatory-induced pain

There is experimental evidence to suggest that migraine arises as a result of the development of a neurogenic inflammatory reaction (Moskowitz & Cutrer 1993). When prior to a migraine attack, for some as yet unknown reason, trigeminal umyelinated C-sensory afferent nociceptors in the walls of blood vessels become activated, a number of vasoactive neuropeptides are released including calcitonin gene-related peptide, substance P and neurokinin A. The effect of this is to cause a sterile inflammatory reaction to develop with, as a consequence, dilatation of the vessels, extravasation of plasma and the leakage of plasma proteins into the dura mater.

The development of this reaction may be blocked by various drugs used to abort migraine attacks including sumatriptan, dihydroergotamine, indometacin and acetylsalicylic acid (Buzzi et al 1989, Buzzi & Moskowitz 1990).

Migraine-induced regional cerebral blood flow changes

Angiographic studies carried out by Olesen et al (1990) on subjects with migraine have shown that initially there is a unilateral regional cerebral blood flow (rCBF) reduction which, beginning posteriorly in the occipital region, gradually spreads anteriorly. This reduction in rCBF starts before the onset of the aura and continues both during it and for some hours after the development of the headache. It is only when the headache has been present for some hours that this hypofusion is replaced by hyperfusion which then persists not only for the rest of the attack but for some time after it.

Therefore, although the aura symptoms develop as a result of hypofusion of the posterior part of the brain, contrary to what was formerly believed, the migraine itself does not arise as a result of a rCBF increase but rather, as stated previously, because of the development of neurogenic inflammation. It is now believed that this sterile inflammatory process, by sensitising trigeminal sensory afferent nociceptors in the walls of blood vessels, causes these nociceptors to respond to previously innocuous stimuli such as the blood vessel pulsations (Strassman et al 1996).

Reasons advanced in favour of migraine being primarily a vascular disorder include the pulsating nature of the pain, its aggravation by physical exertion and the ability of vasoactive drugs to both relieve and exacerbate it. This notwithstanding, it has to be admitted that the pain is not pulsating in about 40% of patients (Olesen 1991).

Generalised muscle tenderness

Controlled studies carried out on patients with migraine have shown that their head and neck muscles in between attacks are more tender than those of headache-free individuals (Lous & Olesen 1982). Furthermore, careful palpation of these muscles shows that there is not only widespread tenderness both during and in between attacks but also, in about 50% of cases, small discrete focal points of exquisite tenderness (Jensen et al 1988, Olesen 1978).

Myofascial tender points

Hay (1976) was one of the first to confirm that intramuscularly situated points of maximal tenderness in migraine are important sources of pain by showing that an injection of a local anaesthetic into them during an attack of migraine aborts it and that in between attacks it reduces the frequency with which they recur.

It is clear, therefore, that the myofascial nociceptive input to the subnucleus caudalis (trigeminal dorsal horn) emanates from activated and sensitised group IV nociceptors in sensory afferent nerve terminals at these sites. Despite this, migraine is not a dull aching type of pain such as that which normally emanates from MTrPs, but a severe throbbing sensation that is often located directly over an extracranial blood vessel. And occasionally it has the lancinating quality of a neurogenic pain (Moskowitz et al 1979).

Furthermore, unlike MTrPs where the application of firm pressure to them causes pain to be referred to distant sites (zones of pain referral), but like fibromyalgia tender points, the application of firm pressure to points of maximal tenderness in the muscles of migraineurs causes pain to be felt locally around them.

Emotional component

Up to 70% of migraineurs consider emotional upsets to be a salient contributory factor in the development of their headaches (Henryk-Gutt & Rees 1973), And, as will be discussed later, the reduction of stress by one means or another is often an essential part of the management of migraine.

Vascular-supraspinal-myogenic model

In the light of clinical and pathophysiological observations, Olesen (1991) has proposed a vascular-supraspinal-myogenic (VSM) model for migraine pain (Box 11.2).

According to this model the intensity of the pain is determined by the sum of a vascular nociceptive input, a myofascial nociceptive input and a supraspinal (emotional) input converging on and being integrated by neurons in the subnucleus caudalis (medullary dorsal horn) with the vascular input predominating over the myofascial input and the emotional one tending to be somewhat variable.

Thus, when the vascular nociceptive input is strong and the myofascial and supraspinal inputs remain weak, only a migraine aura develops. When not only the vascular input is strong but either the supraspinal or myofascial input is moderately strong, migraine with aura develops. And when the vascular input is less strong but the supraspinal and myofascial inputs are appreciable, migraine without aura develops (Fig. 11.6).

Box 11.2 Input to subnucleus caudalis
Migraine Vascular – Supraspinal – Myogenic Tension-type headache Myofascial – Supraspinal – Vascular

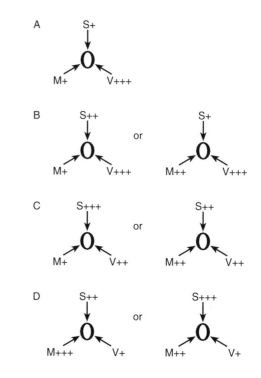

Key: +++ strong, ++ medium, + weak nociceptive input to O (medullary dorsal horn)

Figure 11.6 Illustration of the relative strengths of supraspinal (S), vascular (V) and myofascial (M) inputs to medullary dorsal horn. (A) Aura without headache. (B) Migraine with aura. (C) Migraine without aura. (D) Tension-type headache. Based on Olesen's VSM model of migraine and MSV model of tension-type headache (Olesen 1991).

This VSM model, as will be discussed later, differs from Olesen's model for tension-type headache in that with the latter the myofascial input predominates so that it is a myofascial-supraspinal-vascular (MSV) one.

At the same time it is necessary to emphasise that because the relative strength of these inputs is liable to vary over the course of time, a headache-prone individual is liable to suffer from migraine on some occasions and tension-type headache on others. And, because of this, these two disorders, contrary to what any headache classification might suggest, rather than being two distinct entities are in reality a continuum (see p. 212).

In summary, therefore, migraine is due to a neurogenic inflammatory reaction developing as a result of the release of various vasoactive neuro-peptides including calcitonin gene-related peptide, substance P and neurokinin-A when trigeminal C-sensory afferent nociceptors in the walls of blood vessels for some unknown reason become activated. In addition to this vascular component, there is also a myofascial component due to the activation of group IV sensory afferent nociceptors at points of maximal tenderness in the muscles of the neck, and a supraspinal (emotional) one.

The intensity of the migraine and whether or not an aura precedes it is dependent on the relative strength of these three inputs to the subnucleus caudalis (medullary dorsal horn) for it is following their integration there that migraine-evoking activity is transmitted up the quintothalamic tract to the cerebral cortex.

Influence of biochemical changes on migraine

No discussion concerning the aetiology of migraine would be complete without considering the influence of 5-hydroxytryptamine (serotonin), noradrenaline (norepinephrine) and oestrogen on its development.

Serotonin (5-hydroxytryptamine)

When about 45 years ago it was discovered that 5-hydroxytryptamine is a vasoconstrictor substance that is released from platelets into the serum during blood clotting, the alternative name serotonin was given to it.

Serotonin is not only found in platelets. Large amounts of it are present in cells in the gut wall where it exerts an important influence on intestinal motility. In addition, it is present in the brain, where the main serotonin-producing nucleus is the dorsal raphe nucleus in the midbrain. It is of interest to note that in the experimental animal, activation of this nucleus increases the cerebral blood flow (Underwood et al 1992).

The belief that serotonin is of importance in the development of migraine is supported by a number of studies that suggest an association between an increased production of serotonin in the brain and headache (Marcus 1995). It has, for example, been found that it is possible to bring on migraine by the administration of the serotonin-releasing agent reserpine (Bank 1991) and that this reserpine-induced effect can be blocked by the serotonin receptor antagonist methysergide.

Conversely, headache may be relieved by increasing the blood serotonin level by means of an intravenous infusion of 0.1% serotonin (Goadsby & Lance 1990). It has been postulated that this increase in peripheral serotonin may relieve migraine as a result of it having an autoinhibitory effect on the central serotonin-production structure, the dorsal raphe nucleus (Marcus 1995).

The observation that when a headache is present the platelet serotonin level is reduced to much the same level in both migraine and tension-type headache sufferers (Anthony et al 1967, Rolf et al 1981), and the serotonin metabolite 5-hydroxyindole acetic acid level in the urine is correspondingly raised, confirms that changes in serotonin are of importance in the pathogenesis of both of these two closely related disorders (Curran et al 1965).

Noradrenaline (norepinephrine)

During migraine attacks plasma noradrenaline (norepinephrine) levels decrease and their metabolites increase (Curran et al 1965). Whether these changes are due to this catecholamine being primarily involved in the pathogenesis of migraine or whether they are simply due to a stress reaction to headache is not known.

Oestrogen

That a change in oestrogen level contributes to the development of migraine is shown by 60% of women who have this type of headache reporting an increased incidence of it around the time of a period, and by 14% of women with migraine having headaches only at that time (Marcus 1995). Studies by Somerville (1975) have shown that menstrual-related migraine coincides with a state of oestrogen withdrawal. And, as discussed later, administering oestrogen to counteract this has been shown to be effective in preventing migraine from developing.

Treatment of an acute attack

Soluble aspirin to alleviate the headache and metoclopramide to combat the vomiting is often all that is required. Alternatively, a non-steroidal anti-inflammatory drug such as ibuprofen may prove to be more effective in relieving the pain.

When one or other of these analgesics fails to bring relief a more specific migraine-controlling drug should be employed. Ergotamine is not so widely prescribed as formerly because overuse is liable to lead to the development of severe headaches and serious vascular complications. And also because the triptan group of drugs (sumatriptan, naratriptan, rizatriptan and zolmitriptan) have now been shown to revolutionise the lives of many patients (Goadsby 1999). Their main disadvantages, however, are that they are expensive and they should not be used by anyone with coronary artery disease or uncontrolled hypertension.

Migraine prophylaxis

In view of the multifactorial aetiology of migraine it is necessary to adopt a polytherapeutic approach to its prophylaxis.

All patients (Box 11.3)

With every patient it is necessary to exclude factors liable to trigger off attacks of migraine or make them more frequent and long-lasting. This involves helping each individual patient to identify any ingested substances, such as chocolate, citrus fruits, cheese or red wine, that do this in his or her particular case. Also, to exclude any food allergy and hypersensitivity to either nitrites present in cured meats or sodium glutamate in Chinese food.

It is also essential, as pointed out by Olesen & Bonica (1990), to carry out a psychological assessment and when emotional factors are found to be of significance, to teach the patient coping strat-

---

Box 11.3 Migraine prophylaxis for all patients

Exclude trigger factors:
  Foods (chocolate, citrus fruits, cheese, red wine, etc.)
  Sodium glutamate (Chinese food)
  Nitrites (cured meats)
Identify psychogenic factors and:
  Teach coping strategies
  Employ relaxation techniques.

---

egies and relaxation techniques. With respect to the latter, my personal preference is to employ hypnotherapy and to show the patient how to practise autohypnosis for 5–10 minutes each day. Relaxation tapes, in my experience, are not as helpful. Hilgard & Hilgard (1994) have provided a comprehensive review of hypnosis for the relief of various types of pain, including migraine.

Selected patients (Box 11.4)

Whilst every patient needs an effective treatment regimen for individual attacks only a minority require prophylactic treatment in between attacks to reduce their incidence and severity. Circumstances that warrant this include either two or more severe attacks a month which do not readily respond to abortive medication, or the need to employ such treatment more than twice a week .

The types of treatment available include pharmacotherapy, traditional Chinese acupuncture and superficial dry needling at points of maximal tenderness. Any decision as to which method to use must depend on a number of considerations.

Box 11.4 Migraine prophylaxis for specific groups

- For those having two or more attacks a month, producing disability lasting 3 or more days:
- For those who require abortive medication more than twice a week:
Either administer a drug or employ a needling technique or a combination of both (needling technique includes either traditional Chinese acupuncture or dry needling of tender points)

These include each individual patient's personal preference, bearing in mind that some people are averse to taking drugs, whilst others fear having needles inserted into them. Also, that some people react idiosyncratically to drugs whilst others find that excessively strong needle stimulation of nerve endings brings on migraine.

Drug therapy and one or other of these needling techniques, however, are not mutually exclusive and, in view of the multifactorial aetiology of this disorder, it is often best for a drug and needling technique to be employed concomitantly.

Drug therapy (Table 11.1)

There are several groups of drugs to choose from, each having its own relative indications and contraindications.

Beta-adrenoceptor blocking agents

Beta-adrenergic blockers are the drugs of first choice with side-effects from them usually occurring only with high doses. Experimental work suggests that these agents may act by dilating constricted cerebral vessels and preventing dilatation of extracranial ones. Propranolol is the one most widely used although atenolol, because its longer half-life permits it to be given once a day, is sometimes preferred.

The use of this group of agents, however, has to be avoided in patients with asthma, congestive heart failure, Raynaud's disease and diabetes mellitus.

Calcium-channel blockers

A calcium-channel blocker such as verapamil is a useful alternative to a beta-blocker when the latter is contraindicated because of the above disorders.

Antiserotonergic agents

Pizotifen (Sanomigran), an antiserotonergic drug, is another widely used drug, particularly as, because of a long half-life, it only requires to be taken as a single morning dose. A disadvantage, however, is that it is liable to cause drowsiness and an increased appetite with the eventual development of obesity. Its use also has to be avoided in patients with either urinary retention or glaucoma.

An even more effective serotonin antagonist is methysergide. This is not much used because rarely it gives rise to retroperitoneal, pulmonary or endocardial fibrosis, but as Silberstein et al (1998) have pointed out, this may be avoided by having a medication-free interval of 4 weeks after each 6-month course.

Tricyclic antidepressants

Tricyclic antidepressants are also helpful. Amitriptyline in a sub-antidepressant dose has

Table 11.1 Choice of prophylactic drugs

Drug	Especially useful in	Contraindicated in
Beta-blockers: e.g. propranolol (3 times a day), atenolol (once a day)	Hypertension, angina	Asthma, Raynaud's disease, heart failure, diabetes
Calcium channel blockers: e.g. verapamil	Hypertension, angina, beta-blocker contraindications	Constipation
Serotonin antagonists: e.g. pizotifen, methysergide	Orthostatic hypotension	Obesity, angina, peripheral vascular disease
Tricyclic antidepressants: e.g. amitriptyline	Depression, insomnia	Glaucoma, prostate enlargement
Anticonvulsants: e.g. sodium valproate	Epilepsy	Liver disease, bleeding disorders
Oestrogens: e.g. percutaneous estradiol	Menstrual migraine	

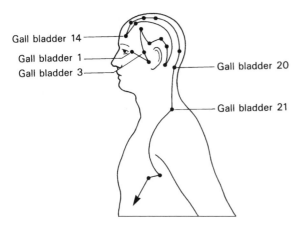

Figure 11.7 The upper part of the traditional Chinese Gall Bladder meridian. The lower part, not shown, extends down the outside of the trunk, leg and foot to terminate at the base of the fourth toe.

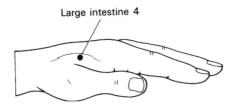

Figure 11.8 The traditional Chinese acupuncture point Large Intestine 4 (Hoku or Hegu) in the first dorsal interosseous muscle.

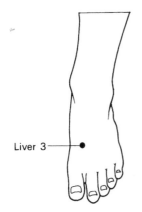

Figure 11.9 The traditional Chinese acupuncture point Liver 3.

been shown to be as effective as propranolol (Zeigler et al 1987). In addition, the anticonvulsant sodium valproate is useful when the pain is lancinating in character. A double-blind trial has

shown it to be superior to a placebo (Hering & Kuritsky 1992).

Oestrogens

There is considerable controversy concerning the use of oestrogens for the prophylaxis of menstrual migraine. Olesen & Bonica (1990) are of the opinion that 'oestrogen treatment more often worsens migraine than not, particularly when given cyclically'.

De Lignières et al (1986), however, in a double-blind placebo-controlled crossover trial during three consecutive cycles, showed that percutaneous estradiol 'had a considerable preventive effect on pure menstrual migraine in women with regular cycles'.

Traditional Chinese acupuncture

With this technique needle stimulation of nerve endings is carried out at points recommended to be used for migraine prophylaxis in textbooks of traditional Chinese acupuncture. Most of these are in the head and neck along the Gall Bladder (GB) meridian (Fig. 11.7). They include one just medial to the mastoid process (GB 20), one over the middle of the upper border of the trapezius (GB 21) and points on this meridian in the temporal region (Campbell 1987). Other points sometimes employed include Large Intestine 4 in the first dorsal interosseous muscle in the hand (Fig. 11.8) and Liver 3 in the foot (Fig. 11.9).

This method employed by Loh et al (1984), in a controlled trial carried out at the National Hospital for Neurology and Neurosurgery, London, UK, gave results which led them to conclude that 'acupuncture is a beneficial treatment for . . . some patients, and that its more widespread use is justified'.

Vincent (1989) also carried out a controlled trial of this technique at University College London, UK. The results led him to conclude that 'true acupuncture was significantly more effective than the control procedure in reducing the pain of migraine'.

The disadvantage, however, of this technique is that the selection of traditional Chinese acupuncture points is perforce an empirical one based on esoteric principles not readily reconcilable with those upon which the practice of Western medicine is based. Also, knowing where to locate them requires a certain amount of specialised training.

The reasons for traditional Chinese acupuncture seeming to be of value for migraine prophylaxis are not certain but must presumably include the evocation of activity in opioidergic pain-modulating mechanisms considered to be responsible for the development of acupuncture induced analgesia in general (Bowsher 1998).

Markelova et al (1984) and Starr (1994) have suggested that the effectiveness of this technique in suppressing migraine may also be due to its ability to control fluctuations in blood serotonin levels.

Superficial dry needling at points of maximal tenderness

This technique involves stimulating with a needle A-delta nerve fibres in the cutaneous and subcutaneous tissues overlying intramuscularly situated points of maximal tenderness. One advantage of this method over traditional Chinese acupuncture is that it not only brings into action the same pain-modulating mechanisms as the latter but it also has the specific effect of blocking the intra-dorsal horn passage of migraine-inducing activity generated in activated and sensitised nociceptors at these tender point sites. Another is that the selection of points to be needled is solely governed by what is found on clinical examination of each individual patient.

A controlled trial carried out by Hesse et al (1994), comparing the efficacy of this technique with that of administering the beta-blocker metoprolol for migraine prophylaxis, showed that both are equally effective.

Migraineurs, like patients with fibromyalgia, tend to be strong responders to dry needle stimulation of A-delta nerve fibres in the tissues overlying intramuscularly situated points of maximal tenderness (Baldry 2000). Therefore, it only requires a very light stimulus to abolish the exquisite tenderness at these points and by doing this at regular intervals it is often possible to reduce the frequency and severity of the migraine. Moreover, it is important not to exceed this minimal stimulation as too strong a one, as Hesse and his co-workers discovered, is liable to bring on an attack of migraine.

For these reasons a needle should be inserted to a depth of about 5 mm at these points and left in situ for not more than 5–10 seconds, both for migraine prophylaxis and when deactivating neck muscle TrPs for the alleviation of pain of any other type in someone with a history of migraine.

Needling of distal traditional Chinese acupuncture points

In carrying out acupuncture for migraine prophylaxis there is much to be said for supplementing the effects produced by needling either traditional Chinese acupuncture points or points of maximum tenderness in the head and neck region with those brought about by needling distal points such as Large Intestine 4 in the hand (Fig. 11.8) and Liver 3 in the foot (Fig. 11.9). This is because the neospinothalamic tract up which noxiously generated information is conveyed following needle stimulation of A-delta nerve fibres in the skin not only has a collateral which projects to the midbrain's periaqueductal grey area at the upper end of the serotonin-mediated descending inhibitory system but also a collateral that projects to the subnucleus reticularis dorsalis. And the latter, when stimulated as a result of the development of activity in the neospinothalamic tract, is responsible for the development of a diffuse noxious inhibitory effect (Le Bars et al 1979).

It is possible that this effect of stimulating the subnucleus reticularis dorsalis may be of particular relevance with respect to migraine suppression because this structure is situated in close proximity to lamina V of the medullary dorsal horn (subnucleus caudalis) which, as stated earlier, has as one of its functions the integration of migraine-arousing stimuli.

> **Box 11.5** Tension-type headache characteristics
>
> At least two of following:
> 1. Pressing/tightening non-pulsating pain
> 2. Mild or moderate intensity (i.e. may inhibit but not prohibit activities)
> 3. Bilateral location
> 4. No aggravation on walking upstairs or similar activity
>
> Plus both of following:
> 5. No nausea or vomiting
> 6. Either no photophobia or phonophobia or one but not the other present

---

TENSION-TYPE HEADACHES

Tension-type headaches (T-THs) may be either episodic or chronic. The cephalalgia characteristically takes the form of a dull aching non-pulsatile feeling of pressure, tightness or constriction. In contrast to the severe pain of migraine the discomfort is only mild to moderate in severity (Box 11.5). It usually takes the form of a vice-like constriction that affects the whole of the head, but it may be localised to one or other region of it.

Pathogenesis

For long it was believed that T-TH develops because the scalp and neck muscles are held in a persistently contracted state as a result of emotional tension. And that the compression of small blood vessels brought about by this results in ischaemia-induced activation of nociceptors at MTrP sites.

This theory, however, became discredited once electromyographic studies had shown that whilst muscle activity may be moderately increased in T-THs this is not nearly as much as it is with migraine (Bakal & Kaganov 1977); additionally, it was shown that muscle spasm and any increased electromyographic activity that might be associated with this is not the cause of the pain (Jensen 1995, Olesen & Jensen 1991). It also became untenable once it was realised that any muscle contraction that may be present is never sufficient to constrict blood vessels (Olesen &

Bonica 1990). Two possible reasons for the development of anxiety-induced MTrP activity, including that which arises in patients with T-TH, were discussed at some length in Chapter 3.

Migraine and tension-type headaches – a continuum

In the past T-TH was considered to be a separate entity but it is now realised that it is so closely related to migraine that the two together form a continuum. Hopkins (1993), during the course of discussing this has stated:

... a number of researchers have instructed their computers to try to sort out a taxonomic classification of headaches. With the exception of so-called cluster headaches such attempts at classification have failed. The present-day concept is that there is no clear-cut combination of symptoms of headache, or associated symptoms, that allows a separation into clearly distinct entities. A consensus has developed that patients with chronic recurrent headaches have at different times varying amounts of the features that have, in the past, been called migrainous (unilateral headaches of a throbbing type, associated with nausea) and at other times features of headaches that have, in the past, been called tension headaches or muscle-contraction headaches (pain at the back of the head, a headache described as like a band, or like a feeling of pressure on top of the head).

Similarly, Loh et al (1984), during the course of explaining why they included patients with both migraine and tension-type headache in a trial comparing the relative effectiveness of acupuncture and standard medical treatment stated: 'patients commonly have both kinds of headache and they frequently do not differentiate them when they report their progress. Although there are clear-cut examples of migraine and of muscle tension headaches, there are many headaches where it is artificial to assign them to one or other of these two categories'.

In view of all this it is hardly surprising to find that both of these disorders have the following features in common:

1. More muscle tenderness than controls do (Olesen 1991)
2. Abnormal EMG activity

3. A platelet serotonin content significantly lower than in normal controls (Rolf et al 1981)
4. A decreased cerebrospinal fluid beta-endorphin level.

Also, in both migraine without aura (Makashima & Takahashi 1991) and T-TH (Schoenen et al 1987), there is inhibition of voluntary EMG activity of the temporalis muscle in response to trigeminal nerve stimulation. Thus, whereas normally there are two successive extroceptive suppression silent periods (ES1 and ES2), with T-TH ES2 is absent, and with migraine without aura it is reduced (Silberstein et al 1998).

Myofascial-supraspinal-vascular model of tension-type headache

Olesen (1991) is of the opinion that what determines whether a patient at any particular time develops migraine or a tension-type headache is the relative amounts of three inputs (supraspinal, myofascial and vascular) to the trigeminal subnucleus caudalis (medullary dorsal horn) for, as he states:

... according to our model, patients develop migraine because of a primary vascular nociception. In tension-type headache the primary nociception is probably myofascial. In both conditions supraspinal facilitation may be large or small although it is probably relatively more important in tension-type headache. We can now explain the interrelationship between the two disorders. Patients with chronic tension-type headache often develop migraine-like episodes. A possible explanation is continuous myofascial nociceptive input increasing the sensitivity of caudalis neurons which then respond to episodic moderate (normal) perivascular nociceptive input resulting in migraine-like headache.

It therefore follows that, whereas migraine has a vascular-supraspinal-myogenic input to the subnucleus caudalis, T-TH has a myofascial-supraspinal-vascular one.

Myofascial nociceptive input

Systematic palpation of the pericranial muscles in T-TH invariably reveals the presence of MTrPs (Simons & Mense 1998). And it is clearly from these that the myofascial input to the subnucleus caudalis arises.

Prophylaxis

Prophylactic measures should be employed in any case where the frequency of headache attacks is more than two a week, their duration is for more than 3–4 hours and their severity is such that there is a risk of analgesia-induced chronic daily headaches developing.

Pharmacotherapy

Any of the drugs used for migraine prophylaxis may be used. Of these, however, amitryptyline is probably the one most commonly administered with 10–20 mg/day often being sufficient for T-TH prophylaxis. However, a serotonin-specific reuptake inhibitor such as fluoxetine may be preferred as it has fewer side effects. In one controlled trial fluoxetine was more effective than a placebo (Saper et al 1994).

Deactivation of myofascial trigger points

As a nociceptive input to the subnucleus caudalis from TrPs in the neck muscles is a prime cause of T-TH developing, their deactivation is clearly essential. And as my experience has shown that this only requires minimal stimulation of A-delta nerve fibres in the tissues overlying them, superficial dry needling, carried out in exactly the same manner as for migraine prophylaxis is recommended.

Traditional Chinese acupuncture for the prophylaxis of T-TH cannot be recommended. This is because Vincent (1990), in a crossover study involving 14 patients, found that it was superior to sham acupuncture in only 4 of them. And because Tavola et al (1992), in a similar study, found that it was no more effective than a placebo.

Psychotherapy

As a supraspinal input to the subnucleus caudalis is also of importance in the development of

T-TH, it is essential in all cases to carry out a detailed psychological assessment and, depending on what is learnt from this, to formulate stress-coping strategies and to employ one or other form of relaxation therapy. My personal preference, as in the treatment of migraine, is to use hypnotherapy and to teach the patient how to carry out autohypnosis on a regular daily basis.

TEMPORO-FACIAL PAIN

Myofascial trigger point pain

Pain may develop in the temporo-facial region as a result of the activation and sensitisation of TrP nociceptors in one or more of the following – the temporalis, masseter, and the lateral and medial pterygoid muscles. Each of these will therefore be considered in turn.

Temporalis muscle (Fig. 11.10)

Anatomical attachments

This fan-shaped muscle, the action of which is to close the mouth by elevating the mandible, is attached above to the temporal bone. From this attachment its fibres converge to end in a tendon which is inserted into the coronoid process of the mandible.

Factors responsible for development of TrP activity

Reasons for TrP activity developing in this muscle include occlusal disorders, persistent grinding of the teeth (bruxism), directly applied trauma to the temporal region and exposure of the temple to a current of cold air. In addition, traction carried out in an attempt to relieve neck pain may, by overloading the temporalis muscle, cause activity to develop in its TrPs and thereby give rise to yet more pain.

In addition, TrP nociceptors in this muscle may become activated as a secondary event when pain from TrPs in either the upper part of the trapezius or the sternocleidomastoid muscle is referred to the temporal region.

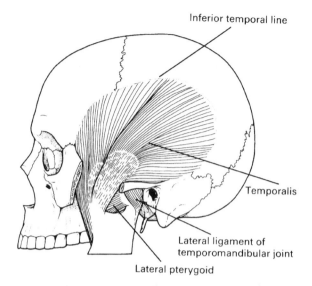

Figure 11.10 Left temporalis. The zygomatic arch and masseter have been removed.

TrP activity may also be found to be present in this muscle in tension-type headaches (p. 212) and in the temporomandibular myofascial pain-dysfunction syndrome (p. 222).

TrP sites and pain referral patterns

When searching for TrPs in this muscle it should be placed on the stretch by propping the mouth open. A cylindrical cardboard air-tube used for respiratory function testing is very useful for this purpose (Fig. 11.11).

The sites at which TrPs are likely to be found include:

1. the anterior part of the temple at the lateral end of the supraorbital ridge;
2. midway between this point and the ear along the line of the zygomatic arch;
3. on the same line just in front of the ear;
4. just above the ear.

The referral of pain from a TrP at site 1 is along the supraorbital ridge and on occasions towards the upper incisors; that from a TrP at sites 2 and 3 is locally in the region of the temple and sometimes downwards into the teeth of the upper jaw; that from a TrP at site 4 is in a backwards and upwards direction from it (Fig. 11.12 A, B, C and D).

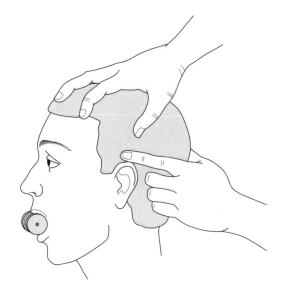

Figure 11.11 Searching for TrPs in the temporalis muscle with the mouth propped open.

Temporal giant cell arteritis

Pain which arises as a result of temporalis muscle TrP activity has to be distinguished from pain in the temporal region that develops as a result of giant cell arteritis, a disorder which may involve any large artery but which usually affects either the temporal branch or the occipital branch of the external carotid artery.

Differentiating between arteritis pain and MTrP pain in the temporal region may at times be difficult. They both may take the form of a persistent severe ache. Arteritis pain, however, in some cases has an electric-shock-like character. In addition, there is tenderness of the tissues with both types of pain. Moreover, an artery affected by giant cell arteritis may initially feel normal. It is only at a later stage that it becomes thickened, pulseless and tender.

An important distinguishing feature is that the erythrocyte sedimentation rate (ESR) in giant cell arteritis is invariably markedly elevated (70 mm/h or more).

If from the character of the pain, the physical signs and the presence of a high ESR, giant cell arteritis is suspected, prednisolone (40–60 mg a day) should be started immediately without waiting for a biopsy of the artery to be carried out because, should this disorder be the cause of pain, it not only affords immediate relief, thus helping to confirm the diagnosis, but also prevents irreversible blindness from developing which, in an untreated case, is liable to do so at an early stage.

Deactivation of trigger points

Before deactivating TrPs in the temporalis muscle Simons et al (1999a) recommend deactivating any TrPs that may be present in the masseter muscle because otherwise any TrP-induced tautness of it, by impeding the flow of venous blood from the temporalis muscle, is liable to cause a haematoma to develop following the insertion of a needle.

The deactivation of TrPs should be carried out with the mouth propped open as putting the muscle on the stretch makes it easier to locate them (see p. 214).

With any of the deeply applied techniques discussed in Chapter 7 there is a risk of damaging the temporal artery. The use of superficial dry needling is therefore recommended.

Preventative measures

When malocclusion is present some type of dental corrective procedure may have to be carried out. Before embarking on this, however, an occlusal splint should be fitted and TrPs in the temporalis and other masticatory muscles deactivated.

In cases where bruxism is present an occlusal splint should be worn at night. Also, hypnotherapy should be used and autohypnosis taught in order to reduce the emotional tension responsible for the bruxism developing.

In addition, the muscle should be stretched by opening the mouth wide several times a day.

Masseter muscle (Fig. 11.13)

Anatomical attachments

The masseter muscle consists of a superficial and a deep part. The superficial part, which is the

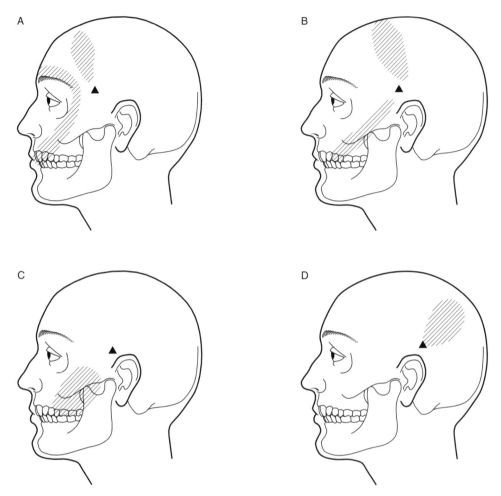

Figure 11.12 The pattern of pain referral from TrPs in the temporalis muscle in its anterior part (A); in its intermediate part (B and C); and in its posterior part (D).

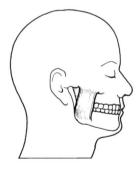

Figure 11.13 The masseter muscle.

larger of the two, arises from the zygomatic process of the maxilla and the zygomatic arch. Its

fibres pass downwards and backwards to be inserted into the angle and the lower half of the ramus of the mandible. The deep part, much of which is concealed by the superficial part, arises from the zygomatic arch and its fibres pass vertically downwards to be inserted into the lateral surface of the coronoid process and upper half of the ramus of the mandible.

Factors responsible for the development of TrP activity

Reasons for TrP activity developing in this muscle include bruxism, occlusal disorders produced by a wearing down of natural or artificial teeth, stress-induced contraction of the muscle, prolonged overstretching of it during dental surgery and directly applied trauma to the side of the face. Satellite TrPs in it may also become activated when pain is referred to the jaw region from TrPs in the sternocleidomastoid muscle.

The secondary activation of TrP nociceptors is liable to take place in this muscle's synergists, the temporalis and medial pterygoid muscles, and also in the contralateral masseter muscle TrP activity in this muscle also occurs in the temporomandibular MTrP pain syndrome (see p. 222).

Trigger point examination

In order to locate TrPs in this muscle it is necessary to put it on the stretch by propping open the mouth in the same way as when searching for TrPs in the temporalis muscle. TrPs in its superficial part usually occur near to either the upper or lower attachments. TrPs in its deep part are located by palpating over the posterior part of the ramus of the mandible immediately in front of the external auditory meatus.

Patterns of pain referral (Fig. 11.14A and B)

TrPs in the superficial part of the muscle refer pain along both the maxilla and mandible, around the molar teeth and to the region of the temporomandibular joint.

Those in its deep part refer pain to the region of the temporomandibular joint and ear. And when this happens tinnitus may also develop.

Deactivation of trigger points

Any of the methods described in Chapter 7 may be used but again superficial dry needling is the easiest and would seem to be just as effective as the others.

Preventative measures

Bruxism requires to be treated by reducing stress with some form of relaxation technique such as hypnotherapy and teaching the patient to practise autohypnosis on a regular basis each day.

Any occlusal disorder present needs to be dealt with. Before embarking upon any procedure to correct this permanently the fitting of an occlusal splint provides worthwhile temporary relief.

Lateral (external) pterygoid muscle
(Fig. 11.15)

Anatomical attachments

The lateral pterygoid muscle has a superior and inferior division. The superior division is attached in front to the sphenoid bone and behind to the capsule of the temporomandibular joint. The inferior division is attached in front to

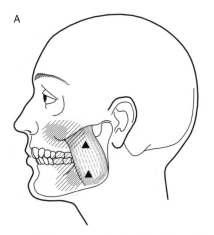

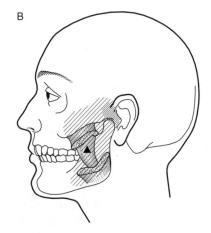

Figure 11.14 A: The pattern of pain referral from trigger points (▲) in the superficial part of the masseter muscle; B from a trigger point (▲) in its deep part.

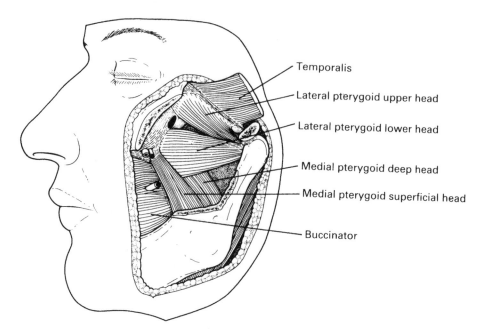

Figure 11.15 The left ptyerygoid muscles. The zygomatic arch and part of the ramus of the mandible have been removed.

the lateral pterygoid plate and behind to the neck of the mandible.

Factors responsible for the development of TrP activity

This may be due either to malocclusion of the teeth or anxiety-induced bruxism or both. It may also occur in the temporomandibular MTrP pain syndrome (see p. 222). In addition, it may develop as a secondary event when pain from TrPs in the sternocleidomastoid muscle is referred to the region in which this muscle is situated.

TrP pattern of pain referral

TrPs in this muscle refer pain to around the temporomandibular joint and in the region of the maxillary sinus (Fig. 11.16).

TrP examination

An intraoral examination of this muscle for the purpose of locating TrPs in it is both technically difficult and only allows the anterior attachment of its inferior division to be examined.

External palpation is therefore preferable. This entails separating the jaws about 3 cm and then applying firm pressure through the masseter muscle. Before doing this, however, it is essential for all TrPs in the masseter and temporalis muscle to have been deactivated as active TrPs in either or both of these prevents the mouth from being opened wide enough for a satisfactory examination to be carried out.

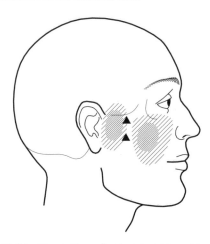

Figure 11.16 The pattern of pain referral from trigger points (▲) in the lateral pterygoid muscle.

Deactivation of trigger points

Local anaesthetic injection into or deep dry needling of trigger points   An intraoral approach is not recommended because the position of the muscle makes needling of it by this route difficult.

However, the extraoral route through the coronoid notch provides good access to both bellies of the muscle. With the mouth propped open the needle is passed through the coronoid notch in an upwards direction until contact is made with the lateral pterygoid plate. The needle is then withdrawn slightly in order to allow TrPs in various parts of the muscle to be penetrated (Cohen & Pertes 1994).

It needs to be stressed however that anyone attempting to carry out the extraoral approach requires to have much manual dexterity as the needle has to be accurately directed in the limited space occupied by the muscle. Also, there has to be a detailed knowledge of the region's anatomy for there are numerous nerves and vessels, including the maxillary artery and pterygoid plexus of veins, that are liable to be damaged.

Superficial dry needling   Although the lateral pterygoid muscle lies beneath the masseter muscle, it is possible, as with any other deeply situated muscle in the body, to deactivate a TrP in it by means of stimulating with a needle A-delta nerve fibres in the skin and subcutaneous tissues immediately overlying the maximally tender TrP site.

Therefore, because the deeply applied procedure just described is both hazardous and technically difficult to carry out, there is much to be said for only using it should superficial dry needling fail to relieve the pain.

Preventative measures

Malpositioning of the teeth when the jaws are closed should be corrected by the fitting of an occlusal splint. Bruxism should be treated in the same way as when it is a cause of TrP activity developing in the temporalis or masseter muscles.

A search for TrPs in the sternocleidomastoid muscle should also be carried out and when found to be present, deactivated.

Medial (internal) pterygoid muscle
(Fig. 11.15)

Anatomical attachments

The medial pterygoid muscle is attached below to the angle of the jaw and above to the lateral pterygoid plate.

TrP activation and pain referral patterns

TrP activity in this muscle rarely occurs alone. It almost invariably arises secondary to the development of TrP activity in the lateral pterygoid and masseter muscles. Therefore, if after deactivating TrPs in the latter two muscles, opening the mouth is still painful and restricted with, in addition, difficulty in swallowing, the possibility that TrP activity in the medial pterygoid may be the cause has to be considered.

Pain is referred from TrPs in this muscle to the tongue, the hard palate, the pharynx, the temporomandibular joint and the ear. As is the case with the lateral pterygoid, the pain is not referred to the teeth (Fig. 11.17).

TrP examination

This is carried out with the patient placed in the supine position and a prop placed between the teeth to open the jaw as far as possible without causing unacceptable discomfort. This is necessary because, due to there being marked restriction of mouth opening, it would not otherwise be possible to carry out an intraoral examination. Also, the effect of a prop is to place the muscle on the stretch and, as a result, any TrPs present are more readily located.

The muscle is first palpated from the outside by pressing a finger against the inner surface of the mandible at its angle. At this site the lower end of the muscle is just within reach of the finger. An intraoral examination is then carried out in order to reach parts of the muscle higher up.

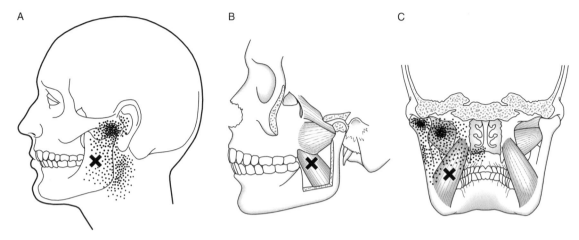

Figure 11.17   Referred pain pattern (stippled) and location of trigger point (x) in the left medial pterygoid muscle. A: External area of pain to which the patient can point. B: Anatomical cut-away to show the location of the trigger point area in the muscle which lies in the inner side of the mandible. C: Coronal section of the head through the temporomandibular joint. (Reproduced with permission from Simons D G, Travell J G, Simons L 1999 Travell & Simons Myofascial pain and dysfunction. The trigger point manual, vol. 1, upper half of the body, 2nd edn. Wiliams & Wilkins, Baltimore.)

With the pad of the finger facing outwards, it is inserted into the mouth and slid behind the lower molar teeth until it encounters the bony edge of the ramus of the mandible, and just behind this, it comes up against the muscle running in a vertical direction.

Deactivation of trigger points

As the intra- and extraoral methods of deactivating TrPs in this muscle are technically difficult and somewhat hazardous (Cohen & Pertes 1993), it is fortunate that Simons et al (1999b) have found that pain emanating from TrPs in this muscle is readily alleviated by stretching the muscle and applying a vapocoolant spray to it.

For this purpose the patient is placed in the supine position and encouraged to stretch the muscle by placing two fingers behind the lower incisor teeth and the thumb under the chin and then pulling the mandible forwards and downwards to open the jaws fully. Whilst this is being done a vapocoolant spray is swept from the neck below upwards to the temporomandibular joint. It is important to ensure that the spray does not go into the eye by placing a pad over it.

Before carrying out this procedure it is essential to deactivate TrPs in other masticatory mus-

cles as otherwise it may not be possible to open the mouth sufficiently widely.

Preventative measures

Measures similar to those discussed when considering the lateral pterygoid muscle should be employed.

Differential diagnosis

MTrP pain affecting the temporo-facial region has to be distinguished from trigeminal neuralgia, atypical facial pain and migrainous neuralgia.

Trigeminal neuralgia

This common condition usually has its onset in elderly people. Its development in a younger person makes it necessary to exclude the possibility of there being underlying multiple sclerosis.

Its diagnosis should never be made if the distribution of the pain does not correspond to that of one or more of the divisions of the trigeminal nerve. The mandibular and maxillary divisions are affected in about 40% of cases. The mandibular division alone affects about 20% and all three divisions about 15% of cases. It is rare for the ophthalmic division to be affected by itself (Hopkins 1993).

The pain is quite unlike MTrP pain because rather than being a persistent dull ache it takes the form of severe stabbing or shooting electric-shock-like paroxysms. Each bout only lasts for about 30 seconds but they keep recurring at short intervals. Stimuli which are particularly likely to bring them on include lightly touching the face, shaving and washing – also, eating and talking when the third division is involved. The course taken by the disorder and its treatment has already been discussed in Chapter 5.

Atypical facial pain

Atypical facial pain (syn: atypical facial neuralgia) is the name given to a disorder that has none of the characteristics of trigeminal neuralgia (Weddington & Blazer 1979), is not due to disease in structures such as the teeth, bones or sinuses (Sharav 1994), and cannot be shown to emanate from TrPs in muscles.

The diagnosis of this disorder is therefore reached by a process of exclusion (Loeser 1990).

Depression is considered to be an important contributory factor. And two double-blind studies (Feinmann et al 1984, Sharav et al 1987) have shown that the efficacy of a tricyclic antidepressant is superior to that of a placebo in alleviating the pain. Sharav et al (1987) have shown that the analgesic effect of a drug of this type is independent of its antidepressive action.

Migrainous neuralgia

This disorder is also known as cluster headache because of the characteristic cluster of attacks which are liable to recur for days or weeks followed by remissions lasting months or years.

The pain, which at its height is very severe and lasts for up to an hour, mainly affects the eye region, but is liable to spread to the temple, forehead and face. During each paroxysm of pain lacrimation, redness of the conjunctiva and nasal congestion are prominent features.

It is predominantly a disorder of males and most commonly comes in during the fourth and fifth decades. Treatment is far from straightforward. Each attack of pain is too transient for it to be influenced by an orally administered analgesic. Two forms of treatment during attacks that have proved to be helpful are inhalation of oxygen and subcutaneous injections of sumatriptan.

Ergotamine suppositories, lithium carbonate and nifedipine have been found to be effective prophylactic agents (Silberstein et al 1998).

INTRA-ARTICULAR TEMPOROMANDIBULAR JOINT PAIN

The commonest reason for pain developing in the temporomandibular joint (TMJ) is internal derangement (Sharav 1994).

Patients with rheumatoid arthritis commonly have abnormal radiographic appearances of the disorder in the TMJ but pain is rare (Chalmers & Blair 1973). Similarly, radiographic evidence of osteoarthritis in the joint is usually no more than a chance finding (Mayne & Hatch 1969).

Internal derangement of the temporomandibular joint

Aetiology

In this disorder there is an abnormal relationship between the articular disc and mandibular condyle with most commonly displacement of the disc in an anteromedial direction. Possible factors that may contribute to this include jaw trauma, muscle hyperactivity and hyperextension of the mandible.

Symptoms

These include pain, usually confined to the temporomandibular region, limited or deviated mouth opening and a clicking or snapping sound on opening and closing the mouth. There is sometimes an increase in intensity of the pain prior to the click and a decrease following it.

Signs

Both the temporomandibular joint and the masticatory muscles are tender to touch. In addition, crepitus and scraping sounds are heard when a stethoscope is placed over the joint whilst the patient opens and closes the mouth.

Investigations

Disc displacement may be demonstrated by injecting a radiopaque contrast material into the joint space. The presence of this disc abnormality, up until recently, has been considered an essential diagnostic finding, but there are now reservations about it because Nitzan & Dolwick (1991) found that more than half of their patients at a late stage of this disorder had normally shaped discs. Also, Westesson et al (1989) have shown that 15% of asymptomatic people have radiographically demonstrable disc displacement.

Treatment

Various conservative measures to be discussed when considering the management of the temporomandibular myofascial pain dysfunction syndrome are mainly employed. In certain selected cases, however, surgical intervention is considered necessary (Nitzan et al 1991).

EXTRA-ARTICULAR TEMPOROMANDIBULAR PAIN

Three causes of this will be considered: partially erupted wisdom teeth, giant cell arteritis and the temporomandibular MTrP pain syndrome.

Partially erupted wisdom teeth

In late adolescence the commonest cause of pain in the region of the TMJ is infection and acute inflammation round a partially erupted wisdom tooth.

Giant cell arteritis

In the elderly an important cause of pain in the region of the temporomandibular joint is ischaemia of the muscles caused by giant cell arteritis (Cawson 1984). Because the pain is brought on by mastication, it is sometimes referred to as jaw claudication (Latin, claudicare – to limp). As, however, a jaw cannot limp! the term is etymologically incorrect and should therefore be avoided.

Temporomandibular MTrP pain syndrome

TrP activity in the masticatory muscles is a common reason for pain developing in the temporomandibular region in this disorder (syn: temporomandibular joint pain-dysfunction syndrome; TMPDS).

The syndrome arises in people age 15–40 with up to 80% of sufferers being women.

Aetiological factors

There is much controversy concerning the aetiology of this syndrome. It was for long thought that an occlusal disturbance is an important contributory factor. Krogh-Poulsen & Olsson (1966), for example, stated that this, by upsetting the proprioceptive feedback, is liable to give rise to bruxism and spasm of masticatory muscles. However, there is little or no support for this belief because, as Greene & Marbach (1982) have pointed out in their review of the subject, the incidence of occlusal disturbances in patients with this disorder is no higher than it is in asymptomatic controls.

Furthermore, bruxism is now considered to be a stress-related disorder (Clark et al 1980) that may or may not be accompanied by temporomandibular pain (Rugh & Harlan 1988). Therefore, although bruxism and occlusal disharmony are both often present in the disorder they are no longer considered to be causes of it.

Sharav (1994) believes that research into the causes of this syndrome should concentrate more on central generators of pain mechanisms rather than peripheral inputs such as occlusal interferences and 'muscle hyperactivity' (Lund et al 1991). And the role of trigeminal neurogenic inflammation and the contribution of the sympathetic nervous system should be more closely studied (Basbaum & Levine 1991).

All this notwithstanding it has to be remembered that as long ago as 1954 Schwartz & Tausig made the important observation that pain in the temporomandibular region may be relieved by injecting tender masticatory muscles with procaine; that Schwartz in 1958, after treating a large number of such cases, concluded that the pain is primarily myogenic; also that Travell in a classic paper published in 1960 entitled 'Temporomandibular joint dysfunction' confirmed that pain perceived to be arising from the temporomandibular joint is not infrequently referred to it from TrPs in masticatory muscles and other muscles in the head, neck and shoulder region. Furthermore the pain may be relieved by injecting procaine into these TrPs and/or by the application of a vapocoolant spray to the muscles whilst at the same time gently stretching them.

It was formerly believed that this syndrome arises in emotionally unstable people but subsequent studies have failed to confirm this. Salter et al (1983) compared the emotional state of patients with this syndrome with that of patients with other facial disorders and concluded that there was little or no evidence of neuroticism in either group. And Schnurr et al's (1990) study of the disorder led them to conclude that the personality traits of patients with it are not significantly different from those of people who suffer from other pain disorders or from those of healthy controls.

Nevertheless, it has to be admitted that persistent pain from TMPDS, like persistent pain from any other cause, is apt to give rise to anxiety and depression (Fine 1971), and these emotional reactions to pain not infrequently have to be treated.

Finally, the relationship between TMPDS and tension-type headache (T-TH) has to be considered as the incidence of the latter in patients with TMPDS is higher than it is in controls (Magnusson & Carlsson 1978). The 1986 International Association for the Study of Pain Classification includes both disorders under the collective term *craniofacial pain of musculoskeletal origin*. However, the important difference is that most patients with TMPDS have pain and muscle tenderness confined to one side in contrast to patients with T-TH where both of these tend to be bilateral.

Symptoms

The syndrome mainly develops in otherwise fit females age 15–40. The predominant symptom is pain. This is usually unilateral and takes the form of a persistent dull ache in the region of the ear, the temple and the angle of the jaw with exacerbations of it occurring either spontaneously or in response to movements of the jaw. Mastication therefore makes it worse. In addition, movements of the jaw may produce a clicking noise but this is not a distinctive feature as it is also common in asymptomatic people. Other symptoms include sensations of fullness in the ear and dizziness.

Signs

On examination there is limited mouth opening with, in some cases, an accompanying deviation of the mandible as a result of pain and muscle shortening.

The two muscles most commonly involved are the lateral pterygoid and masseter. Greene et al (1969), in a study of 277 patients with TMPDS, found that 84% had tenderness of the lateral pterygoid muscle and 70% had tenderness of the masseter muscle. Sharav et al (1978) observed much the same in a series of 42 patients.

TrP activity, however, is not confined to these two muscles. It is also liable to develop in the temporalis, medial pterygoid, upper part of the trapezius and sternocleidomastoid muscles.

Treatment

This includes the deactivation of MTrPs; the use of muscle stretching exercises; the administration of simple analgesics, anxiolytics and antidepressants; and, in some cases, the wearing of an occlusal splint. In addition, the reduction of emotional tension by means of hypnosis and teaching the patient to carry out short periods of autohypnosis on a regular daily basis is often helpful.

REFERENCES

Anthony M, Hinterberger H, Lance J W 1967 Plasma serotonin in migraine and stress. Archives of Neurology 16:544–552

Baldry P E 2000 Superficial dry needling. In: Chaitow L (ed) Fibromyalgia syndrome: a practitioner's guide to treatment. Churchill Livingstone, Edinburgh, pp 77–90

Bakal D A, Kaganov J A 1977 Muscle contraction and migraine headache: psychophysiologic concepts. Headache 17:208–215

Bank J 1991 Brainstem auditory evoked potentials in migraine after Rausedyl provocation. Cephalalgia 11:277–279

Basbaum A I, Levine J D 1991 The contribution of the nervous system to inflammation and inflammatory disease. Canadian Journal of Physiology and Pharmacology 69:683–694

Bowsher D 1998 Mechanisms of acupuncture. In: Filshie J, White A (eds) Medical acupuncture: a western scientific approach. Churchill Livingstone, Edinburgh, pp 69–82

Buzzi M G, Moskowitz M A 1990 The antimigraine drug sumatriptan blocks neurogenic extravasation from blood vessels in duramater. British Journal of Pharmacology 99:202–206

Buzzi M G, Sakas D E, Moskowitz M A 1989 Indomethacin and acetylsalicyclic acid block neurogenic plasma protein extravasation in rat duramater. European Journal of Pharmacology 165:251–258

Campbell A 1987 Acupuncture. The modern scientific approach. Faber & Faber, London

Cawson R A 1984 Pain in the temporomandibular joint. British Medical Journal 288:1857–1858

Chalmers I M, Blair G S 1973 Rheumatoid arthritis of the temporomandibular joint. Quarterly Journal of Medicine 42:369–386

Clark G T, Rugh J T, Handleman S L 1980 Nocturnal masseter muscle activity and urinary acid catecholamine levels in bruxers. Journal of Dental Research 59:1571–1576

Cohen H V, Pertes R A 1994 Diagnosis and management of facial pain. In: Rachlin E S (ed) Myofascial pain and fibromyalgia. Trigger point management. Mosby, St Louis, p 378

Curran D A, Hinterberger H, Lance J W 1965 Total plasma serotonin 5-hydroxyindolacetic acid and p-hydroxy-m-methoxymandelic acid excretion in normal and migrainous subjects. Brain 88:997–1009

De Lignières B, Vincens M, Mauvais-Jarvis P et al 1986 Prevention of menstrual migraine by percutaneous oestradiol. British Medical Journal 293:1540

Feinmann C, Harris M, Cawley R 1984 Psychogenic facial pain: presentation and treatment. British Medical Journal 288:436

Fine E W 1971 Psychological factors associated with non-organic temporomandibular joint pain dysfunction syndrome. British Dental Journal 131:402–404

Goadsby P J 1999 Mechanisms and management of headache. Journal of the Royal College of Physicians of London 33:228–234

Goadsby P J, Lance J W 1990 Physiopathology of migraine. Revue du Practicien 40:389–394

Greene C S, Marbach J J 1982 Epidemiologic studies of mandibular dysfunction. A critical review. Journal of Prosthetic Surgery 48:184–190

Greene C S, Lerman M D, Sutcher H D, Leskin D M 1969 The TMJ pain-dysfunction syndrome: heterogeneity of the patient population. Journal of American Dental Association 79:1168–1172

Hay K M 1976 The treatment of pain in trigger areas in migraine. Journal of the Royal College of General Practitioners 26:372–376

Headache Classification Committee of the International Headache Society 1988 Classification and diagnostic criteria for headache disorders, cranial neuralgias and facial pain. Cephalalgia Supplement 7:1–96

Henryk-Gutt R, Rees W L 1973 Psychological aspects of migraine. Journal of Psychosomatic Research 17:141–153

Hering R, Kuritsky A 1992 Sodium valproate in the prophylactic treatment of migraine. A double-blind study versus placebo. Cephalalgia 12:81–84

Hesse J, Mogelvang B, Simonsen H 1994 Acupuncture versus metoprolol in migraine prophylaxis: a randomized trial of trigger point inactivation. Journal of Internal Medicine 235:451–456

Hilgard E R, Hilgard J R 1994 Hypnosis in the relief of pain. Brunner/Mazel, New York

Hopkins A 1993 Clinical neurology. A modern approach. Oxford University Press, Oxford, p 117

Jensen K 1995 Mechanism of spontaneous tension-type headache. An analysis of tenderness, pain thresholds and EMG. Pain 64:251–256

Jensen K, Taxen C, Olesen J 1988 Pericranial muscle tenderness and pressure-pain threshold in the temporal region during common migraine. Pain 35:65–70

Krogh-Poulsen W E, Olsson A 1966 Occlusal disharmonies and dysfunction of the stomatognathic system. Dental Clinics of North America, November: 627–635

Le Bars D, Dickenson A, Besson J M 1979 Diffuse noxious inhibitory control parts I & II. Pain 6:283–327

Loeser J D 1990 Cranial neuralgias. In: Bonica J J (ed) The management of pain, 2nd edn. Lea & Febiger, Philadelphia, pp 676–686

Loh L, Nathan P W, Schott G D, Zilkha K J 1984 Acupuncture versus medical treatment for migraine and muscle tension headaches. Journal of Neurology, Neurosurgery and Psychiatry 47:333–337

Lous I, Olesen J 1982 Evaluation of pericranial tenderness and oral function in patients with common migraine, muscle contraction headache and 'combination headache'. Pain 12:385–393

Lund J P, Tonka, R, Widmer C G, Stohler C S 1991 The pain adaptation model: a discussion of the relationship between chronic musculoskeletal pain and motor activity. Canadian Journal of Physiology and Pharmacology 69:683–694

Magnusson T, Carlsson G E 1978 Comparison between two groups of patients in respect of headache and mandibular dysfunction. Swedish Dental Journal 2:85–92

Makashima K, Takahashi K 1991 Extroceptive suppression of the masseter temporalis and trapezius muscles produced by mental nerve stimulation in patients with chronic headache. Cephalalgia 11:23–28

Marcus P 1995 Interrelationships of neurochemicals estrogen and recurring headache. Pain 62:129–139

Markelova V F, Vesnina V A, Malygina S I, Dubovkaia L A 1984 Changes in blood serotonin levels in patients with migraine headaches before and after a course of reflexology. Journal of Neuropathology and Psychiatry 84:1313–1316

Mayne J G, Hatch G S 1969 Arthritis of the temporomandibular joint. Journal of the American Dental Association 79:125–130

Moskowitz M A, Cutrer F M 1993 Sumatriptan: a receptor-targeted treatment for migraine. Annual Review of Medicine 44:145–154

Moskowitz M A, Reinhard J F Jr, Romero J, Melamed E, Pettibone D J 1979 Neurotransmitters and the fifth cranial nerve. Is there a relationship to the headache phase of migraine? Lancet ii:883–885

Nitzan D W, Dolwick M F 1991 An alternative explanation for the genesis of closed-lock symptoms in the internal derangement process. Journal of Oral and Maxillofacial Surgery 49:810–815

Nitzan D W, Dolwick M F, Martinez G A 1991 Temporomandibular joint arthrocentesis. A simplified treatment for severe limited mouth opening. Journal of Oral and Maxillofacial Surgery 49:1163–1167

Olesen J 1978 Some clinical features of the acute migraine attack. An analysis of 750 patients. Headache 18:268–271

Olesen J 1991 Clinical and pathophysiological observations in migraine and tension-type headache explained by integration of vascular, supraspinal and myofascial inputs. Pain 46:125–132

Olesen J, Bonica J J 1990 Headache. In: Bonica J J (ed) The management of pain, 2nd edn. Lea & Febiger, Philadelphia, vol 1, pp 687–726

Olesen J, Jensen R 1991 Getting away from simple muscle contraction as a mechanism of tension-type headache. Pain 46: 123–124

Olesen J, Friberg L, Skyhoj-Olsen T et al 1990 Timing and tomography of cerebral blood flow, aura and headache during migraine attacks. Annals of Neurology 28:791–798

Rolf L H, Wiele G, Brune G G 1981 5-Hydroxytryptamine in platelets of patients with muscle contraction headache. Headache 21:10–11

Rugh J D, Harlan J 1988 Nocturnal bruxism and temporomandibular disorders. Advances in Neurology 49:329–341

Salter M, Brooke R L, Merskey H et al 1983 Is the temporomandibular pain and dysfunction syndrome a disorder of the mind? Pain 17:151–166

Saper J R, Silberstein S D, Lake A E, Winters M E 1994 Double-blind trial of fluoxetine: chronic daily headache and migraine. Headache 34:497–502

Schnurr R F, Brooke R I, Rollman G B 1990 Psychosocial correlates of temporomandibular joint pain and dysfunction. Pain 42:153–165

Schoenen J, Jamart B, Gerard P et al 1987 Extroceptive suppression of temporalis muscle activity in chronic headache. Neurology 37:1834–1836

Schwartz L L 1958 Conclusions of the temporomandibular joint clinic at Columbia. Journal of Periodontology 29:210–212

Schwartz L L, Tausig D P 1954 Temporomandibular joint pain – treatment with intra-muscular infiltration of tetracaine hydrochloride: a preliminary report. New York State Dental Journal 20:219–223

Sharav Y 1994 Orofacial pain. In: Wall P D, Melzack R (eds) Textbook of pain, 2nd edn. Churchill Livingstone, Edinburgh, ch 31

Sharav Y, Tzukert A, Rafaeli B 1978 Muscle pain index in relation to pain dysfunction and dizziness associated with the myofascial pain-dysfunction syndrome. Oral Surgery 46:742–747

Sharav Y, Singer E, Schmidt R, Dionne R A, Dubner R 1987 The analgesic effect of amitryptyline on chronic facial pain. Pain 31:199–202

Silberstein S D, Lipton R B, Goadsby P J 1998 Headache in clinical practice. Isis Medical Media, Oxford

Simons D G, Mense S 1998 Understanding and measurement of muscle tone as related to clinical muscle pain. Pain 75:1–17

Simons D G, Travell J G, Simons L 1999a,b Travell & Simons Myofascial pain and dysfunction. The trigger point manual, vol. 1, upper half of the body, 2nd edn. Williams & Wilkins, Baltimore, p 360 (a), p 374 (b)

Somerville B W 1975 Estrogen-withdrawal migraine. Duration of exposure required and attempted prophylaxis by premenstrual estrogen administration. Neurology 25:239–244

Starr M S 1994 5-HT: The story so far. Acupuncture in Medicine 12(2):100–102

Strassman A M, Raymond S A, Burstein R 1996 Sensitization of meningeal sensory neurons and the origin of headaches. Nature 384:560–563

Tavola T, Gala C, Conte G, Invenizzi G 1992 Traditional Chinese acupuncture in tension-type headache: a controlled study. Pain 48:325–329

Travell J 1960 Temporomandibular joint dysfunction. Temporomandibular joint pain referred from the muscles of the head and neck. Journal of Prosthetic Dentistry 10:745–763

Underwood U D, Bakalian M J, Arango V, Smith R W, Mann J J 1992 Regulation of cortical blood flow by the dorsal raphé nucleus: topographic organization of cerebrovascular regulatory regions. Journal of Cerebral Blood Flow Metabolism 12: 664–673

Vincent C A 1989 A controlled trial of the treatment of migraine by acupuncture. Clinical Journal of Pain 5(4):305–312

Vincent C A 1990 The treatment of tension headache by acupuncture: a controlled single case design with time series analysis. Journal of Psychosomatic Research 34(5):553–561

Weddington W N, Blazer D 1979 Atypical facial pain and trigeminal neuralgia: a comparison study. Psychosomatics 20:348–356

Westesson P L, Eriksson L, Kurita K 1989 Reliability of negative clinical temporomandibular joint examination. Prevalence of disc displacement in asymptomatic temporomandibular joints. Oral Surgery, Oral Medicine and Oral Pathology 68:551–554

Zeigler D K, Hurwitz A, Hassanein R S, Kodanaz H A, Preskorn S H, Mason J 1987 Migraine prophylaxis. A comparison of propranolol and amitryptyline. Archives of Neurology 44:486–489

12

The lower back

INTRODUCTION

Low-back pain is extremely common. It has been estimated that each year in Great Britain 7% of the adult population present to general practitioners with this disability at a cost of £500 million to the National Health Service (United Kingdom Department of Health 1994). The pain is of two types, non-mechanical and mechanical.

Non-mechanical type low-back pain

With pain of this type the onset is usually insidious. It tends over the course of time to increase gradually in intensity. It is as severe at rest as it is during the course of activities, and may even seem worse at night because there is nothing to distract the mind from it. Also, unlike with mechanical type pain, it cannot be eased by a change in position.

Causes include neoplastic, infective, inflammatory and metabolic diseases of the spine. In addition, it may be referred to the lumbar region as a result of disease in the abdomen or pelvis.

Mechanical type low-back pain

In the vast majority of patients with low-back pain the pain is mechanically determined. Thus it tends to be relieved by rest and to be aggravated by movements, particularly when they are carried out following sitting or lying down for some time. Various activities which make it worse include twisting, lifting, bending and coughing.

Its onset may be either sudden or gradual. And the course taken by it may be acute (pain 0–7 days' duration), subacute (pain lasting from 7 days to 3 months) or chronic (pain persisting for more than 3 months).

Adverse prognostic factors

The variables that affect the course taken by low-back pain of this type in any particular individual are extremely complex for, apart from any influence underlying structural disorders may have on it, there is evidence to show that its liability to become chronic is determined by a large number of other factors.

Thomas et al (1999), in a prospective study designed to predict who, among 180 patients with low-back pain followed up for 12 months, would develop long-term pain found that chronicity occurred in one-third of them. And that the factors responsible for this outcome could be divided into those of a general nature and those which are episode-specific.

Their study showed that women, the elderly and those with a past history of low-back pain all have an increased likelihood of poor outcome. Other adverse factors included high levels of psychological distress, low levels of physical activity, unemployment, dissatisfaction with either working conditions or employment status and current or previous cigarette smoking. This latter observation served to confirm the close relationship between smoking and low-back pain reported by others (Battié et al 1991, Kelsey et al 1984).

Their findings also confirmed that the prognosis tends to be poor when low-back pain is part of a more widespread pain syndrome such as fibromyalgia. Also, that other predictors of a poor outcome include a long duration of symptoms before consultation; restricted spinal movements; and the radiation of pain down the leg such as may occur with compression of a nerve root or irritation of the spinal canal.

Multifactorial aetiology

There has been considerable controversy over the years concerning the pathogenesis of mechanical type low-back pain. One important but all too frequently overlooked site from which such pain may arise is a myofascial trigger point (MTrP). This is well illustrated by Rosomoff et al (1990), who found MTrPs to be the source of pain in 96% of 283 patients referred to them with 'chronic intractable benign back pain'.

In this chapter therefore particular attention will be drawn to low-back pain, with or without pain down the leg, that arises as a result of MTrP activity in what will be referred to as the lumbar MTrP pain syndrome.

Other mechanical type low-back pain disorders that will be considered include the lumbar facet joint syndrome, lumbar disc prolapse, lumbar spondylosis, degenerative spondylolisthesis, lateral canal stenosis and neurogenic claudication, as it is essential to be able to distinguish them from the MTrP pain syndrome, particularly as with each of them, for various reasons to be discussed, MTrP activity may develop as a secondary event.

It must be made clear, however, from the outset that it is not always possible to be certain as to the cause or causes of mechanical type low-back pain in any particular individual (Nachemson 1976, 1979) as its aetiology is often multifactorial with not only physical but also occupational and psychological factors contributing to it.

Occupational factors

Magora (1970), from extensively investigating the relationship between mechanical type low-back pain and occupational factors, found that the incidence of pain is far greater in those whose work forces them to sit for prolonged periods than it is in those who constantly move about. Heavy lifting, particularly when this is only occasional, is a frequent cause of it. He also found that this type of low-back pain occurs with about the same frequency in those with sedentary occupations as in those doing heavy labour, but that the sedentary workers' symptoms come on more often after weekend athletic activities.

Occupational factors may also contribute to its persistence. For this reason, when such pain develops as a result of the activation of MTrPs, it is not sufficient simply to deactivate these points by one or other of the methods described in Chapter 7 without at the same time determining whether any adjustments to the working conditions have to be made in order to prevent them from becoming repeatedly reactivated.

Psychological factors

Turk & Flor (1984), in a comprehensive review of the aetiological factors responsible for the development of mechanical type low-back pain, pointed out that chronic back pain is increasingly viewed as a psychophysiological and a psychosocial problem stemming from the interaction of physical, psychological and social factors.

With respect to this it is interesting to note that although Magora (1970) found a high incidence of absence from work amongst manual workers because of the pain preventing them from carrying out their duties, the incidence of back pain correlated best with how physically demanding workers perceived their work to be rather than how objectively demanding it was. Furthermore, he discovered that its incidence is more closely related to psychological problems at the workplace or at home rather than to objective physical factors.

Westrin (1973) in his study of low-back pain concluded that its incidence is especially high in those not happy with their jobs, or who are divorced or have problems with alcohol.

Anxiety and depression therefore may not only arise as a result of low-back pain having been present for some considerable time but may also contribute to its development.

LUMBAR MTrP PAIN SYNDROME

Factors responsible for development of TrP activity

Trauma

Direct or indirect trauma to the muscles of the lower back is liable, as elsewhere in the body, to cause tearing of their fibres and bleeding into the tissues. The pain from damage of this kind should only last for a relatively short period of time as spontaneous healing of the tissues is likely to be completed within a few weeks. Not infrequently, however, the pain persists for much longer than this due to trauma-induced activation and sensitisation of nociceptors at TrP sites in these muscles.

It is because a search for TrP activity regrettably tends not to be carried out as part of the routine examination of trauma-evoked low-back pain that this particular cause is often overlooked.

It is, for example, due to this that all too commonly doctors engaged in medico-legal work assume that the persistence of post-accident low-back pain in the absence of radiographic or magnetic resonance imaging (MRI) evidence of structural damage must be entirely psychological and associated with an unconscious or even at times a conscious desire for compensation. And from having served for many years on an industrial accident appeal tribunal it has become evident to me that those who seek redress for injury-induced low-back pain are liable to suffer serious injustices as a result.

Anxiety

People of an anxious temperament are liable to suffer from low-back MTrP pain at times of stress. Possible mechanisms responsible for bringing this about were discussed in Chapter 3.

Structural disorders of the spine

TrPs may become active as a secondary event in lumbar muscles situated in an area affected by pain that has arisen because of some spinal lesion such as. for example, a disc prolapse, a facet joint disorder or vertebral metastases. And this TrP activity is particularly likely to develop if these muscles are in such severe spasm as to cause them to become ischaemic.

Lumbar radiculopathy

Secondary TrP activity may develop in the lower back and leg when a lumbar nerve root becomes entrapped for one reason or another. This is because of the effect motor nerve compression has on motor endplates at TrP sites in the muscles supplied by the nerve root.

Characteristics of the pain

MTrP pain in the lumbar region, as elsewhere in the body, takes the form of a persistent dull ache. It may remain confined to the lower part of the back or be felt both in the low-back and leg. In addition, it may at times be referred anteriorly. And conversely, pain from MTrPs in the anterior abdominal wall may on occasions be referred to the lumbar region (Ch. 15).

The pain may be either intermittent or persistent. It tends to be made worse by movements such as twisting, lifting or bending. It is also liable to become worse on walking. With respect to this, it has to be remembered that pain in the buttock and thigh brought on by walking may also be vascular in origin and develop either as a result of aorto-iliac occlusion (Leriche's syndrome) or as a result of atheromatous obstruction in the internal iliac artery causing ischaemia of the sciatic nerve (Lamerton et al 1983). It is therefore essential when investigating the cause of persistent low-back pain for good history-taking to be supplemented by a careful physical examination that includes palpation of the femoral pulses.

Moreover, when a patient with low-back pain complains of leg pain that is brought on by walking and relieved by resting, another possibility that has to be taken into consideration is that this is due either to intermittent claudication (Ch. 13) or neurogenic claudication (p. 256).

Pain emanating from lumbar MTrPs tends to disappear on lying down. However, sleep may be disturbed as a result of the weight of the body exerting pressure on them.

The search for myofascial trigger points

In all cases of persistent low-back pain down the leg a systematic search for MTrPs is mandatory.

In order to do this the patient should lie on the unaffected side with the knees well drawn up.

The following muscles should then be systematically palpated: the thoracolumbar paravertebral muscles from the level of the tenth dorsal vertebra above to the coccyx below; the quadratus lumborum; the glutei and the piriformis. Following this, the patient should turn into the supine position in order that the anterior abdominal wall muscles (Ch. 15) and the iliopsoas muscle (p. 241) may be palpated.

The thoracolumbar paravertebral muscles (Fig. 12.1)

Anatomical relationships

These comprise a superficial and a deep group of muscles. The superficially situated group are known collectively as the erector spinae. The deeply situated group in order of depth include the semispinalis, the multifidi and the rotatores.

Factors responsible for development of TrP activity

TrP activity is liable to develop in the paravertebral muscles when they are suddenly strained as a result of lifting a heavy load with the back held in an awkward position or when they are subjected to sustained overloading during prolonged stooping.

In addition, pain from a spinal lesion such as a ruptured intervertebral disc may cause TrP activity to develop in these muscles. This is particularly liable to happen should they have gone into spasm severe enough to cause them to become ischaemic.

Erector spinae

MTrP sites and patterns of pain referral

The muscles in the superficially placed erector spinae group most likely to develop TrP activity are the longissimus thoracis and, lateral to this, the iliocostalis lumborum (Fig. 12.1).

Pain from TrPs in the iliocostalis lumborum muscle in the upper lumbar region (Fig. 12.2) and from TrPs in the longissimus thoracis at the

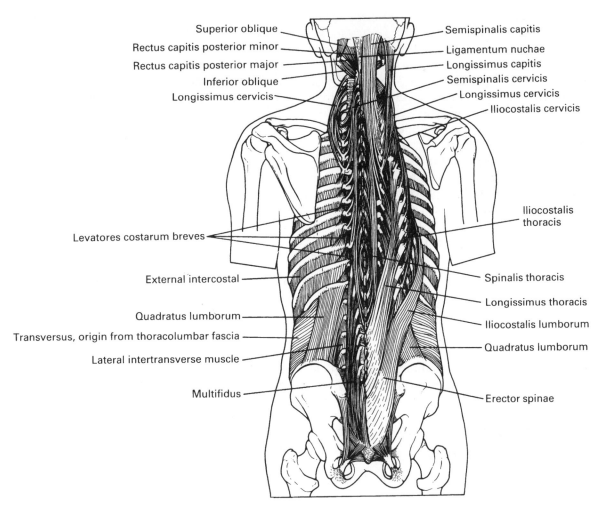

Figure 12.1   The deep muscles of the back. On the left side the erector spinae and its upward continuations (with the exception of the longissimus cervicis, which has been displaced laterally) and the semispinalis capitis have been removed.

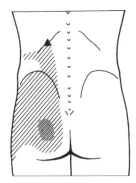

Figure 12.2   The pattern of pain referral from a trigger point (▲) in the iliocostalis lumborum muscle.

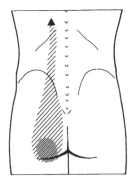

Figure 12.3   The pattern of pain referral from a trigger point (▲) in the longissimus thoracis muscle.

lower thoracic level (Fig. 12.3) is referred to the buttock (Simons et al 1999a).

Pain referred to the buttock from TrPs in one or other of these paravertebral muscles may cause satellite TrPs in the gluteal muscles to become activated. Pain from these satellite TrPs is then referred down the leg with, as a consequence, the development of satellite TrPs in thigh muscles. A muscle in which this frequently happens is the tensor fasciae latae (Ch. 13). Examination of this for TrP activity should be carried out routinely in all patients with MTrP low-back pain.

Similarly, satellite TrP activity may develop in the hamstring muscles (Ch. 13). When this happens, pain is referred down the back of the leg as far as the knee. And as a result of TrP-induced shortening of this group of muscles, straight leg raising becomes limited. The clinical manifestations then simulate those of a prolapsed intervertebral disc except that, with the latter, the pain tends to extend down as far as the ankle. Also, it either has a shooting electric-shock-like character or is a burning type of discomfort; and it is made worse by coughing, laughing or sneezing.

Deep paraspinal muscles

MTrP sites and patterns of pain referral

Pain from a TrP in either the multifidi or rotatores muscles in the lumbar region is referred locally to the tissues around the spinous process of the vertebra adjacent to it (Fig. 12.4). Pain from a TrP in one or other of these muscles in the sacral region is referred to the coccyx and causes it to become very tender (Fig. 12.5).

As Simons et al (1999b) have pointed out, TrPs in the iliocostalis thoracis muscle in the lower part of the thorax and in the multifidi anywhere along the length of the lumbar spine may also refer pain anteriorly to the abdomen. It is then liable to be misinterpreted as being of visceral origin.

Nerve entrapment

The spinal nerves' dorsal primary rami, before reaching the skin, pass through the paravertebral muscles and TrP-induced shortness of these muscles is liable to lead to entrapment of the nerves with the consequent development of sensory changes in the form of hypoaesthesiae, paraesthaesiae and occasionally dysaesthesiae. These sensory changes quickly disappear once MTrP deactivation has been carried out.

Deactivation of the paraspinal muscles' TrPs

Deactivation of TrPs in the superficial erector spinae group presents no difficulty and this may be achieved most simply by means of superficial dry needling.

TrP activity in more deeply situated muscles, however, often gives rise to considerable muscle spasm and to overcome this, it is often necessary to carry out deep dry needling. For this, Gunn (1996) advises using a 3-inch needle and leaving it in situ for 10–20 minutes.

Prevention of trigger point reactivation

Postural modifications Anyone prone to low-back pain, particularly those with TrPs in the paraspinal muscles, should learn to pick up objects from the floor with the knees bent and the back kept absolutely straight.

When sitting in a chair there must be sufficient lumbar support to maintain the normal lumbar lordotic curve. This may necessitate placing a cushion at waist level.

The use of a mattress that is too soft should be avoided as the lack of support aggravates tendons in the back muscles. Also, when sleeping on the side a person with low-back pain should place a pillow between the knees in order to prevent the uppermost knee from dropping forward onto the bed and causing rotating torsion of the spine.

Muscle stretching exercise The exercise described by Simons et al (1999c) should be carried out on a daily basis. This consists of sitting in a bath filled with comfortably hot water and leaning forwards with the knees straight until the hands reach the legs. The fingers are then

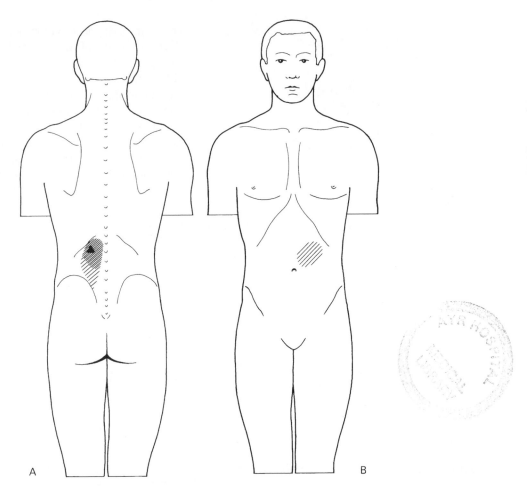

Figure 12.4   A and B: The pattern of pain referral from a trigger point (▲) in the deep group of paraspinal muscles (multifidi and rotatores) in the upper lumbar region.

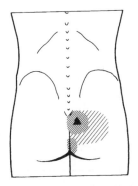

Figure 12.5   The pattern of pain referral from a trigger point (▲) in the deep group of paraspinal muscles (multifidi and rotatores) in the sacral region.

pushed down the shins until slight discomfort is experienced from stretching the paraspinal muscles. This degree of stretch is maintained for several seconds. The patient then relaxes for a short time before repeating the manoeuvre. The eventual aim is to reach as far as the feet.

Quadratus lumborum muscle
(Fig. 12.6)

Anatomical attachments

This quadrilateral-shaped muscle, which is made up of a superficially placed lateral part and a deeper lying medial part, arises below from the

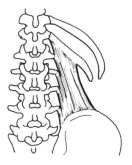

Figure 12.6 The quadratus lumborum muscle.

iliolumbar ligament and the adjacent part of the iliac crest and is attached above to the medial one-half of the twelfth rib and the transverse processes of the upper four lumbar vertebrae.

Actions

When the muscle on one side contracts it elevates the pelvis on that side. And when the muscles on both sides contract they help to extend the lumbar part of the spine. Another action of this muscle is to draw down the lower ribs during inspiration.

Factors responsible for the development of TrP activity

TrP activity in this muscle is liable to be brought about as a result of bending down to pick up an object from the floor with the trunk twisted to one side. It may also develop if the muscle is subjected to some form of direct trauma, for example a car accident, or when it is repeatedly strained carrying out some activity such as gardening or housework. In addition, TrP activity is liable to develop as a result of sleeping on a mattress that is not firm enough to provide adequate support for the back.

TrP-related physical signs

Physical signs brought about as a result of TrP activity in this muscle include restricted movements between the lumbar vertebrae and sacrum both when walking and when getting up from a

chair or bed; the development of scoliosis; the disappearance of the normal lumbar lordosis; tilting of the pelvis towards the contralateral side; and restriction of flexion, extension and side-bending of the lumbar spine. In addition, shortening of the muscle as a result of TrP activity has the effect of elevating the pelvis on the affected side with, as a consequence, the limb on that side seeming to be shorter than the contralateral one. This apparent leg length inequality (LLI), unlike true LLI (see p. 242), disappears once the TrPs in this muscle have been deactivated.

TrP activity in this muscle is also responsible for tenderness in the loin. Although this may be quite marked it is easily overlooked because of the relatively small space between the lower ribs and the iliac crest, and also because a large part of this muscle is covered by the paraspinal musculature.

The search for trigger points

When searching for TrPs in this muscle it is essential for the patient to lie on the uninvolved side with the arm on the affected side stretched upwards over the head in order to elevate the thoracic cage. In addition, the knee on the affected side should be positioned behind the knee on the opposite side in order to pull the iliac crest downwards. Also, the space between the ribs above and the iliac crest below should be opened still further by having the patient lying stretched across a pillow. The muscle should then be examined by means of vertically applied deep palpation of the flank (Fig. 12.7).

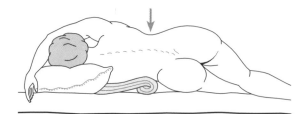

Figure 12.7 To show position in which the patient should be placed when palpating the flank (↓) for the purpose of searching for trigger points in the quadratus lumborum muscle.

MTrP sites and patterns of pain referral

Active TrPs in the superficial lateral part of this muscle refer pain to the iliac crest and greater trochanter (Fig. 12.8). In this latter region it may be confused with that caused by trochanteric bursitis. Pain from these TrPs may also be referred anteriorly towards the groin.

Active TrPs in the deeper medial part of this muscle refer pain to around the sacroiliac joint, where it has to be distinguished from that which arises as a result of a disorder in the joint itself, and also to the buttock (Fig. 12.9).

The referral of pain to the buttock is liable to lead to the development of satellite TrP activity in the gluteal muscles including the gluteus minimus. From satellite TrPs in this latter muscle, pain is then referred down the leg in a distribution similar to that of the pain of a first sacral nerve radiculopathy such as, for example, may develop as a result of the prolapse of an intervertebral disc.

As one of the actions of the quadratus lumborum muscle is to draw down the lower ribs during inspiration (see p. 234), should this muscle contain active TrPs any sudden inspiratory-induced tension in it such as may be caused by coughing or sneezing is liable to bring on a paroxysm of MTrP pain in the buttock. And should there already be satellite TrPs in the gluteus minimus pain from these is liable to shoot down the leg in a referral pattern similar to that taken by pain brought on by coughing or sneezing in someone with a prolapsed disc (see p. 249).

Diagnostic distinguishing features are that when pain with this pattern of referral develops as a result of a radiculopathy there is an accompanying neurological deficit, restricted straight leg raising and evidence of a disc lesion at a corresponding segmental level on magnetic MRI. When such pain arises as a result of a sudden surge of satellite TrP activity in the gluteus minimus, deactivation of the TrPs in this muscle temporarily alleviates it and deactivation of the primary TrPs in the quadratus lumborum muscle provides long-term relief from it.

Perpetuation of TrP activity

Factors liable to cause TrP activity in the quadratus lumborum muscle to be perpetuated

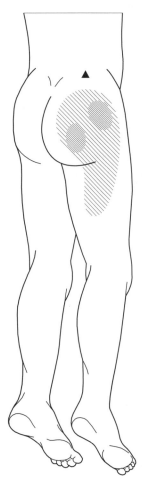

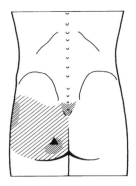

Figure 12.8 The pattern of pain referral from a trigger point (▲) in the gluteus maximus muscle.

Figure 12.9 The pattern of pain referral from a trigger point (▲) in the gluteus medius muscle.

include a lower limb length inequality, a small hemipelvis, short upper arms and a poor sleeping posture. Sleeping flat on the back with the knees straight should be avoided because this causes shortening of the quadratus lumborum. And, as a result, the pelvis is tilted forwards with an increased lumbar lordosis.

Sleeping, therefore, should be carried out lying on the unaffected side with a mattress firm enough to provide adequate support. For should this be too soft undesirable shortening of the muscle containing the TrPs takes place. In addition, a pillow should be placed between the knees and legs to prevent the uppermost one from dropping forwards on to the bed and placing undue tension on an already taut muscle.

Deactivation of myofascial trigger points

Those who carry out a deeply applied deactivating technique that involves penetration of the TrPs (see Ch. 7) not surprisingly find this easier to do with ones in the superficial part of the muscle. However, no matter whether the TrPs are in the superficial or deep part of the muscle, superficial dry needling with needles inserted into the skin and subcutaneous tissues immediately overlying them is usually sufficient to relax the muscle and relieve the pain.

Muscle stretching exercises

Travell & Simons (1992a) describe a useful number of corrective exercises but the one my patients are routinely taught to carry out following deactivation of TrPs in this muscle involves lying on the back and pushing the hip downwards on one side whilst at the same time elevating the hip on the other side – and then reversing the process. This has the effect of tilting the pelvis and by so doing stretching each of the two quadratus muscles in turn.

The effectiveness of this manoeuvre is enhanced by breathing in whilst elevating the hip on the affected side and breathing slowly out whilst pushing it downwards.

Gluteus maximus, medius and minimus

These three muscles make up the musculature of the buttock with the gluteus maximus overlying the gluteus medius, and this in turn overlying the gluteus minimus.

Factors responsible for the development of TrP activity

TrP activity in a gluteal muscle is liable to be brought about should it be subjected to directly applied acute trauma or to indirect trauma such as, for example, when it becomes overloaded during the course of sporting activities. In addition, satellite TrP activity in the gluteal muscles is liable to develop when pain is referred to the buttock from TrPs in the paravertebral muscles or quadratus lumborum muscle.

Gluteus maximus

Anatomical attachments The gluteus maximus, which is the largest and most superficial of the three glutei muscles, is attached above to the posterior iliac crest, the sacrum and the coccyx. Its fibres then run obliquely downwards and laterally with most of them converging to form a thick tendinous lamina which inserts into the iliotibial tract and the remainder converging to form a tendon which inserts into the gluteal tuberosity just below the greater trochanter.

Actions Its main action is to raise the trunk after stooping and, in association with the iliotibial tract, it holds the femur steady during standing.

MTrP sites and patterns of pain referral TrPs in this muscle may occur anywhere in it. Three common sites are adjacent to the sacrum, around the ischial tuberosity and in the region of the coccyx.

Because this muscle lies so near to the surface palpable bands at TrP sites are readily felt and local twitch responses easily elicited.

Pain referred from these MTrPs is mainly localised to the buttock itself (Fig. 12.8).

Associated trigger points TrP activity in this muscle is not infrequently accompanied by TrP activity in the other two gluteal muscles.

Gluteus medius

Anatomical attachments This thick fan-shaped muscle is attached above to the iliac crest and its lower part tapers down to be inserted into the greater trochanter. It is situated deep to the gluteus maximus and overlies the gluteus minimus.

Actions The gluteus medius is an extremely powerful abductor of the thigh. Its anterior fibres also assist with medial rotation of the thigh.

MTrP sites and patterns of pain referral TrPs in this muscle are most commonly located just below its attachment to the iliac crest.

Because this muscle lies deep to the gluteus maximus the locating of TrPs in it requires the application of firmer pressure than that required when examining this latter muscle. Also, palpable bands and local twitch responses are not usually evident.

Pain from these TrPs is referred both to the buttock and to the upper part of the back of the thigh (Fig. 12.9).

Associated trigger points TrP activity in this muscle is often accompanied by TrP activity in the gluteus minimus, piriformis and tensor fasciae latae.

Gluteus minimus

Anatomical attachments This muscle, which is the deepest of the three gluteal muscles, is fan-shaped and, like the gluteus medius, is attached above to the iliac crest, and below, its fibres converge to form a tendon which attaches to the greater trochanter.

Actions Like the gluteus medius, it is an abductor of the thigh.

MTrP sites and patterns of pain referral Because this muscle is so deeply situated TrPs in it are likely to be overlooked unless extremely firm palpation is used when searching for them. For the same reason it is not possible to feel palpable bands in this muscle or to elicit local twitch responses.

When palpating the buttock it is often difficult to be certain whether deep-lying TrPs are situated in the gluteus medius or minimus. Their TrP pain referral patterns, however, have been shown to be different (Travell & Simons 1992b).

TrPs in the anterior part of the gluteus minimus refer pain to the lower outer part of the buttock, the lateral aspects of the thigh and the outer side of the leg as far as the ankle (Fig. 12.10A). TrPs in the posterior part refer pain to the buttock and the back of the thigh and calf (Fig. 12.10B).

Radiculopathy pain and gluteus minimus TrP pain As Rubin (1981) and Reynolds (1981) have pointed out, the distribution of pain in the leg from sciatic nerve entrapment and from TrPs in the gluteus minimus is similar. The path taken by pain from TrPs in the anterior part of this muscle coincides with that taken by pain arising as a result of a L5 radiculopathy. And the path taken by pain from TrPs in the posterior part of the muscle coincides with that taken by the pain of a S1 radiculopathy. The character of the pain from these two sources, however, tends to be different. MTrP pain takes the form of a persistent dull ache whereas a radiculopathy pain has a burning electric-shock-like quality. Also, with the latter there is likely to be a neurological deficit. At the same time it has to be remembered that, because of the effect motor nerve compression has on motor endplates at a TrP site, entrapment of a nerve root may lead to the development of TrP activity as a secondary event in muscles supplied by it.

Associated TrP activity TrP activity in this muscle rarely occurs alone. There is liable to be similar activity in the gluteus medius, vastus lateralis, quadratus lumborum and piriformis.

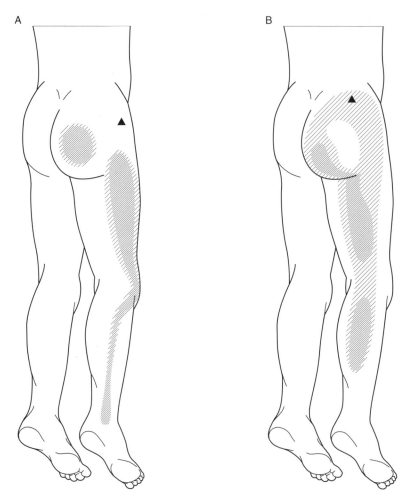

Figure 12.10   A: Pattern of pain referral from a trigger point (▲) in the anterior part of the gluteus minimus. B: Pattern of pain referral from a trigger point (▲) in its posterior part.

Deactivation of trigger points in gluteal muscles

TrPs in the gluteus maximus and the gluteus medius immediately beneath it may be readily deactivated by any of the methods described in Chapter 7.

For the deactivation of TrPs in the gluteus minimus any technique that involves TrP penetration of the TrP may need a 5–6 cm (2–2½ inch) needle. Furthermore, if a local anaesthetic such as 0.5% procaine solution is injected, weakness of the leg may develop so that on standing immediately

following treatment, the patient may fall. No such problem arises when superficial dry needling is employed, and fortunately, despite the depth at which this muscle lies, this is often all that is required.

Piriformis muscle (Fig. 12.11)

Anatomical attachments

The piriformis muscle, a thick well-developed muscle, is so-called because it is pear-shaped

(Latin *pirium* – pear plus *forum* – shape). Attached medially to the sacrum it leaves the pelvic cavity via the greater sciatic foramen to become inserted laterally into the greater trochanter.

Actions

This muscle, together with the quadratus femoris, the obturator externus, the obturator internus and the gemelli which lie immediately below it, are external rotators of the thigh when the hip is extended. They also assist with abduction when the hip is flexed.

The piriformis syndrome

In the disorder known as the piriformis syndrome (Synek 1987) pain arises for several reasons. One is because of trauma-induced activation of nociceptors at MTrP sites in the piriformis muscle. A second is that this muscle becomes shortened and thickened as a result of the TrP activity with, as a consequence, compression of various nerves that pass through the greater sciatic notch, including in particular, the sciatic nerve (Pace 1975, Pace & Nagle 1976). And a third is because dysfunction of the sacroiliac joint frequently develops in this syndrome and contributes to any pain that may be felt in the

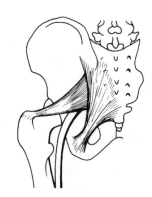

Figure 12.11 The outer part of the piriformis muscle with its attachment to the greater trochanter. The sciatic nerve is shown in its normal position behind this muscle.

region of this joint (Kirkaldy-Willis & Hill 1979, Travell & Travell 1946).

Trauma responsible for piriformis TrP activation

TrP activity in the piriformis muscle is liable to develop should it become overloaded such as when twisting the trunk sideways whilst bending to pick up a heavy object. Also, when it is held in a shortened position for some considerable time, as for example may happen, when lying with the hips flexed and knees spread apart during the course of some surgical procedure. TrPs are also liable to develop activity in this muscle when it is subjected to direct trauma as, for example, in a motor vehicle accident. Baker (1986) examined 100 patients with injuries incurred in this manner and found that a large number of them had TrPs in the piriformis muscle.

MTrP sites and patterns of pain referral

The upper border of the piriformis muscle is located by drawing a line (the piriformis line) from the proximal end of the greater trochanter to the sacroiliac junction. Active TrPs near to its medial attachment are found to be exquisitely tender when pressure is applied to the region of the greater sciatic foramen during the course of a rectal or vaginal examination (Barton et al 1988, Thiele 1937). TrPs may also become activated in the laterally situated part of the muscle near to its attachment to the greater trochanter. These may be readily located on external examination.

The search for both these medially and laterally situated TrPs should be carried out with the patient lying in the semi-prone position with the affected side uppermost. From nociceptors at either of these two MTrP sites pain is referred to the sacroiliac region, across the buttock, the hip and the posterior part of the thigh (Fig. 12.12). It is made worse by sitting for any length of time, also by prolonged standing and by walking.

Associated TrP activity

TrP activity in this muscle rarely occurs alone but usually in association with similar activity in the gluteal muscles and the other lateral rotators of the thigh that lie immediately below it.

Pace abduction test

Pain and weakness on resisted abduction–external rotation of the thigh is a sign of the piriformis syndrome (Pace & Nagle 1976).

The test consists of the examiner placing his hands on the outer sides of the knees and ask-

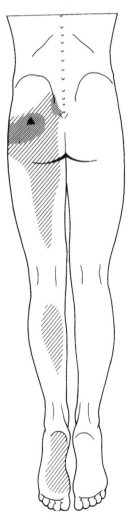

Figure 12.12 The pattern of pain referral from a trigger point (▲) in the piriformis muscle.

ing the patient to push the hands apart. The test is positive should this manoeuvre give rise to pain and weakness on the affected side (Pace 1975).

Nerve compression pain

A piriformis muscle that has become shortened as a result of MTrP activity is liable to compress one or other of the various nerves that pass through the greater sciatic foramen.

Compression of the sciatic nerve causes pain to be felt down the back of the leg from the thigh to the calf and sometimes as far as the foot. It may also give rise to numbness and paraesthesiae in the foot.

Compression of the gluteal nerves contributes to the pain felt in the buttock in this disorder.

Compression of the pudendal nerve causes pain to be felt in the perineum and gives rise to sexual dysfunction in the form of dyspareunia in the female and impotence in the male.

Differential diagnosis

The piriformis syndrome may develop as a primary event or secondary to a sacroiliitis due to either ankylosing spondylitis in HLA-B27 positive young adults, psoriatic arthropathy or Reiter's disease. Therefore the erythrocyte sedimentation rate should always be measured and when found to be raised, radiographic examination of the sacroiliac joint is mandatory.

It is necessary to remember that nerve entrapment at the greater sciatic foramen may not only occur as part of the piriformis syndrome but also may be caused by a tumour. Therefore, in cases where this possibility exists a computed tomographic (CT) scan is essential.

The pain from a prolapsed intervertebral disc may be similar to that which develops in the piriformis syndrome. A sensory or motor deficit is in favour of a disc lesion. Motor denervation shown on electromyography also suggests a disc lesion. However, slowing of the conduction velocity in the sciatic nerve where it passes through the pelvis is in favour of the piriformis syndrome.

Magnetic resonance imaging may or may not be helpful because the discovery of a disc lesion by this means does not imply that it is responsible for any pain that may be present unless, in addition to this, there are appropriate neurological signs of nerve root compression at the same segmental level.

Therefore, in all cases of sciatic nerve entrapment a search for TrPs in the piriformis muscle is essential and when these are found to be present it is first necessary to observe the effect deactivating them has on the pain.

Methods of treating the piriformis syndrome

Thiele (1937) recommended massaging the piriformis muscle with a finger inserted into the rectum. The massage is initially carried out lightly but on subsequent occasions the pressure applied can be gradually increased as the muscle tenderness subsides.

Other methods employed include ultrasound treatment applied to the muscle for 5–6 minutes a day over a period of 1–2 weeks (Hallin 1983). Barton et al (1988) have reported the use of a combination of ultrasound therapy and muscle stretching.

Alternatively, one of the MTrP deactivating procedures described in Chapter 7 may be employed.

Pace (1975) injected a local anaesthetic/corticosteroid (triamcinolone) mixture into the TrPs. Travell & Simons (1992c) recommend injecting a 0.5% solution of procaine into them. Rachlin (1994) advises inserting either 0.5% procaine, 1% lignocaine (lidocaine), saline or dry needles into them. However, despite the muscle being a deeply lying one, superficial dry needling is frequently all that is required.

Identifying a TrP prior to carrying out one of these deactivating procedures presents no difficulty when it is situated in the outer part of the muscle. However, locating a TrP in its medial part is best done with the tip of a finger of the left hand inserted into the rectum. And then, with the right hand, a needle can be inserted externally through the tissues in the direction of the intrarectally placed finger tip.

Prevention of TrP reactivation

It is essential to look for and, if present, to correct any lower limb length inequality (p. 242); similarly for a Morton foot disorder (mediolateral rocking of the foot) (p. 245).

Psoas major and iliacus muscle (syn: iliopsoas muscle)

Anatomical attachments

The psoas major muscle is a long fusiform muscle that arises from attachments to the 12th thoracic vertebra and all the lumbar vertebrae. From these attachments it descends across the brim of the pelvis to become attached by means of a tendon to the lesser trochanter of the femur.

The iliacus muscle is a flat triangular muscle which arises from the upper two thirds of the iliac fossa. At its lower end most of its fibres converge to be inserted into the lateral side of the psoas tendon.

Because the primary action of the psoas major and iliacus muscles is to flex the hip, functionally they act as one muscle and therefore the alternative collective name for them is the iliopsoas muscle.

Factors responsible for the development of iliopsoas muscle TrP activity

TrP activity is liable to develop in this conjoint muscle whenever it is overloaded such as may happen during the course of a fall or while carrying out some athletic pursuit. Also, when it is strained as a result of prolonged sitting with the hips acutely flexed. Truck drivers are said to be particularly likely to develop backache because of this (Travell & Simons 1992d).

Because of the shortening of the iliopsoas muscle that takes place as a result of TrP activity in it there is a tendency to stand with the weight on the contralateral leg with the knee on the affected side slightly bent, and also to stand with the trunk inclined to the affected side. The reason for adopting this posture is because it helps to reduce the tension in the muscle and as a consequence to alleviate the pain.

TrP activity in this muscle is often associated with similar activity in other muscles, including the thigh adductors and various posteriorly situated ones including the glutei and hamstrings.

MTrP sites and patterns of pain referral

The search for TrPs in the iliopsoas muscle should be conducted with the patient lying supine. There are two sites in this muscle where active TrPs may readily be located. One is just above its distal attachment to the lesser trochanter. The other is inside the brim of the pelvis in the region of the anterior superior iliac spine. In order to be able to locate TrPs at this site it is essential for the anterior abdominal muscles to be well relaxed.

Pain from TrPs in the iliopsoas muscle is referred mainly to the back along the paravertebral gutter on the affected side and in some cases to the front of the thigh (Fig. 12.13A and B).

It should be noted that TrPs in the iliopsoas muscle and TrPs in the rectus abdominis muscle (see Ch. 15) may refer pain to the lumbar region. It therefore follows that in all cases of low-back pain it is necessary to search for TrPs not only in the muscles of the back but also in both of these anteriorly situated ones.

Deactivation of myofascial trigger points

Locating and deactivating TrPs at the two sites already discussed present no particular problems. However, TrPs may also occasionally develop activity in the upper part of the psoas muscle near to its attachment to the lumbar vertebrae. These TrPs may easily be overlooked and even when they are found their position makes deactivation extremely difficult.

ACUTE, RECURRENT AND CHRONIC LUMBAR MTrP PAIN

Acute lumbar MTrP pain

Acute mechanical type low-back pain brought about as a result of direct trauma to or overloading of the lumbar muscles causing MTrPs to become active is common and usually spontaneously disappears within 2–6 weeks. Should the pain be very severe bed rest may initially be required but this should not be continued for more than 2 days (Deyo et al 1986). After this, physical activity including the regular carrying out of muscle stretching exercises should be encouraged. And in order to assist with alleviating the pain, deactivation of any MTrPs that may be present should be carried out every other day.

Persistent lumbar MTrP pain

Low-back pain is recurrent or chronic in up to 39% of adults (Papageorgiou et al 1995). A common reason for this is the perpetuation of MTrP activity.

One or more of the following factors may contribute to this.

Lower limb length inequality

Relative shortness of one leg is not uncommon. Friberg (1983) radiographically determined the length of limbs in 359 symptom-free soldiers and found that 56% of them had a lower limb length inequality (LLLI) of 0–4 mm; 30% had a LLLI of 5–9 mm and 14% had one of 10 mm or greater.

LLLI may be a congenital deformity in which case not infrequently one side of the body is smaller than the other so that not only is one lower limb shorter than the other but there is also slight, but discernible, facial asymmetry, unequal length of the two arms, one half of the pelvis smaller than the other and one foot a little smaller than the other. Alternatively the deformity may be acquired, for example, because

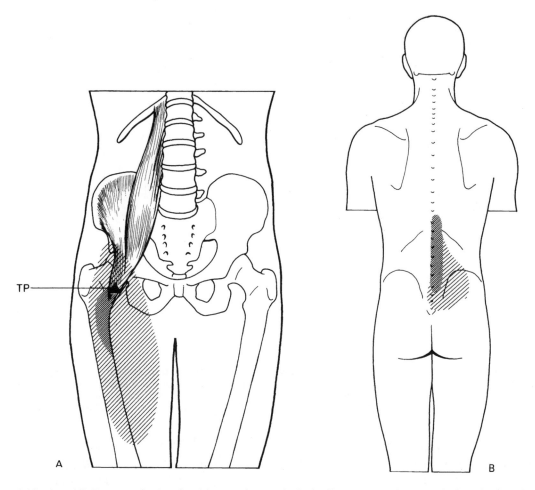

Figure 12.13   A and B: Patterns of pain referral from a trigger point in the iliopsoas muscle near to its insertion into the lesser trochanter.

of an injury or as a result of a badly fitting hip prosthesis.

A person with LLLI tends to stand with the weight of the body shifted to the side of the shorter limb and the knee on the side opposite to this slightly flexed. The torso will also be tilted when walking.

There is, in addition, likely to be a scoliosis. When the leg-length difference is 6 mm ($\frac{1}{4}$ inch) or less, a C-shaped scoliosis develops with, as a consequence, sagging of the shoulder on the side opposite to the short leg. In order to counteract this it is necessary to raise the heel on the short side (Fig. 12.14A and B). When

the leg-length difference is 1.3 cm ($\frac{1}{2}$ inch) or more an S-shaped scoliosis develops and, as a result of this, there is sagging of the shoulder on the same side as the short leg (Gerwin 1991, Travell & Simons 1992e). Again, raising the heel on the affected side corrects this (Fig. 12.15 A and B).

Examination   Should LLLI be suspected the undressed patient should be asked to stand with both legs straight with, in particular, no bending of the knees and the feet brought together. An estimate as to whether or not there is any LLLI may then be made by comparing the relative heights of

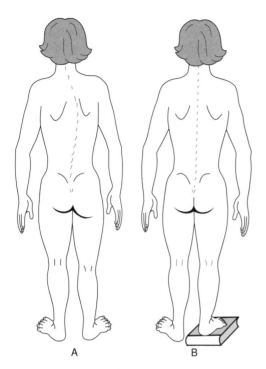

A   B

Figure 12.14   A: Diagram to show C-shaped scoliosis and sagging of the left shoulder produced by right leg being 6 mm ($\frac{1}{4}$ inch) or less shorter than the left one. B: Correction of scoliosis by raising the right heel.

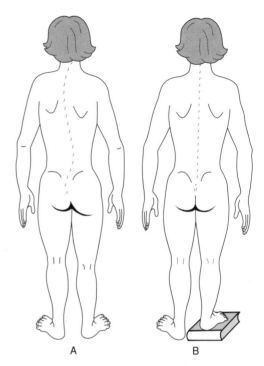

A   B

Figure 12.15   A: Diagram to show S-shaped scoliosis and sagging of the right shoulder produced by right leg being being 1.3 cm ($\frac{1}{2}$ inch) or more than the left one. B: Correction of scoliosis by raising the right heel.

the iliac crests and the greater trochanters. A more accurate method, but one which tends not to be undertaken routinely, is to carry out a radiological assessment employing the technique described by Travell & Simons (1992f).

Once a difference in length between the two legs has been identified it is first necessary to ascertain whether this is an apparent LLLI brought about as a result of TrP activity in the quadratus lumborum muscle (see p. 234) and therefore correctable by deactivating TrPs in it, or whether it is a true LLLI that needs to be corrected by raising the heel on the shorter side. The amount that this has to be done is most conveniently determined by seeing how many filing cards or pages of a journal have to be placed under the foot on the shorter side. A cobbler can then increase the thickness of the heel of the shoe on the shorter side accordingly.

Small hemipelvis

A lower limb length inequality is often accompanied by a smaller hemipelvis and an

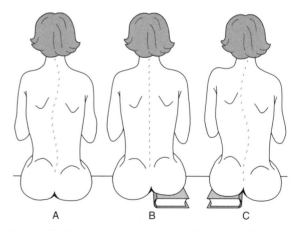

A   B   C

Figure 12.16   A: Hemipelvis on the right side smaller than on the left side causing S-shaped scoliosis. B: Scoliosis corrected by raising right buttock. C: Scoliosis made worse by raising left buttock.

abnormally short upper limb on the side of the short leg. When one side of the pelvis is smaller than the other there is a compensatory S-shaped scoliosis and a corresponding downward tilt of the shoulder girdle on the affected side. The scoliosis may be corrected by placing a cushion under the ischial tuberosity on the affected side (Fig. 12.16).

Short upper arms

Shortness of the upper arms relative to the height of the torso is not looked for as often as it should for this deformity puts a strain on muscles in the shoulder girdle, particularly the upper trapezius and levator scapulae (see Ch. 8). In addition, short upper arms predispose to the development and perpetuation of TrP nociceptor activity in the quadratus lumborum muscle.

Morton's foot deformity

A short first metatarsal bone with, as a consequence, a relatively long second one, a disorder first described by Morton (1935), has been found to be present in approximately 40% of individuals (Harris & Beath 1949). The effect of this deformity is to cause medio-lateral rocking of the foot so that on walking the weight of the body is transferred from the second to the first metatarsal head with pronation of the foot at the ankle and internal rotation of the leg at the knee and hip. And, as a result of the strain produced by these postural changes, TrP activity is liable to develop in various muscles. These include the peroneal group (Ch. 13), the vastus medialis (Ch. 13), the gluteus medius (p. 237) and the gluteus minimus (p. 237).

Deactivation of the MTrPs in these muscles only gives a relatively short period of relief unless this underlying disorder is corrected by placing a pad under the first metatarsal head (Ch. 13).

Fibromyalgia

Low-back pain is invariably chronic when it is part of the generalised muscle pain disorder fibromyalgia.

In order to make this diagnosis, however, it is essential for the diagnostic criteria laid down by the American College of Rheumatology to be fulfilled (Wolfe et al 1990). It certainly cannot be made simply because there is widespread myofascial pain as the concomitant development of several MTrP pain syndromes is not uncommon. To add to the confusion fibromyalgia may develop in someone already suffering from the MTrP pain syndrome (Bennett 1986a, 1986b, 1990). The reason for this is not known but should it happen in a person already engaged in seeking compensation for a regional MTrP pain disorder it is liable to engender considerable medico-legal controversy (see Ch. 8).

Furthermore, it has been shown that patients with chronic low-back pain may ultimately develop fibromyalgia. In a retrospective study of 53 patients who had had pain in the lumbar region for more than 3 months with no severe pathology on spinal X-rays and no radicular symptoms or signs to account for it, Làpossy et al (1995) found that after an average of 18 years (11–40), no less than 25% of them (all females except one) had developed this generalised muscle pain disorder.

Biochemical deficiencies

As already discussed in Chapter 7, lumbar MTrP pain, in common with similar pain in other regions of the body, may become chronic as a result of a failure to recognise and correct various underlying biochemical deficiencies (Gerwin 1995).

Concomitant complex regional pain syndrome and MTrP pain syndrome

Both MTrP pain (Ch. 6) and disc prolapse pain (Maigne et al 1996) are liable to become chronic as a result of the concomitant development of the complex regional pain syndrome type 1 (RSD).

Neurophysiological changes responsible for pain chronicity

As discussed in Chapters 2 and 4, MTrP pain in any region of the body, including the low-back, may become chronic as a result of the setting up of self-perpetuating ischaemic changes at MTrP sites and self-perpetuating circuits between MTrPs and the spinal cord. Also, as Jason (1997) has pointed out, because of the development of dorsal horn neuroplasticity.

Psychological and occupational factors

Psychological and occupational factors that may also be responsible for the persistence of mechanical type low-back pain, including that due to MTrP activity, were discussed earlier when considering its multifactorial aetiology (p. 228).

LUMBAR FACET JOINT PAIN

The possibility that the facet joints in the spine could be a source of pain was first put forward by Goldthwait in 1911. Diagnostic radiology had only just recently been introduced and it was from observing asymmetry of the facet joints in X-rays of the spine that led him to suggest that this could be 'an explanation for many cases of lumbago, sciatica and paraplegia'.

In 1927 the Italian surgeon Putti lent support to this idea by expressing the view that radiographically demonstrable degenerative changes in the facet joints are a cause of sciatic pain. And in 1933 Ghormley stated that sciatica is caused by facet joint-induced nerve pressure and introduced the term 'the facet syndrome'.

However, following Mixter & Barr's historic discovery in 1934 that the commonest reason for sciatica developing is the rupture of an intervertebral disc, interest in the facet joints was to wane for some considerable time.

It was therefore thirty years before anything further was written on the subject. Then in 1963 Hirsch et al reported that they could bring on pain in the back and lower extremities by injecting hypertonic saline into the tissues around a facet joint. And soon after this Skirm Rees (1971), somewhat surprisingly as he was a general practitioner working alone in a small Australian town, announced that he could relieve low-back pain by denervating the facet joints. For this he employed a specially hooked bladed knife which he inserted percutaneously into the region of a facet joint under local anaesthesia.

The cutting of nerves in this way was clearly a somewhat hazardous procedure but Rees's results appeared to be so good that the neurosurgeon Norman Shealy decided to visit him in order to learn more about the technique. He eventually attempted to carry out the procedure himself, but because it caused so much bleeding he very soon abandoned the use of a knife and employed instead firstly thermocoagulation of the nerves and later on radiofrequency denervation. In addition, he considerably reduced the risks of the procedure by carrying it out under fluoroscopic control (Shealy 1975).

The importance of all this was quickly recognised by the Californian orthopaedic surgeon Vert Mooney for, as he has since said (Mooney 1992),

In 1972 when I first visited Dr Shealy and observed patients in obvious pain and distress being brought to the fluoroscopy unit for the procedure I was quite impressed at the remarkable reversal of symptoms following the apparent obliteration of innervation at the various facet levels. It seemed quite apparent that denervation of these joints was effective in relieving the patients' pain. Also, that localisation of the joints under fluoroscopy was quite simple.

It was because of what Mooney had observed on visiting Shealy that he and his colleague James Robertson decided to repeat the work carried out by Hirsch and his co-workers in the 1960s. However, instead of injecting hypertonic saline into the region of a facet joint, as had previously been done, they inserted it directly into the joint itself using both fluoroscopy and the injection of a contrast material (Conray 60) to ensure the accurate placement of the needle within the joint capsule.

They did this on 5 normal individuals and 15 patients with chronic back pain and sciatica. In both of these groups the hypertonic saline provoked an almost immediate onset of pain at the injection site followed a few seconds later by pain which extended from there into the lower part of the back and down the leg. The only difference between the normal individuals and those suffering from back and leg pain was that the pain artificially induced in the latter group radiated over a wider area.

Their next important observation was that the hypertonic saline-induced pain in these two groups was abolished by injecting 2–5 cc of 1% xylocaine into the facet joint. Following this, they injected a steroid/local anaesthetic mixture into the facet joints of 100 patients with low-back and leg pain which, on clinical grounds, was considered might possibly be emanating from a facet joint.

Their original intention was to carry out a 'Shealy type' rhizotomy on those whose pain was relieved by this steroid/local anaesthetic mixture, but as they found that the latter itself gave long-term relief in one fifth of the patients and partial relief in another third, they decided there was no need to do this and introduced the injection technique as a combined diagnostic–therapeutic procedure (Mooney & Robertson 1976).

Although Mooney & Robertson's combined diagnostic–therapeutic injection procedure is still widely employed for what is now called the facet joint syndrome, there continues to be considerable controversy concerning its causation, clinical manifestations and treatment.

LUMBAR FACET JOINT SYNDROME

Possible aetiological factors

Apart from when facet joint pain occasionally arises as a result of some inflammatory disorder such as ankylosing spondylitis or rheumatoid arthritis there are no generally agreed reasons for it developing.

It certainly cannot be due to the degenerative changes that develop in the joints as a secondary event following degeneration of the intervertebral discs (Butler et al 1990), as these combined disc and facet joint degenerative changes of what is called lumbar spondylosis (p. 254) are observed radiographically as commonly in those without a history of low-back pain as they are in those with one (Lawrence et al 1966, Magora &

Schwartz 1976, 1978). These degenerative changes are also frequently seen in CT scans carried out on asymptomatic patients (Wiesel et al 1981).

When considering the pathogenesis of this syndrome it furthermore has to be remembered that Revel et al (1992), from the carrying out of diagnostic facet joint nerve blocks, have provided evidence to suggest that pain is liable to emanate from facet joints that have normal appearances on plain X-rays, CT and MRI.

One theory is that the pain may arise because of the entrapment of meniscoid fragments of cartilage avulsed from the articular surface as a result of trauma. Bogduk & Jull (1985) have suggested that this may be one of the main causes of an acute locked back. Other possible causes include synovial impingement, joint subluxation, chondromalacia and capsular inflammation (Dreyfuss et al 1995); also trauma-induced fractures, capsular tears, articular cartilage disruption and haemarthrosis, all of which have been observed in post-mortem examinations of people killed in motor vehicle accidents (Twomey et al 1989).

Clinical manifestations

There is nothing in the history or physical examination that is uniquely characteristic of this syndrome.

The distribution of the pain is widely variable. It may be confined to the back or may in addition be referred to the buttock and upper thigh and may in some cases even extend down as far as the calf and foot. It may also be felt in the groin.

There are in addition no distinctive physical signs. Admittedly, tenderness on deep palpation of the tissues overlying the facet joint is sometimes found but this is not a constant feature. Jackson et al (1988), from a study of 390 consecutive patients, and Schwarzer et al (1994a), from a study of 176 patients who underwent fluoroscopically controlled diagnostic facet joint nerve blocks, concluded that there are no features in either the history or clinical examination that are predictive of the response likely to be obtained with this procedure.

Diagnosis

It is generally agreed that the only way of establishing that pain emanates from a facet joint is to alleviate it by injecting a local anaesthetic, under fluoroscopic control, either into the joint itself or into the medial branches of the dorsal rami that innervate it.

This diagnostic procedure is carried out on any facet joint which, on deep palpation, is found to be markedly tender, or one which, when put through movements, is found to be painful. When no such localising signs are present the L4–L5 and L5–S1 joints should first be blocked as it is these which are most commonly affected (Dreyfuss et al 1995).

When the diagnostic facet joint block procedure was first introduced it was customary to carry it out using only one anaesthetic substance. Unfortunately, this gave an unacceptably high false-positive responder rate and in an attempt to reduce this the injection of a short-acting anaesthetic substance followed by a longer-acting one is now recommended.

Schwarzer et al (1994a) studied 176 consecutive patients with chronic low-back pain who were firstly given a facet joint block using lignocaine (Lidocaine). Those who responded positively to this were then given an injection of the longer-acting bupivacaine. Analgesia had to be achieved with both of these substances for a patient to be considered a true responder. Nevertheless, even using this two-block procedure there was a false-positive rate of 38%. This, however, is in keeping with the result obtained in a previous study (Schwarzer et al 1992) for in that a placebo rate of 32% was reported.

From use of this dual diagnostic procedure it has been estimated that the prevalence of chronic low-back facet joint pain is only 15% (Schwarzer et al 1994b). Unfortunately the diagnostic technique has not as yet been applied to a group of patients with acute low-back pain and so the frequency with which this emanates from a facet joint is presently unknown (Dreyfuss et al 1995).

Treatment

The current method of treating pain considered to be emanating from a facet joint pain is to inject a corticosteroid/local anaesthetic mixture into the affected joint.

There have been many uncontrolled trials to assess the efficacy of these forms of treatment and two controlled ones.

The first controlled trial was carried out by Lillius et al (1989). In that study, patients judged from a facet joint diagnostic block to have facet joint pain were randomly divided into three treatment groups. One group was treated with an intra-articular steroid and local anaesthetic injection, a second group was treated with pericapsular injections of those two substances and a third control group was given injections of saline into the affected joint.

There was no statistically significant difference in the response rate in the three groups and overall only 36% of the patients achieved pain relief lasting 3 months.

The second trial was carried out by Carette et al (1991). In their study, 97 patients who had achieved more than 50% pain alleviation with a diagnostic facet joint block were divided into a treatment group and a control group. The treatment group received an intra-articular injection of methylprednisolone. The control group was given an intra-articular injection of saline.

Forty-two per cent in the treatment group and 33% in the control group reported significant pain relief both immediately and 3 months later. Furthermore, 22% in the treatment group and 10% in the control group had sustained improvement for 6 months following treatment.

It may therefore be seen in these two controlled trials that neither a steroid injection, nor a combined steroid and local anaesthetic injection has been shown to be particularly effective in relieving facet joint pain. And Deyo (1991), having studied these findings, was forced to conclude: 'The poor results of these studies may have occurred because, despite careful diagnostic efforts, many patients had sources of pain other than the facet joints, or because a corticosteroid injection is inefficacious even when facet joints are the source of pain. In either event, the form of treatment appears to be over-used and minimally effective'.

Jackson (1992), who has had considerable experience in this particular field, has gone even further by provocatively asking – 'the facet syndrome, myth or reality?', and by concluding that this question can only be answered by the carrying out of further prospective randomised controlled clinical studies.

LUMBAR DISC HERNIATION PAIN

Predisposing factors

Degenerative changes in the discs begin to take place in the first year of life when adoption of the upright posture causes pressure to be created on them. This degenerative process gradually progresses from then onwards so that by the time adolescence is reached it is not uncommon for bulging of the annulus fibrosus to be observed on MRI (Kraemer 1995).

It is not, however, until early adult life or even more commonly the fourth or fifth decade that disc herniation takes place. By that stage of life the annulus fibrosus is likely to have developed fissures in it and to have become sufficiently weakened for it to rupture and allow degraded nuclear material to flow through it when subjected to some form of mechanical pressure.

Disc herniation is far less likely to occur at a later stage of life than this because although the annulus fibrosus has had a greater chance of rupturing, the nucleus pulposus by then is too desiccated to be readily extruded through it.

Character and causation of the pain

There is often a history of recurrent episodes of low-back pain before the eventual sudden onset of sciatica with a severe shooting type of pain that radiates from the lower part of the back, down the leg to the foot. The distribution of this pain varies according to which root is affected. About 70% of disc herniations occur at the L5/S1 level with compression of the first sacral root.

The pain which develops as a result of this radiates from the lumbar region down the back of the thigh, the outer side of the lower leg and the outer side of the foot to as far as the fifth toe. Twenty-five per cent are at the L4/L5 level with compression of the fifth lumbar root. With this, the pain radiates from the lower back down the posterolateral part of the thigh, the lower leg and the front of the foot as far as the big toe. With the rarer L2 and L3 root lesions pain radiates down the front of the thigh.

Disc prolapse pain is aggravated by sitting, lifting and twisting the torso. It is usually relieved by lying down. It is also characteristically made worse by coughing, sneezing, laughing and straining to open the bowels.

There are two main causes for the pain. One is mechanical compression of the nerve root. The other is an inflammatory reaction in the neural tissue produced by phospholipase A-2 (PLA-2) and other enzymes that are liberated from the nucleus pulposus following its extrusion (Saal et al 1990). The pain is always at its worst during the first 3 weeks after the prolapse has taken place. This is because the extruded disc material, no longer influenced by the osmotic system present in an intact disc, absorbs water and, as a consequence, temporarily increases in size. Also, because it is during this period that the inflammatory reaction is at its height.

Eventually the extruded disc material becomes smaller due to a decrease in its fluid content and because of enzymatic resorption and phagocytosis. Also, because the inflammatory reaction in the neural tissue gradually abates. It is because of this natural healing process that after a period of time ranging from a few weeks to several months discogenic pain tends to disappear spontaneously (Kraemer 1995).

There may also be superimposed MTrP pain. This may arise as a result of activity developing as a secondary event when inflammatory discogenic pain causes lumbar muscles to go into spasm severe enough to make them become ischaemic. It may also arise when radiculopathy pain in the back and leg develops. This is because TrP activity is liable to develop in muscles innervated by the entrapped nerve root or roots as a result of the effect of motor nerve compression on motor endplates at TrP sites.

All this notwithstanding it is necessary to bear in mind that disc rupture is not necessarily painful. Boden et al (1990), in a study employing MRI, have shown that although 20% of people have disc protrusions by the age of 60 most of these are symptomless. Porter et al (1978) have shown that an important factor in determining whether or not a disc herniation causes pain to develop is the size and shape of the vertebral canal. Porter (1993a), from comparing the vertebral canal measurements in 173 patients with disc protrusion and 671 volunteers, found that nearly half of the patients with root symptoms and signs of acute disc protrusion had particularly small canal measurements.

It is therefore now well recognised that it is possible for a person with a capacious canal to accommodate a disc protrusion without pain developing. It is, however, not only the size of the canal that matters but also its shape, A small trefoil-shaped canal being particularly disadvantageous (Porter 1993b).

Nerve root entrapment: physical signs

With a S1 root lesion there is a depressed or absent ankle tendon reflex; also tingling and sensory loss along the outer aspect of the foot. And with severe lesions there may be some wasting of the gastrocnemius and soleus muscles.

With a fifth lumbar root lesion there is a certain amount of foot drop and weakness of the extensor hallucis longus. In some cases there may be sensory impairment on the outer aspect of the leg and dorsum of the foot. The tendon reflexes are not affected (Hopkins 1993).

With the rarer L2 and L3 root lesions there is a weakness of the quadriceps muscle and depression of the knee jerk.

Straight leg raising test

Although restricted straight leg raising on the affected side is always present with a disc-induced radiculopathy, it has to be stressed that it is not pathognomonic of this as it is also present when MTrP activity in the hamstrings causes these muscles to become shortened.

However, reproduction of the pain on raising the contralateral leg only occurs with a radicular lesion and when present is indicative that treatment employing conservative measures alone will not be sufficient.

Investigations

A plain X-ray of the spine is of no help in the diagnosis of disc prolapse for all that it is capable of revealing are the radiographic appearances produced by the loss of disc height and by the presence of osteophytes, both of which are frequently seen in asymptomatic people. It is, however, of considerable value in excluding other causes of low-back pain such as vertebral metastases, ankylosing spondylitis and degenerative spondylolisthesis.

In order to confirm that low-back pain is due to an intervertebral disc rupture it is necessary to carry out either MRI, CT or myelography. However, with respect to this it is essential to remember that disc protrusion can take place without giving rise to symptoms and signs. Jensen et al (1994) in a MRI study of the lumbar spine in people without back pain found an appreciable incidence of protruding discs. Therefore evidence of a disc prolapse on MRI does not necessarily imply that any pain which may happen to be present is due to it unless, in addition, there is limited straight leg raising and, in particular, clinical signs of entrapment of a nerve root at the same segmental level as that indicated on the scan.

Management of disc prolapse

For many years after Mixter & Barr (1934) had shown that the commonest cause of sciatica is rupture of an intervertebral disc and that the pain may be relieved by a discectomy, the operation was carried out far too frequently and often with disastrous results. Some of these surgical catastrophes were due to technical errors at the time of operating (Greenwood et al 1952) but in the main they were due to inaccuracies in the diagnosis of the disorder and, in particular, to a poor selection of cases for operation (Nachemson 1976, Spengler & Freeman 1979).

Gradually, over the years it has become increasingly evident that sciatica occurring as a result of disc herniation can usually be brought under control without recourse to surgery and that it is only a minority of patients that require this.

This change in attitude has largely come about as a result of studies showing that for the majority of patients the results with conservative treatment are ultimately as good as those obtained using surgery. Friedenberg & Shoemaker (1954) were among the first to show that a substantial number of patients with ruptured disc-evoked back pain and sciatica successfully lose their pain and are enabled to return to full-time employment with conservative treatment alone.

Weber (1983) came to a similar conclusion from a controlled prospective study in which 126 patients were divided into two groups: a group treated conservatively and a group treated surgically. The results in these two groups 1 year, 4 years and 10 years later were then compared. After 1 year the surgically treated group did significantly better; and again at 4 years, but by this time the difference between the two groups was no longer statistically significant. At the end of 10 years no patients in either group had sciatica and the incidence of low-back pain in the two groups was similar.

As a result of surveys such as these it is now realised that immediate surgery is only required for those with dysfunction of the bladder or bowel brought about by cauda equina compression from a large midline disc rupture. All other patients should be treated conservatively and only the relatively small number who do not respond to this need surgery.

Conservative treatment

This includes 1–2 weeks' bed rest followed by gradually increasing mobilisation with, after a time, the carrying out of an intensive progressive exercise programme (Manniche et al 1991, Wynn Parry 1994).

Saal & Saal (1989) studied 64 patients with objectively proven disc prolapse subjected to an aggressive physical rehabilitation regime in order to see whether treatment of this type obviated the need for surgery. At an average of 31 months' follow-up 90% of these patients were found to have done well, with nearly all of them being able to return to work and only 6 needing a discectomy.

Pain control requires the use of analgesics. In addition, steroids are widely used for their anti-inflammatory effect. Also, as will be explained, there is a limited place for the deactivation of MTrP deactivation and the use of transcutaneous nerve stimulation (TENS).

Corticosteroids

As stated previously, the pain of a disc prolapse-induced radiculopathy is partly due to an inflammatory reaction in the neural tissues brought about by the release of the enzyme phospholipase A2 from extruded disc material and, as a result of this, the liberation of the arachidonic acid derivates prostaglandins and leukotrienes.

The recent discovery of receptor sites for substance P and other neuropeptides in the outer part of the annulus fibrosus and in the posterior longitudinal ligament has led to the belief that it is these neuropeptides that sensitise disc nociceptors to the effects of prostaglandins and leukotrienes (Weinstein et al 1995).

The rationale for using a corticosteroid is the belief that its anti-inflammatory effect includes inhibiting either the synthesis or action of these neuropeptides, and blocking phospholipase A2 activity. It may in addition alleviate the pain by having a C-fibre sensory afferent conduction blocking effect (Johansson et al 1990).

The successful use of orally administered corticosteroids has been reported by Johnson & Fletcher (1981) and of intramuscularly administered ones by Green (1975). It is, however, epidural steroid injections that are most widely employed despite the value of this form of treatment having recently been questioned by Bogduk (1995), Rowlingson (1994), and Weinstein et al (1995).

Bogduk (1995), stated that 'there is no compelling data from double-blind controlled trials that vindicate the use of lumbar or caudal epidural steroids'. He pointed out that when the National Health and Medical Research Council in Australia assessed the results of epidural steroid trials it could find no evidence to support the belief that an injection of this type is efficacious and for this reason could neither proscribe nor endorse it. Because it remains an unproven procedure the Council considered it essential to obtain fully informed consent from every patient prior to it being carried out.

Nevertheless, epidural steroid injections continue to be widely used for the treatment of nerve root inflammation (Rowlingson 1994) with it being generally agreed that in order to ensure the accurate placing of the steroid in the epidural tissues it is essential for the injection to be carried out under fluoroscopic control (Dreyfuss 1993, El-Khoury et al 1988, Mehta & Salmon 1985).

MTrP pain-relieving procedures

As previously stated, following the prolapse of a lumbar intervertebral disc, prior to the development of low-back and leg sciatic nerve entrapment pain there is often episodic pain in the lumbar region. As much of this latter pain emanates from MTrPs, significant relief from it may be obtained by deactivating them. In those cases where there is little or no muscle spasm, this may be achieved by carrying out superficial dry needling. However, should there be considerable muscle spasm then the deactivation of the MTrPs requires the very much stronger stimulus provided by deep dry needling. And, once lumbar radiculopathy pain has developed, relief from any superimposed MTrP pain also requires the employment of this latter technique (Chu 1995, Gunn 1996). Transcutaneous nerve stimulation (Ch. 2) is also useful in palliating both the sciatic and the MTrP pain.

Responsiveness to conservative treatment

The varying responsiveness of patients to conservative treatment allows them to be divided into three groups.

One group consists of those who quickly lose all their symptoms and are able to return to work in a few weeks.

A second group consists of those whose progress is slower but who nevertheless gradually recover over a period of some months. With patients in this group the degree to which the straightened leg on the affected side can be raised steadily increases week by week and the vast majority ultimately recover without recourse to surgery (Alaranta et al 1990).

Nevertheless, amongst this group there are some who have to have the disc removed. These include patients for whom it is imperative to get back to work as quickly as possible, patients who, despite having adequate conservative treatment, suffer from intolerable pain and in particular those who, because of it, develop emotional disturbances (Spangfort 1994).

Before surgery is carried out on this latter group of patients it is necessary to determine that the pain complained of is typical of that which arises as a result of disc prolapse. Drawings need to be completed by the patient showing the distribution and character of the pain (Ransford et al 1976). Bizarre symptoms and signs should be regarded with suspicion and may necessitate a psychological assessment. However, provided the physical signs and investigations including MRI confirm that the pain is due to a disc lesion, surgery may have to be carried out at a relatively early stage.

The third group is made up of those who, because of a failure to respond to conservative treatment, eventually need to have an operation.

Indications for surgical intervention

Indications for surgery following a period of adequately carried out conservative treatment include increasingly limited straight leg raising, loss of diurnal changes in straight leg raising, and a 'trunk list'.

Persistently limited straight leg raising

Porter (1993c), from long experience in the treatment of disc lesions, is of the opinion that surgery should be carried out in all cases where despite conservative treatment there is a worsening of symptoms over the months together with a progressively increased restriction of straight leg raising. Surgery should also be carried out in those patients who, after having had 3 weeks' rest in a hospital bed for a confirmed disc lesion, continue to have straight leg raising limited to 50° or less.

Contralateral straight leg raising-evoked pain

Pain in the affected leg brought about by raising the contralateral one is indicative of a possible need for surgical intervention. Khuffash & Porter (1989) found that, of their patients with disc symptoms and the evocation of pain in the affected leg by this means, 51% required discectomy compared with 15% in which this phenomenon was not present.

Diurnal changes in straight leg raising

With a partial disc protrusion diurnal changes in straight leg raising may be as much as 30°. However, once the annulus has completely ruptured this diurnal change is no longer observed and the prognosis with conservative treatment alone is poor (Porter & Trailescu 1990).

Deviation of lumbar spine

About one-third of patients with lumbar disc prolapse have deviation of the lumbar spine to one side – the so-called 'trunk list'. This is caused by reflex muscle spasm that is abolished either by lying down or by hanging from a bar. Khuffash & Porter (1989) have found that of their patients with disc symptoms and this spine abnormality, 40% eventually required surgery compared with 20% of patients without it.

Effects of delayed surgical intervention

From what has been said it follows that in the face of steadily worsening symptoms, together with a gradual reduction in straight leg raising and other signs now recognised to be predictors, conservative measures are unlikely to be sufficient, and a traditional open discectomy or, in less severe cases, a percutaneous discectomy, should be carried out without delay. The reason for this is that should a nerve be allowed to remain severely entrapped for an unduly long period of time irreversible changes take place in it and in the central nervous system and these cause long-term persistence of the pain even should the nerve eventually be surgically decompressed (Wyn Parry 1989).

Post-laminectomy pain

Spangfort (1972) reviewed the results of 2504 laminectomies carried out because of clear-cut neurological signs of nerve root entrapment and found that complete relief of both leg and back pain occurred in only 60% of cases.

It has for long been generally agreed that some of the main causes for surgery failing to relieve disc prolapse pain include exploration carried out at the wrong site, the overlooking of a second disc prolapse, and the development of adhesions or bony encroachments (Greenwood et al 1952). There may also be irreversible nerve damage because of delay in carrying out surgery (Wynn Parry 1989). In addition, it has recently become evident that there are two disorders which are occasionally the cause of postoperative pain developing. These are discitis and arachnoiditis (Spangfort 1994). However, what is still not sufficiently well recognised is that the back pain which often persists following a sciatic pain-relieving discectomy frequently emanates from overlooked MTrPs. These three causes of post-laminectomy pain will therefore be discussed.

Postoperative discitis

This complication of disc surgery is relatively rare with an incidence probably not exceeding 1–2%. Most cases are caused by a low-grade infection of the disc space but a few appear to be of an aseptic type (Fouquet et al 1992).

Its outstanding feature is the development of very severe spasmodic pain during the second week following the operation. This pain, which is quite unlike the original disc prolapse pain, affects the lower abdomen, the groin, the hips and upper thighs.

Fever may or may not be present but the erythrocyte sedimentation rate, which is normally only temporarily elevated following a discectomy, remains persistently high.

Radiographic abnormalities are liable to appear within 3–4 weeks. These include changes in the vertebral endplates, vertebral cavitation, vertebral sclerosis and marked narrowing of the disc space. MRI is the best means of demonstrating these.

Needle aspiration provides a positive culture in less than half the cases.

The treatment of this condition includes complete bed rest and the prescribing of an antibiotic. The acute pain then usually disappears in 6–12 weeks but in some cases it is replaced by a less intense chronic low-back pain.

Spinal arachnoiditis

Arachnoiditis not infrequently developed when myelography was carried out using an oil-based contrast medium but its incidence fell considerably once a water-soluble one was introduced for this purpose.

There is evidence to show that this disorder may also sometimes arise as a complication of disc surgery (Symposium 1978). There are several possible reasons for this. These include an inflammatory reaction produced by substances such as local anaesthetics, blood, infected material, disc fragments in the arachnoid space, and also the irritant effect of surgically induced trauma (Ransford & Harries 1972).

The pain, which is often of a very severe burning type, affects the back and one or both legs, is unrelieved by rest and is not readily responsive to analgesics. In addition to this there may also be exceedingly painful cramp in the leg muscles.

The difficulty in treating arachnoiditis pain and, because of this, the persistence of it over a

long-term period, frequently leads to much psychological distress.

Post-discectomy MTrP pain

It is not uncommon in cases where discectomy has been successful in relieving the sciatic pain in the leg for low-back pain to persist postoperatively. One important and all too often overlooked cause for this is the presence of active TrPs in the lumbar muscles (Gerwin 1991). These MTrPs may have become activated preoperatively or during the course of the operation as a result of surgically induced trauma to the muscles. In addition, persistent pain following discectomy or any other form of surgery may emanate from active MTrPs in incisional skin scars.

Deactivation of these MTrPs by means of superficial dry needling carried out at weekly intervals for a few weeks is usually all that is required to relieve the pain.

LUMBAR SPONDYLOSIS

There are several reasons for believing that lumbar spondylosis only gives rise to low-back and leg pain in the relatively small number of patients where the degenerative disc and facet joint changes present in this disorder give rise to nerve root entrapment. And that in the majority of people it is asymptomatic.

One of the reasons for coming to this conclusion is that Schmorl & Junghanns (1932), in their classic study of over 4000 spines, showed that degenerative changes in the discs and facet joints are present in 50% of people by the end of the fourth decade, in 70% of them by the end of the fifth decade and in 90% by the seventh decade. And yet despite this there is no evidence to show that low-back pain becomes increasingly common and more severe with advancing years. On the contrary, its highest incidence is in middle-aged people.

Another is that numerous comparative studies by radiologists have shown that the radiographic features of disc and facet joint degeneration are as commonly present in asymptomatic people as they are in those with low-back pain (Horal 1969,

Hult 1954, Hussar & Guller 1956, Magora & Schwartz 1976, Splithoff 1952).

A third is that there is no evidence to suggest that the intensity of low-back pain is in direct proportion to the amount of degenerative changes seen on a straight radiograph. It is not uncommon for a person with severe pain to have only slight radiographic changes and conversely for someone who is symptomless to have advanced ones.

It therefore follows that finding evidence of degenerative changes in the discs and facet joints on straight X-rays of the spine does not of itself imply that any low-back and leg pain which may be present is due to them. And that pain can only with any certainty be attributed to such changes in the small minority of cases where they have led to the development of a radiculopathy.

DEGENERATIVE SPONDYLOLISTHESIS

Pathogenesis

In this disorder there is forward displacement of a vertebra in relation to the one immediately below it together with degenerative changes in the facet joints and margins of the vertebral bodies. Osteophytes that form as a result of these degenerative changes may encroach upon a root canal. It should be noted that with this type of spondylolisthesis, unlike with others which develop earlier in life, the neural arch remains intact.

The displacement of the vertebra takes place relatively late in life with symptoms usually developing about the sixth decade.

Symptomatology

Discomfort in the back and leg is brought on by postural changes such as when getting up from a chair or straightening up from a stooped position. Both standing and walking also tend to be painful.

In addition, fourth or fifth lumbar nerve root entrapment pain may develop. In men this disorder may lead to the onset of neurogenic claudication.

Investigations

Confirmation of the diagnosis comes from observing characteristic changes of the disorder in lateral radiographs of the spine. CT or MRI is required to determine which nerve root is entrapped.

Secondary MTrP activity

The muscle pain, its attendant postural changes and any motor nerve compression that may develop in this disorder are all liable to lead to the secondary development of MTrP activity and the superimposition of MTrP pain.

Management

Conservative measures including, where necessary, the deactivation of MTrPs is usually all that is required. It is only occasionally that the severity of the root entrapment pain makes surgical intervention necessary.

LATERAL CANAL STENOSIS

Factors responsible for its development

With lateral canal stenosis there is usually an antecedent disc rupture. The disc prolapse may have occurred some considerable time before symptoms and signs of lateral canal stenosis nerve root entrapment develop and over the years is liable to have given rise to episodes of low-back pain and sciatica, or to bouts of back pain alone. Alternatively, in those cases where the central canal is sufficiently wide the prolapse may have been entirely symptomless.

Lateral canal stenosis following a disc prolapse develops as a result of the organisation and fibrosis of sequestrated disc material together with thickening and ossification of ligaments. Osteophytes arising from the disc and facet joint margins may also contribute to the narrowing of the canal.

Rarer causes of lateral canal stenosis include tumours and aneurysms. Degenerative spondylolisthesis (see p. 255) may also produce the same symptoms.

Symptoms

The predominant symptom, as with a disc prolapse, is low-back and sciatic-type pain which extends from the buttock, down the back of the leg, to the foot. The pain, however, is more severe than that caused by a disc prolapse and, unlike with the latter where relief is obtained by lying down, it is present all the time so as to severely disrupt sleep. Sitting is also uncomfortable and in particular travelling in a car for any length of time becomes impossible. Fortunately, unlike with a disc rupture, coughing and sneezing do not make the pain worse. Relief from it can be obtained by flexing the body forwards as the adoption of this particular posture increases the space in the root canal.

The pain, which initially is invariably severe, may be constantly present and cause the patient to become physically and emotionally exhausted. Alternatively, it may be episodic and brought on by certain physical activities such as standing or walking. Its natural history is widely variable. It may, after a period of time, ranging from a number of weeks to several years, gradually decrease in intensity and eventually spontaneously subside. Alternatively, it may not only persist indefinitely but over the years get progressively worse.

Signs

The physical signs in this disorder are remarkably few. What is particularly surprising is that despite the sciatic pain being so severe, straight leg raising is usually not restricted. Getty et al (1981) found that only one-third of their cases had any significant restriction of this. And in a series of cases studied by Porter (1993d) straight leg raising was 80° or more in 74% of them.

In addition, tendon reflexes are usually normal, sensation is rarely affected and muscle wasting or weakness is very exceptional.

Diagnosis

A clinical diagnosis of this disorder has to be made from the character of the pain because despite its severity there is a paucity of physical signs. Straight X-rays of the spine are also of no help in confirming the diagnosis because, although there is usually evidence of L5/S1 disc space reduction and other degenerative changes, similar appearances are common in asymptomatic people over the age of 40. However, both CT and MRI provide valuable diagnostic information and it is essential to carry out one or other of these as soon as a decision to operate has been made in order to establish the precise level at which surgery should be performed.

Management

Most patients need no more than pain-relieving medication and reassurance that over the course of time the pain is likely to gradually become less before eventually disappearing. During this time of waiting for spontaneous improvement to take place, epidural injections of a local anaesthetic/steroid mixture are sometimes helpful. It is only in the exceptional case that surgical decompression of a root canal is required. Following operation, the pain is usually less severe but unfortunately not uncommonly it continues to persist. Sometimes this is the result of irreversible nerve damage but when it is mainly confined to the lower back it is always worthwhile looking for MTrPs that have become secondarily activated for when present, deactivation of them may provide a certain amount of symptomatic relief.

NEUROGENIC CLAUDICATION

Neurogenic claudication is a disorder in which pain, brought on by walking and relieved by resting, develops in one or both legs as a result of cauda equinal ischaemia.

Pathogenesis

The disorder predominantly affects males. The male/female ratio is 9:1. Moreover, it commonly develops in men over the age of 50 who, during their working lives, have been engaged in heavy manual labour.

One constant feature is a narrow lumbar central canal (Verbiest 1954). And because of this, the terms neurogenic claudication and central canal stenosis have tended to be employed synonymously. This, however, is misleading as central canal stenosis cannot be the sole cause for the disorder developing. One reason for saying this is because it has been found to be present in 21% of asymptomatic people over 60 years of age (Boden et al 1990). Another is because a spinal tumour and a large central disc prolapse can considerably narrow the central canal without producing claudication.

Central canal stenosis therefore can only be one of the aetiological factors although admittedly a vital one. And, moreover, as Porter & Ward (1992) have pointed out, there is a high incidence of multiple-level stenosis and also of combined central and lateral root canal stenosis.

Another important contributory factor is severe widespread degenerative changes in the discs and facet joints in several segments of the spine. Associated with this there is not uncommonly a degenerative spondylolisthesis, a condition in which there is vertebral displacement, but unlike with other forms of this disorder, an intact neural arch (see p. 255). This disorder, when present, also serves to reduce the size of the already narrowed canal. The symptoms would seem to be due to these various structural changes causing inadequate oxygenation of the cauda equina but exactly how they bring this about remains a matter for conjecture (Porter 1993e).

Symptoms

The patient complains of discomfort in one or both legs. This may take the form of either a numbness, a burning sensation or a painful cramp. The affected limb is said to feel abnormally heavy and tired. The discomfort is brought on by walking but the amount of exercise required varies widely over the course of a day.

A characteristic feature is that the distance walked can be increased by bending forwards with both hips and knees flexed in an ape-like posture, the so-called simian stance (Fig. 12.17). And it is because this flexed position reduces the pain that it is more comfortable to walk up a hill bending forwards than downhill leaning backwards.

Once the condition has become established the distance that can be walked before symptoms develop is never more than a mile and may be as little as 20 yards. Sleep is frequently disturbed by restless legs and cramps that cause the patient to get out of bed and walk about. Low-back pain is often present and not infrequently has been present for some considerable time prior to the onset of the claudication.

Clinical examination

Physical signs are remarkably few. Palpation of the lumbar spine may reveal a certain amount of

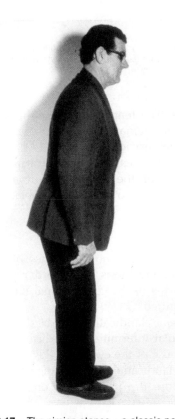

Figure 12.17 The simian stance – a classic posture adopted by patients with neurogenic claudication, with flexed hips and knees. (Reproduced with permission from Porter 1987.)

A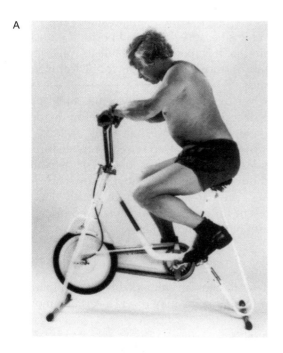

B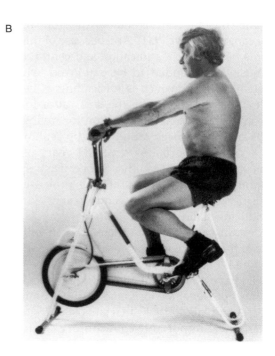

Figure 12.18 The cycle test. The cycling distance is the same in vascular intermittent claudication whether the spine is flexed (A) or upright (B). The extended spine in (B) limits the cycling distance in neurogenic claudication. (Reproduced with permission from Porter 1987.)

tenderness. The tendon reflexes, muscle power and sensation remain normal. Also, straight leg raising is not restricted.

The use of a treadmill is helpful in assessing the severity of the disorder as it allows the exercise tolerance to be measured objectively.

Investigations

A plain X-ray may show evidence of degenerative spondylolisthesis but in order to demonstrate stenosis of the central canal either CT or MRI is required.

Neurogenic claudication may be distinguished from vascular intermittent claudication (see Ch. 13) by the use of the cycle test (Fig. 12.18). With vascular claudication the distance that can be cycled before the pain comes on is the same

whether the spine is flexed or extended. But with neurogenic claudication the distance before the onset of pain is less with the spine extended than it is with it flexed.

Management

In those whose symptoms are not particularly severe simply reducing their activities may be all that is required to make their lives tolerable. It may also prove helpful to give calcitonin for about 8 weeks as this, for some unexplained reason, often significantly increases the pain-free walking distance (Porter 1993e).

When, however, the disorder is causing considerable disability surgical decompression is required.

REFERENCES

Alaranta H, Hulme M, Einola S et al 1990 A prospective study of patients with sciatica. A comparison between conservatively treated patients and patients who have undergone operation part ii: results after one year follow-up. Spine 15:1345–1349

Baker B A 1986 The muscle trigger: evidence of overload injury. Journal of Neurology, Orthopaedics, Medicine and Surgery 7:35–44

Barton P M, Grainger R W, Nicholson R L et al 1988 Towards a rational management of piriformis syndrome. Archives of Physical Medicine and Rehabilitation 69:784

Battié M C, Videman T, Gill K et al 1991 Volvo award in clinical sciences. Smoking and lumbar intervertebral disc degeneration. Spine 16:1015–1021

Bennett R M 1986a Current issues concerning management of the fibrositis/fibromyalgia syndrome. American Journal of Medicine 81(suppl 3A):15–18

Bennett R M 1986b Fibrositis: evolution of an enigma. Journal of Rheumatology 13(4):676–678

Bennett R M 1990 Myofascial pain syndromes and the fibromyalgia syndrome. A comparative analysis. In: Friscton R, Awad E (eds) Advances in pain research and therapy. Raven Press, New York, vol 17, pp 43–65

Boden S D, Davis D, Dina T, Patronas N J, Weisel S W 1990 Abnormal magnetic resonance scans of the lumbar spine in asymptomatic subjects. A positive investigation. Journal of Bone and Joint Surgery 72A:403–408

Bogduk N 1995 Spine update, epidural steroids. Spine 20(7):845–848

Bogduk N, Jull G 1985 The theoretical pathology of the acute locked back: a basis for manipulative therapy. Manual Medicine 1:78–82

Butler D, Trafimow J H, Andersson G B J, McNeill T W, Huckman M S 1990 Discs degenerate before facets. Spine 15(2):111–113

Carette S, Marcoux S, Truchon R et al 1991 A controlled trial of corticosteroid injections into the facet joints for chronic low back pain. New England Journal of Medicine 325:1002–1007

Chu J 1995 Dry needling (intramuscular stimulation) in myofascial pain related to lumbosacral radiculopathy. European Journal of Physical Medicine and Rehabilitation 5(4):106–121

Deyo R A 1991 Fads in the treatment of low back pain. New England Journal of Medicine 325:1039–1040

Deyo R A, Diehl A K, Rosenthal M 1986 How many days of bed rest for acute low back pain? A randomised clinical trial. New England Journal of Medicine 315:1064–1070

Dreyfuss P 1993 Epidural steroid injections. A procedure ideally performed with fluoroscopic control and contrast media. International Spinal Injection Society Newsletter 1:34–40

Dreyfuss P H, Dreyer S J, Herring S A 1995 Contemporary concepts in spine care. Lumbar zygapophysial (facet) joint injections. Spine 20(18):2040–2047

El-Khoury G, Ehara S, Weinstein S, Montgomery W J, Kathol M H 1988 Epidural steroid injections. A procedure ideally performed with fluoroscopic control. Radiology 168:554–557

Fouquet B, Goupille P, Jattiot F et al 1992 Discitis after lumbar disc surgery. Features of 'aseptic' and 'septic' forms. Spine 17:356–358

Friberg O 1983 Clinical symptoms and biomechanics of lumbar spine and hip joint in leg length inequality. Spine 8:643–651

Friedenberg Z B, Shoemaker R C 1954 The results of non-operative treatment of ruptured lumbar discs. American Journal of Surgery 86:933–935

Gerwin R 1991 Myofascial aspects of low back pain. Neurosurgery Clinics of North America 2(4):761–784

Gerwin R 1995 Myofascial back and neck pain. Spine: State of the Art Reviews 9(3):1–15

Getty C J M, Johnson J R, Kirwan E O'G, Sullivan M F 1981 Partial undercutting facetectomy for bony entrapment of the lumbar nerve root. Journal of Bone and Joint Surgery 63–B:330–335

Ghormley R K 1933 Low back pain with special reference to the articular facets, with presentation of an operative procedure. Journal of the American Medical Association 101:1773–1777

Goldthwait J E 1911 The lumbosacral articulation. An explanation of many cases of 'lumbago, sciatica and paraplegia'. British Medical and Surgical Journal 164:356–372

Green L N 1975 Dexamethasone in the management of symptoms due to herniated lumbar disc. Journal of Neurology, Neurosurgery and Psychiatry 38:1211–1217

Greenwood J, McGuire T, Kimbell F 1952 A study of the causes of failure in the herniated intervertebral disc operation. Journal of Neurosurgery 9:15–20

Gunn C C 1996 The Gunn approach to the treatment of chronic pain. Churchill Livingstone, Edinburgh

Hallin R P 1983 Sciatic pain and the piriformis syndrome. Postgraduate Medicine 74:69–72

Harris R I, Beath T 1949 The short first metatarsal: its incidence and clinical significance. Journal of Bone and Joint Surgery (Am) 31:553–565

Hirsch C, Inglemark V E, Miller N 1963 The anatomic basis for low back pain: studies on the presence of sensory endings in ligamentous capsular and intervertebral disc structures in the human lumbar spine. Acta Orthopaedica Scandinavica 33:1–17

Hopkins A 1993 Clinical neurology. A modern approach. Oxford University Press, Oxford, pp 337–338

Horal J 1969 The clinical appearance of low-back pain disorders in the city of Gothenburg, Sweden. Acta Orthopaedica Scandinavica Supplement 118: 8–73

Hult L 1954 Cervical dorsal and lumbar spinal syndromes. A field investigation of a non-selected material of 1200 workers in different occupations with special reference to disc degeneration and so-called muscular rheumatism. Acta Orthopaedica Scandinavica Supplement 17: 1–102

Hussar A E, Guller E J 1956 Correlation of pain and the roentgenographic findings of spondylosis of the cervical and lumbar spine. American Journal of Medical Science 232:518–527

Jackson R P 1992 The facet syndrome, myth or reality? Clinical Orthopaedics and Related Research 279:110–120

Jackson R P, Jacobs R R, Montesano P X 1988 Facet joint injection in low back pain. A prospective statistical study. Spine 13:966–971

Jason M I V 1997 Why does acute back pain become chronic? Chronic back pain is not the same as acute back pain lasting longer. British Medical Journal 314:1639–1640

Jensen M C, Brant-Zawadzki M N, Obuchowski N et al 1994 Magnetic resonance imaging of the lumbar spine in people without back pain. New England Journal of Medicine 331:69–73

Johansson A, Hao J, Sjolund B 1990 Local corticosteroid application blocks transmission in normal nociceptor C-fibres. Acta Anaesthesiologia Scandinavica 34:335–338

Johnson E W, Fletcher E R 1981 Lumbosacral radiculopathy. Review of 100 consecutive cases. Archives of Physical Medicine and Rehabilitation 62:321–323

Kelsey J L, Githens P B, O'Conner T et al 1984 Acute prolapsed intervertebral disc. An epidemiological study with special reference to driving automobiles and cigarette smoking. Spine 9:605–613

Khuffash B, Porter R W 1989 Cross leg pain and trunk list. Spine 14:602–603

Kirkaldy-Willis W H, Hill R J 1979 A more precise diagnosis for low-back pain. Spine 4:102–109

Kraemer J 1995 Presidential Address: Natural course and prognosis of intervertebral disc diseases. Spine 20(6):635–639

Lamerton A J, Bannister R, Wittington R, Seifert M H, Eastcott H H G 1983 'Claudication' of the sciatic nerve. British Medical Journal 286:1785–1786

Làpossy E, Maleitzke R, Hrycaj P, Mennet W, Müller W 1995 The frequency of transition of chronic low back pain to fibromyalgia. Scandinavian Journal of Rheumatology 24:29–33

Lawrence J S, Sharp J, Ball J, Bier F 1966 Osteoarthritis: Prevalence in the population and relationship between symptoms and x-ray changes. Annals of the Rheumatic Diseases 25:1–24

Lillius G, Laasonen E M, Myllynen P, Harilainen A, Gronlund G 1989 Lumbar facet joint syndrome. A randomized clinical trial. Journal of Bone and Joint Surgery (British) 71:681–684

Magora A 1970 Investigation of the relation between low-back pain and occupation to age, sex, community, education and other factors. Industrial Medicine and Surgery 39:465–471

Magora A, Schwartz A 1976 Relation between the low back syndrome and x-ray findings. 1. Degenerative osteoarthritis. Scandinavica Journal of Rehabilitation Medicine 8:115–125

Magora A, Schwartz A 1978 Relation between the low back syndrome and x-ray findings. 2. Transitional vertebra (mainly sacralization). Scandinavica Journal of Rehabilitation Medicine 10:135–145

Maigne J-Y, Treuil C, Chatellier G 1996 Altered lower limb vascular perfusion in patients with sciatica secondary to disc herniation. Spine 21:1657–1660

Manniche C, Lundberg E, Christensen I, Bentzen L, Hasselsoe G 1991 Intensive dynamic back exercises for chronic low-back pain. A clinical trial. Pain 47:53–63

Mehta M, Salmon N 1985 Extradural block. Confirmation of the injection site by x-ray monitoring. Anaesthesia 40:1009–1012

Mixter W J, Barr J S 1934 Rupture of the intervertebral disc with involvement of the spinal canal. New England Journal of Medicine 211:210–215

Mooney V 1992 Facet joint syndrome. In: Jayson M I V (ed) The lumbar spine and back pain, 4th edn. Churchill Livingstone, Edinburgh, pp 291–306

Mooney V, Robertson J 1976 The facet syndrome. Clinical Orthopaedics and Related Research 115:149–156

Morton D J 1935 The human foot. Its evolution, physiology and functional disorders. Columbia University Press, New York

Nachemson A L 1976 The lumbar spine – an orthopaedic challenge. Spine 1:59–71

Nachemson A 1979 A critical look at the treatment for low-back pain. Scandinavian Journal of Rehabilitation Medicine 11:143–149

Pace J B 1975 Commonly overlooked pain syndromes responsive to simple therapy. Postgraduate Medicine 58:107–113

Pace J B, Nagle D 1976 Piriform syndrome. Western Journal of Medicine 124:435–439

Papageorgiou A C, Croft P R, Ferry S, Jayson R I V, Silman A S 1995 Estimating the prevalence of low-back pain in the general population. Spine 20:1889–1894

Porter R W 1987 The lumbar spine and back pain. Churchill Livingstone, Edinburgh

Porter R W 1993a–e Management of back pain, 2nd edn. Churchill Livingstone, Edinburgh, p. 169 (a), p. 168 (b), p. 179 (c), p. 191 (d), pp 197–215 (e)

Porter R W, Trailescu I F 1990 Diurnal changes in straight leg raising. Spine 15:103–106

Porter R W, Ward D 1992 Cauda equina dysfunction: the significance of multiple level pathology. Spine 17:9–15

Porter R W, Wicks M, Hibbert G 1978 The size of the lumbar spinal canal in the symptomatology of disc lesions. Journal of Bone and Joint Surgery 60B:485–487

Putti V 1927 New conceptions in the pathogenesis of sciatic pain. Lancet 2:53–60

Rachlin E S 1994 Injection of specific trigger points. In: Myofascial pain and fibromyalgia. Trigger point management, Mosby, St Louis, pp 232–235

Ransford A O, Harries B J 1972 Localised arachnoiditis complicating lumbar disc lesions. Journal of Bone and Joint Surgery 54B:656–665

Ransford A O, Cairns D, Mooney V 1976 The pain drawing as an aid to the psychological evaluation of patients with low back pain. Spine 1:127–134

Rees W E S 1971 Multiple bilateral subcutaneous rhizolysis of segmental nerves in the treatment of the intervertebral disc syndrome. Annals of General Practice 26:126–127

Revel M E, Listrat V M, Chevalier X J et al 1992 Facet joint block for low back pain: Identifying predictions of a good response. Archives of Physical Medicine and Rehabilitation 73:824–828

Reynolds M D 1981 Myofascial trigger point syndrome in the practice of rheumatology. Archives of Physical Medicine and Rehabilitation 62:111–114

Rosomoff H L, Fishbain D, Goldberger M et al 1990 Myofascial findings in patients with 'chronic intractable benign pain' of the back and neck. Pain Management 3(2):114–118

Rowlingson J C 1994 Epidural steroids. Do they have a place in pain management? American Pain Society Journal 3(1):20–27

Rubin D 1981 An approach to the management of myofascial trigger point syndrome. Archives of Physical Medicine and Rehabilitation 62:107–110

Saal J A, Saal J S 1989 Non operative treatment of herniated lumbar intervertebral disc with radiculopathy. An outcome study. Spine 14:431–437

Saal J S, Franson R C, Dobrow R et al 1990 High levels of inflammatory phospholipase A2 activity in lumbar disc herniations. Spine 15:674–678

Schmorl G, Junghanns H 1932 Die gesunde und kranke Wirbelseule im Roentgenbild. Thieme, Leipzig

Schwarzer A C, Wang S, Laurent R, McNaught P, Brooks P M 1992 The role of the zygapophysial joint in chronic low back pain. Australian and New Zealand Journal of Medicine 22:185

Schwarzer A C, Aprill C N, Derby R, Fortin J, Kine G, Bogduk N 1994a Clinical features of patients with pain stemming from lumbar zygapophysial joints. Is the lumbar facet syndrome a clinical entity? Spine 19:1132–1137

Schwarzer A C, Aprill C N, Derby R, Fortin J, Kine G, Bogduk N 1994b The relative contributions of the disc and zygapophysial joint in chronic low back pain. Spine 19:801–806

Shealy C N 1975 Percutaneous radiofrequency denervation of spine facets and treatment for chronic back pain and sciatica. Journal of Neurosurgery 43:448–451

Simons D G, Travell J G, Simons L 1999a–e Travell & Simons myofascial pain and dysfunction. The trigger point manual, 2nd edn. Williams & Wilkins, Baltimore, vol 1, p. 914 (a), p. 916 (b), p. 936 (c)

Spangfort E V 1972 The lumbar disc herniation – a computer-aided analysis of 2504 operations. Acta Orthopaedica Scandinavica Supplement 142: 1–95

Spangfort E 1994 Disc surgery. In: Wall P D, Melzack R (eds) Textbook of pain, 3rd edn. Churchill Livingstone, Edinburgh, pp 1067–1074

Spengler D M, Freeman C W 1979 Patient selection for lumbar discectomy – an objective approach. Spine 4:129–134

Splithoff C A 1952 Lumbosacral junction. Roentgenographic comparison of patients with and without backaches. Journal of the American Medical Association 110: 106–112

Symposium 1978 Lumbar arachnoiditis: nomenclature, etiology and pathology. Spine 3:21–92

Synek V M 1987 The piriformis syndrome. Review and case presentation. Clinical and Experimental Neurology 23:31–37

Thiele G H 1937 Coccygodynia and pain in the superior gluteal region. Journal of the American Medical Association 109:1271–1275

Thomas E, Silman A J, Croft P R, Papageorgiou A C, Jason M I V, Macfarlane G J 1999 Predicting who develops chronic low back pain in primary care: a prospective study. British Medical Journal 318:1662–1667

Travell J G, Simons D G 1992a–f Myofascial pain and dysfunction. The trigger point manual. Williams & Wilkins, Baltimore, vol. 2, pp 82–84 (a), pp 151–169 (b), pp 207–209 (c), p. 96 (d), pp 47–48 (e), pp 59–63 (f)

Travell J, Travell W 1946 Therapy of low back pain by manipulation and of referred pain in the lower extremities by procaine infiltration. Archives of Physical Medicine 27:537–547

Turk D C, Flor H 1984 Etiological theories and treatments for chronic back pain. 11. Psychological models and interactions. Pain 19:209–233

Twomey L T, Taylor J R, Taylor M M 1989 Unsuspected damage to lumbar zygapophyseal (facet) joints after motor vehicle accidents. Medical Journal of Australia 151:210–217

United Kingdom Department of Health, Clinical Standards Advisory Group 1994 Epidemiology review: the epidemiology and cost of low back pain. HMSO, London

Verbiest H 1954 A radicular syndrome from developmental narrowing of the lumbar vertebral canal. Journal of Bone and Joint Surgery 36B:230

Weber 1983 Lumbar disc herniation: a controlled prospective study with ten years' observation. Spine 8:131–140

Weinstein S M, Herring S A, Derby R 1995 Contemporary concepts in spine care: epidural steroid injections. Spine 20(16):1842–1846

Westrin C G 1973 Low back sick-listing. A sociological and medical insurance investigation. Scandinavian Journal of Social Medicine Supplement 7

Wiesel S W, Tsourmas N, Feffer H L et al 1981 A study of computer assisted tomography 1: the incidence of positive CAT scans in asymptomatic group of patients. Spine 9:549–551

Wolfe F, Smythe H A, Yunus M B et al 1990 The American College of Rheumatology 1990 criteria for the classification of fibromyalgia: a report of the multi-center criteria committee. Arthritis and Rheumatism 33:160–172

Wynn Parry C B 1989 The failed back. In: Wall P D, Melzack R (eds) Textbook of pain, 2nd edn. Churchill Livingstone, Edinburgh, pp 341–353

Wynn Parry C B 1994 The failed back. In: Wall P D, Melzack R (eds) Textbook of pain, 3rd edn. Churchill Livingstone, Edinburgh, p 1082

13

The lower limb

INTRODUCTION

As pain referred to the lower limb from myofascial trigger points (MTrPs) in the lumbar and
gluteal regions has already been dealt with, the
main purpose of this chapter is to consider the
diagnosis and management of pain arising as a
result of the primary activation of MTrP nociceptors in the thigh, leg and foot.

Other topics that will be discussed include
pain around the knee as a result of it being
referred there from MTrPs in the thigh; knee
pain from structural disorders in and around
the joint; ischaemia-induced MTrP activity as a
complication of intermittent claudication; the
possible role of MTrP activity in the development

of leg cramps and restless legs (Ekbom's syndrome); pain referred to the foot from MTrPs in the leg; and pain arising as a result of various structural disorders that affect the foot itself.

PAIN FROM MTrPs IN THE ANTERIOR, LATERAL AND MEDIAL ASPECTS OF THE THIGH

The muscles to be discussed include the tensor fasciae latae, the hip adductors and the quadriceps group.

Tensor fasciae latae muscle (Fig. 13.1)

Anatomical attachments

The tensor fasciae latae muscle is situated subcutaneously in the upper lateral aspect of the thigh. Proximally it has attachments to the anterior iliac crest, the anterior superior iliac spine and the deep surface of the fascia lata. Distally, the tendinous fibres of its anteromedial half extend down the thigh to insert into a retinaculum on the lateral aspect of the patella. And the tendinous fibres of its posterolateral half at the junction of the upper and middle thirds of the thigh insert into the thickened band of the fascia lata known as the iliotibial tract which, distally, attaches to the lateral condyle of the tibia (Paré et al 1981).

Actions

This muscle assists with the abduction, medial rotation and flexion of the thigh at the hip. It also assists, above, in stabilising the pelvis and below, in stabilising the knee (Paré et al 1981).

Factors responsible for the development of TrP activity

TrP activity is liable to develop in this muscle when it is subjected either to direct trauma or to chronic overloading, such as when a poor posture is adopted, either because of persistent low-back pain or a painful disorder of the foot.

In addition, satellite TrPs are liable to become active in this muscle when pain is referred down

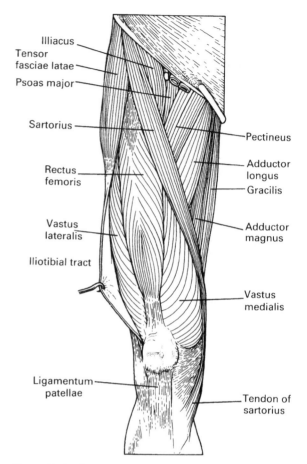

Figure 13.1 Superficial muscles of the thigh. Extensor aspect.

the outer side of the thigh from TrPs in either the gluteus minimus, gluteus medius or quadratus lumborum.

For these reasons, as stated in Chapter 12 and reiterated here because of its importance, the physical examination in all cases of low-back pain must include a search for MTrPs not only in the lumbar musculature but also in the muscles on the outer side of the thigh.

MTrP sites and patterns of pain referral

TrPs are liable to be found anywhere along the length of this muscle, particularly in its upper and middle part. Pain from these TrPs is referred mainly to the region of the greater trochanter but also down the outer side of the thigh. Because of the tenderness over the greater trochanter and at the TrP sites themselves it is painful to lie on the affected side.

The locations and patterns of pain referral of these TrPs are similar to those liable to be found in the vastus lateralis muscle.

Differential diagnosis

Trochanteric bursitis Should TrPs in this muscle be overlooked the pain is liable to be attributed to a trochanteric bursitis.

Meralgia paraesthetica Pain in a similar distribution to that from TrPs in the tensor fasciae latae muscle may develop as a result of entrapment of the lateral femoral cutaneous nerve where it passes through the inguinal ligament. It is, however, different in character, for it is of a burning type and the patient complains of paraesthesiae. Also, on examination, sensory changes in the distribution of the nerve are found. The disorder tends to occur in people who are overweight, particularly if they wear tight, constricting clothing. It may also develop in those who have one leg longer than the other.

An injection of a local anaesthetic to block the nerve at the inguinal ligament is often all that is necessary to control the pain (Teng 1972). In addition, weight should be reduced and tight clothing avoided. Also, where necessary any lower limb-length inequality should be corrected. Occasionally surgical release of the nerve is found to be necessary.

Hip adductors

The adductor muscles of the hip are situated in the upper medial part of the thigh between the quadriceps group of muscles anteriorly and the hamstring muscles posteriorly.

The most anterior of the adductors is the adductor longus, and beneath this is the closely associated adductor brevis. And deep to these lies the adductor magnus.

The principal hip adductors from which TrP pain is liable to arise are the adductor magnus and adductor longus.

Factors responsible for the development of TrP activity

TrP activity in these two hip adductor muscles may develop as a result of the hip joint being subjected either to prolonged adduction or to excessive abduction. It therefore may occur, for example, as a result of gripping tightly with the thighs whilst balancing on a horse (Travell 1957) or the pillion seat of a motor cycle (Baldry 1993). It may also occur when the thighs are widely abducted such as when an anaesthetised patient is placed in the lithotomy position for the purpose of carrying out a lengthy surgical procedure.

TrP activity may also develop in these muscles when they are suddenly overloaded as a result of a loss of balance leading to a fall with the legs wide apart such as may happen during skating.

In addition, it may develop in patients with osteoarthritis of the hip and following surgery for a hip disorder.

Adductor magnus muscle (Fig. 13.1)

Anatomical attachments

The upper attachments of this muscle are to the inferior ramus of the pubis, the ischial ramus and the ischial tuberosity. From these insertions it splits into three parts. An upper horizontally situated part, the adductor minimis, inserts laterally into the gluteal tuberosity just below the greater trochanter; a middle part spreads out from its upper attachment to be inserted into the mid-part of the shaft of the femur; and a posteriorly situated ischiocondylar part runs vertically downwards from the ischial tuberosity to be inserted by means of a tendon to the adductor tubercle on the medial condyle of the femur.

MTrP sites and patterns of pain referral

TrP activity is liable to develop close to where this muscle attaches to the ischial tuberosity.

Pain from TrPs at this site is referred upwards into the pelvic cavity. It may be localised to the vagina or rectum or take the form of a more diffuse, ill-defined, deeply situated intrapelvic dull ache (Fig. 13.2).

TrPs may also become active in the middle part of this muscle near to its insertion into the mid-part of the femur. Pain from these is referred to the upper part of the thigh and groin (Fig. 13.3).

Because the adductor magnus muscle is covered by a number of other muscles TrPs in it are easily overlooked and deep palpation is required in order to locate them.

Adductor longus muscle (Fig. 13.1)

Anatomical attachments

This superficially placed triangular-shaped muscle is attached at its apex to the pubic bone. From there its broad, fleshy belly passes diagonally downwards and laterally to become attached at its base to the mid-point of the femur.

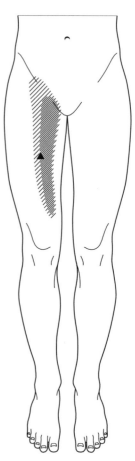

Figure 13.3 The pattern of pain referral both up and down the front of the thigh from an adductor magnus TrP (▲) in the mid thigh.

MTrPs: their sites, patterns of pain referral and deactivation

TrPs are liable to develop activity close to where this muscle inserts into the pubic bone (Fig. 13.4). Pain from these is referred up to the groin and down the anteromedial aspect of the thigh as far as the inner side of the knee. There may also be a spillover pattern that extends downwards over the tibia (Long 1956, Travell 1950).

Quadriceps femoris group of muscles

The quadriceps femoris group of muscles include the rectus femoris, vastus intermedius, vastus lateralis and vastus medialis.

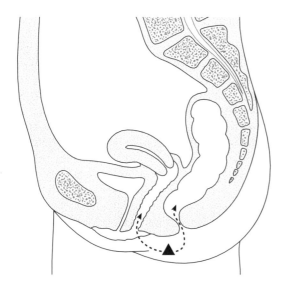

Figure 13.2 The pattern of pain referral to the vagina or rectum from a TrP (▲) high up in the adductor muscle close to its attachment to the ischial tuberosity.

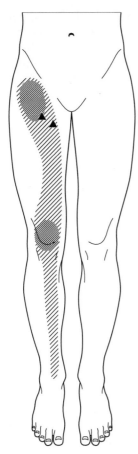

Figure 13.4   The pattern of pain referral from a TrP (▲) in the adductor longus. The pain is invariably referred upwards to the groin. And in some cases distally, particularly to the knee region and to a lesser extent downwards over the tibia.

Rectus femoris (Fig. 13.1)

Anatomical attachments

This muscle, which lies between the vastus medialis and vastus lateralis and overlies the vastus intermedius, arises proximally by two tendons, one attached to the anterior inferior iliac spine and the other to the groove just above the acetabulum.

It is a broad muscle that covers most of the front of the thigh. Distally it is attached to the patella and via the patellar ligament to the tibial tuberosity.

Factors responsible for the development of TrP activity

TrPs in this muscle may become active as a result of direct trauma to the front of the thigh and when a fall causes it to become suddenly overloaded. Also, as a result of the application of prolonged pressure to the thigh such as may happen when sitting for a long time with a heavy weight resting on the thighs.

MTrP sites and patterns of pain referral

TrPs are liable to be found just below this muscle's upper attachment. From these, pain is referred to the lower part of the thigh and knee joint (Fig. 13.5). The pain in this latter region is particularly likely to be troublesome at night and to disturb sleep. It should be noted that pain referred from a TrP in the adductor longus has a similar distribution.

Vastus intermedius

The vastus intermedius muscle is situated immediately behind the rectus femoris. Proximally, it attaches to the upper part of the shaft of the femur. Distally, it attaches to the patella and via the patellar ligament to the tibial tuberosity.

Reasons for TrPs developing in the rectus femoris and vastus intermedius and their pain referral patterns are similar. Because TrPs in the vastus intermedius lie some distance beneath the rectus femoris muscle very firm pressure is required to palpate them. And for the same reason, their deactivation by any technique which requires a needle to be inserted directly into them is technically difficult. It may, however, be achieved by the use of superficial dry needling (see Ch. 7).

Vastus lateralis (Fig. 13.1)

Anatomical attachments

This muscle, which is the largest of the quadriceps group, occupies the outer aspect of the thigh. Above, it arises by a broad aponeurosis that attaches to the upper part of the femur.

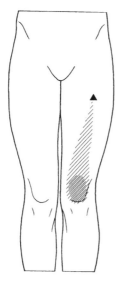

Figure 13.5 The pattern of pain referral from a trigger point (▲) in the rectus femoris muscle.

Below, it attaches to the patella and to the tibial tuberosity via the patellar ligament.

Factors responsible for the development of TrP activity

TrPs in this muscle are liable to become active as a result of trauma to the outer side of the thigh. Also, when the muscle is suddenly overloaded by falling awkwardly during some sporting activity, or as a result of injections given into the lateral aspect of the thigh such as, for example, by diabetics.

MTrP sites and patterns of pain referral

TrPs are liable to be found anywhere along the length of the muscle. As they tend to be situated some distance from the surface it is necessary to employ deep palpation when searching for them.

Pain is referred from these TrPs along the outer side of the thigh upwards towards the greater trochanter and downwards to the outer side of the knee. Pressure applied to these TrPs when lying on them during sleep often aggravates the pain (Fig. 13.6).

Activity in a TrP in the distal part of the muscle close to its attachment to the lateral border of the patella causes this part of the muscle to contract with restriction of the patella's movement so as to make it difficult to bend the knee or to get up from a chair. This disorder has been called the 'stuck patella' by Travell & Simons (1992a).

Associated trigger points

Pain referred down the outer side of the thigh from TrPs in the gluteus minimus is liable to lead to the development of satellite TrP activity in the vastus lateralis muscle.

Therefore, with pain down the lateral aspect of the thigh it is necessary to search for TrPs not only at that site but also higher up in the buttock.

Vastus medialis (Fig. 13.1)

Anatomical attachments

The vastus medialis muscle has proximal attachments to the upper part of the femur, the tendons of the adductor longus and magnus, and the medial intermuscular septum. Distally, it

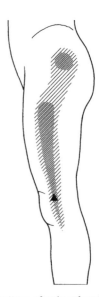

Figure 13.6 The pattern of pain referral from a trigger point (▲) in the vastus lateralis muscle.

attaches to the medial border of the patella and, via the patellar tendon, to the tibial tuberosity.

Factors responsible for the development of TrP activity

TrP activity in this muscle is particularly liable to develop in someone with instability of the foot because of a relatively short first metatarsal bone and a long second one (Morton's deformity, see p. 282). Also, whenever the muscle is acutely overloaded such as during athletic pursuits and when the inner side of the thigh is subjected to direct trauma.

MTrP sites and patterns of pain referral

Pain from a TrP just above the knee is referred to the front of the knee joint and often disturbs sleep (Fig. 13.7). A person with TrP activity at this site may have unexpected falls due to it causing intermittent weakness of the knee joint, a disorder called by Travell & Simons (1992b) 'the buckling knee syndrome'.

There may also be TrP activity halfway down the inner side of the thigh. Pain from a TrP at this

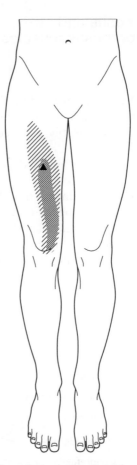

Figure 13.8 The pattern of pain referral from a TrP (▲) halfway down the thigh in the vastus medialis muscle.

site is referred along the medial aspect of the lower part of the thigh to the knee (Fig. 13.8).

Deactivation of myofascial trigger points

The deactivation of TrPs both in deeply lying muscles and in muscles situated just below the skin surface in the anterior medial and lateral aspects of the thigh may readily be achieved by carrying out superficial dry needling (see Ch. 7).

PAIN FROM TRIGGER POINTS IN THE POSTERIOR THIGH MUSCLES

The muscles to be discussed include the semitendinosus, semimembranosus and biceps femoris (hamstring muscles), and also the popliteus.

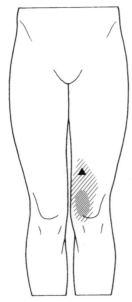

Figure 13.7 The pattern of pain referral from a trigger point (▲) in the vastus medialis muscle.

Semitendinosus and semimembranosus muscles

(Fig. 13.9)

Anatomical attachments

These two muscles are situated on the inner side of the posterior thigh with the semitendinosus overlying the more deeply situated semimembranosus.

Proximally they are attached to the ischial tuberosity.

Distally, the semitendinosus muscle is attached by a tendon that curves around the posteromedial aspect of the tibia's medial condyle to the tibia. This tendon, together with the tendons of the gracilis and sartorius muscles, form what has somewhat fancifully been called the goose's foot (pes anserinus).

Distally, the semimembranosus muscle is attached by a tendon to the medial condyle of the tibia just below the joint capsule.

MTrP sites and pain referral patterns

TrPs in these two muscles are liable to be found in their bellies in the lower part of the posterior thigh. From these, pain is mainly referred upwards to the buttocks. This upward referral is similar in direction to that of pain from TrPs located just above the elbow in the biceps muscle (see Ch. 10). Some pain may also be referred downwards towards the back of the knee (Fig. 13.10).

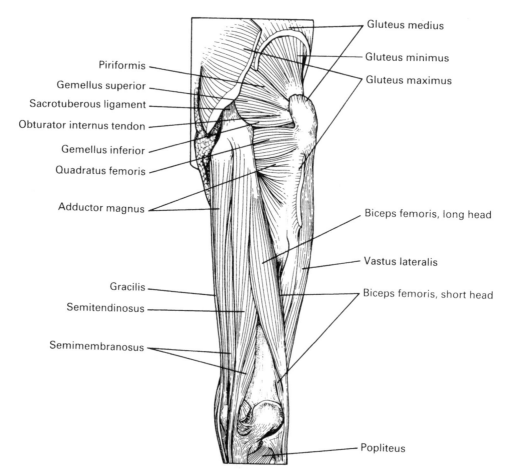

Piriformis
Gemellus superior
Sacrotuberous ligament
Obturator internus tendon
Gemellus inferior
Quadratus femoris
Adductor magnus
Gracilis
Semitendinosus
Semimembranosus

Gluteus medius
Gluteus minimus
Gluteus maximus
Biceps femoris, long head
Vastus lateralis
Biceps femoris, short head
Popliteus

Figure 13.9 The muscles of the gluteal region and flexor aspect of the right thigh. Posterior aspect.

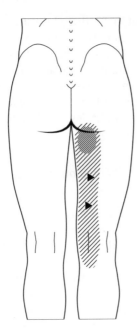

Figure 13.10 Composite pattern of pain referral from TrPs (▲) in the semimembranosus and semitendinosus muscles.

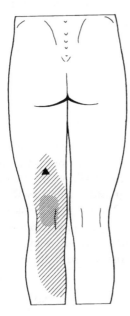

Figure 13.11 The pattern of pain referral from a trigger point (▲) in the belly of the biceps femoris muscle.

Biceps femoris muscle (Fig. 13.9)

Anatomical attachments

The biceps femoris, the laterally situated hamstring muscle, has a long head and a short head. The long head attaches proximally to the ischial tuberosity by a tendon that is common to it and the semitendinosus muscle.

The short head of the muscle, which is attached proximally to the femur, joins the long head halfway down the thigh and together they are attached distally to the lateral aspect of the fibula.

MTrP sites and pain referral patterns

TrPs in this muscle are liable to be found in its belly in the mid to lower part of the thigh. Pain is referred from these to the back of the knee (Fig. 13.11).

Factors responsible for the development of hamstring TrP activity

Primary activity TrPs in these muscles may become active when the posterior aspect of the thigh is subjected to trauma. This may happen during the course of a fall. Also, when the edge of a chair is allowed to press against it for a prolonged period. In addition, Sherman (1980) has noted that when the hamstring muscles are used to cover the end of an above-knee amputation stump, trauma-induced activation of TrP nociceptors in these muscles is liable to occur, with, as a consequence, the development of phantom limb pain which requires the deactivation of these TrPs for its relief.

Secondary activity When pain radiates down the back of the thigh as a result of sciatic nerve entrapment from, for example, a ruptured intervertebral disc, TrP activity is liable to develop in the hamstring muscles as a secondary event. There are two possible reasons for this.

One is that should the radiculopathic pain cause these muscles to go into spasm severe enough to render them ischaemic, the ischaemia may be responsible for TrP activity developing in them.

The other, and probably the commoner reason in view of electromyographic studies carried out by Chu (see Ch. 4) is that because these hamstring muscles are supplied by branches of the sciatic nerve (L4, 5 and S1 nerve roots) the motor nerve compression, by its effect on motor endplates at TrP sites in these muscles, leads to the development of TrP activity in them.

Hamstring TrP-induced pain

TrP activity in the hamstrings gives rise to pain both on walking and on sitting; also, when getting up from a chair.

The weight of the body pressed against TrPs in the laterally situated biceps femoris muscle often leads to the development of sleep-arousing pain at night.

TrP-induced shortening of the hamstring muscles is liable to cause overloading of the quadriceps group of muscles with, as a consequence, the development of TrP activity in them. When this happens the pain from TrPs in this latter group of muscles may become the dominant symptom and the primary TrP activity in the hamstring muscles may be overlooked unless specifically looked for. It therefore follows that whenever TrP activity is found in the quadriceps group, a search for TrPs in the hamstrings should be carried out and vice versa.

Hamstring TrP-evoked restricted straight leg raising

Because pain from TrPs in the hamstring muscles extends down the back of the thigh in the distribution of sciatic nerve entrapment pain, and because TrP activity in these muscles causes them to become shortened with, as a result, limited straight leg raising, it all too frequently happens that pain caused by the primary activation of MTrPs in the hamstrings is erroneously considered to have arisen as a consequence of sciatic nerve radiculopathy.

It cannot be too strongly emphasised that an abnormal straight leg raising test is not pathognomonic of sciatic nerve entrapment. It is one

cause of it but TrP-induced tightness of the hamstrings is another. Therefore, in any case where pain down the back of the thigh is accompanied by limited straight leg raising, a search for TrPs in the hamstrings is essential, and should they be found to be present, the effect deactivating them has on the straight leg raising test should be observed.

Deactivation of hamstring muscles' trigger points

There may at any one time be a large number of TrPs in the hamstring muscles that require to be deactivated. And as the technique of injecting a local anaesthetic into each of these TrPs requires much widespread probing with the cutting edge of a hollow needle it inevitably causes damage to blood vessels. Much bleeding into the tissues with consequent post-injection soreness is therefore a frequent complication. And it is because of this that Travell & Simons (1992c) advise: 'when injecting hamstring TrPs, it is wise to limit treatment to only one side of the body on one visit. The patient may experience sufficient post-injection soreness to make weight bearing on the treated limb temporarily painful. Two sore limbs could unnecessarily restrict mobility.'

It is possible to avoid this complication by using the superficial dry needle technique described in Chapter 7.

Avoidance of hamstring TrP reactivation

When TrPs in the hamstrings have been successfully deactivated it is important that any chair used by the patient allows the feet to rest on the ground without undue pressure being exerted on the back of the thighs. Also, prolonged sitting in one position such as may happen on a long car journey should be avoided by having frequent leg-stretching breaks from driving.

Hamstring stretching exercise

It is helpful for those liable to develop TrP activity in the hamstrings to carry out a stretching exercise on a regular basis. This consists of sitting on the floor and repeatedly reaching as far as possible down the shins with the outstretched hands.

Popliteus muscle (Fig. 13.9)

Anatomical attachments

This thin, flat, triangular-shaped muscle which derives its name from the Latin word *poplus* (the ham of the knee) forms the floor of the popliteal fossa behind the knee. Above and laterally its apex is attached by a tendon to the lateral condyle of the femur and the head of the fibula. Below and medially its base is attached to the back of the upper end of the tibia.

Factors responsible for the development of TrP activity

TrPs in this muscle are liable to become active during the carrying out of athletic pursuits, particularly those that involve sudden twisting movements of the body.

MTrP sites and patterns of pain referral

TrPs are liable to be found along the muscle's medial attachment to the tibia. Also, at its apical tendinous attachment to the lateral condyle of the femur and the fibula.

This TrP activity gives rise to pain at the back of the knee during the course of running or walking, particularly when going downhill or downstairs. The pain is also exacerbated by any attempt to fully extend the knee (Fig. 13.12).

MTrP examination

In order to search for TrPs in this muscle, the patient should lie on the affected side with the knee flexed and positioned on the edge of the couch so that the leg can be rested on the seated examiner's lap with the foot plantar flexed. The purpose of flexing the knee and the foot is to relax the overlying gastrocnemius and plantaris muscles.

The lower medial part of the muscle along its attachment to the upper part of the tibia has to be palpated by directing a finger between the semitendinosus muscle and the medial head of the gastrocnemius muscle.

The upper laterally placed apical part of the muscle is covered by the lateral head of the gastrocnemius, the soleus and the plantaris muscles. It can, however, be examined by palpating between the tendon of the biceps femoris laterally and the lateral head of the gastrocnemius medially.

Deactivation of myofascial trigger points

When deactivating TrPs in this muscle by any method that involves penetration with a needle there is a risk of damaging such structures as the popliteal artery and peroneal nerve. These complications can be avoided by employing the superficial dry needling technique described in Chapter 7. However, even with this technique, care has to be taken to avoid rupturing a Baker's cyst and, as a consequence, causing the pseudo-thrombophlebitis syndrome to develop.

Differential diagnosis

Quadriceps femoris, adductor longus, hamstring and popliteus MTrP pain that is referred to the

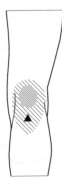

Figure 13.12 The pattern of pain referral from a TrP (▲) in the popliteus muscle.

knee has to be distinguished from pain which develops there as a result of various locally occurring disorders including osteoarthritis of the knee joint. The other disorders that have to be included in the differential diagnosis are chondromalacia patellae, patellar tendinitis, anserine bursitis, pes anserinus tendinitis, medial ligament syndrome, Pellegrini–Stieda disease and iliotibial band friction syndrome. Each of these will therefore now be discussed.

Osteoarthritis of the knee joint

Predisposing factors

Middle-aged men and women are equally liable to be affected by osteoarthritis of the knee. From age 50 onwards, however, its incidence in women is considerably higher and it is particularly prevalent in obese women (Felson et al 1988). Ageing alone, however, is not responsible for its development. There are grounds for believing that there is a genetic predisposition. Also, joint injury and mechanical stresses are contributory factors. This is why relatively young people, particularly men, develop the disease following damage to the knee sustained during sporting activities or following an operation such as meniscectomy.

Pathology

Firstly, destruction of the cartilage takes place. This causes the subchondral bone to become sclerotic and intraosseous cysts to develop. Other characteristic changes include the formation of osteophytes at the joint's margins, synovial inflammation, capsular thickening and the development of tender points in the periarticular tissues.

Symptoms

Pain is the main symptom. At the onset it is no more than a mild aching. Gradually, however, it increases in intensity and becomes particularly severe following weight bearing. Eventually the joint movements become increasingly restricted

partly because of pain and partly because of contraction of the joint capsule.

Synovial inflammation causes pain to be present at rest as well as on movement and is responsible for the development of early morning stiffness.

The disorder is episodic (Massurdo et al 1989) with symptoms that have been present for several months being followed by a spontaneously developing long-term remission.

Physical signs

Joint enlargement At an early stage the contours of the joint are normal. Over the course of time, however, there is an increase in joint size. Initially this is because of bony enlargement at the joint's margins but at a later stage it is also due to swelling of the soft tissues and the development of an effusion.

Restricted movements Over the course of time all movements of the joint become increasingly restricted.

Periarticular tender points Palpation of the periarticular tissues, particularly around the upper anteromedial aspect of the tibia, the patella and the popliteal fossa, reveals the presence of well-defined tender points. As will be discussed, there are reasons for believing that it is from these tender points that much of the pain emanates.

Dysfunction of the quadriceps group of muscles There is increasing weakness and wasting of the quadriceps muscle.

Quadriceps wasting rapidly develops in any disorder which causes the movements of the knee joint to become restricted. The vastus medialis is often the first muscle in this group to be affected. The circumference of the thigh a hand's breadth above the patella should be measured and compared with the other side in order to obtain objective evidence of muscle wasting.

Reasons for the development of osteoarthritic knee pain

Osteoarthritic pain cannot be due to destruction of the articular cartilage as this tissue is devoid of nerve endings. Sites, however, from which the pain may arise include subchondral bone, the synovium, the joint capsule and the periarticular tender spots as all of these have a plentiful supply of group IV nociceptors.

Subchondral bone pain Changes in bone such as subchondral sclerosis and the marginal proliferation of it that leads to the development of osteophytes are responsible for stimulating nociceptors situated in the densely innervated periosteum and in the walls of blood vessels that permeate bone.

In addition, Arnoldi et al (1971, 1980) have shown that, in osteoarthritis of the hip joint, intraosseous hypertension leads to the development of the intraosseous engorgement-pain syndrome (Lemperg & Arnoldi 1978). Recent work indicates that the same mechanism probably also operates at the knee joint (McCarthy et al 1994).

Synovial and capsular pain Group IV nociceptors in the free nerve endings present in the synovium and capsule become mechanically stimulated when the pressure in the joint increases. And they become chemically stimulated when inflammation-induced tissue damage leads to the liberation of nociceptor sensitising substances such as bradykinin, prostaglandins, serotonin, histamine and neuropeptides.

In addition, pain may develop as a result of the calcium crystal-induced inflammatory changes which are believed to be a not uncommon complication in osteoarthritis (Dieppe et al 1976).

Periarticular tender point pain A deformed, unstable osteoarthritic knee joint causes a strain to be imposed on various periarticular structures with, as a result, the activation and sensitisation of nociceptors at small, well-defined sites which, because of their characteristic tenderness, have come to be known as tender points.

Dixon (1965) was one of the first to draw attention to the presence of these periarticular tender points after he had analysed the cause of pain in 120 osteoarthritic knees. He demonstrated that

these tender points are important sources of pain by showing that it is possible to alleviate it by injecting substances such as local anaesthetics and steroids into them.

Anteriorly, tender points are commonly found in the anteromedial aspect of the upper part of the tibia where the lower part of the collateral ligament and, superficial to this, the tendons of the sartorius, gracilis and semitendinosus muscles (pes anserinus – goose's foot) insert into the tibia.

It should be noted that tenderness at this site may also occasionally be due to inflammation of the anserine bursa situated between the ligament and these tendons. Tender points may also be located along the edges of the patella, particularly along its lateral upper border.

Posteriorly, tender points are frequently found to be present in the popliteal fossa, particularly at the centre of it and on its inner side.

It is of considerable interest that these periarticular tender points have a close spatial correlation with traditional Chinese acupuncture points in this region of the body.

Investigations

Osteophytes, sclerotic subchondral bone and cysts in bone may be seen on a plain radiograph. However, it has for long been known that there is no correlation between the intensity of the pain and the amount of knee joint damage seen on a radiograph. It is this discrepancy between the amount of pain felt and the extent of the pathological changes seen on a radiograph in this disorder that led Hadler (1992) to entitle a paper on the subject, 'Knee pain is the malady – not osteoarthritis'.

With magnetic resonance imaging (MRI) it is possible to observe changes in the soft tissues and subchondral bone not demonstrable on plain radiographs. And by the use of scintigraphy it has been possible to confirm the phasic nature of the disorder (McCrae et al 1992). Arthroscopy is also useful because it allows not only direct inspection of the knee joint but also the carrying out of lavage for the removal of joint debris.

Medical forms of treatment

Drug therapy Simple analgesics taken on a regular basis may prove helpful.

Non-steroidal anti-inflammatory drugs (NSAIDs) continue to be widely employed despite not being as useful as initially anticipated. Furthermore, there is recent evidence to show that they not only have more serious side-effects than simple analgesics do but that they are also no more effective (McCarthy et al 1994).

The toxicity of NSAIDs has been shown to be particularly high in elderly women, the group most affected by osteoarthritis (Bradley et al 1991). It also has to be remembered that NSAIDs interact with other drugs. For example, they decrease the effect of diuretics and increase the effect of anticoagulants.

NSAIDs, too, by inhibiting the synthesis of prostaglandins are liable to aggravate late-onset asthma. And in conditions such as the nephrotic syndrome, hepatocellular failure and cardiac failure, in which glomerular filtration is prostaglandin-dependent, their use is liable to precipitate uraemia and increase oedema. Also, because of their effect on prostaglandins they are liable to cause gastro-intestinal bleeding, either from an erosive gastritis or peptic ulcer, which is a particularly serious complication in an elderly arteriosclerotic person.

Physiotherapy Wasted quadriceps muscles should be strengthened by exercises.

The weight should be taken off the affected side by the use of a walking stick held in the contralateral hand. Local heat and hydrotherapy provide a certain amount of symptomatic relief. Shock-absorbing insoles may also prove helpful. In addition, Kovar et al (1992), in a randomised controlled trial, have shown that group exercise therapy is of assistance in controlling the pain.

Deactivation of periarticular tender point nociceptors There are usually several tender points on the upper anteromedial aspect of the tibia (pes anserinus). There is sometimes one, or more, around the edge of the patella. Also, above the knee in the vastus medialis muscle. In addition, there may also be several in the popliteal fossa, particularly on its inner side.

Deactivation of nociceptors at these tender points may be achieved by injecting a local anaesthetic into each of them. Dixon (1965) found that adding a steroid improved the results and stated that by doing this the pain relief obtained may last for weeks, months or even years.

Superficial dry needle stimulation of A-delta nerve fibres at these tender point sites may also satisfactorily relieve the pain and has much to recommend it, as this procedure can be repeated as often as necessary without fear of any side-effects developing. However, for long-term relief from the pain, it may have to be carried out initially once a week for a few weeks and then every 4–6 weeks until such a time as the disorder spontaneously remits.

When deactivating tender points in the popliteal fossa, care needs to be taken to avoid inserting the needle into a popliteal cyst, because it may cause this to rupture with the development of leg pain and swelling, similar to that which occurs with a deep vein thrombosis.

Chondromalacia patellae

Aetiology

In this disorder the articular cartilage of the patella undergoes a trauma-induced degenerative process. The trauma may be of a repetitive type incurred during the course of some athletic activity or it may be an isolated event incurred as, for example, when the knee is violently rammed against the dashboard of a car in a road traffic accident. The disorder may also develop following fracture of the patella and when it has been immobilised for an appreciable time in a plaster cast.

Symptoms

There is a gradual onset of severe aching in the region of the patella. This is made worse by any movements that cause the patella to become compressed against the femur, such as when going up or down stairs. The aching may also be noticed after sitting for an appreciable time with the knee bent.

Signs

On examination, crepitus is elicited when the joint is palpated whilst the patient actively flexes and extends it.

Investigations

When, on clinical grounds, the diagnosis of this disorder is suspected it should be confirmed by arthroscopic examination.

Treatment

This includes quadriceps strengthening exercises and, in some cases, surgical intervention.

Patellar tendinitis

This disorder, which usually affects athletes, may also affect those who, because of advancing years, have given up sporting activities. It leads to the development of pain at the inferior pole of the patella during any activity which involves knee movements, particularly climbing stairs, jumping and running.

It is a degenerative condition of the patellar tendon which usually responds to rest and analgesia. Occasionally, a steroid injection into the tendon area is necessary but care must be taken not to inject more than 0.2 ml, as otherwise necrosis of the tendon may occur. An operation to excise the damaged part of the tendon is sometimes necessary.

Anserine bursitis, pes anserinus tendinitis and medial ligament syndrome

As previously stated, pain and tenderness in the anteromedial aspect of the upper end of the tibia may be a manifestation of the MTrP

pain syndrome, or develop as a result of osteoarthritis of the knee. In addition, it may be due to anserine bursitis, pes anserinus tendinitis or the development of the medial ligament syndrome.

Therefore, when there is no clinical evidence to suggest that pain and tenderness at this site is due either to MTrP activity or osteoarthritis, the possibility that it is due to one of these three other disorders has to be considered. Clinically, there is no way of distinguishing between them but this is of no particular consequence as treatment is the same. This includes rest and heat and, if necessary, a steroid injection.

Pellegrini–Stieda disease

In this disorder, following an injury to the inner side of the leg, pain develops in the region of the upper tibia where the medial collateral ligament attaches to it (Bonica & Lanzer 1990, Graham & Fairclough 1995). On examination, the ligament is found to be thickened and an X-ray reveals the presence of calcified deposits in the ligament. The disorder would seem to be due to calcification of a trauma-induced haematoma. The treatment includes the use of analgesics, and if necessary, the injection of a steroid.

Iliotibial band friction syndrome

In this disorder pain and tenderness develops over the lateral epicondyle of the femur in athletes whilst running. It is believed that the pain occurs as a result of friction between the iliotibial tract and the femur. The pain usually disappears with rest but if not, a steroid should be injected into the tender area.

PAIN FROM MTrPS IN THE ANTERIOR COMPARTMENT OF THE LEG

Muscles in this compartment include the tibialis anterior, extensor digitorum longus and extensor hallucis longus.

Tibialis anterior muscle (Fig. 13.13)

Anatomical attachments

This subcutaneous muscle, which is situated on the lateral side of the tibia, has proximal attachments to its lateral condyle and the upper half of its shaft. In the lower third of the leg it becomes tendinous. This tendon passes across the front of the tibia to reach the medial side of the foot where it attaches to the medial cuneiform and first metatarsal bones. The function of this muscle is to dorsiflex the ankle joint and raise the medial border of the foot; i.e. to invert the foot.

TrP site and pattern of pain referral

TrP activity in this muscle is liable to develop in its upper part near to its proximal attachment (Bonica & Sola 1990). Pain which develops as a result of this is referred downwards and is felt particularly intensely around the ankle and in the big toe (Fig. 13.14).

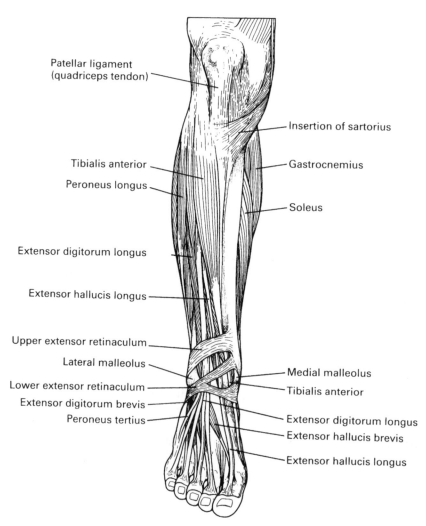

Figure 13.13   Muscles on extensor aspect of right leg.

TrP activity in this muscle causes it to become weakened, with impairment of dorsiflexion and, as a consequence, the development of a foot-drop.

Extensor digitorum longus (Fig. 13.13)

Anatomical attachments

This muscle is situated at the lateral part of the front of the leg in between the tibialis anterior and the peroneus longus. Proximally, it has attachments to the lateral condyle of the tibia, the head of the fibula, the shaft of the fibula and the intramuscular septa.

The part of the muscle attached to the lateral condyle of the tibia and head of the fibula crosses the deep peroneal nerve just below where the latter branches from the common peroneal nerve and wraps around the head of the fibula.

Distally, the muscle forms a tendon which, on the dorsum of the foot, divides into four tendinous slips that attach to the middle and distal phalanges of the four lesser toes. The function of this muscle is to extend the toes at the metatarsophalangeal joints and to dorsiflex the ankle joint.

MTrP sites and pattern of pain referral

TrP activity is liable to take place in the upper part of the muscle approximately a hand's breadth below the head of the fibula. From a TrP at that site pain is referred along the dorsum of the foot to reach the three middle toes (Fig. 13.15).

Nerve entrapment

Taut bands in this muscle are liable to compress the deep peroneal nerve against the head of the fibula with, as a consequence, the development of weakness of the toes and a foot-drop.

Extensor hallucis longus (Fig. 13.13)

Anatomical attachments

This muscle, which lies between the tibialis anterior and exterior digitorum longus, and is largely covered by them, attaches above to the medial surface of the fibula and the interosseous membrane. Below, it is attached by means of a tendon to the distal phalanx of the great toe. The function of this muscle is to extend the phalanges of the great toe and to dorsiflex the ankle joint.

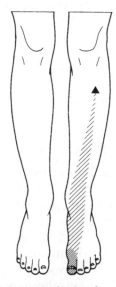

Figure 13.14 The pattern of pain referral from a trigger point (▲) in the tibialis anterior muscle.

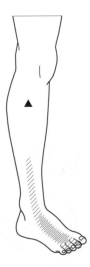

Figure 13.15 The pattern of pain referral from a TrP (▲) in the extensor digitorum longus muscle.

TrP site and pattern of pain referral

TrP activity is liable to take place in this muscle about a hand's-breadth above the ankle. Pain from a TrP at this site is referred to the dorsum of the foot as far as the first metatarsal bone and base of the great toe (Fig. 13.16).

Factors responsible for the development of TrP activity in the anterior compartment muscles (tibialis anterior, extensor digitorum longus and extensor hallucis longus)

These include direct trauma to these muscles. Also, overloading of them such as by long distance running, prolonged walking on rough ground, sitting for long periods with the ankles markedly dorsi- or plantar-flexed, and stubbing the toes against the ground when kicking a ball. Other causes are ischaemia of the muscles as a result of the development of the anterior compartment syndrome, and stress fracture of the tibia and fibula.

An L4–L5 radiculopathy may also lead to the development of TrP activity in the long extensors of the toes (Travell & Simons 1992d). There is reason to believe that this is because of the effect motor nerve compression has on MTrPs' motor endplates (Ch. 4).

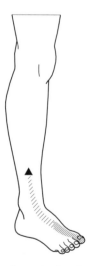

Figure 13.16   The pattern of pain referral from a TrP (▲) in the extensor hallucis longus muscle.

Muscles with similar TrP pain referral patterns

Muscles in the foot with similar TrP pain referral patterns to those in the anterior compartment of the leg include the extensor digitorum brevis on the dorsal surface of the foot and the interossei muscles. It therefore follows that in all cases of dorsal foot pain it is necessary to search for TrPs both locally in the foot and higher up in the muscles of the leg's anterior compartment.

Foot-drop

There are four reasons for foot-drop developing.

One is TrP-induced weakness of the leg's anterior compartment dorsiflexors of the ankle.

A second is compression of the common peroneal nerve as it wraps round the head of the fibula. Factors responsible for this include the application of direct pressure to the nerve as a result of sitting with the knee pressed against the edge of a desk; fracture of the tibia or fibula; prolonged squatting such as, for example, may happen when gardening; and the development of TrP activity in the peroneus longus muscle (see p. 281).

A third is TrP-induced shortening of the extensor digitorum longus giving rise to compression of the deep peroneal nerve.

A fourth is an L4–L5 root lesion occurring as a result of the prolapse of an intervertebral disc. However, the low-back and sciatic pain that accompanies this helps to distinguish it from the other causes mentioned.

Anterior compartment syndrome

In this disorder, which affects athletes, pain develops during the course of running as a result of the tibialis anterior, extensor digitorum longus and extensor hallucis longus muscles becoming swollen and causing the pressure within the anterior compartment of the leg to rise. Because this increased pressure obstructs the venous circulation, the muscles swell still more and ultimately because of this interference with their blood supply they are liable to become necrotic.

Symptoms of this disorder include not only anterior leg pain but also widespread tenderness of the affected muscles and nerve damage-induced paraesthesiae. Treatment includes bed rest and the application of cold to reduce the pain and lessen the metabolic demands of the tissues. In some cases surgical intervention for the purpose of reducing the raised anterior compartment pressure becomes necessary.

Deactivation of trigger points in anterior compartment muscles

When deactivating a TrP in any of these muscles by a method that involves inserting a needle into the TrP there is a risk of penetrating the deep peroneal nerve and/or the anterior tibial artery. In the case of the tibialis anterior muscle this risk may be reduced by directing the needle towards the tibia at a 45° angle to the skin. And similar care has to be taken when injecting a TrP in the extensor digitorum longus. The risk of damaging these structures, however, when injecting a TrP in the extensor hallucis longus is even greater, and for this reason the procedure is not recommended.

Superficial dry needling of TrPs in these muscles is not only much easier and safer but seemingly equally effective (see Ch. 7).

PAIN FROM MTrPs IN THE LATERAL COMPARTMENT OF THE LEG

Muscles in this compartment include the peroneus longus and brevis.

Peroneus longus (Fig. 13.13)

Anatomical attachments

The peroneus longus muscle, which is situated at the upper part of the lateral side of the leg, overlies the peroneus brevis. Proximally, it has two main attachments, one to the head and the other to the upper lateral surface of the shaft of the fibula. Between these two attachments there is a gap through which the common peroneal nerve passes just before it divides into the deep and superficial peroneal nerves. The muscle is also attached proximally to intermuscular septa.

Approximately halfway down the leg the muscle becomes tendinous and the tendon, at the ankle, passes behind the lateral malleolus of the fibula. On reaching the side of the foot, it crosses to the medial side to become attached to the outer side of the first metacarpal bone and the outer side of the medial cuneiform bone. The peroneus longus plantar-flexes the ankle joint and everts the foot. And because of the oblique direction of its tendon across the sole of the foot, it helps to maintain the transverse and longitudinal arches of the foot.

Peroneus brevis (Fig. 13.17)

Anatomical attachments

The peroneus brevis muscle arises from the lower two-thirds of the shaft of the fibula and adjacent intermuscular septa. Initially, it lies behind the peroneus longus but distally its belly extends beyond that of the latter muscle to end in a tendon which, together with the peroneus longus tendon, runs behind the lateral malleolus of the fibula, and in the sole of the foot becomes attached to the outer side of the fifth metatarsal bone.

The peroneus brevis, like the peroneus longus, plantar-flexes the foot upon the leg and in addition assists the peroneus longus to evert the foot.

Factors responsible for the development of TrP activity

TrP activity in one or other of these two muscles is liable to develop should it become overloaded. Reasons for this happening include a fall which results in the ankle becoming twisted and the foot everted; wearing shoes with high heels; weakness of an ankle joint brought about by it being immobilised in

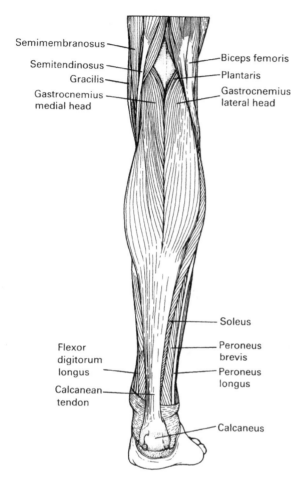

Figure 13.17 Muscles of the right calf; superficial layer.

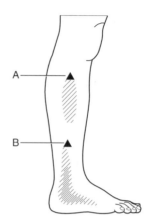

Figure 13.18 The pattern of pain referral from a TrP (▲) in (A) the peroneus longus muscle and (B) the peroneus brevis muscle.

the peroneus brevis are liable to be found just above the ankle.

From these TrPs pain is referred to the outer side of the ankle and for a short distance along the outer side of the foot (Fig. 13.18).

Morton's foot deformity

This consists of a relatively short first metatarsal bone and a long second metatarsal bone with a web between the second and third toes (Morton 1935). It is said to be present in approximately 40% of people (Harris & Beath 1949).

This deformity gives rise to instability of the ankle with mediolateral rocking of the foot. And because of the latter, calluses frequently develop under the heads of the first, second and fifth metatarsals, and also on the medial side of the great toe.

Treatment necessitates placing a felt pad under the first metatarsal head. In addition, tightly fitting shoes should be avoided and, in particular, they should not have narrow pointed toes.

Peroneus longus TrP activity-induced peroneal nerve entrapment

The common peroneal nerve after leaving the popliteal fossa wraps around the head of the fibula to enter the lateral compartment of the leg where it immediately divides into a superficial and a deep branch.

a plaster cast for a prolonged period; and the development of TrP activity in these muscles' antagonist, the tibialis anterior muscle.

Satellite TrP activity may take place in these two muscles when pain is referred to the lateral aspect of the leg from TrPs in the gluteus minimus muscle.

This TrP activity may also be perpetuated in people with a Morton's foot deformity.

TrP sites and pattern of pain referral

TrPs in the peroneus longus are liable to be found immediately below the head of the fibula. TrPs in

TrP activity in the peroneus longus muscle leads to the development of taut bands in it and these are liable to compress the common peroneal nerve and/or its superficial and deep branches against the fibula. Compression of motor fibres in one or other of these nerves causes a foot-drop to develop. In addition, numbness and tingling may be experienced on the dorsum of the foot between the first and second toes.

Deactivation of peroneus longus and brevis trigger points

In order to deactivate a TrP in the peroneus longus muscle just below the head of the fibula, the patient should lie in a semi-prone position with the affected side uppermost. When injecting a local anaesthetic into this TrP there is a risk of producing a peroneal nerve block. This possibility, however, does not arise when employing superficial dry needling.

When deactivating a TrP in the peroneus brevis muscle approximately a hand's-breadth above the ankle there are no structures of importance to avoid.

PAIN FROM MTrPS IN THE SUPERFICIAL POSTERIOR COMPARTMENT OF THE LEG

Muscles in this compartment include the gastrocnemius and the soleus.

Gastrocnemius muscle (Fig. 13.17)

Anatomical attachments

This muscle, which is the most superficial one in the calf, arises by two heads. These are attached to the medial and lateral condyles of the femur by strong well-developed tendons. These two fleshy heads constitute the back of the calf. Towards the ankle they merge to form a tendon which, together with the tendon of the soleus muscle, forms a common tendon – the tendo Achillis (syn: Achilles tendon).

The actions of this muscle include plantar flexing the ankle joint and, acting from below, flexing the knee joint.

Factors responsible for the development of TrP activity

TrPs in this muscle are liable to become active when persistent shortening of it takes place as a result of prolonged plantar flexion at the ankle with the knee bent. The following are circumstances in which this may happen: hill and rock climbing; wearing high heels; and either sitting on a high stool or sleeping without the feet being adequately supported.

Impairment of the blood supply to this muscle may also lead to TrP activity developing in it. Possible causes of this include wearing socks with tight elastic tops; pressure exerted on the calf as a consequence of sitting with it pressed against the edge of a reclining chair; and, in particular, arterial obstruction sufficient to give rise to intermittent claudication.

With intermittent claudication caused by atheromatous narrowing or embolisation of an artery in either the lower abdomen or leg, exercise-induced cramp develops in the calf, thigh or buttock muscles depending on where the obstruction is situated.

The distance a patient with this disorder can walk before the cramp and limping (Latin *claudicatio* – limping or lameness) comes on remains remarkably constant. This is in contrast to when pain in the leg develops as a result of trauma-induced activation of TrPs. For, in that circumstance, the amount of exercise required to bring on the pain varies widely from day to day.

The diagnosis of intermittent claudication depends on eliciting the characteristic history and finding evidence of arterial insufficiency on clinical examination.

The muscle in which ischaemia-induced TrP activity most often takes place is the gastrocnemius. Other muscles in which it may do so include the gluteus medius, soleus and tibialis

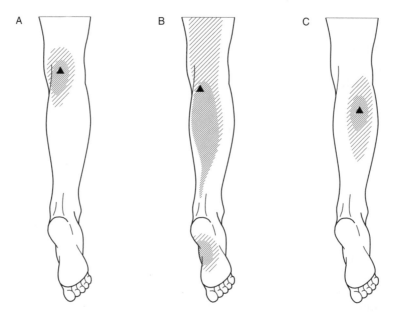

Figure 13.19 The patterns of pain referral from TrPs (▲) in the gastrocnemius muscle. A: TrP (▲) near to the femoral condyle. B: TrP (▲) in the medial head. C: TrP (▲) in the lateral head.

anterior (Arcangeli et al 1965, 1976, Dorigo et al 1979, Travell et al 1952).

Dorigo et al (1979) have shown that when patients with intermittent claudication have active TrPs in their ischaemic muscles, deactivation of these TrPs by injecting a local anaesthetic into them improves their exercise tolerance despite having no effect on the underlying circulatory insufficiency. In my experience the same effect may be obtained with the superficial dry needling MTrP deactivating technique described in Chapter 7.

Gastrocnemius TrP sites and patterns of pain referral

TrP activity is liable to develop in the upper part of this muscle, either where one or other of its bellies inserts into a femoral condyle or at a site a short distance beneath this.

Pain from a TrP near to a femoral condyle is felt mainly in the popliteal fossa (Fig. 13.19A).

Pain from a TrP at a site somewhat distal to this in the medial head of the muscle is referred down the inner side of the back of the leg to the sole of the foot (Fig. 13.19B). A TrP at the same level in the lateral head of the muscle refers pain locally around the TrP itself (Fig. 13.19C).

Deactivation of gastrocnemius trigger points

TrPs in this muscle may be deactivated with the patient lying prone. When deactivating TrPs in this muscle by injecting a local anaesthetic into them there is a high incidence of post-injection soreness that often lasts for as long as 5–6 days (Travell & Simons 1992f). Furthermore, when employing this technique in the popliteal region care has to be taken to avoid damaging the popliteal artery. Both these potential complications can be avoided by using the superficial dry needling technique described in Chapter 7.

Calf cramp

Pathogenesis

Cramp is liable to develop in any of the muscles in the thigh, leg or foot. One of the commonest, however, is the gastrocnemius.

Muscle cramp is a multifactorial disorder. Some of the well-recognised causes include dehydration and salt loss usually from excessive sweating, diarrhoea-induced hypokalaemia; and hypocalcaemia arising as a result of one or another of a number of different disorders. It is also liable to occur as a complication of Parkinson's disease.

As pointed out by Travell & Simons (1992e) another common but not sufficiently well-recognised cause is MTrP activity. In the gastrocnemius muscle TrP-induced cramp often develops following sitting or lying with the foot held in a plantar-flexed position for a prolonged period. This is particularly liable to happen when sleeping with the feet inadequately supported. Nocturnal calf cramp brought about in this manner is particularly liable to develop should the gastrocnemius muscle have been overloaded during the course of activities carried out the previous day.

Treatment

Drugs Muscle cramp due to an electrolyte imbalance clearly needs to be treated by correction of this. There are, in addition, various drugs employed for its symptomatic relief. The one most commonly used is quinine which, by decreasing the excitability of the motor endplate region, increases the refractory period of the muscle (Travell & Simons 1992e). The usual dose is 300 mg just before going to sleep (Whiteley 1982). Hope-Simpson (1976), however, has found 60 mg to be just as effective. Its efficacy has, however, been questioned recently with three studies showing it to have little or no influence on the condition (Baltodano et al 1988, Eaton 1989, Warburton et al 1987). Chloroquine has a similar action and good results with this have been reported by Parrow & Samuelsson (1967).

Aminophylline has also been found to be helpful. This is presumably because of its ability to increase the blood flow through the affected muscle. And there is evidence to suggest a combination of aminophylline and quinine is more effective than quinine alone (Rawls 1966).

Trigger point deactivation In cases where TrPs are found to be present in a muscle affected by cramp deactivation by one method or another should be carried out. Superficial dry needling (see Ch. 7), in my experience, is helpful in the treatment of this disorder but it is often necessary to repeat the procedure two to three times at weekly intervals before any long-lasting relief from it is obtained.

Muscle stretching In order to relieve cramp the gastrocnemius muscle should be stretched by slowly dorsiflexing the ankle whilst standing with the knee extended.

Prophylaxis Warmth from an electric blanket helps to reduce the irritability of TrPs and hence lessens the tendency for muscles containing them to go into cramp. In addition, anyone who suffers from the condition should sleep with the feet pressed against a firm support in order to prevent prolonged plantar flexion.

Restless legs (Ekbom's syndrome)

In this disorder first described by Ekbom (1960), an intolerable discomfort in the legs comes on when sitting down to relax at the end of a day's work. It also prevents getting off to sleep. Repeatedly changing the position of the legs brings some relief but eventually this is only obtained by walking around the room.

In the small number of cases seen by me over the years there has almost invariably been TrP activity in various muscles of the leg including the gastrocnemius.

The deactivation of these TrPs at regular intervals has been said by my patients to have been beneficial but a trial comparing the effect of this form of therapy with that of other forms of treatment, such as the administration of diazepam or carbamazepine, needs to be carried out.

Yunus & Aldag (1996) have also found a significant incidence of both the restless leg syndrome and leg cramps in patients with fibromyalgia.

Soleus muscle (Fig. 13.17)

Anatomical attachments

This broad flat muscle is situated immediately behind the gastrocnemius muscle. Proximally, its main attachments are to the head and upper third of the posterior surface of the shaft of the fibula and to the middle third of the medial border of the tibia and fibula. Distally, its tendon joins with that of the gastrocnemius tendon to form the tendo Achillis (Achilles tendon).

Factors responsible for the development of TrP activity

There are three main factors: muscle overloading, prolonged muscle shortening and muscle ischaemia.

Muscle overloading Activities in which this is liable to happen include skating, skiing and jogging. Also, prolonged walking on an uneven or sloping surface and attempting to keep one's balance when walking across a slippery tiled or highly polished wooden floor wearing shoes with smooth leather soles.

Prolonged muscle shortening Examples of circumstances in which this is liable to happen include wearing high heels, sitting on a high stool with the feet inadequately supported and sleeping with the feet in a persistently plantar-flexed position.

Muscle ischaemia The muscle may become ischaemic as a result of the application of sustained pressure to the calf as, for example, when sitting with it resting against the end of a reclining chair. Also, by the wearing of socks with unduly tight elastic tops and most importantly of all as a consequence of peripheral vascular disease.

TrP sites and patterns of pain referral

TrP activity most commonly develops just above and medial to the upper end of the Achilles tendon. Pain from a TrP at this site is referred to the heel and plantar surface of the foot (Fig. 13.20).

When searching for TrPs in the soleus muscle the patient should lie prone with the knee flexed in order to relax the gastrocnemius.

Deactivation of trigger points

Travell & Simons (1992g) state that deactivating TrPs in the soleus muscle by injecting a local anaesthetic into them is followed by such severe post-injection soreness that the procedure should never be carried out in both legs at the same time. This complication may be avoided by using superficial dry needling (see Ch. 7).

Prevention of TrP reactivation

Avoidance of persistent plantar flexion Persistent plantar flexion should be avoided. At night this may be avoided by sleeping with the feet resting against a firm pillow.

Shoes People with a tendency to develop gastrocnemius and soleus TrP activity have to be careful with regard to their choice of shoes. They should avoid wearing shoes that have either slippery soles or high heels.

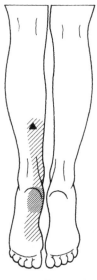

Figure 13.20 The pattern of pain referral from a trigger point (▲) in the soleus muscle.

Reclining chair leg rest They should also avoid using a reclining chair with a leg rest that compresses the calf or causes the feet to be persistently plantar-flexed.

Soleus pedal exercise Whenever it is necessary to sit for an appreciable period of time, such as on a long plane flight, the soleus pedal exercise described by Travell & Simons (1992g) should be carried out as it both stretches the soleus muscle and improves the venous return from the lower limbs.

In this exercise one foot is first fully dorsiflexed and then fully plantar-flexed; and then following a rest the other foot is put through the same movements. These movements should be repeated about six times every half hour.

Differential diagnosis

Pain referred to the heel and sole of the foot from TrPs in either the gastrocnemius or soleus muscle has to be distinguished from the pain of either Achilles tendinitis or plantar fasciitis (see p. 297).

Achilles tendinitis

Inflammation of the peritendinous tissues in the vicinity of the calcaneal insertion of this tendon is a cause of pain developing in the posterior aspect of the heel. The disorder is sometimes referred to as a tenosynovitis (Grennan 1984) but this is a misnomer as the tendon has no synovial sheath. The inflammatory reaction takes place in the loose connective tissue around the tendon. It is liable to affect athletes who subject themselves to over-zealous training (Clement et al 1984), and also those such as military recruits who have to wear heavy ill-fitting boots.

On examination, palpation reveals marked peritendinous tenderness. There may also be some swelling of the tissues and crepitus may be elicited on moving the ankle. The pain is characteristically worse when the patient attempts to stand on tiptoe. Resisted plantar flexion is also painful.

When the condition is acute it is usually possible to control the pain with a non-steroidal anti-inflammatory drug. If not, a corticosteroid/local anaesthetic mixture should be injected into the tissues around the tendon. It is essential to avoid injecting the steroid into the tendon itself as it may rupture and have to be repaired surgically.

In some cases pain at the back of the heel persists long after the acute inflammation has subsided. One not well-recognised cause of this is increased tension in the Achilles tendon brought about by TrP-induced shortening of the soleus and gastrocnemius muscles.

Soleus periostalgia syndrome (syns: medial tibial stress syndrome; soleus syndrome; shin splints)

Athletes and dancers who engage in much strenuous physical activity are liable to develop pain and tenderness along the inner side of the tibia where the soleus muscle attaches to it. It has been shown histologically that the overloading of this muscle causes the periosteum to become partially or completely separated from the tibial cortex and, in the light of this, Detmer (1986) has called the disorder 'chronic periostalgia'.

Stress fracture

Soleus periostalgia syndrome has to be distinguished from a stress fracture giving rise to pain and tenderness along the inner aspect of the lower third of the tibia.

A stress fracture is not evident on a straight X-ray until it has been present for a few weeks. However, a radionuclide scan reveals its presence almost immediately (Rupani et al 1985). Athletes with stress fractures need to give up all strenuous activities for some weeks.

PAIN FROM MTrPs IN THE DEEP POSTERIOR COMPARTMENT OF THE LEG

Muscles in this compartment include the tibialis posterior, flexor digitorum longus and flexor hallucis longus.

Tibialis posterior (Fig. 13.21)

Anatomical attachments

This muscle is situated between the tibia and fibula deep to the soleus muscle. It has on its outer side the flexor hallucis longus and on its inner side the flexor digitorum longus.

Proximally, its main attachments are to the medial surface of the fibula and the interosseous membrane. It also has attachments to the lateral surface of the tibia and intermuscular septa.

Distally, its tendon passes behind the medial malleolus to attach to most of the bones that make up the arch of the foot on its plantar aspect.

Actions

This muscle plantar-flexes the ankle joint and pulls up the medial border of the foot; i.e. it inverts the foot. It is of importance in maintaining the longitudinal arch of the foot.

Factors responsible for the development of TrP activity

Circumstances in which TrP activity is liable to develop in this muscle include running on rough, sloping or uneven ground. TrP activity is also likely to develop when the muscle is overloaded as a result of the foot becoming hyperpronated

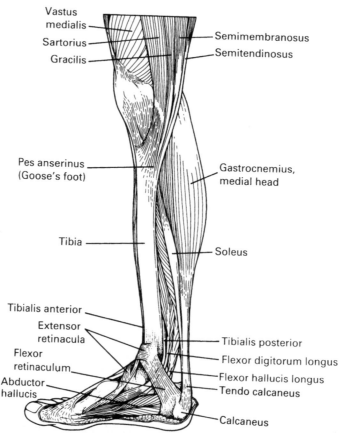

Figure 13.21   Muscles of the right leg, medial aspect.

because of, for example, a Morton's deformity (see p. 245).

TrP sites and patterns of pain referral

TrP activity is liable to develop in the upper third of the muscle. From a TrP at this site pain is referred mainly to the region of the Achilles tendon. It is also felt in the calf and plantar surface of the foot (Fig. 13.22).

Associated trigger points

The tibialis posterior, flexor digitorum longus and flexor hallucis longus are liable to develop TrP activity concomitantly. Somewhat surprisingly there is not usually concurrent TrP activity in the gastrocnemius and soleus muscles. However, TrP activity may develop in the peroneal muscles at the same time.

Clinical examination

Because the tibialis posterior muscle is a foot inverter, TrP activity, by weakening it, causes the patient to walk with the foot everted and abducted; i.e. with a hyperpronated flat-footed gait.

In order to locate TrPs in this muscle the patient should be placed in the prone position and TrP tenderness sought by applying very firm pressure to the upper part of the calf between the tibia and fibula.

Differential diagnosis

Shin splints An unfit person who attempts to carry out some strenuous athletic activity is liable to develop pain along the distal two-thirds of the tibial shaft as a result of damaging the periosteum where the tibialis posterior muscle attaches to the bone. This periostalgia at an early stage may respond to conservative treatment but if the pressure becomes too high (i.e. more than 15 mmHg at rest, with an increase during exercise and a delayed return to the post-exercise level) fasciotomy of the deep posterior compartment is necessary (Rorabeck et al 1988).

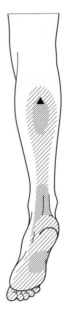

Figure 13.22 The pattern of pain referral from a TrP (▲) in the tibialis posterior muscle.

Tibialis posterior tendon dysfunction Pain and tenderness along the length of this muscle's tendon, particularly where it is situated behind the medial malleolus, may be due to the development of a tenosynovitis. The diagnosis and management of this disorder has been comprehensively reviewed by Johnson & Strom (1989).

Deactivation of trigger points

Because the muscle lies at such a deep level any deactivation technique involving the insertion of a needle into the muscle is hazardous. Therefore, superficial dry needling is preferable (see Ch. 7).

Preventative measures

Any physical activities found to bring on the pain should be given up and exercise obtained by other means such as swimming. Also, Morton's foot deformity if present may require to be treated (see p. 282). And it is important in all cases for attention to be paid to the type of shoes worn. These should provide good ankle support and should not have high heels.

Flexor digitorum longus (Fig. 13.21)

Anatomical attachments

This muscle, which is situated at the back of the tibia, deep to the soleus and gastrocnemius and medial to the tibialis posterior, attaches proximally to the shaft of the tibia. Distally, its tendon passes behind the medial malleolus, and then divides into four separate tendons which attach to the distal phalanx of each of the second, third, fourth and fifth toes.

Actions

This muscle flexes the four lesser toes and in conjunction with the flexor hallucis longus assists with plantar flexion and inversion of the foot.

Both of these muscles assist other plantar flexors in transferring weight to the forefoot and in maintaining equilibrium when this has been achieved. They are also of importance in maintaining the longitudinal arch of the foot.

Factors responsible for the development of TrP activity

These are the same as for the tibialis posterior muscle (see p. 288).

TrP sites and patterns of pain referral

TrP activity is liable to develop in the upper part of the muscle with pain from a TrP there being referred to the central and lateral aspects of the sole of the foot (Fig. 13.23).

Trigger point examination

With the patient lying on the involved side, the knee is bent and the foot plantar-flexed in order to allow the gastocnemius muscle to be pushed to one side, deep firm pressure is applied toward the back of the tibia.

Deactivation of trigger points

Because of the depth at which the muscle lies any method that involves inserting a needle into the muscle itself is hazardous. Superficial dry needling is therefore preferable (see Ch. 7).

Flexor hallucis longus (Fig. 13.21)

Anatomical attachments

This muscle, which mainly arises from the posterior surface of the fibula lateral to the tibialis posterior and deep to the soleus and gastrocnemius, has at its distal end a tendon which crosses over to the medial side and, on the plantar surface of the foot, becomes attached to the base of the terminal phalanx of the great toe.

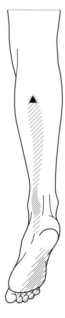

Figure 13.23 The pattern of pain referral from a TrP (▲) in the flexor digitorum longus muscle.

Factors responsible for the development of TrP activity

These are the same as for the tibialis posterior muscle (see p. 288).

TrP sites and pattern of pain referral

TrP activity is liable to develop about a hand's breadth above the ankle. From there pain is referred to the plantar surface of the great toe and first metatarsal (Fig. 13.24).

Trigger point examination

With the patient lying prone deep pressure is applied to the lower part of the calf against the back of the fibula.

Deactivation of trigger points

As with the other two muscles in this compartment, deeply applied techniques are hazardous. Superficial dry needling (see Ch. 7) is therefore preferable.

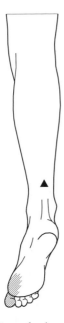

Figure 13.24 The pattern of pain referral from a TrP (▲) in the flexor hallucis longus muscle.

Preventive measures

Shoes should be worn with soles that are flexible enough to allow the metatarsal joints of the toes to move fully. Also, the wearing of high heels should be avoided.

If, despite treatment, an athlete finds that the pain quickly recurs, any activity such as running should be given up for a time and exercise obtained by other means, such as by swimming or cycling. And then when running is eventually resumed it should initially only be carried out for short distances and on flat even surfaces.

PAIN FROM MTrPs IN THE FOOT

There are nine muscles in the foot that have distinctive TrP pain referral patterns (Table 13.1). Because the muscles are small and some of their patterns of pain referral overlap, initially identifying each muscle's individual zone of TrP pain referral must have required considerable clinical acumen. Much credit therefore is due to Travell & Simons (1992h) for not only having done this but for also having given such a clear and comprehensive account of the diagnosis, differential diagnosis and treatment of MTrP foot pain. The following is a brief review of the subject mainly based on this.

Firstly, pain referral patterns from TrPs in the dorsal and plantar muscles will be described. Following this, factors responsible for the development of TrP activity in foot muscles will be considered. And then some general remarks will be made concerning the deactivation of MTrPs in the foot. Finally, some causes of heel pain will be discussed including in particular plantar fasciitis.

DORSAL SURFACE OF THE FOOT

Extensor digitorum brevis (Fig. 13.13)

Anatomical attachments

This thin muscle is the only one on the dorsum of the foot. It is situated deep to the tendons of the extensor digitorum longus. Proximally, it is attached to the calcaneum. Distally it ends in

Table 13.1   Muscles of the foot

Dorsal surface			
Extensor digitorum brevis			

Plantar surface	Medial	Centre	Lateral
First layer	Abductor hallucis	Flexor digitorum brevis	Abductor digiti minimi
Second layer		Flexor digitorum accessorius (quadratus plantae) Lumbricales	
Third layer	Flexor hallucis brevis Adductor hallucis		
Fourth layer		Interossei	

four tendons. The medial part of the muscle with its tendinous insertion into the proximal phalanx of the great toe is sometimes described as a separate muscle, the extensor hallucis brevis (Fig. 13.13). The other three tendons are inserted into the outer sides of the tendons of the extensor digitorum longus.

TrP sites and patterns of pain referral

Pain from TrPs in this muscle is referred to the proximal part of the dorsum of the foot in the vicinity of these TrP sites (Fig. 13.25). This, it should be noted, is in contrast to pain from TrPs in the extensor digitorum longus, which is referred along the whole length of the dorsum of the foot including the toes, and also to pain from TrPs in the extensor hallucis longus, which is referred to the distal aspect of the first metatarsal bone and great toe (p. 280).

TrP activity in the short extensor and the long extensor muscles of the toes often develops concomitantly.

PLANTAR SURFACE OF THE FOOT

The muscles in the plantar region of the foot may be conveniently divided into four layers (Table 13.1).

The first layer

The muscles in the first layer include the abductor hallucis, flexor digitorum brevis and abductor digiti minimi (Fig. 13.26).

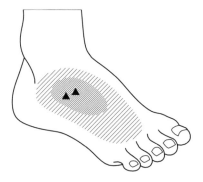

Figure 13.25   The pattern of pain referral from a TrP (▲) in the extensor digitorum brevis muscle.

Abductor hallucis

Anatomical attachments

This muscle is situated subcutaneously on the posterior half of the medial border of the foot. Proximally, its main attachment is to the calcaneum. Distally, its tendon inserts, together with the medial tendon of the flexor hallucis brevis (see third layer), into the medial side of the proximal phalanx of the great toe.

TrP sites and pattern of pain referral

TrPs are liable to be found anywhere along the belly of this muscle. Pain is referred from these TrPs to the posterior half of the medial border of the plantar surface of the foot (Fig. 13.27).

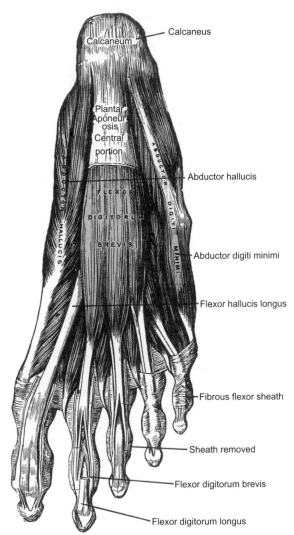

Figure 13.26   The superficial plantar muscles of the right foot.

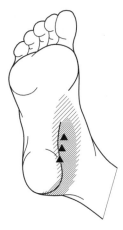

Figure 13.27   The pattern of pain referral from a TrP (▲) in the abductor hallucis muscle.

TrP sites and pattern of pain referral

TrPs in the bellies of this muscle refer pain transversely across the ball of the foot. This, it should be noted, is in contrast to the flexor digitorum longus pain pattern, which is along the lateral side of the sole of the foot (Fig. 13.28). TrP activity in the flexor digitorum brevis and flexor digitorum longus not uncommonly develop concomitantly.

Abductor digiti minimi

Anatomical attachments

The belly of this subcutaneous muscle is situated along the length of the lateral border of the foot.

Flexor digitorum brevis

Anatomical attachments

This muscle, which is situated in the middle of the sole of the foot, has four bellies. Proximally, these are attached to the medial tubercle of the calcaneum and the centre part of the plantar fascia. Distally, each of its four tendons is attached to one of the lesser toes.

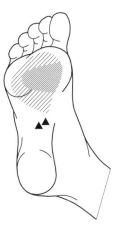

Figure 13.28   The pattern of pain referral from a TrP (▲) in the flexor digitorum brevis muscle.

Proximally, it attaches to the calcaneum and plantar fascia. Distally, its tendon, together with the flexor digiti minimi brevis, is inserted into the proximal phalanx of the fifth toe.

TrP sites and pattern of pain referral

TrPs in the belly of this muscle refer pain to the plantar aspect of the fifth metatarsal bone (Fig. 13.29).

The second layer

The muscles in the second layer include the flexor digitorum accessorius (syn: quadratus plantae) and the lumbricales (Fig. 13.30).

Flexor digitorum accessorius (syn: quadratus plantae)

Anatomical attachments

This muscle has two heads. These arise from the medial and lateral sides of the calcaneum deep to the plantar fascia. These two heads join to form a flattened band which is inserted into the tendon of the flexor digitorum longus before the latter divides into four tendons that become attached to the plantar surfaces of the bases of the distal phalanges of the second, third, fourth and fifth toes.

The function of the flexor digitorum accessorius is to assist in converting the oblique pull of the tendons of the flexor digitorum longus into a direct backward pull on the toes.

TrP sites and pattern of pain referral

TrPs in the heads and main belly of this muscle refer pain to the plantar surface of the heel (Fig. 13.31). This is in contrast to TrPs in the gastrocnemius and flexor digitorum longus, which refer pain to the instep in front of the heel. Also, to TrPs in the soleus muscle, which refer pain not only to the plantar surface of the heel but also to the back of the heel and into the Achilles tendon. And to TrPs in the tibialis

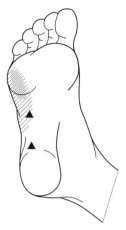

Figure 13.29   The pattern of pain referral from a TrP (▲) in the abductor digiti minimi muscle.

posterior, which refer pain mainly to the Achilles tendon but also to a lesser extent into the calf and sole of the foot.

The lumbricales

These four muscles, which serve as accessories to the tendons of the flexor digitorum longus, are too small to have distinctive TrP pain referral patterns.

The third layer

The muscles in the third layer include the flexor hallucis brevis, adductor hallucis and flexor digiti minimi brevis (Fig. 13.32).

Flexor hallucis brevis

Anatomical attachments

This muscle, which lies on the medial side of the foot, is for the most part covered by the plantar fascia. Proximally, it arises by a pointed tendinous process from the cuboid bone, the cuneiform bone and from the part of the tendon of the tibialis posterior which is attached to that bone. It divides into a medial and lateral belly and the tendons of these are inserted into the corresponding sides of the base of the proximal phalanx of the great toe.

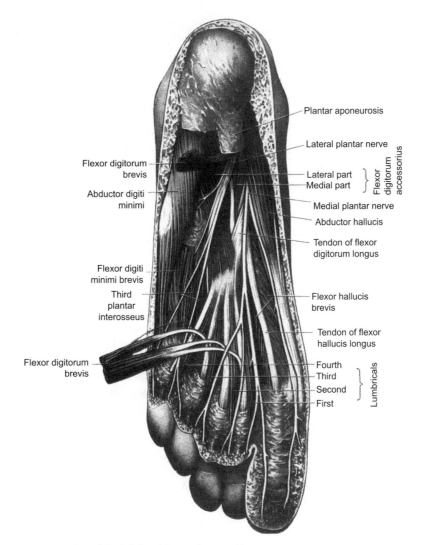

Figure 13.30 The plantar muscles of the left foot: first and second layers.

TrP sites and pattern of pain referral

As the lateral belly of this muscle is deeply situated beneath the plantar fascia deep palpation is required in order to locate TrPs in it. In contrast to this, TrPs in the medial belly may be located by lighter palpation through the thinner skin along the inner side of the sole of the foot. TrPs in either of these two parts of the muscle refer pain to the head of the first metatarsal bone both on its plantar and dorsal aspects. Also, to a lesser extent, to the great toe and second toe (Fig. 13.33).

Adductor hallucis

Anatomical attachments

This muscle has two heads: an oblique one, which arises from the base of the second, third and fourth metatarsal bones and which is inserted, together with the lateral belly of the flexor hallucis brevis, into the lateral side of the proximal phalanx of the great toe; and a transverse one, which arises from the plantar metatarsophalangeal ligaments of the third, fourth and fifth toes and which is also inserted into the lateral side of the proximal phalanx of the great toe.

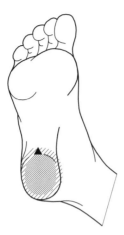

Figure 13.31   The pattern of pain referral from a TrP (▲) in the flexor digitorum accessorius (quadratus plantae) muscle.

TrP sites and pattern of pain referral

TrPs in this muscle refer pain to the sole of the foot in the region of the first to the fourth metatarsal heads (Fig. 13.34), i.e. in a similar distribution to that of pain referred from TrPs in the flexor digitorum brevis.

Flexor digiti minimi brevis

This flexor of the little toe, which arises from the base of the fifth metatarsal bone and is inserted into the proximal phalanx of the fifth toe, is too small to have a distinctive MTrP pain referral pattern.

The fourth layer

The muscles in the fourth layer include the dorsal and plantar interossei (Fig. 13.35).

Anatomical attachments

The dorsal interossei, four in number, are situated between the metatarsal bones. They arise by two heads from the adjacent sides of the metatarsal bones between which they are placed. The first is inserted into the medial side of the second toe, the other three into the lateral sides of the second, third and fourth toes.

The plantar interossei, three in number, arise from the shafts of the third, fourth and fifth metatarsal bones and insert into the medial sides of the same toes.

TrP sites and pattern of pain referral

A TrP in the belly of an interosseous muscle refers pain forwards from the TrP site along either the dorsal or plantar surface of the foot in a narrow band towards the toe into which the muscle is inserted (Fig. 13.36).

Factors responsible for the development of TrP activity in foot muscles

TrPs in these muscles are liable to become active as a result of trauma such as may be incurred by a fall that results in stubbing the toes or bruising the dorsal or plantar aspect of the foot, particularly when the trauma is severe enough to sprain an ankle or fracture a bone in the foot. Restricting movements of the foot by placing it in a cast for the treatment of a fracture also tends to encourage the development of TrP activity.

In addition, TrP activity is liable to develop when movements of the toes are restricted as a result of wearing shoes that are either too tightly fitting or too short.

Also, a Morton's foot deformity that causes mediolateral rocking of the foot may lead to the development of TrP activity, particularly in the abductor digiti minimi and abductor hallucis muscles.

Deactivation of trigger points in foot muscles

Because the extensor digitorum brevis on the dorsal surface of the foot lie superficially the deactivation of TrPs in it is straightforward using any of the methods described in Chapter 7.

Particular care, however, has to be taken in deactivating TrPs on the plantar aspect of the foot. It is of considerable importance to avoid infection developing by thoroughly cleaning the skin and applying an antiseptic prior to inserting a needle through it. As the insertion of a needle

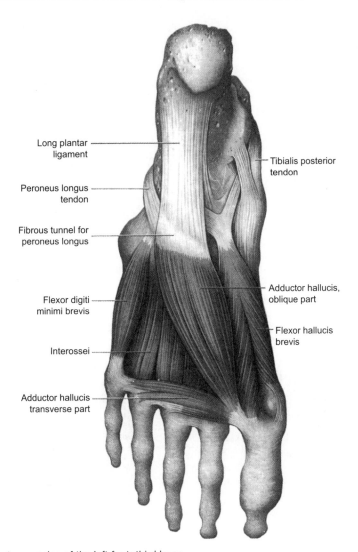

Long plantar
ligament

Peroneus longus
tendon

Fibrous tunnel for
peroneus longus

Flexor digiti
minimi brevis

Interossei

Adductor hallucis
transverse part

Tibialis posterior
tendon

Adductor hallucis,
oblique part

Flexor hallucis
brevis

Figure 13.32   The plantar muscles of the left foot: third layer.

into the plantar surface of the foot is particularly liable to cause bleeding into the tissues, it is essential on withdrawing the needle to secure haemostasis by applying firm sustained pressure. Because needling the plantar surface of the foot is very painful, superficial dry needling at the TrP site is, in my opinion, the treatment of choice.

HEEL AND SOLE OF FOOT PAIN

Finally, it is necessary to consider some of the common causes for pain developing in the heel and the sole of the foot. These include Achilles tendinitis (p. 287); referral from TrPs in the gastrocnemius (p. 283), soleus (p. 286), flexor digitorum accessorius (p. 294) and abductor hallucis (p. 292); and plantar fasciitis.

Plantar fasciitis

Pathogenesis

The aetiology of this disorder is uncertain. There are grounds for believing that it is most

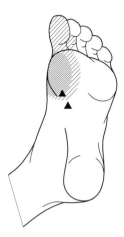

Figure 13.33 The pattern of pain referral from a TrP (▲) in the flexor hallucis brevis muscle.

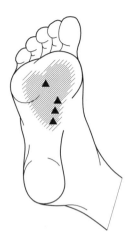

Figure 13.34 The pattern of pain referral from TrPs (▲) in the transverse and oblique heads of the adductor hallucis muscle.

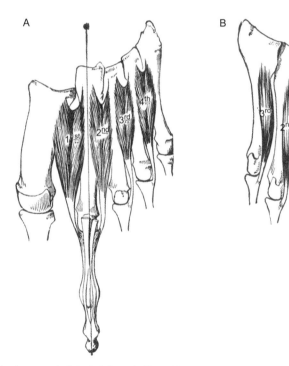

Figure 13.35 The interossei of the left foot. A, Dorsal interossei viewed from the dorsal aspect. B, Plantar interossei viewed from the plantar aspect. The axis to which the movements of abduction and adduction are referred is as indicated.

commonly due to traction-induced microtears in the plantar fascia causing it to become inflamed. Occasionally it is part of a more widespread inflammatory condition such as Reiter's disease. Granulomatous changes and fibroblastic prolif-

eration have been observed in biopsy specimens of the fascia.

Traction on the plantar fascia may occur as a result of a tight Achilles tendon limiting dorsiflexion. Causes for Achilles tendon tightness

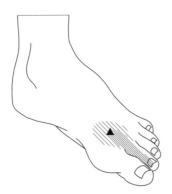

Figure 13.36 The pattern of pain referral from a TrP (▲) in the first dorsal interosseous muscle.

developing include TrP-induced shortening of the gastrocnemius and soleus muscles. Traction on the plantar fascia may also be brought about because of TrP-induced shortness of muscles that have attachments to it. These include the abductor hallucis, flexor digitorum brevis and abductor digiti minimi.

Obesity would seem to be a predisposing factor as it has been found to be present in 40% of men and 90% of women suffering from this disorder (De Maio 1993).

Age and sex

The disorder may develop at any age but does so mainly in young adult male athletes and middle-aged women.

Symptoms

The pain may initially be diffuse but with time it usually becomes localised around the insertion of the plantar fascia into the medial calcaneal tubercule.

The pain in the heel is most marked when first putting the foot to the floor on waking. Then after a few steps it becomes less intense. However, it again becomes worse following either strenuous activity or sitting down.

Heel pain that is worse on initial weight-bearing after getting out of bed is typical of plantar fasciitis. This is in contrast to the pain of a calcaneal stress fracture, which is usually worse on walking.

Heel pain that comes on during the night is liable to be due to some other cause such as the tarsal tunnel syndrome, infection or neoplasm.

Signs

There is invariably a point of maximum tenderness on the anteromedial aspect of the heel at the site where the fascia attaches to the medial tubercle of the calcaneum. The point is deep-seated and requires firm palpation to elicit it.

Tightness of the Achilles tendon with, as a consequence, restricted dorsiflexion of the ankle, is present in 78% of patients (De Maio et al 1993).

Tenderness on squeezing the Achilles tendon raises the possibility of a stress fracture of the calcaneum. A plain lateral radiograph of the heel is required to exclude this. A heel spur may also be seen on the radiograph but, as stated, when considering Achilles tendinitis this is of no diagnostic value as it is not uncommonly found in asymptomatic feet.

Treatment

Non-steroidal anti-inflammatory drugs (NSAIDs)

An oral NSAID, by decreasing the inflammatory response, reduces the pain.

Steroid/local anaesthetic injections

If an oral NSAID does not give sufficient relief the injection of a steroid/local anaesthetic mixture into the point of maximum tenderness on the anteromedial aspect of the heel should be carried out.

The needle is inserted into the medial side of the heel and advanced in a lateral and slightly upwards posterior direction as close as possible to the plantar surface of the calcaneum (Fam 1995). One injection may be sufficient but not infrequently it has to be repeated. This, however, is not without risk because the steroid may cause fat pad atrophy with, as a consequence, a loss of cushioning of the heel. And when this happens the plantar fascia is liable to rupture (Sellman 1994). Also, osteomyelitis of the calcaneum has been reported (Gidumal & Evanski 1985).

Local anaesthetic injections

In view of these possible complications the routine use of steroid injections cannot be recommended, particularly as a prospective randomised study has shown that there is no significant difference with respect to pain relief between injecting lignocaine (Lidocaine) alone and a steroid/lignocaine mixture (Blockey 1956). In view of this Singh et al (1997) recommended that a steroid injection should be reserved for the occasional patient with refractory symptoms.

Footwear

It is essential for shoes to have an arch support and cushioned heels. An orthosis should also be used. A sponge rubber cushion with its centre removed can be fitted under the heel. However, because the plantar fascia is stretched during flattening of the foot Singh et al (1997) prefer an orthosis designed to maintain the medial longitudinal arch during ambulation and prescribe a full-length or three-quarter length accommodative inlay of medium density plastazote.

Search for myofascial trigger points

Because, as previously explained, MTrP activity may develop in association with plantar fasciitis, a search for MTrPs is essential and, when found to be present, they should be deactivated. Imamura et al (1998) have invariably found TrPs to be present in calf muscles of patients with the disorder and have confirmed that treatment of these speeds up recovery.

Exercises for relieving Achilles tendon tightness

Because the majority of patients with plantar fasciitis have tightness of the Achilles tendon and this, by putting a strain on the fascia, perpetuates the disorder, it is essential for the patient to be taught how to relieve this tendon tightness by stretching the gastrocnemius and soleus muscles.

The gastrocnemius is stretched by dorsiflexing the foot whilst keeping the knee extended. The soleus is stretched by dorsiflexing the foot whilst keeping the knee flexed. The patient should be told to carry out sustained stretching of these muscles several times a day.

REFERENCES

Arcangeli P, Corradi F, D'Ayala-Valva 1965 Alterations of skin and muscle sensibility in chronic obliterating arteriopathy of the lower limbs and their importance in determining intermittent claudication. Acta Neurovegetativa 27:511–545

Arcangeli P, Digiesi V, Ronchi O, Dorigo B, Bartoli V 1976 Mechanisms of ischaemic pain in peripheral occlusive arterial disease. In: Bonica J J, Albe-Fessard D (eds) Advances in pain research and therapy. Raven Press, New York, vol 1, pp 965–973

Arnoldi C C, Lemperg R K, Linderholm H 1971 Immediate effect of osteotomy on the intramedullary pressure of the femoral head and neck in patients with degenerative osteoarthritis. Acta Orthopaedica Scandinavica 42:357–365

Arnoldi C C, Djurhuus J C, Heerfordt J, Karte A 1980 Intraosseous phlebography, intraosseous pressure measurements and Tc-polyphosphate scintigraphy in patients with various painful conditions in the hip and knee. Acta Orthopaedica Scandinavica 51: 19–28

Baldry P E 1993 Acupuncture, trigger points and musculoskeletal pain, 2nd edn. Churchill Livingstone, Edinburgh, p 335

Baltodano N, Gallo B V, Weidler D J 1988 Verapamil vs quinine for recumbent nocturnal leg cramps in the elderly. Archives of Intensive Medicine 148: 1969–1970

Blockey N J 1956 The painful heel. British Medical Journal ii:1277–1278

Bonica J J, Lanzer W L 1990 Painful disorders of the thigh and knee. In: Bonica J J (ed) The management of pain, 2nd edn. Lea & Febiger, Philadelphia, pp 1557–1584

Bonica J J, Sola A 1990 Other painful disorders of the lower limb. In: Bonica J J (ed) The management of pain, 2nd edn. Lea & Febiger, Philadelphia, p 1627

Bradley J D, Brandt K D, Katz B P, Kalasinski L A, Ryan S I 1991 Comparison of an anti-inflammatory dose of ibuprofen, an analgesic dose of ibuprofen and acetaminophen in treatment of patients with osteoarthritis of the knee. New England Journal of Medicine 325: 87–91

Clement D B, Taunton J E, Smart G W 1984 Achilles tendinitis and peritendinitis: etiology and treatment. American Journal of Sports Medicine 12:179–184

De Maio M, Paine R, Maugire R, Diez D J R 1993 Plantar fasciitis. Orthopedics 16:153–163

Detmer D E 1986 Chronic shin splints. Classification of and management of medial tibial stress syndrome. Sports Medicine 3:436–446

Dieppe P A, Huskisson E C, Crocker P, Willoughby D A 1976 Apatite deposition disease: a new arthropathy. Lancet i:266–268

Dixon A St J 1965 Progress in clinical rheumatology. J A Churchill, London, pp 313–329

Dorigo B, Bartoli V, Gristillo D, Beconi D 1979 Fibrositic myofascial pain in intermittent claudication. Effect of anaesthetic block of trigger points on exercise tolerance. Pain 6:183–199

Eaton J M 1989 Is this really a muscle cramp? Postgraduate Medicine 86:227–232

Ekbom K A 1960 Restless leg syndrome. Neurology 10:868

Fam A G 1995 The ankle and foot. In: Klippel J H, Dieppe P A (eds) Practical rheumatology. Mosby, London, p 120

Felson D, Anderson J, Naimark A et al 1988 Obesity and knee osteoarthritis. The Framingham Study. Annals of Internal Medicine 109:18–24

Gidumal R, Evanski P 1985 Calcaneal osteomyelitis following steroid injection. Foot and Ankle 6:44–46

Graham G P, Fairclough J A 1995 The knee. In: Klippel J A, Dieppe P A (eds) Practical rheumatology. Mosby, London, pp 97–110

Grennan D M 1984 Rheumatology. Baillière Tindall, London, p 152

Hadler N M 1992 Knee pain is the malady – not osteoarthritis. Annals of Internal Medicine 116(7): 598–599

Harris R I, Beath T 1949 The short first metatarsal: its incidence and clinical significance. Journal of Bone and Joint Surgery (Am) 31:553–565

Hope-Simpson R E 1976 Night cramp. British Medical Journal ii:1563

Imamura M, Fischer A A, Imamura S T et al 1998 Treatment of myofascial pain components in plantar fasciitis speeds up recovery. In: Fischer A A (ed) Muscle pain syndromes and fibromyalgia. Haworth Medical Press, New York, pp 91–110

Johnson K A, Strom D E 1989 Tibialis posterior tendon dysfunction. Clinical Orthopaedics 239:196–206

Kovar P A, Allegrante J P, Mackenzie C R, Peterson M G, Gutin B, Charlson M E 1992 Supervised fitness walking in patients with osteoarthritis of the knee. A randomized controlled trial. Annals of Internal Medicine 116:529–534

Lemperg R K, Arnoldi C C 1978 The significance of intraosseous pressure in normal and diseased states with special reference to the intraosseous engorgement-pain syndrome. Clinical Orthopaedics and Related Research 136:143–156

Long C 1956 Myofascial pain syndromes. Part III. Some syndromes of the trunk and thigh. Henry Ford Hospital Medical Bulletin 4:102–106

McCarthy C, Cushnaghan J, Dieppe P 1994 Osteoarthritis. In: Wall P D, Melzack R (eds) Textbook of pain, 3rd edn. Churchill Livingstone, Edinburgh, pp 387–396

McCrae F, Shouis J, Dieppe P, Watt I 1992 Scintigraphic assessment of osteoarthritis of the knee joint. Annals of the Rheumatic Diseases 51:938–942

Massurdo Z L, Watt I, Cushnaghan J, Dieppe P 1989 An eight-year prospective study of osteoarthritis of the knee joint. Annals of the Rheumatic Diseases 48:893–897

Morton D J 1935 The human foot: its evolution, physiology and functional disorders. Columbia University Press, New York

Paré E B, Stern J T, Schwartz J M 1981 Functional differentiation within the tensor fasciae latae. Journal of Bone and Joint Surgery (Am) 63:1457–1471

Parrow A, Samuelsson S-M 1967 Use of chloroquinine phosphate – a new treatment for spontaneous leg cramps. Acta Medica Scandinavica 181:237–244

Rawls W B 1966 Management of nocturnal leg cramps. Western Journal of Medicine 7:152–157

Rorabeck C H, Fowler P J, Nott L 1988 The results of fasciotomy in the management of chronic exertional compartment syndrome. American Journal of Sports Medicine 16:224–227

Rupani H D, Holder L E, Espinola D A et al 1985 Three-phase radionuclide bone imaging in sports medicine. Radiology 156:187–196

Sellman J R 1994 Plantar fascia rupture associated with corticosteroid injection. Foot and Ankle 15:376–381

Sherman R A 1980 Published treatments of phantom limb pain. American Journal of Physical Medicine 59: 232–244

Singh D, Angel J, Bentley G, Trevino S G 1997 Plantar fasciitis. British Medical Journal 315:172–175

Teng P 1972 Meralgia paresthetica. Bulletin of the Los Angeles Neurological Society 37:75–83

Travell J 1950 The adductor longus syndrome: a cause of groin pain. Bulletin of the New York Academy of Medicine 26:284–285

Travell J 1957 Symposium of mechanism and management of pain syndromes. Proceedings of the Rudolf Virchow Medical Society 16:126–136

Travell J G, Simons D 1992a–h Myofascial pain and dysfunction. The trigger point manual. The lower extremities. Williams & Wilkins, Baltimore, vol 2, p 266 (a), p 262 (b), p 334 (c), p 480 (d), p 408 (e), p 416 (f), p 452 (g), pp 501–539 (h)

Travell J, Baker S J, Hirsch B B et al 1952 Myofascial component of intermittent claudication. Federation Proceedings 11:164

Warburton A, Royston J P, O'Neill J et al 1987 A quinine a day keeps the leg cramps away? British Journal of Clinical Pharmacology 23:459–465

Whiteley A M 1982 Cramps, stiffness and restless legs. Practitioner 226:1085–1087

Yunus M B, Aldag J C 1996 Restless leg syndrome and leg cramps in fibromyalgia syndrome: a controlled study. British Medical Journal 312:1339

14

The chest wall

INTRODUCTION

It is still not sufficiently well recognised that chest pain, with or without pain down the arm, commonly emanates from trigger points in muscles of the chest wall despite it now being over 50 years since three American physicians, Janet Travell, Myron Herman and Seymour Rinzler, first wrote about this (Travell et al 1942).

In this chapter attention will first be drawn to the anterior chest wall myofascial trigger point (MTrP) pain syndrome and various other pain disorders from which it has to be distinguished. And following this the posterior wall MTrP pain syndrome and its differential diagnosis will be discussed.

ANTERIOR CHEST WALL MTrP PAIN SYNDROME

Factors responsible for the development of MTrP activity

The factors responsible for the development of TrP activity in anterior chest wall muscles include trauma and anxiety. The trauma in some cases is brought about as a result of a direct injury to the chest wall. In others it takes the form of either acute or chronic overloading of the muscles. Possible reasons for anxiety causing TrP activity to develop in these and other muscles in the body have been described in Chapter 3. TrPs may also become active as a secondary event when the muscles containing them happen to lie in a part of the chest wall to which the pain of coronary heart disease is referred. In addition, TrP activity is liable to develop in these muscles for some as yet unexplained reason in patients with mitral valve prolapse.

Muscles liable to be involved

Anterior chest wall TrP pain is liable to develop in one or more of the following muscles – sternocleidomastoid, scalene, sternalis, subclavius, pectoralis major, pectoralis minor and the intercostals.

Sternocleidomastoid muscle

As stated in Chapter 8, TrP activity in the lower end of the sternal division of this muscle may cause pain to be referred over the upper part of the sternum (Fig. 8.12A). This pain may then in turn cause satellite TrPs to develop in the sternalis muscle.

Scalene muscles

As also stated in Chapter 8, pain from TrPs in one or other of the scalene muscles is liable to be referred both down an arm and anteriorly over the pectoral region (Fig. 8.14) and, because of this, on the left side its distribution and that of coronary artery disease (CAD) pain may be similar. Also, to add to the confusion, scalene TrP pain, like CAD pain, is liable to be brought on by exertion.

It also has to be remembered that scalene TrP pain, when referred over the anterior chest wall, is liable to cause satellite TrPs in the pectoralis major muscle to become activated, with pain from these then also being felt in the pectoral region and arm (Fig. 14.4).

Sternalis muscle

Anatomical attachments

This anomalous muscle, which is only present in one person in twenty, usually takes the form of a long thin strip covering one of the lateral borders of the sternum. Sometimes there are two covering them both. And occasionally the two strips join together to cover the whole of the sternum.

Factors responsible for development of TrP activity

TrP activity in this muscle is liable to develop as a primary event when the sternal region of the chest wall is subjected to trauma, and as a secondary event when coronary heart disease pain is referred to that region or when TrP pain is referred there from either the lower end of the sternocleidomastoid muscle (Fig. 8.12A) or a scalene muscle (Fig. 8.14).

TrP sites and patterns of pain referral

TrPs are liable to be found anywhere along the length of this muscle. Pain from them is felt substernally and in some cases in the pectoral region and arms (Fig. 14.1).

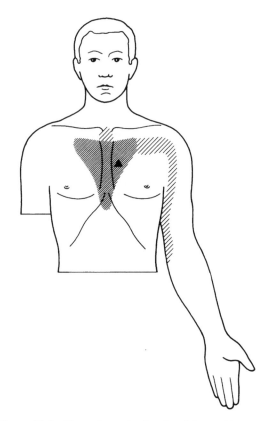

Figure 14.1 The pattern of pain referral from a trigger point or points (▲) in the sternalis muscle.

Associated trigger points

TrP activity in this muscle is rarely an isolated event. It usually occurs in conjunction with the development of this in the pectoralis major muscle. And, as stated earlier, pain from TrP activity in either the sternal division of the sternocleidomastoid muscle or a scalene muscle may be referred downwards over the sternum and cause satellite TrPs in the sternalis muscle to become activated.

Pectoralis major (Fig. 14.2)

Anatomical attachments

This large thick superficially situated anterior chest wall muscle has an extensive origin from the inner half of the clavicle, the sternum and the rib cartilages. Its posterior surface is in contact with the sternum, ribs, subclavius, pectoralis minor, serratus anterior and the intercostals. It

has a clavicular, a sternocostal and a costo-abdominal section. It is this latter section which laterally forms the anterior axillary fold. On the outer side of the chest wall the fibres of these three sections converge to form a tendon that is inserted into the bicipital groove of the humerus.

Factors responsible for the development of TrP activity

The factors which may cause primary TrP activity to develop in this muscle include lifting a heavy weight, or holding it for a sustained period; any task involving repeated adduction of the arm, such as when cutting a hedge with manually operated shears, or sustained adduction, such as when the arm is placed in a sling for any length of time; exposure of the muscle to draughts or damp; persistent contraction of the muscle from chronic anxiety; and in particular when a faulty slouching posture is adopted

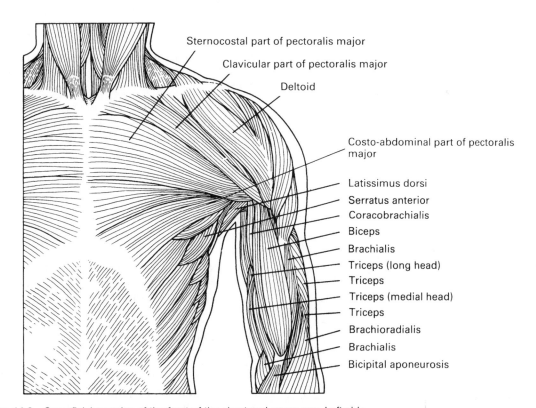

Figure 14.2 Superficial muscles of the front of the chest and upper arm. Left side.

when reading, writing or carrying out some task at a work bench.

TrPs in this muscle may also develop activity as a secondary event when pain from coronary artery disease is referred to the left anterior chest wall.

TrP sites and patterns of pain referral

The pattern of pain referral varies according to the particular section affected.

TrPs in the clavicular section of the muscle refers pain both locally and even more markedly over the shoulder as far as the anterior part of the deltoid muscle (Fig. 14.3).

TrPs in the sternal section are located mainly along the parasternal and mid-clavicular lines. TrPs along the parasternal line refer pain locally and over the sternum. TrPs in the mid-clavicular

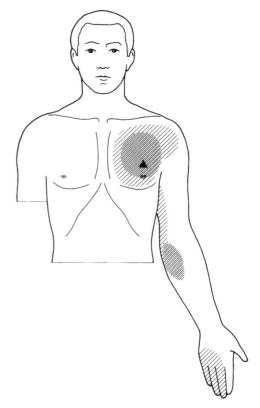

Figure 14.4 The pattern of pain referral from a trigger point or points (▲) in the sternal section of the pectoralis major muscle.

line give rise to severe pain over the anterior part of the chest and thus, on the left side, over the praecordium. It also radiates down the inner aspect of the arm where it is felt particularly strongly over the medial epicondyle and terminates in the ring and little fingers (Fig. 14.4).

TrP activity in the lateral free margin of the muscle, where it forms the anterior axillary fold, gives rise to pain and tenderness in the breast, as well as tenderness of the nipple. In women this not infrequently leads to an erroneous diagnosis of mastitis in spite of the texture of the breast being normal (Fig. 14.5).

Associated trigger points

TrP activity in the pectoralis major may occur in conjunction with this developing in the sternalis, sternocleidomastoid, and scalene muscles. The anterior deltoid may also develop satellite TrP

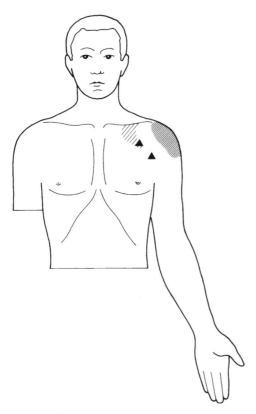

Figure 14.3 The pattern of pain referral from a trigger point or points (▲) in the clavicular section of the pectoralis major muscle.

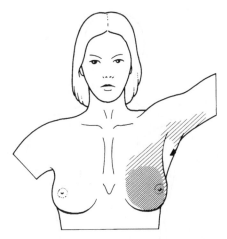

Figure 14.5 The pattern of pain referral from a trigger point or points (▲) in the lateral free margin of the pectoralis major muscle.

activity as it lies within this muscle's pain referral zone.

Subclavius muscle (Fig. 14.6)

Anatomical attachments

This small triangular muscle, placed between the clavicle and first rib behind the upper part of the

pectoralis major, has a thick tendinous attachment to the junction of the first rib and first costal cartilage. And from there its fibres pass obliquely upwards and laterally to be inserted into a groove on the under surface of the intermediate third of the clavicle.

Factors responsible for the development of TrP activity

TrPs in this muscle are liable to become activated for the same reasons as, and often in conjunction with, TrPs in the pectoralis major muscle.

TrP sites and patterns of pain referral

TrPs are liable to be found at the medial end of this muscle near to its attachment to the first rib. Pain from these TrPs is referred across the front of the shoulder, down the front of the upper arm in the midline, the front of the forearm on the radial side, and the radial side of the palmar surface of the hand and fingers (Fig. 14.7). It should be noted that the pain for some reason is not felt at either the elbow or the wrist (Simons et al 1999).

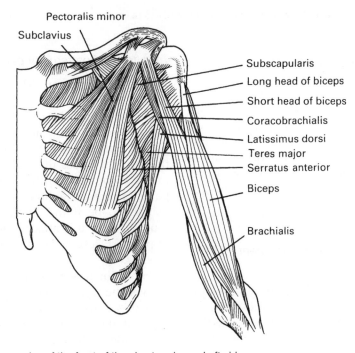

Figure 14.6 The deep muscles of the front of the chest and arm. Left side.

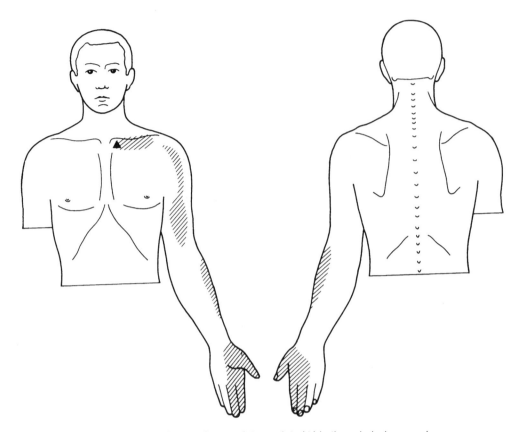

Figure 14.7 The pattern of pain referral from a trigger point or points (▲) in the subclavius muscle.

Pectoralis minor (Fig. 14.6)

Anatomical attachments

This thick triangular muscle, which is situated in the upper part of the thorax deep to the pectoralis major, arises from the third, fourth and fifth ribs near to their cartilages. From these its fibres pass upwards and laterally to form a flat tendon that is inserted into the coracoid process.

Factors responsible for the development of TrP activity

The factors responsible for TrP activity developing in this muscle are similar to those which cause it to occur in the pectoralis major muscle. And for this reason it often develops in these two muscles concomitantly.

TrP sites and patterns of pain referral

When searching for TrPs in this muscle the patient may either be seated or lying in the supine position. In either case the pectoralis major should be slackened by having the patient's arm lying comfortably to the side with the forearm across the abdomen. The pectoralis minor is then put on the stretch by getting the patient to brace the shoulder backwards. TrPs are usually to be found in the lower part of the muscle where it is attached to the ribs, or in the upper part close to its attachment to the coracoid process.

Pain from TrPs in this muscle is referred widely over the front of the chest so that, on the left side, this is over the praecordium. Also, over the front of the shoulder, and at times down the ulnar side of the arm into the middle, ring and little fingers (Fig. 14.8).

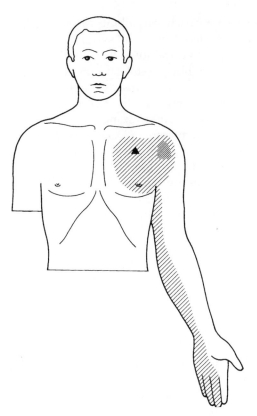

Figure 14.8 The pattern of pain referral from a trigger point or points (▲) in the pectoralis minor muscle.

Intercostal muscles

Anatomical attachments

An intercostal muscle arises from the lower border of each rib and is inserted into the upper border of the rib below. As the name implies it wraps around the chest wall and occupies the whole of an intercostal space.

TrP sites and patterns of pain referral

TrP activity is liable to develop anywhere along the length of an intercostal muscle. The pain which arises as a result of it is localised to the TrP site. As the factors responsible for the development of this TrP activity are the same for both the anterior and posterior parts of the muscle, in order to avoid repetition, discussion of this will be deferred until considering the posterior chest wall MTrP pain syndrome later in the chapter (p. 323).

DIFFERENTIAL DIAGNOSIS

The pain which emanates from anterior chest wall MTrPs has to be distinguished from that which arises in various musculoskeletal, psychological and oesophageal disorders. Furthermore, the pain from all of these sources has to be distinguished from that of coronary heart disease. Each of these disorders will therefore be considered in turn. Following this the development of MTrP pain as a complication of mitral valve prolapse will be discussed. And then attention will be drawn to methods of investigating anterior chest wall pain.

Musculoskeletal pain disorders

Musculoskeletal disorders which, because of the distribution of their pain and the presence of focal areas of exquisite tenderness, have to be distinguished from the anterior chest wall MTrP pain syndrome include pathological fractures, sternoclavicular joint arthropathy, manubrosternal arthropathy, the painful xiphoid syndrome, and in particular, costochondritis and fibromyalgia.

Pathological fractures

Pathological fractures with focal areas of pain and tenderness are liable to arise in patients with metastases from carcinoma of either the breast, prostate, kidney, lung or thyroid (Condon & Harper 1950); also with osteoporosis, osteomalacia and Paget's disease of bone (Daffner 1978). Elderly patients with osteoporosis may not only fracture their ribs spontaneously but may also do so following bouts of coughing (Mitchell 1951).

Sternoclavicular joint arthropathy

Pain, swelling and severe tenderness of the sternoclavicular joint may develop in patients with osteoarthritis, rheumatoid arthritis, ankylosing spondylitis, psoriatic arthropathy and infective arthritis (Bonica & Sola 1990). The diagnosis therefore is not normally difficult as there is usully evidence of disease elsewhere in the body. However, as sternoclavicular joint pain is liable to radiate from the joint to various parts of the anterior chest wall it is liable to simulate pain of cardiac or pulmonary origin (Yood & Goldenberg 1980). And as it is exacerbated by movements such as shrugging of the shoulders it also has to be distinguished from that of either myofascial or costochondral origin.

Manubrosternal arthropathy

Pain, swelling and tenderness of the manubrosternal joint may develop as a result of rheumatoid arthritis, psoriatic arthropathy and ankylosing spondylitis. It is an uncommon disorder but as the pain does not always remain localised but may radiate widely along the upper part of the chest wall towards the shoulder region, it is liable on the left side to simulate angina and, on either side, to simulate pain emanating from TrPs in the subclavius muscle (Fig. 14.7), or the clavicular section of the pectoralis major muscle (Fig. 14.3).

The painful xiphoid syndrome

This rare condition, also known as the xiphoidalgia syndrome (Wehrmacher 1958) and xiphoid cartilage syndrome (Fam & Smythe 1985), is one in which the xiphoid cartilage is tender with pain radiating from it to the praecordium or to the upper abdomen. It therefore has to be distinguished from MTrP pain and from pain arising as a result of a cardiac or abdominal disorder.

Costochondritis

This common cause of anterior chest wall pain, has over the years, been given a variety of names. These have included costochondritis (Calabro 1977), costosternal chondrodynia (Carabasi et al 1962) and the costosternal syndrome (Wolf & Stern 1970). Also, as Calabro et al (1980) have pointed out, although Epstein et al (1979) did not specifically employ the term costochondritis,

they were clearly describing cases of it in their paper entitled 'Chest wall syndrome'.

There is no certainty as to the aetiology of costochondritis but possibly trauma contributes to its development. In this disorder a number of costal cartilages, usually the second to fifth, become painful and extremely tender.

The pain may remain localised to the parasternal region but frequently it radiates across the chest towards the shoulder, down the arm, and in some cases, up into the neck. The distribution of this pain is therefore similar to that which emanates from TrPs in various muscles including the sternalis muscle (Fig. 14.1), the subclavius muscle (Fig. 14.7), and the pectoralis major (Figs 14.3–14.5) and minor (Fig. 14.8) muscles. Also, on the left side of the chest its referral pattern may simulate that of coronary artery disease pain.

Tietze's syndrome

In 1921 the German physician Tietze described a painful disorder of the costal cartilages that has since been called Tietze's syndrome (Levey & Calabro 1962).

Although this disorder is closely allied to costochondritis it is nevertheless much rarer. A search of the world literature in May 1954 carried out by Kayser (1956) disclosed only 159 reported cases of it.

There are various features which serve to distinguish it from costochondritis. As Kayser (1956) pointed out, firstly, the disorder only affects one or more of the upper four costal cartilages. Secondly, an involved costochondral junction is not only painful and tender but also swollen. And thirdly, unlike with costochondritis, there may be a persistent cough due to an upper respiratory tract infection. With respect to this, Kayser (1956), during the course of discussing precipitating factors in his review of 159 reported cases of this syndrome, stated:

... the trauma of coughing has received considerable attention in the literature on this syndrome. Rib fractures due to coughing are reported from time to time and violent coughing can inflict considerable stress on the costal cartilages and costochondrial junctions. However, in the majority of reported cases a history of a cough was not given ... A statement as to the presence or absence of respiratory infections was found in sixty-four cases. Of these fifty-one patients had either a cough or a respiratory infection. Fourteen patients did not. Common colds, bronchitis and pneumonia were mentioned most frequently.

The pain in this syndrome may remain localised to the affected costal cartilages but not infrequently it radiates widely over the chest wall. Coughing and deep breathing tend to make it worse.

The diagnosis can only be made once other conditions that cause swelling of the costal cartilages such as rheumatoid arthritis have been ruled out on clinical grounds (Fam & Smythe 1985) and cartilaginous tumours (O'Neal & Ackerman 1951) have been excluded by the obtaining of a biopsy specimen that shows the presence of normal costal cartilage (Kayser 1956).

Fibromyalgia

Patients with fibromyalgia are liable to have tender points at their second costochondral junctions (Wolfe et al 1990). These clearly have to be distinguished from MTrPs and from localised areas of costochondritis tenderness. This usually, however, presents no difficulty because, as explained elsewhere (Ch. 16), fibromyalgia is a disorder in which there is generalised pain together with tender points in several parts of the body and various other characteristic manifestations.

Psychogenic pain disorders

Disorders in which psychogenic pain may simulate either MTrP pain or coronary artery disease pain include acute panic attacks, conversion disorder (formally known as conversion hysteria), hypochondriasis and a cardiac neurosis known by various names, including DaCosta's irritable heart syndrome.

Acute panic attacks

An acute panic attack may lead to the development of a variety of somatic symptoms including praecordial pain, tachycardia, sweating and hyperventilation.

Although the attack itself may last for from only a few minutes up to 30 minutes, after it has subsided a dull praecordial ache may persist for some considerable time with, as a consequence, the arousal of apprehension in the patient as to the state of the heart. This, however, is not altogether unwarranted because an acute anxiety state causes a rise in plasma catecholamine levels and this, in someone whose coronary arteries are already narrowed, may lead to the development of angina or even a myocardial infarct (Billings 1977).

Conversion disorder

Conversion disorder is one in which a symptom or symptoms suggestive of organic disease arise as an expression of psychological conflict (see Ch. 3). A common one is pain and because this is usually confined to a single area of the body Walters (1961) has suggested calling it 'psychogenic regional pain'. A frequent site for it to develop is the chest wall and in particular the praecordium.

The pain in this disorder tends to be described in characteristically dramatic terms and when present in the praecordial region has to be thoroughly investigated before the patient will accept that it is not due to heart disease.

Hypochondriasis

As discussed in Chapter 3, a hypochondriac is liable to become unduly concerned about any organ in the body, with one of the commoner of these being the heart, so that should praecordial pain develop for one reason or another the person concerned immediately becomes consumed with worry that it must be some life-threatening cardiac disorder. From the manner in which the pain is described there is usually no reason to believe that it is of any particular significance, but nevertheless in order to convince the patient of this a comprehensive cardiological assessment is often required.

Cardiac neurosis

There is a group of people who, when subjected to occupational or domestic stress greater than they can cope with, develop a cardiac neurosis, or what the 19th century physician Jacob DaCosta called the irritable heart. This has been accorded various synonyms including DaCosta's syndrome, effort syndrome and neurovascular asthenia.

DaCosta published his classic paper entitled 'On irritable heart; a clinical study of a form of functional cardiac disorder and its consequences' in 1871, the year before he was elected Professor of Medicine at Jefferson Medical College, Philadelphia, having observed the manifestations of the disorder in soldiers under his care at a military hospital in Philadelphia during the American Civil War (Major 1945).

He stated that due to the stresses of war these soldiers suffered from 'a functional disorder of the heart to which I gave the name of irritable heart'. Among the symptoms the soldiers complained of were palpitations, cardiac pain, tachycardia and shortness of breath.

The palpitations, he said, came on in severe frequent long-lasting attacks and were 'attended with increased pain in the cardiac region and under the left shoulder'. They were, he continued, 'readily excited by exertion and might be then so violent that the patient would fall to the ground insensible. This happened to some on the march, or field of battle; or they fell in the ranks and were taken prisoner'. His account of the pain in these soldiers under his care was a model of clarity. And because it still remains one of the best descriptions of the type of discomfort suffered by cardiac neurotics it will be quoted in full:

Pain was an almost constant symptom. I cannot recall a single well-marked instance of the complaint in which it was wholly absent; and often it was the first sign of disorder noticed by the patient. It was generally described as occurring in paroxysms, and as sharp and lancinating; a few likened it to a burning sensation, or spoke of it as tearing, or as burning at times, and at others cutting; or as a 'dull sullen' pain, becoming at times acute. In some cases no other pain happened than what occurred in these sharp attacks, or a mere feeling of uneasiness in the

region of the heart existed; but in the large majority there was a substratum, as it were, of discomfort, or of dull heavy pain. In exceptional cases the pain was altogether of this character. Unwonted exercise or exertion would generally produce an attack of sharp pain, and a fit of palpitation was very apt to do the same; but the acute pain also happened without any unusual disturbance of cardiac action, and was, in truth, in rare instances, noticed to be decreased by exercise, or to be most severe when the patient was free from palpitation. Deep breathing was stated to make the pain severe, when it was otherwise but slight; cough produced a kindred result.

From DaCosta's account of the type of chest pain suffered by a patient with a cardiac neurosis it may be seen that it is not of a constricting type like angina but rather is variously described as being of a stabbing, burning or piercing nature. Its location is also different for, as Edmonstone (1995) has stated, a patient with angina demonstrates where it is felt by placing a hand across the sternum, whereas someone with a cardiac neurosis indicates the position of the pain caused by this by pointing with an index finger to an area of the chest wall in the vicinity of the apex of the heart. Also, unlike angina, the duration of the pain varies from a few seconds up to several hours or even days. In addition, its onset is not clearly related to exertion and is not relieved by resting. And, furthermore, the patient does not stand still during an attack of pain but on the contrary tends to be restless and agitated.

Billings (1977) has identified a number of features in the history that are highly suggestive of chest wall pain being psychogenic. He included amongst those pain felt in the region of the cardiac apex, and described in highly emotive terms by someone with overt neurotic traits; pain heralded by emotional upsets; and pain having a variable responsiveness to medicaments. At the same time he emphasised that such features do no more than suggest that the pain may be primarily psychogenic and because they cannot of themselves be taken as proof of it, recommended the use of the Minnesota Multiphasic Personality Inventory (Hathaway & McKinley 1967) or some similar test designed to exclude the presence of an underlying psychological disturbance.

A comprehensive review of such tests has been provided by Chapman & Syrjala (1990).

This notwithstanding it cannot be stressed too strongly that the finding of evidence of neuroticism does not of itself rule out the possibility of underlying coronary artery disease, for as Procacci et al (1994) have warned, distinguishing between cardiac neurosis pain and angina on clinical grounds alone is often extremely difficult, with patients dismissed as being neurotic all too frequently suddenly dying from an acute myocardial infarct. They even went so far as to say: 'It appears, thus, that the criteria of a normal coronary arteriogram and a negative or insignificant effort test are insufficient to discard the diagnosis of myocardial ischaemia in cases of pain habitually considered as non-organic.'

Oesophageal pain disorders

Pain arising as a result of either anterior chest wall musculoskeletal disorders or cardiac disorders may simulate oesophageal pain. For although the latter in some cases is felt posteriorly in the interscapular region, in others it is felt in locations such as the neck, the jaw, the anterior aspect of the chest including the praecordium, the shoulders and the upper arms. Distinguishing features, however, are that with oesophageal pain disorders there are no focal areas of tenderness to be found on examination of the chest wall. Also, the pain is likely to be aggravated by the passage of food and relieved by the taking of milk or antacids.

MTrP pain in association with mitral valve prolapse

Mitral valve prolapse (syn: floppy mitral valve), a disorder first shown by Barlow et al in 1963 to be the cause of late apical systolic murmurs, is deserving of special mention because, for some as yet unexplained reason, patients suffering from it are prone to develop pain including myofascial trigger point pain. Before discussing this, however, it is first necessary to say something about the pathogenesis, pathology and diagnosis of this disorder, and also about the

symptoms other than pain that develop as a result of it.

Pathogenesis

Mitral valve prolapse is a relatively common cardiac disorder occurring in 5–10% of females and in 1–2% of males. Most patients have no identifiable connective tissue disorder but occasionally it is present in those with recognised ones such as Marfan's and Ehlers–Danlos syndromes. There are grounds for believing that it is genetically determined as it is frequently inherited together with other structural abnormalities such as pectus excavatum (Hammermeister 1990).

Pathology

In this disorder the mitral valve's chordae tendinae are excessively long. Also, its cusps are unusually large with myxomatous changes in them. As a result of these abnormalities mitral incompetence develops with the cusps prolapsing into the left atrium during ventricular contraction.

Symptoms

Pain When Maresca et al (1989) looked for evidence of angina pectoris in 30 patients with mitral valve prolapse they found that none of them had pain of this type but that 26 had MTrPs in the chest wall and 12 in this group had MTrP pain.

They also observed that some of those in this group had MTrPs in various other parts of the body but Maresca (1997, personal communication) has recently confirmed that despite this none of them had the criteria laid down by the American College of Rheumatology (Wolfe et al 1990) for a diagnosis of fibromyalgia. They therefore concluded that the chest pain which arises in patients with mitral valve prolapse most commonly occurs as a result of the development of the MTrP pain syndrome. And that occasionally it is due to other causes. Alpert (1993) is also of this opinion for he stated, 'Mitral valve prolapse occurs disproportionately frequently in subjects with various causes of chest pain'. He includes amongst these not only chest wall pain disorders but also coronary artery spasm, oesophageal spasm and panic attacks (Alpert et al 1991, 1992).

Finally, as Procacci et al (1994) have pointed out, patients with mitral valve prolapse are clearly not immune from developing coronary heart disease with typical anginal pain then being present.

Palpitations Palpitations are common due to the development of a dysrhythmia and, because of the latter, there is occasionally a reduction in cardiac output sufficient to give rise to dizziness, syncope or even sudden death.

Physical signs

The diagnosis can be made from the physical examination alone in most cases as there is a characteristic apical mid-systolic click followed by a late systolic murmur. Occasionally there is a pansystolic murmur indistinguishable from that present in other forms of mitral regurgitation. Confirmation of the diagnosis is made by demonstrating the prolapse on an echocardiograph.

Cardiac and non-cardiac anterior chest wall pain – the differential diagnosis

Allison (1950), during the course of writing about patients with non-cardiac chest pain stated, 'the frequency with which such patients are seen in routine out-patient work emphasises the need for a re-orientation towards pain in the chest and suggests that in clinical teaching pride of place is too often given to angina pectoris in explanation of the pain and too little regard is paid to local structural causes'.

This is as true today as when it was written nearly fifty years ago and because it is the MTrP pain syndrome and costochondritis which are the two anterior chest wall disorders whose pain most commonly simulates that of coronary artery disease (CAD) the importance of distin-

guishing between the latter and the other two disorders will now be discussed.

MTrP pain and coronary artery disease pain

Gutstein (1938), Kelly (1944), Mendlowitz (1945) and in particular the two American physicians Travell & Rinzler (1948) showed how closely the distribution of pain occurring as a result of the primary activation of MTrPs in the anterior chest wall may simulate that of coronary artery disease (CAD) pain.

Pain arising as a result of trauma-induced TrP activity in a single muscle such as the pectoralis may do this (Fig. 14.4). And so may pain which develops as a result of TrP activity spreading from one muscle to another until ultimately several muscles are involved in the process. Travell (1976) gave a good example of a chain reaction such as this when she described how TrP activity in the sternal division of the sternocleidomastoid muscle may cause pain to be referred down the length of the sternum. Pain in this distribution may then lead to the development of TrP activity in the sternalis muscle with, as a consequence, the referral of pain to the praecordium and the development of TrP activity in the pectoralis major muscle. This TrP activity may then in turn give rise to pain which is referred to the left shoulder and down the left arm. It may therefore be seen that doing nothing more than straining a muscle in the neck may lead to pain with a pattern of distribution exactly similar to that which arises as a result of CAD.

Furthermore, Rinzler & Travell (1948) recognised that MTrP pain may develop as a secondary event in muscles affected by CAD pain and showed that deactivation of these MTrPs, either by injecting a local anaesthetic into them or by applying an ethyl chloride spray to the skin overlying them, may, in some cases, relieve not only the pain emanating from these points but also the cardiac pain.

They did this in a study of 31 patients which they divided into three groups. Group I consisted of 4 patients with acute myocardial infarction; group II consisted of 18 patients with effort angina and prior myocardial infarction; and group

III consisted of 9 patients with effort angina uncomplicated by myocardial infarction.

They found that deactivation of MTrPs gave prolonged pain relief in patients in groups I and II but negligible, or at best only temporary pain relief, in group III. From these results it may be seen that finding active TrPs in the chest wall muscles and relieving any pain which may be present by deactivating them by one means or another to relieve any pain which may be present does not of itself rule out the possibility that some of this pain may be stemming from underlying CAD.

Rinzler & Travell's observations were clearly of the greatest importance but regrettably they have not received the attention they deserve. Terminological obfuscation over the years may have contributed to this. Wehrmacher (1958), for example, in a wide-ranging review of painful anterior chest wall syndromes included among these one in which pain emanates from 'trigger zones' in the anterior chest wall. He described how this may develop either alone or concomitantly with CAD pain and stated that both may be alleviated by injecting a local anaesthetic into the 'trigger zones'. However, although clearly referring to the same musculoskeletal pain disorder as that previously described by Rinzler and Travell he made no mention of the name given to it by them and somewhat confusingly chose to call it myodynia, or what he said was also known as fibromyositis, despite neither of these terms ever having been widely adopted.

Costochondritis pain and coronary artery disease pain

Costochondritis, like the anterior chest wall MTrP pain syndrome, has a pain referral pattern similar to that of CAD and is a disorder, furthermore, which may develop in conjunction with CAD.

Wolf & Stern (1976) confirmed this in a study of 320 consecutive patients with anterior chest wall pain of at least 3 months' duration seen by them in their hospital outpatient departments in Jerusalem. In this group of patients, the pain was due to costochondritis or what they termed the

costosternal syndrome in 21. In 9 others the pain was due to concomitant costochondritis and CAD, a finding which led them to conclude that the frequency of the costosternal syndrome (costochondritis) is relatively high, both as a sole cause of chest pain and in combination with CAD.

Epstein et al (1979) came to the same conclusion from a study carried out at the National Institutes of Health, Bethesda, on 12 patients with severe incapacitating chest pain initially considered to be cardiac in origin, but which on subsequent evaluation was discovered to be due to costochondritis or what they called the chest wall syndrome in 5 of these patients, and to a combination of this syndrome and various cardiac disorders in the other 7 (2 having a cardiomyopathy, 1 having mitral valve prolapse, 1 having aortic incompetence and 3 having ischaemic heart disease).

METHODS OF INVESTIGATING ANTERIOR CHEST WALL PAIN

As CAD pain, MTrP pain and costochondritis pain may have similar characteristics, similar referral patterns and may in some cases develop concomitantly, it is clearly essential to distinguish between them by taking a detailed history followed by a careful examination of the chest wall and a comprehensive cardiological assessment that includes the employment of various sophisticated diagnostic techniques.

History

When taking the history it is essential to pay particular attention to the following: the location of the pain; the type of pain (e.g. constricting, cramping, stabbing, burning, tingling, aching); aggravating factors (e.g. exertion, movements of the body, climatic changes, deep breathing); pain-relieving factors (e.g. resting, changes in posture, administration of substances such as glyceryl trinitrate (nitroglycerin), analgesics, antacids); symptoms other than pain (e.g. palpitations, shortness of breath, sweating, nausea, vomiting, heartburn); and pain elsewhere in the body such as the head, neck or low-back. In addition, it is necessary to enquire whether there has been any recent injury or the carrying out of a task which may have overloaded the muscles.

Myocardial infarction pain is characteristically of a severe constricting type and is frequently accompanied by other symptoms such as sweating and shortness of breath. Angina (other than crescendo or pre-infarction angina) usually takes the form of a substernal constricting feeling brought on by exertion and relieved by resting. In contrast to these two types of pain, the pain of both the MTrP pain syndrome and costochondritis is typically a dull aching discomfort that is present at rest and aggravated by movements.

There are nevertheless exceptions to all of this. Pain of musculoskeletal origin, like that of cardiac origin, may sometimes only come on with exercise and be relieved by resting. It also, like myocardial infarction pain, may be accompanied by shortness of breath and sweating. To add to the confusion angina of the so-called unstable type comes on at rest and may last up to 30 minutes. Furthermore, it should be noted that the reporting by the patient of a seemingly favourable response to glyceryl trinitrate (nitroglycerin) may be misleading since the placebo effect of this ensures that up to 30% of patients with chest pain from any cause may be improved by it.

Clearly therefore it is often impossible to distinguish between cardiac and non-cardiac pain from the history alone. This is shown by Myers et al (1977) who reported that out of 17 patients with normal coronary arteriograms and clinical evidence of a musculoskeletal pain syndrome called by them 'cerviprecordial angina', 12 complained of shortness of breath including paroxysmal nocturnal dyspnoea and sweating, 14 had pain induced by exercise and relieved by resting, and 12 had rapid and complete relief of their pain following the administration of glyceryl trinitrate (nitroglycerin).

Similarly, Levine & Mascette (1989), in a prospective study of 62 adults referred to them for coronary arteriography, found that of the 5 patients discovered to have normal coronary arteriograms and clinical evidence of a musculoskeletal pain disorder, 3 described their pain as being a pressing squeezing tightness, 3 complained of sweating and 2 reported shortness of breath. In addition, 4 stated that the pain was aggravated by exertion, 3 said it was relieved by rest and 4 reported obtaining relief with glyceryl trinitrate (nitroglycerin).

It was similarly from finding anomalies such as these that led Epstein et al (1979) in their survey of patients with costochondritis, or what they called the chest wall syndrome, to conclude that:

> While the pain of chest wall syndrome often occurs at rest and lasts for many minutes to hours, most patients also complain of exertion-induced pain. In some patients the pain is indistinguishable from typical angina pectoris due to coronary artery disease. This is unusual, however, and careful questioning often discloses that the pain has atypical precipitating features more closely related to postural changes and to stresses imposed on the structures of the chest wall than to physical exertion per se. The posture-related precipitation of chest discomfort also probably accounts for the frequency with which nocturnal chest pain is reported by these patients.

Examination of the anterior chest wall

For the diagnosis of costochondritis it is necessary to apply firm pressure to each of the costal cartilages in turn in order to ascertain whether or not it is abnormally tender and in particular to see whether by means of this palpation it is possible to reproduce the spontaneously occurring pain.

Epstein et al (1979) have also pointed out that, in this disorder, it is usually possible to reproduce pain closely resembling the spontaneously occurring one by means of flexing the arm across the anterior chest with steady prolonged traction applied in a horizontal direction whilst at the same time rotating the head as far as possible towards the ipsilateral shoulder.

In order to ascertain whether or not the pain is emanating from MTrPs it is necessary to carry out a systematic search for these in the neck, shoulder region and anterior chest wall.

It cannot be emphasised too strongly, however, that the eliciting of physical signs of a musculoskeletal pain disorder does not rule out the possibility that some of the pain may be of cardiac origin. Furthermore, it is necessary to reiterate that injecting a local anaesthetic into MTrPs may not only relieve pain emanating from these, but may also alleviate coexisting cardiac pain (Rinzler & Travell 1948). Similarly, carrying out a local anaesthetic block of the superficial tissues in cases of costochondritis may not only relieve the pain of this disorder but also may alleviate any concomitant cardiac pain (Reeves & Harrison 1953).

It therefore follows that with both the anterior chest wall MTrP pain syndrome and costochondritis, no matter whether or not the pain is relieved by some form of locally applied treatment, it is sometimes necessary to carry out specialised investigations for the purpose of excluding underlying heart disease.

Cardiac investigations

These should include not only auscultation of the heart and measurement of the blood pressure but, in addition, chest radiography, electrocardiographic exercise testing and radionuclide cineangiography; also, in some cases, coronary arteriography.

Chest radiography

A chest radiograph is required in order to exclude any underlying disease of the lung and to provide information concerning the size and shape of the heart and to exclude the presence of dextrocardia.

Electrocardiograph exercise testing

Graded exercise on a bicycle or treadmill imposes an increasing workload on the heart and in patients with CAD gives rise to ST segment depression changes on an ECG. This test, however, while of use in the management of confirmed CAD, is of limited value in making a diagnosis of this disorder because even with asymptomatic patients the false-positive rate may be as high as 64% if the single criterion of 1 mm ST segment depression is used (Petch 1986). A negative ECG response to exercise makes it less likely that underlying CAD is present but unfortunately the low sensitivity of the test still leaves the diagnosis in doubt (Redwood et al 1976).

Radionuclide cineangiography

Radionuclide left ventricular angiography using technetium is of considerable use in assessing the ventricular function of patients with CAD. Borer et al (1977) were the first to show that the ventricular function of patients with CAD and many other cardiovascular disorders including hypertension deteriorates during exercise. An exercise-induced abnormality of ventricular function therefore, although non-specific, nevertheless provides objective confirmation of significant underlying cardiac pathology.

It therefore follows that if physical examination confirms the presence of costochondritis or the MTrP pain syndrome and a radionuclide test shows the left ventricular function to be normal then it is highly unlikely that there is any underlying CAD.

Coronary arteriography

The main use of coronary arteriography is in assessing whether or not surgical intervention is required in the treatment of known CAD. It is rarely necessary to carry it out for the purpose of excluding CAD as this can usually be achieved non-invasively with radionuclide angiography.

POSTERIOR CHEST WALL MTrP PAIN SYNDROME

Muscles from which posterior chest wall TrP pain is liable to arise include the levator scapulae (see Ch. 8), trapezius (see Ch. 8), latissimus dorsi, serratus anterior, serratus posterior superior, serratus posterior inferior, rhomboids, the paraspinals and the intercostals.

Latissimus dorsi muscle (Fig. 14.9)

Anatomical attachments

Latissimus dorsi, which translated from the Latin means 'widest of the back', is an appropriate name for this muscle with its extensive fan-shaped attachment which stretches from the spinous processes of the lower six thoracic and all the lumbar vertebrae and sacrum in the midline, to the crest of the ilium, and to the last four ribs; and from which, it sweeps upwards into the axilla, to form with the teres major muscle the posterior axillary fold prior to the tendons of these two muscles then joining together to be inserted into the bicipital groove of the humerus. However, although this muscle covers such a large area of the back, TrPs usually only become activated in the part of it that is situated in the posterior axillary fold.

Factors responsible for the development of MTrP activity

TrPs in the posterior axillary fold are liable to become active should the upper part of this muscle where it inserts into the humerus become subjected to strain. Examples of when this may occur include reaching forwards and upwards with the arm whilst carrying some heavy object; stretching the arm such as when hanging on to a rope; or straining the arm whilst engaging in some unusually heavy task such as digging or weeding.

TrP site and pattern of pain referral

From TrPs in the posterior axillary fold, pain of a dull aching type is referred to the inferior angle of the scapula and the part of the back immediately around this. It may also extend to the posterior aspect of the shoulder, and down the inner side of the arm, forearm and hand, to terminate in the ring and little fingers (Fig. 14.10).

The pain is persistent and is neither aggravated nor relieved by any type of movements. It is probably because this pain is not influenced by movements and because the TrPs responsible for it are tucked away in the posterior axillary fold that its myofascial origin is so often overlooked.

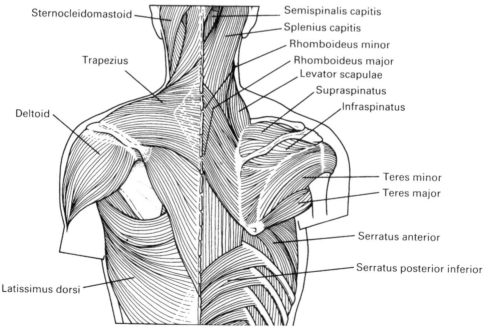

Figure 14.9 Superficial muscles of the back of the neck and upper part of the trunk. On the left, the skin, superficial and deep fasciae have been removed. On the right, the sternocleidomastoid, trapezius, latissimus dorsi and deltoid have been dissected away.

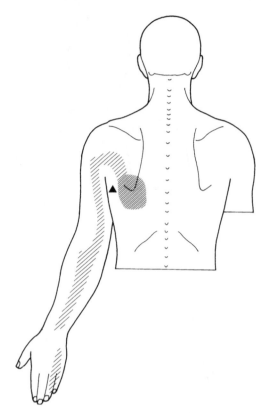

Figure 14.10 The pattern of pain referral from a trigger point or points (▲) in the latissimus dorsi muscle where this muscle together with the teres major muscle forms the posterior axillary fold.

Trigger point examination

The TrPs are most readily found by placing the patient in the supine position, and putting the muscle on the stretch by abducting the arm and placing the hand behind the head.

Both the superficial and deep parts of the muscle in the posterior axillary fold should be examined, because when Simons & Travell (1976) inserted 7.5% saline into the muscle at this site, an injection into the deep fibres referred pain to the back around the lower part of the scapula, whilst an injection into the superficial ones referred pain down the arm.

Associated trigger points

TrPs are likely to develop at the same time in the anatomically closely related teres major (Ch. 9) and the long head of the triceps (Ch. 10).

Serratus anterior muscle (Fig. 14.9)

Anatomical attachments

This muscle, which wraps itself closely around the chest wall, is attached anteriorly to the upper eight ribs and posteriorly to the vertebral border of the scapula.

Factors responsible for the development of MTrP activity

TrP activity may arise in this muscle when it is strained during the course of athletic pursuits or physical training; also, when this happens as a result of severe coughing; and in addition should the muscles of the chest wall be held in a persistently tense state as a result of anxiety.

TrP sites and patterns of pain referral

TrPs in this muscle are usually located in the mid-axillary line at about the level of the fifth and sixth ribs in line with the nipple. There are often accompanying palpable bands with it then being possible to elicit local twitch responses by sharply plucking them with a finger.

Pain from TrP activity in this muscle is referred to the side and back of the chest, and at times down the ulnar aspect of the arm (Fig. 14.11). The patient may also complain that it is painful to take a deep breath – the so-called 'stitch in the side'.

Trigger point examination

With the patient lying down and turned so that the affected side is uppermost, the muscle is put on the stretch by pulling the arm backwards.

Associated trigger points

The TrP activity is often an isolated event but after a time it may also develop in this muscle's main antagonist, the latissimus dorsi.

A

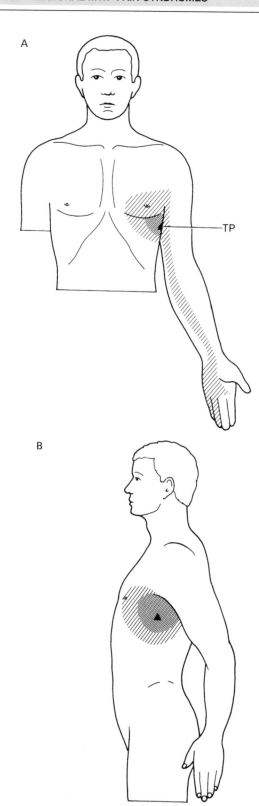

B

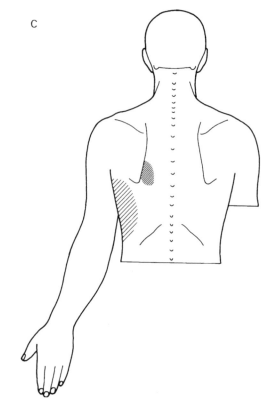

Figure 14.11   A, B and C The pattern of pain referral from a trigger point or points (▲) in the serratus anterior muscle.

Serratus posterior superior muscle
(Fig. 14.12)

Anatomical attachments

This thin quadrilateral muscle, which is situated beneath the trapezius and rhomboids, is attached superomedially to the spines of the seventh cervical vertebra and the first three dorsal vertebrae; and inferolaterally to the second to fifth ribs near to their angles behind the upper part of the scapula.

Factors responsible for the development of MTrP activity

TrP activity in this muscle may develop as a result of protracted bouts of coughing. Also, when the scapula is pressed hard against it as a result of the shoulders being persistently elevated

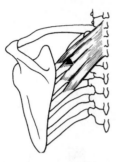

Figure 14.12 With the arm to the side, a trigger point in the inferolateral part of the serratus posterior superior cannot be palpated as it lies behind the upper inner part of the scapula. To palpate a trigger point at this site, therefore, the scapula has to be pulled forwards as shown.

and rotated forwards such as may occur when sitting for long periods at a desk or working surface that is too high. In addition, satellite TrPs may develop in this muscle when TrP activity in

the scalene muscles causes pain to be referred to the posterior chest wall around the inner part of the scapula (see Ch. 8).

TrP sites and patterns of pain referral

TrPs in this muscle are most often found near to its inferolateral insertion. When these develop activity pain is felt as a dull ache around the insertion of the muscle into the ribs behind the scapula. It is also referred to the back of the shoulder and down the back of the arm as far as the medial epicondyle at the elbow. Occasionally it is also felt down the inner side of the forearm and hand as far as the little finger (Fig. 14.13). This pain pattern is similar to the one produced by compression of the eighth cervical nerve root (Reynolds 1981). However, unlike with the latter, there are no objective neurological signs.

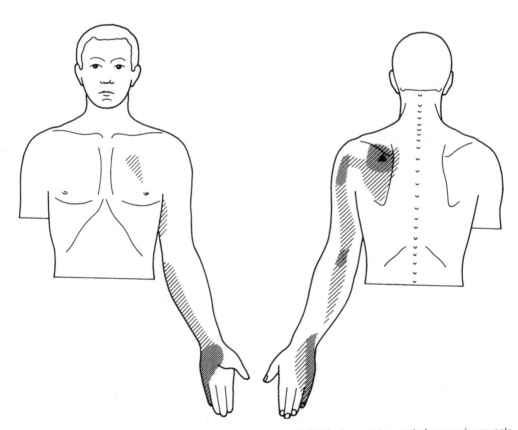

Figure 14.13 The pattern of pain referral from a trigger point or points (▲) in the serratus posterior superior muscle.

Trigger point examination

With the patient sitting forwards and the arm stretched across the front of the chest, in order to bring the scapula out of the way, the muscle which lies behind the upper part of this bone deep to the trapezius and rhomboid muscles can be palpated by rolling a finger over it against the underlying ribs (Fig. 14.12).

Associated trigger points

TrPs in this muscle are often associated with TrP activity in the synergistic inspiratory scalene muscles in the neck, the nearby erector spinae muscles, and overlying rhomboids.

Serratus posterior inferior muscle
(Fig. 14.9)

Anatomical attachments

This muscle, which is situated in the lower part of the posterior chest wall, is attached medially to the spines of the lower two dorsal vertebrae and the upper three lumbar vertebrae and from these attachments it passes obliquely upwards to be inserted into the last four ribs a little beyond their angles.

Factors responsible for the development of TrP activity

TrPs in this muscle and adjacent ones are liable to become activated should these muscles become strained as a result of, for example, twisting the torso during the course of lifting a heavy load.

TrP sites and patterns of pain referral

TrP activity is particularly liable to develop in the outer part of the muscle close to its attachment to the ribs. Pain is then felt locally at the TrP site.

Rhomboids (major and minor)
(Fig. 14.9)

Anatomical attachments

The rhomboideus minor, the smaller of the two, attaches above to the ligamentum nuchae and

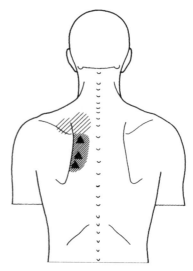

Figure 14.14   The pattern of pain referral from a trigger point or points (▲) in the rhomboid muscles.

spinous processes of the seventh cervical and first dorsal vertebrae, and below to the upper medial border of the scapula.

The rhomboideus major, which is situated immediately below it, attaches above to the spinous processes of the second, third, fourth and fifth dorsal vertebrae and below to the medial border of the scapula between its spine and inferior angle.

Factors responsible for the development of TrP activity

TrP activity is liable to develop in these two muscles as a result of them being strained as, for example, by bending over a desk or table for any length of time.

It may also occur when these muscles, together with the trapezius, become overloaded by having to counteract TrP-induced tension in the pectoralis major and minor.

TrP sites and patterns of pain referral

TrPs in these muscles are commonly located along the medial border of the scapula and pain from these is felt locally in their vicinity in a distribution similar to that of pain from TrPs in the levator scapulae muscle (Fig. 14.14).

Trigger point examination

With the patient seated the arm on the affected side should be brought well forwards in order to get the scapula out of the way. TrPs may then be located (Fig. 14.15) just medial to inner border of the scapula (Sola & Kuitert 1955).

Intercostal muscles

TrP activity is liable to develop in an intercostal muscle should it be subjected to some form of direct injury or become strained as, for example, during a bout of severe coughing. The pain of a dull aching type (Kelly 1944), which arises as a result of this, is usually felt around the TrP site but with TrPs situated in the posterior part of the muscle the pain tends to radiate forwards around the chest wall along the line of the ribs.

Intercostal MTrP pain therefore has to be distinguished from pain around the chest wall which comes on prior to the development of a herpes zoster rash, and from the pain of a burning or electric-shock-like character in the same distribution that develops as a late complication of herpes zoster (post-herpetic neuralgia). It also has to be distinguished from pain resulting from nerve root compression caused by either a neurogenic tumour, vertebral metastases, or the prolapse of an intervertebral disc.

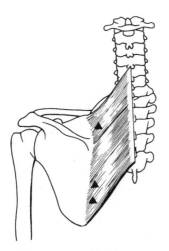

Figure 14.15 Trigger points (▲) along the medial border of the scapula in the rhomboid muscles.

It furthermore has to be remembered that a radiculopathy caused by any of these disorders, because of the effect of motor nerve compression on a MTrP's motor endplates, may lead to the development of MTrP activity as a secondary event in muscles innervated by the entrapped nerve.

Paraspinal muscles (see Fig. 12.1)

The paraspinal muscles include a superficial erector spinae group of longitudinally directed muscles and a deeper group of diagonally arranged ones. In the thoracic region the two muscles in the superficial group most likely to develop TrP activity are the laterally placed iliocostalis thoracis and the medially situated longissimus thoracis. And in the deep group, they are the multifidi and beneath these the rotatores.

Factors responsible for the development of TrP activity

TrP activity in the paraspinal muscles is liable to develop whenever these become strained by, for example, the lifting of heavy objects with the torso twisted, or prolonged stooping.

TrP sites and patterns of pain referral

The pain referral pattern from a TrP in a superficially placed thoracic paraspinal muscle varies according to where it is situated in the muscle. For example, a TrP in the middle part of the iliocostalis thoracis refers pain to the back of the chest wall around the lower angle of the scapula and at times up towards the shoulder (Fig. 14.16). A TrP in its lower part refers pain upwards towards the scapula, downwards towards the iliac crest and laterally towards the iliac fossa (Fig. 14.17). And a TrP in the lower part of the longissimus thoracis refers pain downwards towards the buttock (Fig. 14.18).

Pain from a TrP in either the multifidi or rotatores is referred locally around the TrP site itself (Fig. 14.19).

Trigger point examination

When searching for TrPs in the paraspinal muscles the patient should be placed on the

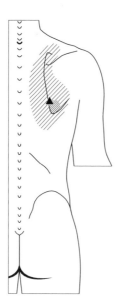

Figure 14.16 Pain referral from a trigger point (▲) in the mid-part of the iliocostalis thoracis.

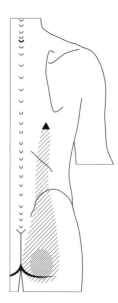

Figure 14.18 Pain referral from a trigger point (▲) in the longissimus thoracis.

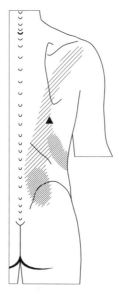

Figure 14.17 Pain referral from a trigger point (▲) in the lower part of the iliocostalis thoracis.

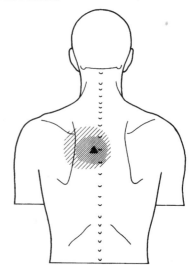

Figure 14.19 The pattern of pain referral from a trigger point (▲) situated deep in the paravertebral gutter in the multifidus muscle at the mid-thoracic level.

unaffected side with the head supported on a pillow and the knees brought up towards the chest.

TrPs in the superficially placed iliocostalis thoracis and longissimus thoracis are readily found by applying firm pressure along the length of the paravertebral gutter. TrPs in the deeper lying multifidi and rotatores muscles are not so readily located. However, because the muscles are attached medially to the base of each successive vertebra's spinous process and laterally to its transverse process, an active TrP somewhere along the length of one of these muscles causes the vertebral spinous process in its immediate vicinity to become tender. And therefore when searching for TrPs in these muscles it is best to first of all palpate the spine of each vertebra in turn and when one is found to be tender, to palpate adjacent deeply situated paraspinal musculature by applying firm pressure in a posteromedial direction at that level.

Secondary paraspinal muscle TrP activity

As TrP activity in the paraspinal muscles may develop as a secondary event in osteoporosis, ankylosing spondylitis, ankylosing hyperostosis disc prolapse and facet joint sprain it is necessary to consider each of these disorders in turn.

Osteoporosis of the spine

Osteoporosis, a disorder which principally affects post-menopausal women and patients on corticosteroid therapy, is a common cause of lumbar and thoracic back pain. Initially the disorder gives rise to a low-grade persistent discomfort but at a later stage a very intense pain is liable to develop when a vertebra affected by it suddenly fractures. The intensity of the pain is such as to cause the paraspinal muscles to go into spasm that is severe enough to lead to the development of ischaemia-induced TrP activity.

The pain from the vertebral fracture initially requires the administration of analgesics but it eventually subsides spontaneously. In contrast to this the MTrP pain is liable to persist and requires deactivation of MTrPs for its relief.

Ankylosing spondylitis

This disorder is liable to arise in anyone possessing the histocompatibility antigen HLA-B27 but most commonly it affects young men who have this genetic marker.

Initially pain develops in the lumbar region as a result of inflammatory changes taking place in the sacroiliac joints and lumbar spine. At a later stage it is liable to extend upwards into the thoracic and cervical spine.

In the thoracic region moderate aching pain from involvement of the costovertebral, costotransverse and facet joints is aggravated by twisting movements of the spine and respiratory movements. And eventually spondylitic changes in these joints leads to restriction of chest expansion.

The pain causes the paraspinal muscles to go into severe spasm with, as in the case of osteoporosis, the secondary development of TrP activity. And when this happens it is often helpful not only to use non-steroidal anti-inflammatory drugs to relieve the spondylitic pain but also to deactivate the TrPs in these muscles (Bonica & Sola 1990).

Ankylosing hyperostosis

This disorder, which not uncommonly affects middle-aged and elderly people, particularly men, gives rise to thoracolumbar pain and stiffness. However, unlike with ankylosing spondylitis, the erythrocyte sedimentation rate (ESR) is normal and radiographic examination of the spine shows gross ossification of the ligaments. After a time the secondary activation of TrP nociceptors may take place.

Dorsal disc prolapse

The incidence of disc prolapse in the dorsal spine is much less than it is in either the cervical or lumbar regions but nevertheless it is now being diagnosed with increasing frequency (Turek 1984, Bonica & Sola 1990).

Dorsal disc prolapse pain, like disc pain elsewhere in the spine, is characteristically made worse by coughing, sneezing and straining, and relieved by lying down. At an early stage pain due to this cause may be confined to the paravertebral region but with fully developed disc herniation nerve entrapment pain is liable to radiate around the chest wall. When this happens, secondary TrP activity may develop not only in the paraspinal muscles but also in one or more of the intercostal muscles.

Dorsal facet joint sprain

Paravertebral MTrP pain in the chest region has to be distinguished from the pain that develops when a dorsal facet joint is sprained as a result of the carrying out of awkward movements such as lifting a load with the body in a twisted position or working with the hands raised above the head.

Thoracotomy-induced pain

Following a thoracotomy persistent pain of a dull aching character may radiate around the chest wall because of trauma-induced TrP activity developing in chest wall muscles, particularly the intercostals. Pain similar in type and distribution may also emanate from TrPs in a surgical scar.

In addition, pain of a burning character or of an electric-shock-like type may radiate around the chest wall when an intercostal nerve is damaged during the course of an operation. An injury of this type may also give rise to hyperaesthesia of the chest wall.

Deactivation of TrPs by one means or another usually readily abolishes the MTrP pain. Post-thoracotomy nerve damage pain, however, is far more difficult to treat. Drugs employed for combating neuropathic pain (see Ch. 5) should be administered. In addition, a posterior intercostal block with a long-acting local anaesthetic may

prove helpful. Transcutaneous electrical nerve stimulation (TENS) is also sometimes of value.

Deactivation of chest wall myofascial trigger points

It has become apparent to me over the years that primary activated chest wall TrPs, no matter whether they are situated in superficially placed muscles or deeply lying ones, are readily deactivated by inserting a needle into the skin and subcutaneous tissues immediately overlying each TrP and then withdrawing it after approximately 30 seconds, with the time, however, varying according to a patient's individual responsiveness (see Ch. 7). Nevertheless, even with this superficial dry needling technique care has to be taken to insert the needle at an oblique angle in order to avoid any possibility of penetrating the pleura and causing a pneumothorax to develop.

In contrast to this, however, a chest wall TrP which has developed activity as a secondary event is invariably situated in a tightly contracted muscle and because of this a far stronger stimulus is required with the needle having to be inserted into the TrP itself – a procedure which in Chapter 7 is called deep dry needling.

REFERENCES

Allison D R 1950 Pain in the chest wall simulating heart disease. British Medical Journal i:332–336
Alpert M A 1993 Mitral valve prolapse. British Medical Journal 306:943–944
Alpert M A, Mukerju V, Sabeti M, Russell J, Beitman B D 1991 Mitral valve prolapse, panic disorder and chest pain. Medical Clinics of North America 75:1119–1133
Alpert M A, Sabeti M, Kushner M G et al 1992 Frequency of isolated panic attacks and panic disorders in patients with mitral valve prolapse. American Journal of Cardiology 69:1489–1490
Barlow J B, Pocock W A, Marchand P, Denny M 1963 The significance of late systolic murmurs. American Heart Journal 66:443–452
Billings R F 1977 Chest pain related to emotional disorders. In: Levene D L (ed) Chest pain: an integrated diagnostic approach. Lea & Febiger, Philadelphia, pp 133–150
Bonica J J, Sola A F 1990 Chest pain caused by other disorders. In: Bonica J J (ed) The management of pain, 2nd edn. Lea & Febiger, Philadelphia, ch 58

Borer J S, Bacharach S L, Breen M V et al 1977 Real-time radionuclide cineangiography in non-invasive evaluation of global and regional left ventricular function at rest and during exercise in patients with coronary artery disease. New England Journal of Medicine 296: 839–844
Calabro J J 1977 Costochondritis. New England Journal of Medicine 296:946–947
Calabro J J, Jeghers H, Miller K A et al 1980 Classification of anterior chest wall syndrome. Journal of the American Medical Association 243:1420–1421
Carabasi R J, Christian J J, Brindley H H 1962 Costosternal chondrodynia: a variant of Tietze's syndrome? Diseases of the Chest 41:559–562
Chapman C R, Syrjala K L 1990 Measurement of pain. In: Bonica J J (ed) The management of pain, 2nd edn. Lea & Febiger, Philadelphia, ch 32
Condon W B, Harper F R 1950 Tumours of the chest wall. Diseases of the Chest 17:741–755
Daffner R H 1978 Stress fractures: current concepts. Skeletal Radiology 2:221–229

Edmondstone W M 1995 Cardiac chest pain: does body language help the diagnosis? British Medical Journal 311:1660–1661

Epstein S E, Gerber L H, Borer J S 1979 Chest wall syndrome. A common cause of unexplained cardiac pain. Journal of the American Medical Association 241(26):2793–2797

Fam A G, Smythe H A 1985 Musculoskeletal chest wall pain. Canadian Medical Association Journal 133:379–389

Gutstein M 1938 Diagnosis and treatment of muscular rheumatism. British Journal of Physical Medicine 1:302–321

Hammermeister K E 1990 Cardiac and aortic pain. In: Bonica J J (ed) The management of pain, 2nd edn. Lea & Febiger, Philadelphia, p 1033

Hathaway S R, McKinley J C 1967 The Minnesota Multiphasic Personality Inventory manual. Psychological Corporation, New York

Kayser H L 1956 Tietze's syndrome. A review of the literature. American Journal of Medicine 21: 982–989

Kelly M 1944 Pain in the chest: observations in the use of local anaesthetics in its investigation and treatment. Medical Journal of Australia 1:4–7

Levey G S, Calabro J J 1962 Tietze's syndrome. Report of two cases and review of the literature. Arthritis and Rheumatism 5:261–269

Levine P R, Mascette A M 1989 Musculoskeletal chest pain in patients with 'angina': a prospective study. Southern Medical Journal 82(5):580–585; 591

Major R H 1945 Biographical review of Jacob M DaCosta (1833–1900) with special reference to his paper published in 1871 'On irritable heart. A clinical study of a form of functional cardiac disorder and its consequences'. In: Classic descriptions of disease, 3rd edn. Charles C Thomas, Springfield, IL, pp 381–385

Maresca M, Galanti G, Castellani S, Procacci P 1989 Pain in mitral valve prolapse. Pain 36:89–92

Mendlowitz M 1945 Strain of the pectoralis minor muscle, an important cause of praecordial pain in soldiers. American Heart Journal 30:123–125

Mitchell J B 1951 Cough fractures. British Medical Journal ii:1492–1493

Myers G, Freeman R, Scharf D et al 1977 Cerviprecordial angina. Diagnosis and management (abstract). American Journal of Cardiology 39:287

O'Neal L W, Ackerman L V 1951 Cartilaginous tumours of ribs and sternum. Journal of Thoracic Surgery 29:71–108

Petch M C 1986 Investigation of coronary artery disease. Journal of the Royal College of Physicians of London 20(1):21–24

Procacci P, Zoppi M, Maresca M 1994 Heart and vascular pain. In: Wall P D, Melzack R (eds) Textbook of pain, 3rd edn. Churchill Livingstone, Edinburgh, p 547

Redwood D R, Borer J S, Epstein S E 1976 Whither the ST segment during exercise? Circulation 54(suppl):703–706

Reeves T J, Harrison T R 1953 Diagnostic and therapeutic value of the reproduction of chest pain. Archives of Internal Medicine 91:8–25

Reynolds M 1981 Myofascial trigger point syndromes in the practice of rheumatology. Archives of Physical Medicine and rehabilitation 62:111–114

Rinzler S, Travell J 1948 Therapy directed at the somatic component of cardiac pain. American Heart Journal 35:248–268

Simons D G, Travell J 1976 The latissimus dorsi syndrome. A source of mid-back pain. Archives of Physical Medicine and Rehabilitation 57:561

Simons D, Travell J G, Simons L S 1999 Travell & Simons myofascial pain and dysfunction. The trigger point manual, 2nd edn. Williams & Wilkins, Baltimore, vol 1, p 821

Sola A E, Kuitert J H 1955 Myofascial trigger point pain in the neck and shoulder girdle. Northwest Medicine 54:980–984

Travell J 1976 Myofascial trigger points: clinical view. In: Bonica J J, Albe-Fessard D (eds) Advances in pain research and therapy, vol 1. Raven Press, New York

Travell J, Rinzler S H 1948 Pain syndromes of the chest muscles: resemblance to effort angina and myocardial infarction, and relief by local block. Canadian Medical Association Journal 59:333–338

Travell J, Rinzler S H, Herman M 1942 Pain and disability of the shoulder and arm: treatment by intramuscular injection with procaine hydrochloride. Journal of the American Medical Association 120:417–422

Turek S L 1984 Orthopaedics: principles and their application, 4th edn. Lippincott, Philadelphia, pp 1519–1521

Walters A 1961 Psychogenic regional pain alias hysterical pain. Brain 84(1):1–18

Wehrmacher W H 1958 The painful anterior chest wall syndromes. Medical Clinics of North America 38:111–118

Wolf E, Stern S 1976 Costosternal syndrome. Its frequency and importance in differential diagnosis of coronary heart disease. Archives of Internal Medicine 136:189–191

Wolfe F, Smythe H A, Yunus M B, Bennett R M et al 1990 The American College of Rheumatology 1990 criteria for the classification of fibromyalgia. Report of the multicentre criteria committee. Arthritis and Rheumatism 33:160–172

Yood R A, Goldenberg D L 1980 Sternoclavicular joint arthritis. Arthritis and Rheumatism 23:232–239

The anterior abdominal wall and pelvic floor

INTRODUCTION

In this chapter the clinical manifestations, differential diagnosis and treatment of myofascial pain arising as a result of trigger point (TrP) activity developing in the muscles of the anterior abdominal wall and pelvic floor will be considered.

The anterior abdominal wall as a source of pain is frequently overlooked. This is because as Renaer (1984) has pointed out, 'when confronted with abdominal pain complaints doctors will automatically think of pain originating in the abdominal viscera'. And yet, as he cogently comments, 'it would appear strange if tissues so abundantly innervated as the skin and the fasciae of the abdominal wall hardly ever caused pain'.

One possible reason for doctors not taking the anterior abdominal wall into account when considering potential sites from which pain may arise is that the majority of books on gastroenterology and most sections on the subject in undergraduate textbooks of medicine give detailed descriptions of diseases of the abdominal viscera and the characteristic patterns of pain associated with these but make little or no reference to the diagnosis and treatment of pain emanating from the wall itself. Thus, for example, although Blendis (1994), in the third edition of Melzack & Wall's *Textbook of Pain*, provides an otherwise comprehensive review of abdominal pain he has no more than a short paragraph on anterior abdominal wall pain, and although admittedly stressing the importance of excluding it gives no guidance as to the type of examination which should be carried out for the purpose.

INCIDENCE

That anterior abdominal wall pain is not rare is shown by Mehta & Ranger (1971) at the United Norwich Hospitals, England, diagnosing it in 103 patients over a period of three and a half years; by Thomson & Francis (1977) at the Gloucester Royal Hospital, England, reporting it to be present in 24 out of 120 patients admitted with acute abdominal pain; and by Gallegos & Hobsley (1989) at the Middlesex Hospital, London, England, finding that, of the patients attending their surgical outpatient department over a seven year period, 26 were suffering from it.

VIEWS CONCERNING PATHOGENESIS
Intercostal neuralgia

Earlier this century it was thought that anterior abdominal wall pain develops as a result of intercostal neuralgia. One of the main supporters of that view was John Carnett, Professor of Surgery at the University of Pennsylvania's School of Medicine.

It was Carnett's belief that the pain is due to a neuralgia involving the lower six intercostal and first lumbar nerves. In his first paper on the subject (Carnett 1926) he expressed the view that this neuralgia develops as a result of various spinal disorders such as syphilitic and tuberculous meningitis; syphilitic, tuberculous, sarcomatous and secondary carcinomatous disease of the vertebrae; osteoarthritis of the spine; and typhoid spondylitis. Also, he said it could be caused by endogenous toxins from carious teeth, infected tonsils and other infections, and by exogenous toxins such as lead, alcohol and arsenic. In his second paper on the subject (Carnett 1934), he stated that the neuralgia may be either acute or chronic and that when the latter, it develops as a

result of either spinal scoliosis, excessive lumbar lordosis, or spinal arthritis. And that these abnormalities also act as predisposing causes of an acute neuralgia brought about either by spinal trauma or some infective disorder such as 'acute tonsillitis, acute sinusitis, an ordinary cold, an abscess or any other acute infection'.

Although Carnett's views concerning the cause of anterior abdominal wall pain are clearly no longer tenable and have for long been relegated to the archives of history there still remains the possibility that it is of neural origin with some believing that it is due to anterior cutaneous nerve entrapment.

Anterior cutaneous nerve entrapment

Mehta & Ranger (1971), Applegate (1972), Doouss & Boas (1975) and Blendis (1994) are amongst those who are of the opinion that anterior abdominal wall pain is due to anterior cutaneous nerve entrapment.

Applegate (1972) pointed out that the anterior cutaneous nerve, together with an artery and vein, form a neurovascular bundle which passes, via a fibrous ring, through the substance of the rectus abdominis muscle to emerge anteriorly through a normally snug opening between the fibres of its anterior sheath (aponeurosis) and that because of this, entrapment of the nerve may be brought about in one or other of three ways. One is because any increase in abdominal pressure is liable to cause the fibrous bands in the rectus muscle's anterior sheath to split apart so as to allow the neurovascular bundle to herniate through it into the subcutaneous tissues. A second is because any involuntary or voluntary contraction of the rectus muscle is liable to compress the nerve in the intramuscular fibrous ring through which it passes. And a third is because any condition which displaces or twists the spine away from the side on which the pain is felt is liable to put undue tension on the nerve and cause it to become compressed against any relatively firm structure through which it passes.

Although entrapment of the anterior cutaneous nerve in the rectus muscle is clearly a possible cause for anterior abdominal wall pain developing, as Thomson & Francis (1977) have pointed out, against it being of neural origin is the absence of sensory changes. Also, it has to be remembered that pain of a similar type is liable to develop in muscles other than the rectus abdominis, such as the external and internal oblique. Therefore whilst not denying that rectus abdominis pain may on occasions be due to anterior cutaneous nerve entrapment other reasons for it developing in this and other abdominal wall muscles have to be considered.

The diagnostic significance of tender points

Applegate (1972), during the course of discussing anterior abdominal wall pain, has stated that 'the prime requisite for making a diagnosis is for the examiner to localise with one finger the maximal point of tenderness and for the patient to confirm that this is the source of the pain'. Doouss & Boas (1975) also drew attention to localised tender points in the muscle. And Mehta & Ranger (1971) who were more guarded than either Applegate or Doouss & Boas concerning the pathogenesis of the pain, and willing to say no more than it may be due to an entrapment neuropathy, also located 'small areas of acute tenderness about the size of a pencil head deep in the rectus sheath' and observed that an injection into such 'trigger areas' relieves the pain. Their assumption was that these tender areas are nerve entrapment sites but the alternative explanation that has to be considered is that they are the same as the tender points found by Balfour (1824) to be present in the muscles of patients suffering from what he called muscular rheumatism.

Muscular rheumatism

One of the first to ascribe anterior abdominal wall pain to rheumatism, or what he termed myofibrositis, was the English physician Murray (1929), who in an address to the Newcastle upon Tyne and Northern Counties Medical Society stated that the 'pain is of a dull aching character generally felt at one spot from which it tends to radiate'.

In 1933, Hunter, a physician in Canada, also drew attention to tender points in the anterior abdominal wall of patients suffering from what he chose to call myalgia. John Kellgren, whilst working with Sir Thomas Lewis at University College Hospital, London, published his important observations on a series of patients suffering from what he also termed myalgia and showed that the pain in that disorder emanates from points of exquisite tenderness in muscle which he simply called tender points (Kellgren 1938), or what two of his contemporary American surgeons, Steindler & Luck (1938), more aptly called trigger points. A number of physicians (Good 1950a, 1950b, Gutstein 1944, Kelly 1942, Long 1956, Melnick 1954) have, over the years, drawn attention to what will be referred to here as the anterior abdominal wall myofascial trigger point (MTrP) pain syndrome.

ANTERIOR ABDOMINAL WALL MTrP PAIN SYNDROME

This syndrome is still not as widely recognised as it should be despite Travell & Simons (1983) having written extensively about it in the first edition of volume one of their trigger point manual.

Factors responsible for the development of MTrP activity

Direct injury

TrP activity may develop in an anterior abdominal wall muscle when it is traumatised either because of a fall or because of an injury such as, for example, may be incurred in a road traffic accident. Also, when it is traumatised as a result of being subjected to sustained or repeated pressure. Examples of the latter amongst my patients include a farmer who developed upper abdominal MTrP pain as a result of cattle on market days constantly banging against the rectus muscle in the epigastric region; a farrier who developed pain of this type because of his practice of shoeing horses with their legs pressed firmly against the external oblique muscle in the left hypochondrial region; and a draughtsman who developed it because of his habit of working for long periods with the lower edge of his drawing board pressed hard against the rectus muscle in the right iliac fossa.

Iatrogenic trauma

TrP activity in the anterior abdominal wall is also liable to develop during the course of a surgical operation. This may happen either when its muscles are traumatised during the course of being retracted or when they are subjected to prolonged pressure against a hard unyielding operating table. TrP activity also not infrequently develops in surgical scars.

Muscle overloading

Another reason for TrP activity developing in an anterior abdominal wall muscle is overloading. Examples of when this may happen include carrying out some vigorous sporting activity, lifting a heavy load, repeated straining at stool and the persistent adoption of a poor posture.

Test to distinguish between extra-abdominal MTrP tenderness and intra-abdominal visceral tenderness

When searching for an anterior abdominal wall TrP it is essential to be able to distinguish between this parietal point of maximal tenderness and a localised area of visceral tenderness by palpating the abdominal wall firstly with its muscles totally relaxed and then with them in a contracted state. This is because in the case of the latter MTrP tenderness is increased, in contrast to visceral tenderness, which is decreased.

The test which should be employed for this purpose is the one first described by Carnett in 1926. His description of the test was as follows:

In order to differentiate between parietal tenderness and intra-abdominal tenderness, I have devised a simple two-stage bedside test which I have not seen mentioned anywhere. (A) In any patient complaining of abdominal pain and tenderness, the examiner

follows the classical advice of gaining the confidence of both the patient and his muscles and then palpates in the usual manner. Irrespective of whether the tenderness is parietal or intra-abdominal, the examiner's fingers, as a rule, will dip fairly deeply into the abdomen before tenderness is elicited. This deep position of the fingers has generally been regarded as proof that the tenderness is intra-abdominal, but in a surprisingly high percentage of cases this assumption will prove to be an error as shown by the next step. (B) The examiner keeps his fingers at the most sensitive area he has discovered on deep pressure and requests the patient to make his abdominal muscles rigid by contracting his diaphragm or by raising and holding his head from the pillow; as the patient tenses his muscles, the examiner relaxes his finger pressure so that his fingers rise out of the abdomen; and then with the patient's abdominal muscles tense the examiner reapplies pressure with his finger tips and he also may exert a little twisting motion with them. If the case under examination is one of intra-abdominal tenderness only, the B stage of the test will fail to elicit any tenderness when strenuous pressure is applied over tense muscles. If the case is one of parietal tenderness, almost or quite as much tenderness will be elicited by the B test as by the A test.

The English physician Murray (1929) who, as mentioned earlier, was one of the first to recognise that anterior abdominal wall pain is of muscular origin, employed Carnett's technique in order to distinguish between visceral tenderness and tenderness occurring as a result of what he called myofibrositis. And once Lewis and Kellgren (1939) had shown that abdominal wall pain emanates from what are now called MTrPs, Carnett's test became increasingly widely adopted.

Clinicians over the years, however, have expressed individual preferences with respect to methods employed for tensing the abdominal wall muscles. For example, Long (1956) advocated doing this by asking the patient to raise both legs. De Valera & Raftery (1976) recommended getting the patient to elevate both feet and head. Travell & Simons (1983) advised getting the supine patient to hold a deep breath. There is clearly little to choose between any of these methods and it is my personal practice to adopt whichever one seems to be the most suitable for any particular individual.

Muscles liable to develop TrP activity

The principal anterior abdominal muscles in which TrP activity is liable to develop include the two rectus abdominis muscles on either side of the midline, and the external oblique muscles in the flanks.

The internal oblique muscle situated deep to the external one may also at times contain TrPs (Fig. 15.1).

Rectus abdominis (Fig. 15.1)

Anatomical attachments

This muscle is attached at its upper end to the cartilage of the fifth, sixth and seventh ribs and at its lower end to the crest of the pubic bone.

Trigger point sites

TrP activity is liable to develop near to its upper attachment to the ribs; in the epigastrium; in the belly of the muscle halfway between the xiphisternum and the umbilicus and halfway between the umbilicus and the pubis; also near to or at the insertion of the muscle into the pubic bone (Fig. 15.2).

Pain referral patterns

TrP activity in this muscle near to its attachments to the ribs gives rise to pain and tenderness in the epigastric region. Pain from TrPs in its outer margin just below the umbilicus tends to be referred to the ipsilateral iliac fossa. Pain from TrPs near to its lower attachment to the pubic bone, like pain from TrPs in the upper part of the adductor longus muscle (see Ch. 13), is referred to the groin. Pain from a TrP in the rectus muscle near to its insertion into the pubic bone may also cause spasm to develop in the detrusor and urinary sphincter muscles (Simons et al 1999).

Finally, it is important to bear in mind that TrPs in the upper part of the rectus muscle may

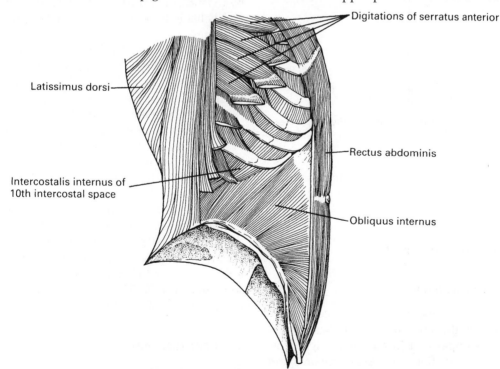

Figure 15.1 Muscles of the right side of the trunk. The external oblique has been removed to show the internal oblique, but its digitations from the rib have been preserved. The sheath of the rectus abdominis has been opened and its anterior lamina removed.

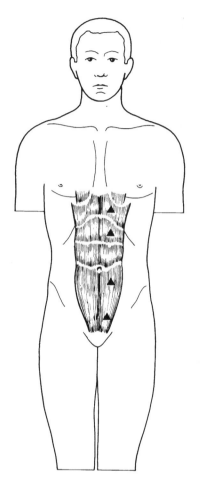

Figure 15.2 Some common trigger point sites (▲) in the rectus abdominis muscle.

refer pain posteriorly to the lower dorsal region. And TrPs in its lower part may refer pain posteriorly to the buttocks.

External oblique muscle
(Fig. 15.3)

Anatomical attachments

The external oblique muscle situated on the outer side of the abdominal wall has attachments at its upper end to the lower eight ribs. And from these its fibres sweep downwards and forwards to be attached to the linea alba medially and the anterior part of the iliac crest at its lower end.

Trigger point sites

TrPs in the muscle are most often found in the vicinity of its upper attachments to the ribs and near to its attachment to the iliac crest (Fig. 15.4).

Pain referral patterns

The referral of pain from TrPs in the upper part of the muscle where it overlies the rib cage is variable. It may either be upwards into the chest, or into the epigastric region, or diagonally down across the abdomen towards the contralateral side.

The referral of pain from TrPs in the lower part of the muscle near its attachment to the iliac crest is to the pubic region.

Symptoms caused by anterior wall MTrP activity

Anterior abdominal wall MTrP pain is usually of a dull aching character, tends to be aggravated by twisting or stretching movements of the trunk and is liable to be aggravated by the pressure of clothing.

Sometimes when TrP activity in an abdominal wall muscle causes it to become lax and distended there is simply a feeling of discomfort (Kelly 1942).

TrP activity in the anterior abdominal wall may also at times be responsible for the development of symptoms other than pain. This is shown by Melnick (1954), who found that out of 54 patients with this, 25% had flatulence and bloating, 11% had vomiting, 11% had heartburn and 4% had diarrhoea. Also, Theobald (1949) reported that dysmenorrhoea may in some cases be relieved by deactivating TrPs in the rectus muscle at a site about halfway between the umbilicus and the pubis. And Hoyt (1953) observed that dysuria is sometimes due to TrP activity in the muscles in the lower part of the abdomen.

Differential diagnosis

Epigastric region

Pain from a TrP in the upper part of the rectus abdominis muscle is felt in the epigastric region

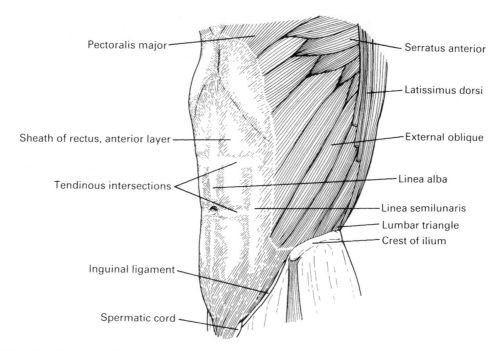

Figure 15.3   The left external oblique muscle.

where it simulates that of a peptic ulcer not only because of its character and location but also because of its tendency to be worse after a meal due to post-prandial abdominal distension stretching the muscle and by so doing increasing the TrP activity.

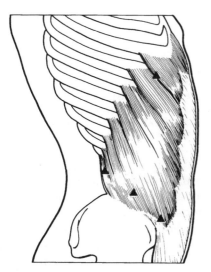

Figure 15.4   Some commonly occurring trigger point sites (▲) in the external oblique muscle.

In addition, as Melnick (1957) has pointed out, TrPs in this muscle are liable to become active as a secondary event when pain from a peptic ulcer causes it to go into spasm. Moreover, the MTrP pain is liable to persist long after the ulcer has healed.

Right hypochondrial region

Pain and tenderness in the right hypochondrial region that develops as a result of TrP activity in either the upper part of the right external oblique muscle or in the lateral upper border of the right rectus muscle is liable to be mistaken for that of gall bladder disease, particularly if ultrasound happens to reveal the presence of gall stones. In addition, MTrP pain in this region is liable to be ascribed erroneously to a hiatus hernia due to it being made worse by bending over as a result of this movement stretching the muscles and, by so doing, increasing the TrP activity.

Left hypochondrial region

Pain and tenderness in the left hypochondrial region that develops as a result of MTrP activity may simulate that produced by various disorders of the lung, heart or gut. And, because the TrPs from which the pain emanates are frequently overlooked, when extensive investigations have failed to reveal any abnormality in one or other of these three organs it is all too often considered to be psychogenic.

Pain from TrPs in the upper part of either the rectus or external oblique muscle may also simulate that present in the slipping rib-cartilage syndrome (see below).

Right iliac fossa

Pain and tenderness in the right iliac fossa may arise as a result of the development of trauma-induced activity in TrPs in the lower lateral border of the rectus abdominis muscle or the external oblique muscle. In the past, when TrPs in muscles in this part of the anterior abdominal wall of an otherwise fit person were overlooked the pain from them was erroneously assumed to be due to a low-grade inflammatory lesion in the appendix, but now that such a diagnosis is no longer tenable, in a female it is liable to be mistakenly attributed to some gynaecological disorder and in a male to neuroticism.

Left iliac fossa

Pain and tenderness in the left iliac fossa of an otherwise fit person may be due to the development of trauma-induced activity in TrPs in the lower part of either the rectus abdominis or external oblique. Failure to identify the presence of TrPs in one or other of these two muscles may lead to various investigations being carried out including a barium enema, and should this show the presence of diverticula, as so often happens in anyone aged 40 or over, the pain is liable to be wrongly attributed to diverticulitis.

Slipping rib-cartilage syndrome

Pain that arises in the upper part of the abdomen and lower part of the chest as a result of the development of TrP activity in the rectus and external oblique muscles near to their attachments to the lower ribs has to be distinguished from that present in a disorder which over the years has been accorded many synonyms, but which perhaps is best called the slipping rib-cartilage syndrome.

The first reference to this syndrome was made by the English psychiatrist Edgar F. Cyriax who, in 1919, reported three cases during the course of reviewing various psychological conditions with pain similar to that of visceral disease. The next was in 1922 when Davies-Colley, a surgeon at Guy's Hospital in London, reported two cases of what he called slipping rib and stated that resection of the cartilage in both cases afforded 'complete relief of the symptoms'. He also expressed the opinion that, 'It is probably not a rare condition and . . . I think it is quite likely that many cases occur in which such an apparently unimportant cause as a movable rib cartilage is unsuspected and the diagnosis missed'.

Subsequently, a number of single cases were reported (Bisgard 1931, Darby 1931, Poynton 1922, Russell 1924, Soltau 1922). However, despite this, Holmes, a surgeon in New Hampshire, USA, came to the conclusion in 1941 that the disorder was not being diagnosed as often as it should, for he said:

Failure to recognize this syndrome has led to needless laparotomies, prolonged suffering and varying degrees of incapacity. Then, too, when the condition has been recognized, there does not appear to be any clear conception of its development. It therefore seems important to present again the primary fundamental features of this syndrome in the hope that it will lead to a more general understanding and stimulate a greater interest in the subject. (Holmes 1941b)

He did this by publishing two detailed accounts of the disorder in each of which he gave a clear description of its pathogenesis, together with precise criteria for its diagnosis and his views concerning its treatment. The first account appeared in May 1941 and the second one in October 1941 (Holmes 1941a, 1941b).

Holmes pointed out that each of the eighth, ninth and tenth costal cartilages is connected to the one above it by a fibrous articulation. And that when, as a result of either direct or indirect trauma the latter becomes weakened, a cartilage, usually the eighth, but sometimes the ninth or tenth, becomes detached from the one above it with, as a result,

... the curling upward of the loosened end, so that on motion the deformed end rubs against the inside of the rib above, causing pain; also on certain motions and manipulation the deformed end slips over the rib border with a click that is felt by the patient, and a pain that is sometimes severe and incapacitating. (Holmes 1941b)

He then discussed the type of trauma responsible for weakening the articulation, the characteristics of the pain, the diagnostic significance of the clicking sound and the treatment of the condition.

The type of trauma

From an analysis of 68 cases including 46 of his own, Holmes concluded that the slipping of a rib cartilage more often results from indirect rather than direct trauma. He pointed out that because the loosening of the cartilage and its ultimate detachment is a gradual process, by the time pain develops, the patient may have forgotten the injury responsible for it particularly if this was of an indirect type.

He gave as an example of a direct injury the impact of a steering wheel against the lower ribs. And as examples of indirect injury he cited:

... sudden flexion, extension, or twisting of the body, by repeated arm pulls, as in golfing, by a sudden pull on the arms in any form of lifting, by pushing, by the act of forced expulsion, as childbirth or coughing, and by many other types of force, any of which may cause or aggravate the condition. (Holmes 1941b)

The character of the pain

Holmes pointed out that the pain usually takes the form of a persistent long-term dull ache but occasionally it is acute, intolerably severe and very incapacitating. And that in addition to it being felt around the rib border, it may also be referred to other sites such as the anterior chest wall, the scapular region, lower back and abdomen.

The diagnostic significance of the click

Holmes considered the click produced by the loosened cartilage slipping over the rib above it to be of such considerable importance as to be pathognomonic of the disorder. He pointed out that it is often apparent to the patient and stressed that the examiner should always attempt to elicit it, for, as he said, 'by manipulation, with the patient in the supine position and the knees flexed, the abnormally loosened and deformed cartilage can be brought out over the rib border with a click and a pain that is diagnostic' (Homes 1941b).

Holmes's views concerning the slipping rib-cartilage syndrome and in particular his criteria for its recognition have been considered at some length because, fifty years later, due to a failure to follow his advice, there is still much confusion concerning its diagnosis. For example, there continues to be a tendency for the pain in this disorder to be ascribed to either pleurisy, myocardial ischaemia or gall bladder disease. And conversely, for pain arising as a result of the development of MTrP activity to be attributed to this syndrome.

One of the main reasons for this confusion is that not sufficient attention is paid to the distinctive click which, as Holmes emphasised, is of such considerable diagnostic significance. Admittedly it is not always heard by the patient and cannot invariably be elicited by the examiner. Nevertheless, when present it is pathognomonic and when not the certainty with which the diagnosis of this disorder can be made is considerably reduced.

Thus, there can be no doubt that patients said by Mynors (1973) to have clicking ribs were suffering from the slipping rib-cartilage syndrome. There can similarly be no dispute that the three patients reported by McBeath & Keene (1975) were suffering from this disorder, or what they chose to call the rib-tip syndrome, for in each case the characteristic click and pain was evoked when the examiner applied digital pressure to the chest wall.

There can be no such certainty, however, that the diagnosis was correct in all of the 46 patients said by Wright (1980) to have the syndrome or in all of the 76 patients said by Scott & Scott (1993) to have it.

The reasons for saying this are as follows. Wright (1980) made no mention of having attempted to evoke a click and only two of his patients were aware of one being present. And it would seem that he based his diagnosis on the single criterion that 'the upper abdominal pain could faithfully be reproduced by pressure at one or more points in the costal margin'.

Similarly, none of the patients reviewed by Scott & Scott (1993) complained of hearing a click and no attempt was made on examination to elicit one. Their diagnostic criteria were restricted to 'pain in the lower chest or upper abdomen, a tender spot (or spots) in the lower costal margin (including the xiphoid) and reproduction of the pain by pressing on that spot'.

The criteria adopted both by Wright and by Scott & Scott were therefore very similar to those which are used for the diagnosis of the MTrP pain syndrome (see Ch. 4). And this is bound to lead to confusion as it is not uncommon for muscles such as the intercostals, the rectus abdominis and the external oblique to develop trauma-induced TrP activity at sites close to their attachments to the lower ribs. And when, as in the case of the slipping rib-cartilage syndrome, tender points are present along the costal margin, pain is referred from these points, and the application of pressure to them causes the spontaneously occurring pain to be reproduced.

Deactivation of anterior abdominal wall myofascial trigger points

It has become evident to me over the years that anterior abdominal wall MTrP pain is so readily alleviated that superficial dry needling (see Ch. 7) carried out at MTrP sites once a week for about 3–4 weeks is often all that is required. This is in marked contrast to MTrP pain in either the neck or low-back, where it is frequently necessary to continue treatment for a much longer period. One possible reason for this is that during the course of everyday living there is a considerably greater mechanical strain imposed upon the muscles in these two regions.

PELVIC MTrP PAIN

Both men and women are liable to develop pain in the pelvic region as a result of it being referred there from TrPs in either the lower back muscles (see Ch. 12) or, as just described, in the anterior abdominal wall muscles.

In addition, there is a gynaecological MTrP pain syndrome and also various pelvic floor MTrP pain syndromes that may affect either sex. Each of these disorders will be considered in turn.

Gynaecological MTrP syndrome

Slocumb (1984, 1990), an American gynaecologist, was one of the first to recognise this syndrome during the course of studying 177 women in a pelvic pain clinic from July 1979 to June 1982. He found that of these 177 women, 131 (74%), had what he called the abdominal pelvic pain syndrome, with pain emanating from TrPs in the abdominal wall (89%), in the vaginal fornices (71%) and in the sacral region (25%).

Pathogenesis

Women develop this syndrome as a result of muscles in the lower abdominal wall and pelvic cavity being subjected to trauma as, for example, may happen during pelvic surgery and childbirth.

With respect to this it is of interest to note that Renaer (1984) when considering what, at that time he called 'pelvic pain without obvious pathology', but which from his description must have mainly if not entirely been that which has subsequently come to be recognised as pelvic myofascial trigger point pain (Beard et al 1994), stated: 'the symptoms frequently start a short time after a delivery. The syndrome is most often seen between 20 and 40 years of age. It is seldom found during the climacteric and never after the menopause.'

Search for trigger points

Slocumb (1984, 1990) has stressed that the traditional bimanual method of examining the pelvis is useless when searching for MTrPs in this syndrome because, due to there being so many tissues between the hand on the abdominal wall and the fingers in the vagina, the clinician is easily misled as from which particular structure any tenderness that may be elicited is arising. He therefore states that TrPs in the abdominal wall should firstly be looked for using Carnett's palpation technique described earlier in this chapter; that the tissues around the vaginal introitus should then be palpated in order to search for TrPs in the pubic region at the insertions of the levator and coccygeus muscles and in areas of previous vaginal trauma such as, for example, an episiotomy scar. After this, a finger should be inserted into the vagina in order to palpate the paracervical region. By these means it is possible to identify the location of any exquisitely tender MTrPs that may be present and by applying sustained pressure to them to reproduce the spontaneously occurring pain.

Characteristics of the pain

The pain, which is of a diffuse, poorly localised, aching type is present in both the lower abdomen and pelvic cavity. It may also be felt in the lower back and thighs.

Pain arising from vaginally situated MTrPs becomes worse during coitus (dyspareunia).

Pain from TrPs in the abdominal wall increases when the muscles containing them become stretched as, for example, by a distended bladder or by twisting movements of the torso; also, when they are compressed by tight clothing.

MTrP activity in the paracervical region is liable to lead to the development of dysmenorrhoea.

Anxiety and depression which so often develop when the pain in this syndrome becomes persistent has the effect of making it worse.

Deactivation of trigger points

Out of 131 patients in the study carried out by Slocumb (1984), 9 were lost sight of, but of 122 patients followed up by him, 89% reported complete or partial relief from the pain 3–36 months after the TrPs had been deactivated by injecting a local anaesthetic into them.

The number of times this had to be carried out was five or less in 92.6% of the cases, with complete pain relief being obtained in 94.8% of the patients who only required two treatments but only in 66.7% of those who had to have six or more treatments. Moreover, patients who only had to have abdominal wall TrPs deactivated had a 100% success rate and 84.6% of those who only had to have vaginal TrPs deactivated were relieved of their pain.

As my own experience of deactivating MTrPs in the pelvic region leads me to believe that equally good results may be obtained from employing the superficial dry needling procedure described in Chapter 7, there is clearly a need for trials to be carried out to compare objectively the efficacy of this technique and the one adopted by Slocumb.

Relaxation therapy

In the management of this syndrome it is necessary not only to deactivate the TrPs, but also to combat the anxiety and depression that is so often present in women with chronic pelvic pain (Beard et al 1994). This is because, as elsewhere in the body, anxiety-induced muscle contraction leads to the persistence of TrP activity (see Ch. 4) so that any TrP deactivating procedure alone is likely to provide no more than short-term pain relief.

My personal preference for combating anxiety in this and any other pain disorder is to employ hypnotherapy and to teach the patient to practise autohypnosis on a regular daily basis (see Ch. 3).

Differential diagnosis

Pain arising from this gynaecological MTrP syndrome has to be distinguished from that which develops as a result of endometriosis, pelvic congestion and chronic pelvic inflammatory disease, particularly when this gives rise to adhesion-induced entrapment of an ovary.

Endometriosis This disorder, in which endometrial tissue arises outside the uterine cavity, may, like the MTrP pain syndrome, give rise to a persistent dull ache in the lower abdomen and pelvic region, and also to dysmenorrhoea and dyspareunia. Commonly, however, it is asymptomatic and therefore finding evidence of it on laparoscopic examination does not of itself mean that it is the cause of any pain which may be present.

Pelvic congestion The symptoms and signs of this disorder have been extensively reviewed by Beard et al (1988).

As with both endometriosis and the gynaecological MTrP pain syndrome, the symptoms in this disorder include a persistent dull ache in the abdomen and pelvic cavity, low-back pain, dysmenorrhoea and dyspareunia. Also, as in the case of the MTrP pain syndrome, prolonged standing brings on the pain and bending forwards exacerbates it.

On examination, deep pressure over the ovarian point (the junction of the upper and middle third of a line drawn from the umbilicus to the anterior superior iliac fossa) commonly elicits pain in the iliac fossa. And examination of the vagina often shows it to be visibly congested with the cervix having a blue or violet colour. In addition, both the uterus and ovaries are liable to be tender (Beard et al 1988).

In any suspected case ultrasound imaging should be carried out as it is possible by this means to detect and measure dilated pelvic veins, but should the findings with this investigation be inconclusive it may be necessary to carry out pelvic venography (Beard et al 1984).

Pelvic infection-induced adhesions

Some women with persistent pelvic pain are found on laparoscopy to have widespread adhesions from some past acute pelvic infection. Nevertheless, as Alexander-Williams (1987) has stated, 'it is a poorly substantiated myth that adhesions can cause abdominal or pelvic pain'. One exception to this, however, is when adhesions cause ovarian entrapment (Christ & Lotze 1975).

Treatment of endometriosis and pelvic congestion

Both endometriosis and pelvic congestion are ovarian hormone-dependent conditions and treatment therefore consists of suppressing the pain with the use of drugs such as naturally conjugated oestrogens, gonadotrophin-releasing hormone and medroxyprogesterone. And in intractable cases, it may be necessary for a bilateral oophorectomy and total hysterectomy to be carried out followed by hormone replacement therapy (Beard et al 1994).

In addition, because anxiety very commonly exacerbates the persistent pain present in disorders such as endometriosis, pelvic congestion and the gynaecological MTrP pain syndrome, treatment with some form of relaxation therapy is helpful.

Pelvic floor muscles (Figs 15.5 and 15.6)

The pelvic floor muscles in which TrP pain may develop include the levator ani and coccygeus, which together form the pelvic diaphragm, as well as various perineal (pelvic outlet) muscles including the external anal sphincter, bulbospongiosus and ischiocavernosus.

Levator ani and coccygeus muscles

These muscles, together with their contralateral counterparts, form a muscular pelvic diaphragm which supports the pelvic viscera and opposes the downward thrust produced by any rise in intra-abdominal pressure. Before considering factors responsible for the development of pain in them their structure and functions will be briefly reviewed.

Each levator ani muscle arises in front from the pubic bone, behind from the ischial spine and between these two insertions from the obturator fascia. It has an outer part, the ileococcygeus muscle, and an inner part, the pubococcygeus.

The two levator ani muscles which together form the greater part of the pelvic cavity provide support for the anus, assist with its contraction

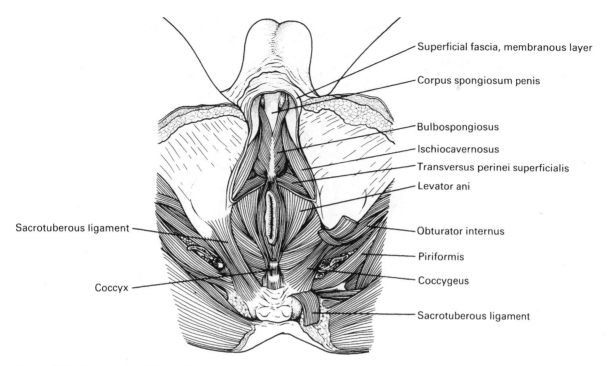

Superficial fascia, membranous layer

Corpus spongiosum penis

Bulbospongiosus

Ischiocavernosus

Transversus perinei superficialis

Levator ani

Obturator internus

Piriformis

Coccygeus

Sacrotuberous ligament

Sacrotuberous ligament

Coccyx

Figure 15.5   The muscles of the male perineum.

and help to pull the coccyx forwards. They also wrap around the urethra and by so doing contribute to its emptying at the completion of urination. In addition, in the male, they provide support for the prostate and in the female act as a vaginal sphincter.

The coccygeus muscle, which is situated behind the levator ani, is triangular in shape. Its apex is attached to the spine of the ischium and its base to the coccyx.

The two coccygeus muscles serve to pull the coccyx forwards after it has been displaced, as may happen, for example, on opening the bowels and during parturition.

Pain syndromes involving the levator ani and coccygeus muscles – a multiplicity of terms

From a review of the literature there might at first sight appear to be several syndromes involving these two muscles, but on closer examination it becomes evident that over the years a multiplicity of terms have been employed in an attempt

to find the most appropriate name for one particular disorder.

It was Sir James Young Simpson, when Professor of Midwifery at Edinburgh University, who, in 1859, introduced the term coccygodynia for the pain which arises when the coccyx, so called because of the likeness of its shape to that of a cuckoo's beak (Greek *kokkus* – cuckoo), is traumatised or inflammation develops in the tissues around it.

The next person to make a special study of coccygeal pain was the American pathologist George Thiele (Thiele 1937). Following this he wrote several papers on the subject culminating in an extensive review based on a study of 324 patients (Thiele 1963). In this review he stated that patients with coccygodynia may be divided into two groups. In 20% of those with this disorder the pain is due to trauma-induced structural damage to the coccyx. In the other 80% the coccyx itself is normal and the pain in the coccygeal region is referred there as a result of spasm developing in the levator ani and

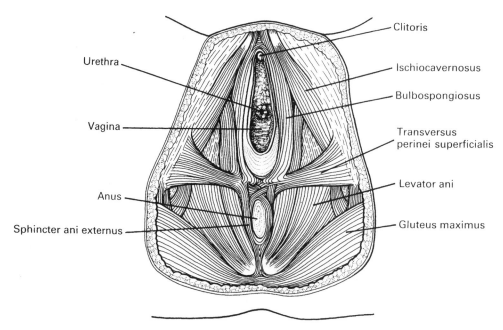

Figure 15.6 The muscles of the female perineum.

coccygeus muscles, either because of a poor sitting posture or because of infection in nearby structures.

This led Smith (1959) to express the opinion that because the aetiology, pathology and clinical manifestations in these two groups are different, it is necessary to distinguish between them by providing names for two separate disorders. He therefore suggested that the term coccygodynia, or what he called coccydynia, should be reserved for the group in which pain is due to trauma-induced structural damage to the coccyx and in which pressure applied to the tip of the coccyx evokes the pain. And that the term levator spasm syndrome should be employed for the group in which the coccyx itself is normal and pain in the coccygeal region arises as a result of spasm developing in muscles in the vicinity of the coccyx.

Others have concurred with this view but somewhat confusingly have chosen to give this latter syndrome a variety of different names. These have included levator syndrome (Grant et al 1975, McGivney & Cleland 1965) and levator ani spasm syndrome (Wright 1969). Also, because it is not only from the levator

ani that the pain arises but also from the coccygeus and in some cases from the piriformis and gluteus maximus, Sinaki et al (1977) decided to call it tension myalgia of the pelvic floor.

However, now that both Long (1956) and Pace (1975) have reported finding MTrPs on rectal examination of patients with this variously-named syndrome, and Travell & Simons (1992) have discussed at length the consequences of TrP activity developing in the levator ani and coccygeus muscles, it would seem more appropriate to call it the pelvic diaphragm MTrP pain syndrome.

Pelvic diaphragm MTrP pain syndrome

Factors responsible for trigger point activation

It would seem that one important factor responsible for TrP activity developing in the levator ani and coccygeus muscles is the overloading of them because of a poor sitting posture. Smith (1959), in discussing the causation of what he called levator spasm syndrome stated: 'many of these people are confirmed slumpers who sit in such a way that the pressure is exerted over the upper buttocks, coccyx and base of the sacrum. It seems that this poor posture may produce undue fatigue and spasm of the supporting pelvic muscles.'

And Thiele (1963), in discussing the causation of what he termed gradual onset coccygodynia, stated:

... prolonged automobile rides or prolonged sitting can produce such severe pain that patients avoid them whenever possible. Since 1950 it has been unusual to treat a woman with coccygodynia who has not spent from one to several hours a day watching television or playing bridge. The severity of the pain is in direct proportion to the amount of time spent sitting.

Surgically induced trauma may also be the cause of TrP activity developing in these muscles for Grant et al (1975), in their analysis of 316 cases of what they termed the levator syndrome, seen during a 15-year period in a proctological practice, found that 'seventeen percent of patients had histories of previous anorectal surgery. Occasionally the syndrome is seen in acute form immediately following anorectal surgery, perineorrhaphy, or in the immediate postpartum state.'

Another suggested reason for the syndrome arising is the development of spasm in these pelvic muscles as a result of disease in some nearby organ. It was this possibility that led the proctologist Thiele (1963) to state that 'men should be questioned about symptoms of posterior urethritis, prostatitis and seminal vesiculitis. In women it is well to ascertain whether there has been bladder irritability or a purulent vaginal discharge.'

He also found that an anal infection was a precipitating cause in 178 of his cases. Other proctologists (McGivney & Cleland 1965, Paradis & Marganoff 1969) have also emphasised the importance of searching for evidence of this in or around the anus. Their experience, however, may reflect a specialty referral bias, as none of the patients who Sinaki et al (1977) investigated in a department of physical medicine were found to have an inflammatory cause.

As anxiety by causing a patient to hold a group of muscles in a persistently contracted state may lead to the development of MTrP activity in other regions of the body such as the neck and low-back (see Chs 8 and 12),there is no reason why it should not have the same effect on muscles in the pelvic floor. Certainly, many of those who have made a special study of this pelvic diaphragm disorder have suggested that emotional disturbances may contribute to its development (Grant et al 1975, Sinaki et al 1977), but as Smith (1959) has said, it is wrong to ascribe the disorder solely to neuroticism.

Age and sex

This disorder, which may arise at any age, most commonly develops in the fourth decade of life and mainly affects women. In Smith's (1959) series of patients 80% were women. Thiele (1963) reported a ratio of 5 women to 1 man. In Grant et al's (1975) analysis of 316 cases, 72% of the patients were women. Also, out of 94 patients reviewed by Sinaki et al (1977), 78 were women and 16 were men.

Symptoms

Persistent rectal pain The main symptom is a persistent ill-defined diffuse aching or throbbing in the rectum made worse by prolonged sitting. The discomfort in some cases radiates to the coccygeal region. And in those in whom there is spasm not only in the levator ani and coccygeus muscles but also in the piriformis muscle, pain is felt in the gluteal region and thigh. Urethral or vaginal pain that comes on during urination is occasionally present. In addition, a minority of women complain of dyspareunia.

Paroxysmal rectal pain (proctalgia fugax) Patients with this syndrome may also develop transient episodes of very severe rectal pain or what Thaysen (1935) termed proctalgia fugax. Grant et al (1975), during the course of reviewing 316 patients with what they called the levator ani syndrome, found that 12% of them had this complication.

These paroxysms of agonising rectal pain usually only last for a few minutes but because of their tendency to come on during the night, they are apt to disturb sleep (Smith 1959).

Because this episodic type of rectal pain is also liable to affect people who are in otherwise good health there has been much speculation as to its cause. It is therefore of interest to note that when 10 doctors who suffered from it carried out rectal examinations on themselves during attacks of pain, they each felt a tender band to one or other side of the rectum and ascribed it to spasm of a levator ani muscle (Douthwaite 1956, 1962).

It may also occasionally arise as a result of colonic spasm in patients with the irritable bowel syndrome (Harvey 1979, Thompson 1984, Thompson & Heaton 1980).

Signs

On rectal examination the levator ani and coccygeus muscles, also in some cases the piriformis muscle, are found to be tender and in a contracted state. And on systematic palpation of an affected muscle it is possible to locate exquisitely tender TrPs with sustained pressure applied to them intensifying the spontaneously occurring pain.

In the majority of cases it is only muscles on one side that are affected and for some unexplained reason this would seem to be most often the left (Grant et al 1975, Smith 1959). As stated previously the coccyx itself is not tender in this disorder.

Treatment

The treatment of this syndrome includes deactivation of the TrPs by means of intrarectal massage with the finger drawn firmly over the bellies of the spastic muscles in a postero-anterior direction. This procedure should be repeated 15–20 times every day for a week and then every other day until improvement takes place. In addition, a muscle relaxant such as diazepam should be administered. Also, the patient should be instructed to immerse the buttocks and hips

in hot water (Sitz baths) on a daily basis. In cases where symptoms persist despite these measures electrogalvanic stimulation of the muscles has been reported to give good results (Nicosia & Abcarian 1985, Oliver et al 1985, Sohn et al 1982).

For the treatment of proctalgia fugax either inhaled salbutamol (Wright 1985) or oral clonidine (Swain 1987) should be tried.

In order to help prevent a recurrence of this MTrP pain disorder the patient should be instructed how to sit properly on a firm surface with the weight of the body distributed equally on the two ischial tuberosities.

External and internal anal sphincter pain

The anal canal is 2–3 cm in length. Its lower half, which is covered with skin, has in its wall the external anal sphincter. This is normally in a state of contraction and keeps the anal orifice closed. Its upper half, which is lined by a mucous membrane, has in its wall the internal anal sphincter. MTrP activity is an often overlooked reason for external anal sphincter pain developing.

External anal sphincter TrP pain

TrPs in the external anal sphincter are liable to become active should this muscle become traumatised. Circumstances in which this may happen include, for example, falling with the legs straddled across a hard surface, anal and perianal surgery, prolonged pillion riding and the unskilled administration of an enema.

The search for trigger points In searching for TrPs in the external anal sphincter it is first necessary to systematically palpate the anal opening externally and then to do so with a well-lubricated gloved finger inserted into it. During this search the patient should be instructed to bear down as this helps to relax the sphincter. In addition to much generalised tenderness, focal areas of exquisite tenderness at TrP sites are found to be present. It may also be possible to palpate taut bands at these sites. And when sustained pressure is applied to these TrPs the spontaneously occurring pain becomes exacerbated.

TrP pain referral Pain from active TrPs in the sphincter is felt around the anus, also in the region of the coccyx and in some cases over the lower half of the sacrum.

Deactivation of trigger points Before attempting this the skin in the perianal area should be scrupulously cleaned. One method of deactivating a TrP is to inject a local anaesthetic into it. This, however, calls for extreme accuracy and is difficult to carry out at this particular site as it entails manipulating the syringe with one hand whilst accurately locating the TrP with a finger of the other hand inserted into the anus (Travell & Simons 1992). My personal preference here, as elsewhere in the body, is to employ the superficial dry needle technique described in Chapter 7. A possible alternative might be to use electrogalvanic stimulation such as that used by Oliver et al (1985) in the treatment of the levator syndrome.

Internal anal sphincter spasm-induced pain

The commonest reason for the internal anal sphincter going into spasm is the development of a fissure in the posterior midline of the anus as a result of the mucosa becoming damaged by a dry hard mass of faecal material. The superficial tear produced by this gives rise to excruciating pain during defecation and in some cases for some hours after it.

On examination there is characteristically a swollen skin tag – a sentinel pile. In addition, a discharge of pus may be observed. Also, the stools may be streaked with blood.

In this disorder any attempt to insert a finger into the anus is often so unacceptably painful and the anal canal along its whole length is so tightly contracted as to make it impossible to carry out a rectal examination. Therefore, in those cases where it is considered necessary to carry this out in order to exclude other causes of anal pain, it may prove necessary to administer a general anaesthetic.

The treatment of the condition should initially be a conservative one with the local application of an anaesthetic gel and the use of bran and bulk laxatives (Bannerjee 1997). There have, in addition, been recent reports suggesting that the local application of a glyceryl trinitrate (nitroglycerin) ointment is helpful in reducing internal anal sphincter pressure (Lund & Scholefield 1997).

Anterior pelvic floor MTrP pain

Muscles in the anterior half of the pelvic floor liable to develop TrP activity include the bulbospongiosus and the ischiocavernosus.

Bulbospongiosus muscle

This muscle is attached posteriorly to the perineal body situated in the centre of the pelvic floor. From there, in the female it divides into two parts which, anteriorly, attach to the clitoris. Contraction of it constricts the vaginal orifice. Also, although erection of the clitoris, like erection of the penis, is primarily an autonomically controlled vascular response, contraction of the bulbospongiosus, by compressing the dorsal vein of the clitoris, assists in its maintenance.

In the male, from its posterior attachment to the perineal body, it also divides into two parts which, in front, wrap around the corpus spongiosum on the posterior aspect of the penis and around the corpus cavernosum on its anterior aspect. The contraction of the muscle assists with the emptying of the urethra at the completion of urination. In addition, contraction of this muscle by compressing the erectile tissue and dorsal vein in the penis assists with the maintenance of an erection.

Ischiocavernosus muscle

There are two ischiocavernosus muscles which together form the lateral boundaries of the perineum. Posteriorly, in both sexes, the muscle is attached to the ischial tuberosity.

Anteriorly, in the female, it inserts into the crus at the base of the clitoris, and, in the male, into the crus at the base of the penis. These muscles, by compressing the crus of the penis and the crus of the clitoris, retard the return of blood from these two organs and by doing so assist in the maintenance of an erection.

Activation of bulbospongiosus and ischiocavernosus trigger points

TrP activity in these muscles is liable to develop whenever they are subjected to direct trauma such as when falling astride a hard surface or when they, together with other muscles in that region of the body, become strained during the course of some sporting activity. It may also happen as in one of my patients as a result of the carrying out of exercises designed to strengthen the lower abdomen and upper thigh muscles.

The search for trigger points in the bulbospongiosus and ischiocavernosus muscles

In the female the bulbospongiosus muscle can only be satisfactorily examined per vaginam. This muscle, together with the levator vaginae part of the levator ani, encircle the vaginal introitus. In searching for TrPs and their associated taut bands in these muscles it is necessary to apply firm pressure to the lateral wall of the introitus. Sustained pressure applied to active TrPs at this site gives rise to the referral of pain locally around the vagina and perineum.

TrPs in the ischiocavernosus muscle are located by applying firm pressure in the region of the clitoris. The clitoris, when compressed, is not normally tender. When, however, TrPs are present in the ischiocavernosus muscle that covers it, firm pressure applied upwards towards the pubic bone elicits both tenderness and the referral of pain from these TrPs to the perineal region.

In the male both the bulbospongiosus muscle and the ischiocavernosus muscles should be examined for TrP activity with the knees drawn upwards and the patient lifting the testicles out of the way. TrPs in the bulbospongiosus muscle are located by palpating along the median line of the perineum over the bulb at the root of the penis.

TrPs in the ischiocavernosus muscle are located by palpating along the laterally placed crus at the root of the penis.

Trigger point deactivation

TrPs in these muscles may be deactivated by injecting a local anaesthetic into them (Travell & Simons 1992). However, in my experience, it is easier and seemingly just as effective to employ the superficial dry needle technique described in Chapter 7.

Pain referred to the scrotum from MTrPs

When pain develops in the scrotum with no obvious pathology to account for it the possibility of it having been referred there from TrPs in nearby muscles has to be considered. These include the lower part of the external oblique just above the inguinal ligament, the upper part of the adductor longus (see Ch. 13), the bulbospongiosus and the ischiocavernosus. Also, as pointed out by Kellgren (1940) over 50 years ago, from TrPs in the muscles and ligaments in the vicinity of the first lumbar vertebra. This referral of pain to the scrotum from TrPs in the lumbar region is possibly associated in some way with the genital branch of the genito-femoral nerve arising from the first and second lumbar nerves (Yeates 1985).

REFERENCES

Alexander-Williams J 1987 Do adhesions cause pain? British Medical Journal 294:659–660

Applegate W V 1972 Abdominal cutaneous nerve entrapment syndrome. Surgery 71:118–124

Balfour W 1824 Illustrations of the efficacy of compression and percussion in the cure of rheumatism and sprains. The London Medical and Physical Journal 51:446–462

Bannerjee A K 1997 Treating anal fissure. British Medical Journal 314:1638–1639

Beard R W, Highman J W, Pearce S, Reginald P W 1984 Diagnosis of pelvic varicosities in women with chronic pelvic pain. Lancet ii:946–949

Beard R W, Reginald P W, Wadsworth J 1988 Clinical features of women with chronic lower abdominal pain and pelvic congestion. British Journal of Obstetrics and Gynaecology 95:153–161

Beard R W, Gangar K, Pearce S 1994 Chronic gynaecological pain. In: Wall P D, Melzack R (eds) Textbook of pain, 3rd edn. Churchill Livingstone, Edinburgh, pp 597–614

Bisgard J D 1931 Slipping ribs: report of case. Journal of the American Medical Association 97:23

Blendis L M 1994 Abdominal pain. In: Wall P D, Melzack R (eds) Textbook of pain, 3rd edn. Churchill Livingstone, Edinburgh, p 587

Carnett J B 1926 Intercostal neuralgia as a cause of abdominal pain and tenderness. Surgery, Gynecology and Obstetrics 42:625–632

Carnett J B 1934 Pain and tenderness of the abdominal wall. Journal of the American Medical Association 102(5):345–348

Christ J L, Lotze E C 1975 The residual ovary syndrome. Obstetrics and Gynecology 46:555–556

Cyriax E F 1919 On various conditions that may simulate the referred pains of visceral disease and a consideration of these from the points of view of cause and effect. Practitioner 102:314–322

Darby J A 1931 Slipping ribs: report of case. Northwest Medicine 30:471

Davies-Colley R 1922 Slipping rib. British Medical Journal i:432

de Valera E, Raftery H 1976 Lower abdominal and pelvic pain in women. In: Bonica J J, Albe-Fessard D (eds) Advances in pain research and therapy. Raven Press, New York, vol 1, pp 933–937

Doouss T W, Boas R A 1975 The abdominal cutaneous nerve entrapment syndrome. New Zealand Journal of Medicine 81:473–475

Douthwaite A H 1956 Proctalgia fugax. British Medical Journal ii:895–900

Douthwaite A H 1962 Proctalgia fugax. British Medical Journal ii:164–168

Gallegos N C, Hobsley M 1989 Recognition and treatment of abdominal wall pain. Journal of the Royal Society of Medicine 82:343–344

Good M G 1950a The role of skeletal muscles in the pathogenesis of diseases. Acta Medica Scandinavica 138:285–292

Good M G 1950b Pseudo-appendicitis. Acta Medica Scandinavica 138:348–353

Grant S R, Salvati E P, Rubin R J 1975 Levator syndrome: an analysis of 316 cases. Diseases of Colon and Rectum 18:161–163

Gutstein R R 1944 The role of abdominal fibrositis in functional indigestion. Mississippi Valley Medical Journal 66:114–124

Harvey R P 1979 Colonic motility in proctalgia fugax. Lancet ii:713–714

Holmes J F 1941a A study of the slipping rib cartilage syndrome. New England Journal of Medicine 224:928–932

Holmes J F 1941b Slipping rib cartilage with report of cases. American Journal of Surgery 54:326–338

Hoyt H S 1953 Segmental nerve lesions as a cause of the trigonitis syndrome. Stanford Medical Bulletin 11:61–64

Hunter C 1933 Myalgia of the abdominal wall. Canadian Medical Journal 28:157–161

Kellgren J H 1938 A preliminary account of referred pains arising from muscle. Clinical Science 3:175–190

Kellgren J H 1940 Somatic simulating visceral pain. Clinical Science 4:303–309

Kelly M 1942 Lumbago and abdominal pain. Medical Journal of Australia 1:311–317

Lewis T, Kellgren J H 1939 Observations relating to referred pain, viscero-motor reflexes and other associated phenomena. Clinical Science 4:47–71

Long C 1956 Myofascial pain syndromes part iii – some syndromes of trunk and thigh. Henry Ford Hospital Medical Bulletin 4:102–106

Lund S N, Scholefield J H 1997 A randomised prospective, double-blind, placebo controlled trial of glyceryl trinitrate ointment in treatment of anal fissure. Lancet 349:11–16

McBeath A A, Keene J S 1975 The rib-tip syndrome. Journal of Bone and Joint Surgery 57:795–797

McGivney J U, Cleland B R 1965 The levator syndrome and its treatment. Southern Medical Journal 58:505–510

Mehta M, Ranger I 1971 Persistent abdominal pain. Anaesthesia 26(3):330–333

Melnick J 1954 Treatment of trigger mechanisms in gastrointestinal disease. New York State Journal of Medicine 54:1324–1330

Melnick J 1957 Trigger areas and refractory pain in duodenal ulcer. New York State Journal of Medicine 57:1037–1076

Murray G R 1929 Myofibrositis as a simulator of other maladies. Lancet i:113–116

Mynors J M 1973 Clicking rib. Lancet i:674

Nicosia J F, Abcarian H 1985 Levator syndrome – a treatment that works. Diseases of Colon and Rectum 28:406–408

Oliver G C, Rubin R J, Salvati E P, Eisenstat T E 1985 Electrogalvanic stimulation in the treatment of levator syndrome. Diseases of Colon and Rectum 28:662–663

Pace J B 1975 Commonly overlooked pain syndromes responsive to simple therapy. Postgraduate Medicine 58(4):107–113

Paradis H, Marganoff H 1969 Rectal pain of extrarectal origin. Diseases of Colon and Rectum 12:306–312

Poynton F J 1922 Memoranda. British Medical Journal i:516

Renaer M 1984 Gynaecological pain. In: Wall P D, Melzack R (eds) Textbook of pain, 1st edn. Churchill Livingstone, Edinburgh, p 373

Russell E N 1924 Memoranda. British Medical Journal i:664

Scott E M, Scott B B 1993 Painful rib syndrome – a review of 76 cases. Gut 34:1006–1008

Simons D G, Travell J G, Simons L S 1999 Myofascial pain and dysfunction. The trigger point manual, 2nd edn. Williams & Wilkins, Baltimore, vol 1, ch 49

Sinaki M, Merritt J L, Stillwell G K 1977 Tension myalgia of the pelvic floor. Mayo Clinic Proceedings 52:717–722

Slocumb J C 1984 Neurological factors in chronic pelvic pain: trigger points and the abdominal pelvic pain syndrome. American Journal of Obstetrics and Gynecology 149:536–543

Slocumb J C 1990 Chronic, somatic, myofascial and neurogenic abdominal pelvic pain. Clinical Obstetrics and Gynecology 33(1):145–153

Smith W T 1959 Levator spasm syndrome. Minnesota Medicine 42:1076–1079

Sohn N, Weinstein M A, Robbins R D 1982 The levator syndrome and its treatment with high-voltage electromagnetic stimulation. American Journal of Surgery 144:580–582

Soltau H K V 1922 Memoranda. British Medical Journal i:516

Steindler A, Luck J V 1938 Differential diagnosis of pain low in the back. Journal of the American Medicine Association 110:106–113

Swain R 1987 Oral clonidine for proctalgia fugax. Gut 28:1039–1040

Thaysen T E H 1935 Proctalgia fugax: a little known form of pain in the rectum. Lancet ii:243–246

Theobald G H 1949 The relief and prevention of referred pain. Journal of Obstetrics and Gynaecology of the British Commonwealth 56:447–460

Thiele G H 1937 Coccygodynia and pain in the superior gluteal region and down the back of the thigh. Causation by tonic spasm of the levator ani, coccygeus and piriformis muscles and relief by massage of the muscles. Journal of the American Medical Association 109: 1271–1275

Thiele G H 1963 Coccygodynia: cause and treatment. Diseases of Colon and Rectum 6:422–436

Thompson W G 1984 Proctalgia fugax in patients with the irritable bowel disease, peptic ulcer or inflammatory bowel disease. American Journal of Gastroenterology 79:450–452

Thompson W G, Heaton K W 1980 Proctalgia fugax. Journal of the Royal College of Physicians of London 14(4):244–248

Thomson H, Francis D M A 1977 Abdominal wall tenderness: a useful sign in the acute abdomen. Lancet ii:1053–1054

Travell J G, Simons D G 1983 Myofascial pain and dysfunction. The trigger point manual. Williams & Wilkins, Baltimore, vol 1, ch 49

Travell J G, Simons D G 1992 Myofascial pain and dysfunction. The trigger point manual, Williams & Wilkins, Baltimore, vol 2, ch 6

Wright J E 1985 Inhaled salbutamol for proctalgia fugax. Lancet ii:659–660

Wright J T 1980 Slipping-rib syndrome. Lancet ii: 632–634

Wright R R 1969 The levator ani spasm syndrome. American Journal of Proctology 20(6):447–451

Yeates W K 1985 Pain in the scrotum. British Journal of Hospital Medicine 33(2):101–104

The fibromyalgia syndrome

16

Clinical characteristics and biopathophysiological mechanisms of fibromyalgia syndrome

Muhammad B. Yunus
Fatma İnanıcı

INTRODUCTION

Fibromyalgia or fibromyalgia syndrome (FMS) is a clinically recognisable condition, which is characterised by chronic musculoskeletal pain and tender points at multiple sites (Yunus et al 1981, Wolfe et al 1990). The purpose of this chapter is to discuss the clinical characteristics, diagnosis and the biopathophysiological mechanisms of FMS.

CLINICAL CHARACTERISTICS

FMS is a common condition (Wolfe 1990) that causes significant disability (Bennett 1996). The population prevalence of FMS by American College of Rheumatology (ACR) criteria has been reported to be 2% in Wichita, Kansas, USA (Wolfe et al 1995a) and 3.3% in London, Ontario, Canada (White et al 1999). In the Wichita study, the prevalence was 3.4% among women and 0.5% among men. The prevalence increased with age, FMS being present most commonly between the ages of 60 and 79 years with more than 7% among women (Wolfe et al 1995a). The prevalence also increased with age in the London,

Ontario study, with <1% in the 18–30 age group to 8% in the peak age group between the ages of 55 and 64 among women (White et al 1999). FMS is more common among females, i.e. 85–90%, and occurs most commonly in the 40–60 age group (Bengtsson et al 1986a, White et al 1999, Wolfe et al 1990).

Pain is the predominant symptom in FMS. Unlike myofascial pain syndrome, a regional pain disorder, the pain in FMS is experienced in widespread locations; about 60–70% of patients complain of 'hurt all over' (Wolfe et al 1990, Yunus et al 1989c, 2000). Stiffness can also be a bothering symptom and is present in most patients. The most common sites of the pain or stiffness symptom in FMS are neck, lower back, hands, knees, shoulder areas, arms, elbows, hips, ankles and feet (Yunus et al 1989c, Yunus & Masi 1993).

Some patients may also have bothersome pain in the chest wall, sometimes as a presenting symptom, with tenderness on palpation by a physician (Mukerji et al 1995, Pellegrino 1990). The pain is constant, but may be aggravated by activities that involve use of the chest wall muscles. The chest pain in these patients may cause great anxiety about having a cardiac or thoracic pain, which should be ruled out by appropriate investigations (if clinically indicated), since FMS may coexist with cardiothoracic pathology.

Pain or stiffness is often aggravated by weather factors, poor sleep, overuse, trauma, mental stress and noise (Campbell et al 1983, Wolfe et al 1990, Yunus et al 1981, 1989c, 2000).

A subset of patients predominantly complain of peripheral arthralgia and present to the physicians with such symptoms (Reilly & Littlejohn 1992). Although tenderness by a physician was not apparently evaluated in this study, our experience has clearly demonstrated that peripheral joints, particularly those in the hands, wrists and feet, may be quite tender on palpation, mimicking an inflammatory arthritis, although objective swelling is absent.

Table 16.1 Symptoms in fibromyalgia syndrome based on several relatively large series of patients seen in rheumatology clinics[a]

Symptoms	% Frequency (mean)[b]	% Frequency (range)
Musculoskeletal		
Pain at multiple sites	100	100
Stiffness	78	76–84
'Hurt all over'	64	60–69
Swollen feeling in soft tissues	47	32–64
Non-musculoskeletal		
Fatigue (most times of the day)	86	75–92
Morning fatigue[c]	78	75–80
Poor sleep[d]	65	56–72
Paraesthesia	54	26–74
Associated symptoms		
Self-assessed anxiety	62	48–72
Headaches	53	44–56
Dysmenorrhoea	43	40–45
Irritable bowel symptoms	40	30–53
Restless legs syndrome	31	
Self-assessed depression	34	31–37
Sicca symptoms	15	12–18
Raynaud's phenomenon	13	9–17
Female urethral syndrome	12	

[a] Adapted from Yunus & Masi (1993), with permission.
[b] Mean values derived from percentage figures reported in multiple studies.
[c] Morning fatigue is a sensitive indicator of non-restorative sleep.
[d] Based on the question 'do you sleep well?' or a similar question.

Other common symptoms of FMS include severe fatigue, sleep difficulties, morning fatigue, paraesthesia and swollen feeling in extremities, as well as several associated features, e.g. headaches, irritable bowel syndrome (IBS), restless legs syndrome, female urethral syndrome and primary dysmenorrhoea (Bengtsson et al 1986a, Wolfe et al 1990, Yunus et al 1981, 1989c, Yunus & Masi 1993, Yunus 1994) (Table 16.1).

Following our initial report that paraesthesia is significantly more common in FMS than in a normal control population (Yunus et al 1981), others have reported that this symptom may be present in as many as 84% of patients with FMS, many having undergone an electrodiagnostic test with normal results in 90% of the cases (Simms & Goldenberg 1988).

FMS has been reported to be associated with several inflammatory diseases, such as rheumatoid arthritis (RA) (Wolfe et al 1984), systemic lupus erythematosus (SLE) (Middleton et al 1994) and Sjögren's syndrome (Bonafede et al 1995). SLE activity was similar between the two groups with and without FMS, but the group with FMS as well as SLE had greater disability (Middleton et al 1994). It is clear that FMS is not 'caused' by these inflammatory conditions, since successful treatment of RA or SLE does not alleviate the symptoms of FMS. The occurrence of FMS in these disorders is much higher than expected, but the actual mechanism of the relationship between FMS and the inflammatory disorders cannot be ascertained from these cross-sectional studies. It is possible that, at least in a subgroup of patients, arthritis or peripheral inflammation acts as a source of continuous nociceptive bombardment that causes central nervous system (CNS) neuroplasticity, causing amplified pain and FMS (see under 'Biopathophysiological mechanism of FMS'). On the other hand, other common factors, such as genetics may also be involved.

Physical examination in FMS shows no joint swelling, but the joints may be quite tender. Range of motion of the neck or other joints may be mildly limited due to pain. However, swelling in the joints may be present due to coexistent arthritis, such as osteoarthritis (OA) or RA.

Despite paraesthesia, neurological examination in FMS is normal. Paraesthesia or swollen feeling is not related to the psychological state of a patient (Yunus et al 1991).

The most remarkable physical finding in FMS is the presence of multiple tender points (TPs) which are reproducible on repeat examination. The large number of TPs differentiates FMS from other musculoskeletal conditions, such as RA, myofascial pain syndrome and OA. Several studies have demonstrated the inter and intra-observer reliability of TPs (Cott et al 1992, Tunks et al 1995). Learning the technique of examination for TPs needs practice, as is the case with mastering any physical finding, e.g. a heart murmur or hepatomegaly. The examiner should use any of the first three fingers to palpate a tender point at an appropriate site (Fig. 16.1) with a moderate digital pressure of 4 kg (roughly the force required to blanch the examining nail when pressed against a hard surface, such as forehead). Elicitation of pain (as contrasted with mere pressure) on palpation at a given site would satisfy the American College of Rheumatology (ACR) criteria for a tender point (Wolfe et al 1990).

It should be remembered that fibromyalgia patients may have TPs at any location, including the so-called control sites (Wolfe et al 1990, Wolfe 1998), and not just among the 18 sites as outlined in the ACR criteria. Skinfold tenderness is also significantly more common in FMS than in other rheumatic diseases (Wolfe et al 1990). Thus, patients with FMS have global hyperalgesia. In many patients, the bones, particularly the tibial shin, are also excessively tender.

The ACR classification criteria of FMS consist of (1) widespread pain for 3 months or longer, and (2) presence of 11 tender points among 18 specified sites (Box 16.1 and Fig. 16.1) (Wolfe et al 1990). Pain in only 3 widespread sites, e.g. left trapezius (left side of the body and above the waist), right leg (right side of the body and below the waist) and neck (axial skeleton) would satisfy the definition of widespread pain in the ACR criteria. However, in clinical practice, pain commonly involves all four limbs as well as the axial skeleton (neck, back or chest wall). In one study, the mean number of sites affected by pain or

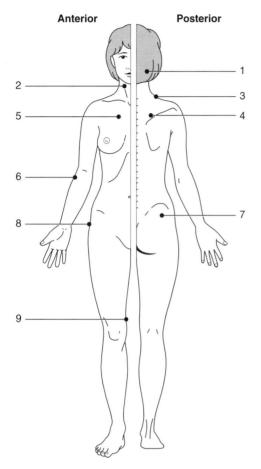

Anterior   **Posterior**

Figure 16.1 Locations of 9 bilateral tender point sites to be palpated for testing American College of Rheumatology criteria for classification of FMS (see Box 16.1 for description). 1, occiput; 2, low cervical; 3, trapezius; 4, supraspinatus; 5, second rib; 6, lateral epicondyle; 7, gluteal; 8, greater trochanter; 9, knee. (Reproduced from Yunus & Masi (1993) with permission.)

stiffness in FMS was 19 as compared with 14 in rheumatoid arthritis (Yunus et al 1989a).

FMS is not a disease or disorder of exclusion and should be diagnosed by its own characteristic features only. Concomitant diseases, such as RA, SLE, Sjögren's syndrome, OA or hypothyroidism, should not influence the diagnosis of FMS, since successful therapy of the treatable diseases, e.g. RA, SLE and hypothyroidism, does not substantially improve the pain or other symptoms of FMS. Co-occurrence of several diseases in the same patient is common in medicine

in general (such as presence of OA and RA in the same patient), and FMS is no exception. Thus, a patient with FMS and RA has two different diseases, and the presence of one does not exclude the diagnosis of the other.

Several diseases may mimic FMS, such as arthritis, polymyalgia rheumatica, hypothyroidism, ankylosing spondylitis, disc herniation and cardiothoracic pain, but none of them have sufficient tender points to satisfy the ACR criteria, and these conditions may be diagnosed by their own characteristic or diagnostic features (Table 16.2). However, it must be remembered that, as stated above, more than one disease may coexist without one causing the other.

Gender differences in FMS have been noted in both community (Wolfe et al 1995b) and rheumatology clinic (Yunus et al 2000) populations. Women, as compared with men, have significantly more fatigue, morning fatigue, irritable bowel symptoms, and a greater number of total symptoms as well as tender points. However, global severity, pain intensity and disability scores were not significantly different between male and female patients.

The clinical characteristics of myofascial pain syndrome (MPS) and FMS overlap. In a study of regional soft tissue pain (RSTP) with tender points, which is likely to be similar to MPS, the frequencies of fatigue, poor sleep, headaches, swollen feeling and paraesthesia were lower in RSTP than in FMS, but higher in RSTP than in normal controls; the total number of TPs was significantly less in RSTP than in FMS (İnanıcı et al 1999). Similar overlap between FMS and RSTP syndrome has been noted by others (Granges & Littlejohn 1993). It has been suggested that MPS and FMS are related syndromes, both clinically and biopathophysiologically (İnanıcı et al 1999, Yunus 1994, Yunus 2000a, 2000b).

BIOPATHOPHYSIOLOGICAL MECHANISMS OF FMS

Although the aetiology or the biopathophysiological mechanisms of FMS are not fully understood, remarkable progress has been made in a

Box 16.1 American College of Rheumatology criteria for classification of fibromyalgia syndrome (from Wolfe et al (1990), with permission)

For classification purposes, patients will be said to have fibromyalgia if both criteria 1 and 2 are satisfied. Widespread pain must have been present for at least 3 months. The presence of a second clinical disorder does not exclude the diagnosis of fibromyalgia.

1. History of widespread pain
   Definition. Pain is considered widespread when all of the following are present: pain in the left side of the body, pain in the right side of the body, pain above the waist, and pain below the waist. In addition, axial skeletal pain (cervical spine or anterior chest or thoracic spine or low back) must be present. In this definition, shoulder and buttock pain is considered as pain for each involved side. 'Low-back' pain is considered lower segment pain.
2. Pain in 11 of 18 tender point sites on digital palpation
   Definition. Pain, on digital palpation, must be present in at least 11 of the following 18 tender point sites:
   Occiput: bilateral, at the suboccipital muscle insertions.
   Low cervical: bilateral, at the anterior aspects of the intertransverse spaces at C5–C7.
   Trapezius: bilateral, at the midpoint of the upper border.
   Supraspinatus: bilateral, at origins, above the scapula spine near the medial border.
   Second rib: bilateral, at the second costochondral junctions, just lateral to the junctions on upper surfaces.
   Lateral epicondyle: bilateral, 2 cm distal to the epicondyles.
   Gluteal: bilateral, in upper outer quadrants of buttocks in anterior fold of muscle.
   Greater trochanter: bilateral, posterior to the trochanteric prominence.
   Knee: bilateral, at the medial fat pad proximal to the joint line.
   Digital palpation should be performed with an approximate force of 4 kg.
   For a tender point to be considered 'positive' the subject must state that the palpation was painful. 'Tender' is not to be considered 'painful'.

Table 16.2 Presenting features of fibromyalgia with confounding diagnosis and key points of differentiation[a]

Presenting features	Confounding diagnosis	Present in confounding disease
Joint pain and subjective swelling	Arthritis	Objective joint swelling
Diffuse muscular aching, stiffness	Polymyalgia rheumatica	$\uparrow$ESR, $\downarrow$Hb, constitutional features
Muscle fatigue, weakness	Myopathy	Objective weakness, $\uparrow$muscle enzymes
Fatigue, sensitivity to cold, muscle pain	Hypothyroidism	$\downarrow T_4$, $\uparrow$TSH
Back pain/stiffness	Ankylosing spondylitis	Sacroiliitis
Sciatica-type pain	Disc herniation	Neurological and radiological findings
Chest pain	Cardiac or pleural pain	Typical history of cardiac pain, pleural rub, ECG, chest film, or laboratory findings of intrathoracic disease

[a] From Yunus & Masi (1993), with permission.
ESR, erythrocyte sedimentation rate; Hb, haemoglobin; T_4, thyroxine; TSH, thyroid-stimulating hormone; ECG, electrocardiogram; $\uparrow$, elevated; $\downarrow$, decreased.

better understanding of this painful and disabling condition since the first controlled clinical description of FMS in 1981 (Yunus et al 1981). It is now clear that FMS has a multifactorial aetiology and pathogenesis, and different aetiology or biopathophysiological mechanisms may be involved in different subgroups.

Because of pain and tenderness in muscles, earlier studies focused on muscle pathology. However, careful, controlled studies have failed to show significant differences between patients and controls in either histopathology or muscle metabolism (Simms 1998, Yunus et al 1989a), or immunochemical and molecular studies of substance P (SP) or serotonin (Sprott et al 1998). Two fine reviews have addressed the issues of muscle abnormalities in FMS (Simms 1998, Olsen & Park, 1998). Blinded and controlled muscle biopsy studies have shown normal histopathology (Yunus et al 1989a).

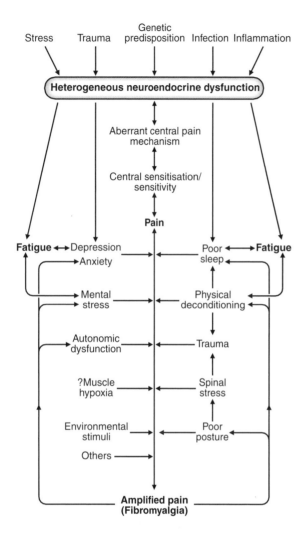

Figure 16.2 A schematic representation of the proposed model for biophysiological mechanisms of FMS showing multiple factors that interact to amplify pain. The primary problem is currently believed to be in the 'box', i.e. a heterogeneous neuroendocrine dysfunction, leading to central sensitisation or sensitivity. (Adapted from Yunus (1994), with permission.)

It was earlier reported that there is a decreased level of adenosine triphosphate (ATP), adenosine diphosphate (ADP), adenosine monophosphate (AMP) and phosphocreatin (PCr) in the muscles of fibromyalgia patients (Bengtsson et al 1986b). Using P-31 magnetic resonance spectroscopy (MRS), Park and associates (1998) found signifi-

cantly decreased levels of PCr and ATP, as compared with normal controls, both at rest and during exercise. However, it is unknown if the controls and the patients were satisfactorily matched in their aerobic fitness. When carefully matched controls with similar aerobic fitness status, as measured by maximal oxygen uptake (VO_2 max), were included in a dynamic study using MRS by Simms and associates (1994), no significant differences were found in the measurements of high-energy phosphate metabolites, PCr and inorganic phosphate between the patients and the controls. By another MRS study, the phosphodiester (PDE) peaks were found to be increased in FMS (Jubrias et al 1994), but this could not be confirmed by other studies (Simms & Hrovat 1995, Simms 1998).

Moreover, multiphase skeletal scintigraphy did not demonstrate subclinical synovitis or indication of inflammation in the soft tissues (Yunus et al 1989b).

An absence of peripheral pathology and a presence of widespread, global tissue hyperalgesia suggested a central mechanism for FMS. Patients with FMS also have allodynia (pain on non-nociceptive stimulus, such as touch), another pointer towards a central mechanism. An aberrant central pain mechanism for FMS has been suggested (Yunus 1992).

Various interacting factors that may cause modulation and amplification of pain leading to fibromyalgia are shown in Figure 16.2, as will be elaborated later. It now seems that the hallmark of diffuse, severe and widespread pain in FMS is an aberrant pain processing at the spinal cord and supraspinal levels.

Substantial evidence has accumulated in recent years that the aberrant central pain mechanism in FMS involves central sensitisation or central sensitivity, as reviewed by Bennett (1999). In the following paragraphs, we will first describe the concept of central sensitisation, provide evidence for it in FMS, and then discuss other neurochemical or neurohormonal perturbations, followed by a discussion of other contributory factors, e.g. non-restorative sleep, psychological distress and environmental modulation. The probable role of genetics, trauma, peripheral inflammation and infections (Fig. 16.2) will also be described.

The concept of central sensitisation

Central sensitisation may be defined as hyperexcitability of the CNS neurons in response to peripheral noxious stimuli, leading to an exaggerated response to a normally painful stimulus (hyperalgesia) and a response of pain following a normally non-nociceptive stimulus, e.g. touch or rubbing (allodynia). Additionally, there is an increased duration of response following a brief stimulus (persistent pain). Animal models have been of great help in understanding the underlying pathophysiological mechanisms of this phenomenon (Coderre et al 1993, Devor 1988, Dubner & Ruda 1992). Following a nociceptive stimulus at the peripheral tissue, either by inflammation (Coderre et al 1993) or nerve injury (Devor 1988, Woolf 1983), a barrage of afferent impulses travel via the C fibres to the dorsal horn with remarkable changes at the synapse and the second order neurons, both in the spinal cord and in supraspinal structures.

Release of substance P at the synapse removes the magnesium block of the N-methyl-D-aspartate (NMDA) receptor channel and allows excitatory amino acids (EAA), e.g. glutamate and aspartate, to activate postsynaptic NMDA receptors. This induces various intracellular and membrane changes, including influx of calcium, activation of second messengers, expression of c-*fos* and alteration of cell membrane permeability (Coderre et al 1993). Besides EAA and substance P, several C-fibre neuropeptides, e.g. neurokinin A, calcitonin gene-related peptide (CGRP), galanin, somatostatin, cholecystokinin and vasoactive intestinal polypeptide, are also involved at the dorsal horn in causing the cellular changes mentioned above (Besson 1999, Coderre et al 1993). The end results of such excessive stimulation at the dorsal horn are striking functional changes in the secondary neurons, including sustained hyperexcitability and sensitivity, amplification of peripheral afferent impulses, expansion of receptive field and 'windup' phenomenon (see below). Supraspinal input is also dynamically involved on an ongoing basis in modulation of the final pain perception, through both inhibition and facilitation (Lima 1998).

Wind-up phenomenon is characterised by a *progressive* increase in the magnitude of response of secondary neurons at the dorsal horn following brief but repeated stimuli of the C fibres, so that responses increase with each repeated stimulus (Woolf & Thompson 1991). This phenomenon is mediated by NMDA receptors and attenuated by NMDA receptor antagonists (Ren 1994). Analogous to 'wind-up' in animals, 'temporal summation' has been observed in humans (Price et al 1994). Human volunteers were subjected to trains of electric shock at a frequency of 1 shock/1.67 second, following which it was observed that the second pain progressively increased. Interestingly, temporal summation was significantly decreased by administration of dextromethorphan, an NMDA receptor antagonist (Price et al 1994).

Evidence for central sensitisation or central sensitivity in FMS

Unlike the animal model wherein central sensitisation is explicable on the basis of a strong peripheral afferent stimulus, i.e. inflammation or nerve injury, as mentioned earlier, such examples of peripheral nociceptive stimulus are not always evident in FMS. One example of an inflammatory stimulus in FMS is peripheral trauma, such as a road accident. FMS following a viral (or bacterial) infection is probably mediated by cytokine-induced nociception at the peripheral tissues, although such an infection may have central neurohormonal effects. FMS also follows an inflammatory arthritis, such as SLE and RA (Middleton et al 1994, Wolfe et al 1984). Even in cases where an obvious source of peripheral nociception is absent, it is likely that the mechanical stress at the cervical and lumbar spine, either because of poor posture, trauma or degenerative changes, may provide a continuous source of noxious stimulus.

It is equally plausible that the central nervous system remains hyperexcitable and hypersensitive in FMS following an initial noxious input at the periphery, irrespective of an ongoing stimulus. Such a model has been suggested in FMS (Kramis et al 1996). This model suggests that, because of an ongoing or ceased inflammation at the peripheral tissues, non-nociceptive fibres, i.e. A-beta fibres, now produce pain on stimulation because of sensitisation of the wide dynamic range neurons at the spinal cord, where these fibres converge along with the nociceptive neurons. In fact, there is evidence from animal studies that the CNS neuroplasticity is sustained even after cessation of inflammation in the peripheral tissues (Coderre et al 1993).

However, we think that there is a possibility of an *intrinsic* central sensitisation in FMS in certain susceptible individuals (central sensitivity as opposed to central sensitisation), even without a peripheral nociceptive stimulus. This may occur because of either a defective inhibitory system or a hyperstimulated facilitatory pathway; a generalised hyperexcitement of peripheral nociceptors may possibly be an additional element. All these factors need to be investigated.

Irrespective of the mechanisms, convincing evidence has accumulated that central sensitisation or central sensitivity is operative in FMS. Related to the concept of central sensitisation in FMS is the fact that other mechanisms of central origin may also be present in FMS. Thus, cognitive functions may influence central sensitivity and hormonal factors may interact with the CNS to further modulate pain.

Granges and Littlejohn (1993) compared 60 patients with FMS, 60 with regional pain syndromes (RPS) and 60 pain-free normal controls. Compared with normal controls and RPS, patients with FMS had significantly greater and more diffuse pain on examination by an algometer, with a strong correlation between the sites of 18 tender points and the control sites. The authors concluded that the pain mechanisms in FMS include a generalised effect on the pain system, reminiscent of central sensitisation or sensitivity. Arroyo & Cohen (1993) studied pain tolerance and perception threshold in 10 patients with FMS and 10 pain-free healthy controls in response to a non-noxious electrocutaneous

stimulation. They found marked and significant reduction in pain tolerance among the patients, which was accompanied by spread and persistence of dysaesthesia – all suggesting a centralisation of peripheral stimulus. The aberrant central pain mechanism in FMS is suggested by another study in which the investigators evaluated stimulus–response function for pressure versus pain in the muscles of 25 women with FMS and 25 female pain-free healthy controls (Bendtsen et al 1997). The muscles of patients with FMS were significantly more tender. Additionally, in contrast with the findings among the controls, stimulus–response function curve among the patients was linear, suggesting a qualitative difference between patients and controls. These findings would suggest a qualitatively different pain in FMS, most likely modulated by a central mechanism. Temporal summation and hyperexcitability have also been demonstrated by repeated electrical stimuli in muscles in FMS (Sorensen et al 1998).

The important role of NMDA receptors in the central pain mechanism of fibromyalgia was demonstrated by a double-blind placebo-controlled test of ketamine versus isotonic saline, administered by intravenous infusion. Following the infusion, ketamine, a non-competitive NMDA receptor antagonist, showed significant reduction of pain intensity as compared with isotonic saline (Sorensen et al 1995).

Kosek & Hansson (1997) investigated 10 patients with FMS and 10 normal healthy controls to assess somatosensory perception from vibration and heterotropic noxious conditioning stimulation (HNCS). HNCS, induced by such methods as noxious heat, noxious cold and submaximal effort tourniquet test, causes potent and widespread, but selective, inhibition of wide dynamic range (WDR) neurons in the dorsal horn of the spinal cord by a mechanism that has been called 'diffuse noxious inhibitory control' (DNIC). Whereas the response to vibratory stimulation (a local increase in pressure pain threshold) was similar in controls and patients, patients with FMS showed an abnormal response to HNCS with the upper extremity tourniquet test. While the controls showed an increased pressure pain threshold, patients with FMS failed to demonstrate such an augmented pressure pain threshold, suggesting an abnormal, central endogenous inhibitory control in fibromyalgia. Additionally, this study (Kosek & Hansson 1997) documented an increased sensitivity to pressure, heat and non-painful cold stimuli among the FMS patients, as compared with the controls.

Studies of cerebral event-related potentials also support a central abnormal sensory processing of pain in FMS. Electroencephalographic waveform changes in the brain following peripheral stimulus provide an index of CNS activation (Gibson et al 1994). Following a painful carbon dioxide stimulation, patients with FMS showed a significant increase in the peak-to-peak amplitude of cerebral potential at pain threshold intensity, as compared with normal controls, but the increase was even greater relative to controls at suprathreshold intensity. This cerebral nociceptive-evoked response (NER) suggests a greater activation of CNS pathways following a noxious stimulus at the periphery in fibromyalgia patients. It has been proposed that the NER represents a physiological correlate of global integration CNS processing of pain perception (Carmon et al 1980, Bromm & Treede 1991). Gibson et al (1994) also demonstrated in their study that the thermal pain threshold is also significantly decreased in FMS compared with controls, apart from the well-established reduced mechanical pain threshold; there was a strong correlation between these two pain modalities. This would suggest that the abnormal pain threshold in FMS is multimodal.

In another controlled study of somatosensory evoked potential in the brain following hand stimulation, Lorenz and associates (1996) demonstrated that patients with FMS had significantly higher amplitudes of laser evoked potential (LEP) in the middle latency N1 (N 170) and the late positivity P2 (P 390) components. An enlargement of the amplitude in the N1 component may indicate an increased nociceptive activation by radiant heat and neuronal synchronisation of the somatosensory cortex. The P2 enlargement may suggest a greater attention or

cognitive integration. Moreover, the distribution of N 170 was broader over the central, vertex and fronto-central leads, in contrast with the healthy controls in whom N 170 was fairly restricted to central and mid-temporal positions, on the contralateral side, suggesting that the nociceptive response in the brain of fibromyalgia patients is widespread, beyond the stimulated hand area. Effects of interspersed auditory stimulus showed that general vigilance was not a factor in the difference for the observed LEP effects. Lorenz and colleagues (1996) also confirmed the hyperalgesic effect of heat in FMS.

Brain functions have been studied by single-photon-emission computed tomography (SPECT) in FMS (Mountz et al 1995), showing that there is decreased regional cerebral blood flow in the thalamus and caudate nucleus (which modulate pain perception) compared with normal controls.

Autonomic nervous system dysfunction

Several studies have demonstrated a disturbance of the autonomic nervous system in FMS. Martinez-Lavin and associates (1997) studied sympathetic–parasympathetic balance in 19 patients with FMS and 19 normal controls by assessing heart rate variability using a high resolution electrocardiogram in both supine and standing positions. Power spectral analysis of heart rate fluctuation provides a quantitative beat-to-beat control of cardiovascular functioning, and such variability around the mean heart rate is a function of the autonomic nervous system. Three components can be identified in a spectrum, i.e. very low frequency, low frequency and high frequency. The low frequency component, when expressed in normalised units, represents the sympathetic function, whereas the high frequency component is contributed mostly by the efferent vagal activity. Results showed significant differences between the patients and the controls in the low frequency band of power spectral analysis after assuming an upright posture, suggesting a deranged sympathetic function.

In another controlled study of autonomic functions, 30 patients with FMS and 30 normal controls were evaluated by 24-hour ambulatory recording of heart rate variability and a power spectral analysis for an assessment of sympatho/vagal balance (Martinez-Lavin et al 1998). FMS patients were found to have decreased accumulated 24-hour heart rate variability and they had lost their circadian variation of sympatho/vagal balance. The diminished 24-hour heart rate variability was accounted for by an increased nocturnal predominance of the low frequency component in the spectral analysis band, suggesting an exaggerated sympathetic modulation of the sinus node. An excessive nocturnal sympathetic activity has been correlated with sleep arousal (Bonnet & Arand 1997), suggesting that a nocturnal sympathetic hyperactivity may contribute to non-restorative sleep and fatigue among fibromyalgia patients.

It has been suggested (Martinez-Lavin et al 1998) that this relentless circadian sympathetic hyperactivity may explain diminished sympathetic response to several forms of stress, such as orthostatic challenge (Martinez-Lavin et al 1997), cold water immersion and acoustic stimulation (Vaeroy et al 1989), as well as exercise (Van Denderen et al 1992), because of a lack of additional sympathetic response to stress. In this context, it is of interest that plasma neuropeptide Y (NPY) is decreased in FMS (Crofford et al 1994). In the sympathetic nervous system, NPY co-localises with noradrenaline (norepinephrine), and a decreased NPY level may represent a diminished sympathoadrenal output (Lundberg et al 1990).

A recent study has shown an exaggerated response of noradrenaline (norepinephrine) to interleukin-6 (IL-6), suggesting an abnormal regulation of the sympathetic nervous system, perhaps secondary to chronic corticotrophin-releasing hormone (CRH) (Torpy et al 2000).

Plasma and urinary catecholamine levels were found to be normal in one study (Yunus et al 1992a), but these parameters may not be a sensitive indicator of sympathetic activity in chronic conditions. Various neurosensory abnormalities in FMS are shown in Box 16.2.

Neurotransmitter/neurochemical dysfunction

Recognising the role of substance P (SP) in pain transmission in FMS, Vaeroy and his associates were the first to measure this neuropeptide in the cerebrospinal fluid (CSF), showing that there was a three-fold elevation in FMS compared with healthy controls (Vaeroy et al 1988a). This finding of increased SP in the CSF of FMS patients has now been confirmed by other independent studies (Bradley at al 1996, Russell et al 1994, Welin et al 1995). There were no significant gender differences in SP, nor was there any correlation between SP level and depression (Russell et al 1994). A related interesting finding is an elevated level of nerve growth factor (NGF) in the CSF of patients with FMS (Giovengo et al 1999); NGF has been shown to promote the growth of SP-containing neurons (Donnerer et al 1992).

The status of CGRP, which co-localises with SP in the afferent neurons, is unknown in FMS. No controlled studies have been published. Russell states that his group did not observe a significant difference between FMS patients and controls in the cerebrospinal fluid CGRP level (Russell 1998).

Among the neurotransmitters involved in pain inhibition, both serotonin and its precursor amino acid, tryptophan, as well as noradrenaline (norepinephrine) and beta-endorphin have been studied in FMS. Serum serotonin level has been found to be low in several controlled studies (Hrycaj et al 1993, Russell et al 1992a). The low serum serotonin level may be attributed to their low levels in the peripheral platelets (Russell 1998).

5-Hydroxyindole acetic acid (5-HIAA), the metabolic product of serotonin, was also found to be low in the CSF of fibromyalgia patients, as compared to normal controls (Houvenagel et al 1990, Russell et al 1992b). Also, 5-HIAA was found to be significantly low in the 24-hour urine of patients with FMS, as compared with controls (Kang et al 1998). Russell et al (1992a) also reported a lower level of 3-methoxy-4-hydroxyphenethylene glycol (MHPG), a metabolite of noradrenaline (norepinephrine), and of homovanillic acid (HVA), a product of dopamine. However, the number of subjects

---

Box 16.2 Neurosensory abnormalities in fibromyalgia syndrome

- Greater and more diffuse pain on mechanical pressure compared with pain-free healthy controls
- Marked reduction of pain tolerance by a non-noxious electrocutaneous stimulation, accompanied by spread and persistence of dysaesthesia
- Qualitatively different pain in muscles by stimulus–response function for pressure versus pain
- Temporal summation and hyperexcitability
- Abnormal central endogenous inhibitory control by noxious stimuli
- Abnormal cerebral somatosensory evoked potentials following a painful peripheral stimulus, suggesting increased central nociceptive activation
- Decreased regional cerebral blood flow in the thalamus and caudate nucleus (which modulate pain) by single-photon-emission tomography (SPECT)
- Deranged sympathetic function by power spectral analysis of heart rate variability
- Exaggerated nocturnal sympathetic activity by spectral analysis of heart rate variability
- Exaggerated response of noradrenaline (norepinephrine) to interleukin-6

---

investigated in this study was rather small, and further studies are indicated.

Low serum tryptophan has been reported by Russell and colleagues (1989). In our study (Yunus et al 1992b), the low serum tryptophan level showed a trend towards significance, but the transport ratio of tryptophan was significantly low, suggesting a decreased brain entry of this amino acid.

The results of ^{3}H-imipramine binding (IB) on platelets, a biochemical indicator of serotonin uptake, were found to be discordant in two studies. Kravitz and colleagues (1992) found a normal binding among 10 non-depressed female patients with FMS, as compared with 10 normal controls. However, IB among the female patients with FMS was significantly lower than that in 6 depressed women. In fact, the findings in FMS and depression were in the opposite direction. Russell and associates (1992b), on the other hand, found a significantly higher imipramine binding among FMS patients compared with healthy controls. Small sample size, patient selection and methodological differences may account for such discrepant results. Further studies in this area are indicated.

With regard to the noradrenaline (norepinephrine) status, decreased MHPG level in CSF (Russell et al 1992a), decreased serum NPY level (Crofford et al 1994), and normal plasma and urinary catecholamine levels (Yunus et al 1992a) have been reported, as mentioned before. However,

there seems to be a sympathetic overactivity during the night, as measured by power spectral analysis of 24-hour heart rate variability, which has been proposed to partially explain the overall diminished sympathetic functions in FMS, as explained above (Martinez-Lavin et al 1998). The sympathetic function is diminished in response to various stimuli, such as cold pressor test, acoustic stimulation and physical exercise, as described under 'Autonomic nervous system dysfunction' above.

So far, investigations of the opioid peptides in FMS have not provided fruitful results. Beta-endorphin levels were found to be normal both in serum (Yunus et al 1986) and CSF (Vaeroy et al 1988b). Since the opioid peptides include enkephalin and pro-dynorphin peptides besides the beta-endorphin, it was important to study these two other peptides. Vaeroy and his collaborators (1991) measured CSF levels of met-enkephalin-arg^6-phe^7, a marker for pro-enkephalin, as well as dynorphin A, the marker for pro-dynorphin. Their results showed that both of these markers for pro-enkephalin and pro-dynorphin, respectively, were elevated, rather than decreased. These combined findings suggest the opioid peptides are unlikely to be involved directly in pain modulation in FMS. In keeping with these observations, Sorensen and colleagues (1995) had noted that neither pain intensity nor the number of tender points improved following intravenous infusion of morphine in a double-blind placebo-controlled test. However, it is possible that the CSF levels of opioid peptides do not necessarily reflect the opioid status in the brain.

Yunus and his associates (1995) investigated the possibility that a combination of biochemical variables (e.g. plasma amino acids and catecholamines) would better classify FMS than either of them alone. Plasma amino acids and plasma catecholamines, as well as urinary catecholamines, from 29 patients with FMS and 30 pain-free controls were subjected to discriminant analysis, yielding seven variables (plasma histidine, methionine, tryptophan, noradrenaline (norepinephrine), isoleucine and leucine, and urinary dopamine) with a sensitivity of 86% and specificity of 77%. Correlation of the discriminant scores showed a significant ($P < 0.001$) relationship with pain severity, fatigue, poor sleep and total tender points. These findings suggest an important new concept that biophysiological mechanisms involved in FMS symptoms may involve more than one chemical or mechanism which are likely to operate synergistically in producing symptoms. However, this study (Yunus et al 1995) included a large number of variables for the discriminant analysis in a relatively few patients, and the results should be interpreted with caution. This tantalising concept of a biophysiological mechanism in FMS involving several synergetic mechanisms needs to be studied further with a larger number of subjects. Neurochemical dysfunctions in FMS are shown in Box 16.3.

Neuroendocrine aberrations

Several studies have documented a perturbation of the hypothalamic-pituitary-adrenal (HPA) axis. A decreased 24-hour urinary free cortisol level in FMS, as compared with normal controls (Crofford et al 1994, Griep et al 1998), as well as patients with rheumatoid arthritis (McCain & Tilbe 1989) has been reported by several investigators. A loss of normal diurnal cortisol fluctuation has been noted, with elevated evening (trough) cortisol level (Crofford et al 1994, McCain & Tilbe 1989). Griep et al (1993, 1998)

have consistently found an exaggerated adrenocorticotrophin hormone (ACTH) response to corticotrophin-releasing hormone (CRH), compared with healthy normal controls, with similar cortisol response between the two groups, which suggested a relative hypocortisolaemia to elevated ACTH in FMS. While basal total plasma cortisol level was decreased, free cortisol level was normal. This would suggest a resistance of glucocorticoid feedback in FMS, since a normal free cortisol level would restrain exaggerated ACTH response to CRH. The cause of exaggerated ACTH response to CRH is speculative.

It seems highly unlikely that there is a primary hypofunction of the adrenal cortex, since the cortisol response to ACTH stimulation was normal (Griep et al 1998). A central mechanism is the most plausible explanation (Crofford & Demitrack 1996, Griep et al 1993, 1998), but the actual nature of such a mechanism is unknown at this time. It has been suggested that there is a central deficiency of CRH and this may be due to multiple factors, such as a perturbation of serotonin or serotonin receptors, glucocorticoid receptors in different areas of the brain, and of the locus coeruleus–noradrenaline (norepinephrine) sympathetic system (Crofford & Demitrack 1996). In fact, a recent study has shown delayed ACTH release after subcutaneous injection of IL-6 (which stimulates hypothalamic release of CRH), suggesting a defect in the hypothalamic CRH neuronal functioning (Torpy et al 2000).

It is clear, however, that the pattern of HPA axis dysfunction in FMS is different from that noted in depression (Lentjes et al 1997). Patients with depression have hyperactivity of the HPA axis in all its components, including an excessive hypothalamic CRH mRNA expression (Raadsheer 1994), an elevated CRH in the CSF (Banki et al 1987, Nemeroff et al 1984), a blunted response of ACTH to CRH administration (Amsterdam et al 1987, Gold et al 1986, Holsboer et al 1984) and a typical hypercortisolaemia that escape dexamethasone suppression (Schatzberg et al 1983). In another study (Maes et al 1998), 24-hour urinary cortisol level was significantly increased in depression, but not in FMS; the difference between fibromyalgia and depression

---

Box 16.3 Neurochemical findings in fibromyalgia syndrome

- Elevated substance P in the cerebrospinal fluid (CSF)
- Decreased serum serotonin level
- Decreased 5-HIAA (metabolite of serotonin) in the CSF
- Decreased 5-HIAA in 24-hour urine
- Low serum tryptophan and low transport ratio of tryptophan
- ^{3}H-imipramine binding on platelets: both normal and increased by two different studies
- Low MHPG (metabolite of noradrenaline (norepinephrine)) in CSF
- Low HVA (metabolite of dopamine) in CSF
- Decreased neuropeptide Y
- Normal pro-enkephalin and pro-dynorphin markers in CSF

---

was highly significant ($P < 0.0002$). Also, in contrast to FMS where glucocorticoid receptors on the lymphocytes have been reported to be normal (Lentjes et al 1997), the number of these receptors is low in depression (Gormley et al 1985, Whalley et al 1986).

Using a different approach, where hypoglycaemia was carefully titrated by using clamps, Adler et al (1999) found reduced ACTH secretion with a normal cortisol response and decreased adrenaline (epinephrine) response among 15 premenopausal women with fibromyalgia and 13 healthy controls. In addition, graded ACTH infusion demonstrated similar cortisol response among patients and controls. Because of the different methodology for inducing hypoglycaemia, the results of this study are not directly comparable to those reported earlier by Griep et al (1993).

Thyroid functions were assessed in 13 patients with FMS and 10 healthy pain-free controls by intravenous injection of thryrotrophin-releasing hormone (TRH) (Neeck & Riedel 1992). While basal thyroid hormone levels were normal, the thyrotrophin or thyroid-stimulating hormone (TSH) as well as thyroid hormone responses in patients with FMS were significantly lower than in controls, whereas the prolactin response was increased in the patients compared with controls. Interestingly, total and free serum calcium as well as calcitonin levels were also significantly decreased among the patients, while the parathyroid hormone (PTH) level was normal. An earlier study had also found a blunted response of TSH with an exaggerated response of prolactin

in response to TRH stimulation in a subgroup of patients with FMS, compared with those with rheumatoid arthritis and low-back pain (Ferraccioli et al 1990). The significance of the blunted response of TSH and of serum T_4 and T_3 to TRH stimulation in FMS remains unknown. Further studies with a larger sample will be useful.

The initial report of a highly significant decrease in insulin-like growth factor-1 (IGF-1), reflecting an integrated secretion of growth hormone (GH), in patients with FMS (Bennett et al 1992) has been subsequently confirmed by the same group of authors employing a larger sample and other rheumatic diseases as controls (Bennett et al 1997), as well as others (Ferraccioli et al 1994), although two other studies employing a small number of patients with FMS did not find a significant difference between patients and controls (Bagge et al 1998, Jacobsen et al 1995). However, a direct measurement of GH has shown a significantly lower level of this hormone than in controls (Bennett et al 1997, Griep et al 1994, Leal-Cerro et al 1999).

Stimulation tests of GH, however, have yielded varying results. In the study by Bennett et al, GH level did not rise following administration of clonidine and L-dopa (both of which normally induce GH secretion by inhibiting hypothalamic somatostatin secretion via alpha-2-adrenergic and dopamine receptors, respectively), whereas a marked and statistically significant increase in GH secretion was found by Griep at al (1994) following hypoglycaemic challenge, suggesting a highly reactive pituitary gland, similar to an exaggerated ACTH secretion secondary to CRH administration as mentioned above (Griep et al 1998). The decreased basal GH level, measured every 20 minutes over a 24-hour period, as reported by Leal-Cerro and colleagues, showed a normal pituitary response to GH-releasing hormone (GHRH), similar to the normal controls. The difference between several investigators with regard to GH secretion following stimulation tests may partly be due to the different stimulating agents used, and perhaps other methodological differences.

GH release involves complex mechanisms involving serotonin, adrenaline (epinephrine), dopamine and alpha-2 noradrenaline as well as gamma-aminobutyric acid (GABA). Many other factors may also influence GH secretion, e.g., exercise, nutritional status, hypoglycaemia, excitement, pain and some drugs (Thorner et al 1998). In their carefully conducted study with an appropriate best-subsets linear regression analysis, Bennett et al (1997) excluded the effects of depression, tricyclic medications, non-steroidal anti-inflammatory medications and obesity on their measured IGF-1 levels.

Although GH deficiency may cause muscle weakness, decreased exercise tolerance and diminished vitality, a correlation of these symptoms in FMS with GH level has not been consistently demonstrated, raising the possibility that a low GH level in FMS may be a secondary phenomenon. In fact, no correlation between pain and low IGF-1 level was found (Bennett et al 1997). Interestingly, however, a double-blind controlled study showed a beneficial effect of subcutaneous injection of GH on overall well-being, functional capacities and number of tender points in a subgroup of patients with significantly low IGF-1 level (Bennett et al 1998).

The mechanism or significance of low GH in FMS remains unclear at this time. Much of the GH is secreted during stage 3 and 4 sleep, which is known to be disturbed in FMS (Moldofsky et al 1975). Also it has been suggested that the low GH level in FMS may be due to a low adrenergic stimulation of the GH axis (Pillemer et al 1997).

Taking all the evidence together, including the dysfunctional HPA axis, it seems likely that the GH deficiency in FMS is central in origin (Griep et al 1994).

Given that FMS is much more common in women than men, appropriate studies of the gonadal steroids in FMS are surprisingly absent in the literature. A brief report of plasma levels of various sex hormones, employing only 10 female patients and 21 controls, showed that only one of the 12 variables (including 10 sex hormones) measured was abnormal. Plasma testosterone level was significantly ($P = 0.01$) higher in FMS than controls. Because of multiple comparisons in a small sample of patients, its significance or reliability remains questionable. Among other hormones measured, plasma oestrone, oestradiol, progesterone, dehydrotestosterone, dehydroepiendrosterone (DHE) and DHE sulphate (DHEAS), follicle-stimulating hormone (FSH) and luteinising hormone (LH) were all normal (Carette et al 1992). Clearly further studies are needed in this important area.

Of three studies reporting on nocturnal secretion of melatonin, two found levels to be normal or elevated, whereas the third showed a decreased nocturnal secretion. Press and colleagues (1998) measured nocturnal urinary melatonin levels from 10 p.m. to 7 a.m. and found them to be similar to those in the controls. In another study, blood was collected every 10 minutes over a 24-hour period for measurement of melatonin among 9 patients with FMS, 8 with chronic fatigue syndrome (CFS) and healthy controls matched for age and menstrual cycle phase. The nocturnal melatonin level was found to be significantly higher among patients with FMS, compared with controls, but the results were not significantly different between CFS patients and the control subjects (Korszun et al 1999). Wikner et al (1998) measured serum melatonin level every 2 hours between 6 p.m. and 8 a.m., and collected urine between 10 p.m. and 7 a.m. for measurement of melatonin in 8 patients and 8 healthy controls, and found that the secretion of melatonin during the dark hours and the peak serum melatonin levels were significantly lower in patients than controls; a tendency towards lower urinary melatonin was also observed. Additionally, these investigators measured serum cortisol, serum TSH and serum ionised calcium and found them to be normal. Overall, melatonin levels seem unremarkable in FMS, given the balance of evidence at this time. Neurohormonal findings in FMS are shown in Box 16.4.

Non-restorative sleep

From many clinical studies, it is clear that sleep difficulties and morning fatigue are common in FMS (Bengtsson et al 1986a, Hyyppa & Kronholm 1995, Wolfe et al 1990, Yunus et al 1981, 1989c). Beginning with the original polysomnographic studies by Moldofsky and colleagues (1975), several objective findings by sleep electroencephalographic (EEG) studies have been documented in FMS as compared with healthy controls. These findings include an increased amount of stage 1 alpha waves (representing arousal), decreased delta waves in stages 3 and 4 (representing restorative sleep), intrusion of alpha waves into the slow delta waves (also called alpha-delta EEG anomaly), decreased total sleep time, higher number of arousals and awakenings (Branco et al 1994, Drewes et al 1995a, 1995b, Perlis et al 1997). A significantly higher number of miniarousals per hour was found among 7 patients with FMS as compared with 6 controls in another study, without any occult sleep apnoea (Molony et al 1986).

However, not all investigators found striking differences between patients with FMS and controls (Horne & Shackell 1991, Jennum et al 1993). Available data should also be interpreted with some caution, because of a relatively small sample of patients in most reports. Moreover, alpha-delta sleep anomaly is not specific for FMS, since patients with rheumatoid arthritis may exhibit the same abnormalities (Moldofsky et al 1983). Carette and associates in a careful study found that only 36% of 22 patients with FMS had alpha-delta anomaly, and this EEG finding did not correlate with disease severity, nor was it affected by amitriptyline treatment (Carette et al 1995). However, other investigators found a beneficial effect of this drug in significantly reducing the alpha-delta wave sleep and improving the non-restorative sleep in 5 patients with FMS (Watson et al 1985). Moreover, controlled clinical trials have shown a beneficial effect of amitriptyline in subjective improvement of sleep quality (Carette at al 1986, Goldenberg et al 1986).

From an observational point of view, there is a relationship between poor sleep and pain intensity as well as attention to pain. Non-restorative sleep in the previous night predicts pain the next day among fibromyalgia patients, which, in turn, is followed by a poor night's sleep (Affleck et al 1996).

It is important to recognise that while non-restorative sleep is an important component of biophysiological mechanisms in FMS, such sleep disturbance is not essential for causation for this disorder. A subgroup of FMS patients do not have sleep difficulties either clinically or by sleep EEG studies. It is also of interest that in a study

---

Box 16.4   Endocrine findings in fibromyalgia syndrome

- Decreased 24-hour urine free cortisol
- Loss of normal diurnal fluctuation of cortisol
- Exaggerated ACTH response to both CRH and hypoglycaemia
- Low total basal plasma cortisol with normal basal free cortisol
- Normal cortisol response to ACTH challenge
- Delayed ACTH release after interleukin-6 administration
- Decreased response of thyroid hormones and TSH to TRH
- Decreased insulin-like growth factor-1 (IGF-1)
- Decreased growth hormone (GH)
- GH response to stimulation studies: both normal and increased in several studies using different agents for stimulation
- Normal nocturnal secretion of melatonin in majority of studies

of 30 patients with sleep apnoea, only 1 patient (3%) had fibromyalgia (Lario et al 1992), and in another study of 108 consecutive patients who had attended a respiratory sleep disorder clinic, only 3 (2.7%) fulfilled the criteria for FMS (Donald et al 1996). Sleep problems in FMS have been well reviewed by Harding (1998).

Additionally, improvement of sleep quality does not necessarily ameliorate pain in these patients (Drewes et al 1991, Moldofsky et al 1996). However, sleep problems must be addressed for a satisfactory management of FMS (see Ch. 17).

Psychological factors

Psychological factors are an important determinant of pain in any disease, irrespective of the disease, and fibromyalgia is no exception. Psychological distress in FMS is characterised by anxiety, depression, mental stress and poor coping skills in a subgroup of patients. Moreover, the frequencies of psychiatric diagnoses are similar to those in other chronic diseases, such as RA, in most studies (Yunus 1994). However, there is a great deal of variability among patients, as reviewed by Yunus (1994), and psychological factors are not necessary for causing FMS (Ahles et al 1991, Campbell et al 1983, Kirmayer et al 1988, Yunus 1994).

Using the National Institute of Mental Health Diagnostic Interview Schedule (DIS), based on the *Diagnostic and Statistical Manual of Mental Disorders III* (DSM III), Hudson et al (1985) found that current major depression was present in 26% of 31 FMS patients compared with none of 14 patients with RA ($P < 0.04$), and that onset of depression preceded FMS in 64%. There was a lifetime history of depression in 71%, compared with 14% in RA. A major criticism of this study by Hudson and his group, which has been overlooked by many reviewers, is that the number of RA patients used as controls is quite small ($N = 14$), raising questions about the reliability of some of its findings. Alfici and associates (1989) also found that depression and obsessive-compulsive traits were significantly more common in FMS than RA. However, other studies using DSM III criteria found no significant difference

in depression or other psychiatric diagnoses between patients with FMS and those with RA (Ahles et al 1991, Kirmayer at al 1988). The study by Ahles and his colleagues (1991), which found major depression in 34% of FMS patients, as compared with 39% of patients with RA, is the only one in the literature that was conducted in a blinded manner.

Significantly increased anxiety disorders were found in the studies of Alfici and associates (1989) and Hudson and colleagues (1985), but not in other studies using either validated questionnaire instruments or DSM criteria.

A good number of investigations have utilised validated questionnaires for evaluation of psychological symptoms and mental stress in FMS, showing no significant difference in anxiety or depression between patients and controls (Ahles et al 1987, Clark et al 1985, Dailey et al 1990). In another study, Uveges et al (1990) found greater psychological distress, including depression, but Hassles scores (that measures daily stress) was a significant covariate. Using the Arthritis Impact Measurement Scales (AIMS) subscale of depression, Hawley & Wolfe (1993) found significantly increased depression scores among patients with FMS, as compared with RA. However, no such difference was found in the AIMS subscales of anxiety and depression in another study (Dailey et al 1990).

With regard to the question of whether FMS is part of a 'spectrum' of depression (Hudson et al 1985, Hudson & Pope 1989, 1990), Yunus (1994) has argued that depression and FMS are different disorders, based on many psychological, therapeutic and neurohormonal studies. It is clear that these two disorders are different biologically, e.g. in their different patterns of HPA axis dysfunction (as described earlier), disturbed sleep architecture and serotonin abnormalities (Yunus 1994), among others. Since 1994, other pieces of evidence have been reported in support of the same conclusion. For example, in one study (Fassbender et al 1997), depressed patients showed a much fewer number of mean tender points than patients with FMS (1.3 vs. 16.5), despite the fact that the two groups shared several common symptoms. In another study, patients with depression demonstrated an increased pain threshold and more stoical responses to pain stimuli (Lautenbacher et al 1994).

Virtually all studies have demonstrated a greater degree of lifetime or daily stresses among patients with FMS as compared with normal controls as well as RA (Ahles et al 1984, Dailey et al 1990, Uveges et al 1990). Stress is an important confounding variable for other psychological distresses, such as anxiety or depression (Dailey et al 1990, Uveges et al 1990). Coping skills in FMS have been reported to be similar to those in RA (Uveges et al 1990).

An important insight has been recently gained regarding the role of psychological factors/psychiatric illnesses in FMS by studies of non-patients (individuals who fulfil the criteria of FMS, but have not consulted a physician). In an important study of patients with FMS, non-patients and healthy, pain-free controls, Aaron et al (1996) found that patients had significantly higher lifetime diagnoses of psychiatric diseases (mood and anxiety disorders), but non-patients did not significantly differ from healthy pain-free controls in any psychiatric diagnoses. The authors conclude that psychiatric disorders determine a patient's consultation with a physician, but are not intrinsically related to the FMS.

In an earlier study, Yunus and associates (1991) studied the relationship between psychological status and clinical features of FMS among 103 patients seen at an outpatient clinic using the Minnesota Multiphasic Personality Inventory (MMPI). They concluded that several core and associated features of FMS, i.e. number of pain sites, number of tender points, fatigue, poor sleep, swollen feeling, paraesthesia, headaches and IBS, were not associated with the psychological status of the patient with FMS. However, pain – along with anxiety, depression and stress – significantly predicted the three MMPI subgroups by discriminant analysis (Yunus et al 1991).

The psychological status of patients with FMS may be summarised by stating that a minority subgroup of patients has significant psychological distress, and irrespective of whether they are related to chronic pain or are independently present, they must be addressed for a proper management of FMS. It is known that psychological status is determined by various factors, such as referral bias, education and social status (Pillay & Sargent 1999, Pincus & Callahan 1995).

Another important consideration is that there are psychological subgroups among the patients with FMS (Turk et al 1996, Yunus et al 1991). Using the Multidimensional Pain Inventory, 87% of FMS patients can be classified into three subgroups, i.e. Dysfunctional, Interpersonally Distressed and Adaptive Copers (Turk et al 1996). Such psychological subgrouping also has important implications for management, since the outcome varies according to pretreatment psychological status (Turk et al 1998).

Genetic factors

Several studies have suggested familial aggregation in FMS (Buskila et al 1996, Pellegrino et al 1989). Studies looking for an association between FMS and HLA are inconsistent, but are generally negative (Branco et al 1996, Burda et al 1986, Horven et al 1992), as reviewed by Yunus (2000c). Moreover, simple association studies with HLA are not as reliable as linkage studies or genomic analysis in establishing a true contribution of genetic elements in a disease, since association may be influenced by several factors, e.g. referral bias.

Our group was the first to report a possible genetic linkage of FMS with HLA (Yunus et al 1999). We studied 40 multi-case families with FMS with HLA typing of B and DR B1 alleles and determining haplotypes without any knowledge of a subject's diagnosis with regard to FMS. Sibship analysis showed a weak but significant ($P < 0.028$) genetic linkage of FMS with HLA. However, we also analysed frequencies of HLA alleles by transmission disequilibrium test (TDT), and found no association of any of the alleles with FMS.

Another recent study revealed a possible association of a polymorphism in the serotonin transporter gene regulatory region with FMS

(Offenbaecher et al 1999). A significantly higher frequency of S/S genotype of the serotonin transporter (5-HTT) was found compared with healthy controls, but the difference disappeared when the confounding effect of the psychologically disturbed group was statistically adjusted. Thus, there was no association of S/S genotype with 'pure' FMS.

Gene mapping, as our group is currently investigating, will help clarify the issue of genetic factors in FMS in the next few years.

An integrated hypothesis for biopathophysiological mechanisms in FMS

It is clear that FMS is a heterogeneous condition and multiple factors are involved in varying degrees in different patients. For example, neither psychological distress nor poor sleep is important in every case; some cases may involve genetic factors and some may be triggered by mental or physical stress, infection, inflammation and physical trauma, which may activate the neurohormonal aberrations (Fig. 16.2), leading to an aberrant central pain mechanism.

As Figure 16.2 depicts, the essential biopathophysiological mechanism lies in the 'box' of heterogeneous neuroendocrine dysfunction. The word 'heterogeneous' implies different mechanisms in different subgroups among FMS patients, as well as the fact that neuroendocrine perturbations in the psychiatric disorders are generally different from those in FMS (although with some overlaps between them). In Figure 16.2, depression and anxiety are shown to be resulting from the same 'heterogeneous neuroendocrine dysfunctions' box, but the dysfunctions are not the same as those found in FMS.

Many other factors, such as poor sleep, continued psychological distress, further trauma, physical deconditioning, mental and physical stress, and many environmental factors (e.g. noise, cold or damp weather, lack of support, unsatisfactory work conditions and a lack of empathy and understanding from physicians and other health care providers) may interact to further amplify thé pain and perhaps, other symptoms, of FMS.

Although physical deconditioning may be an aggravating or perpetuating factor for both pain and fatigue, clinical observations have consistently suggested that many patients describe active exercising habits prior to the onset of their illness.

Our knowledge about what is in the 'heterogeneous neuroendocrine dysfunction box' is quite incomplete at this time. However, to be fair, one must also remember that recognition of, and research in, FMS is quite new compared with many other diseases which are still incompletely understood (such as various connective tissue diseases)

DISABILITY AND QUALITY OF LIFE IN FMS

Disability in FMS assessed by both self-assessed questionnaires and performance of standardised tasks is similar to that found in other rheumatic diseases. Using both AIMS (Burckhardt et al 1993) and the Health Assessment Questionnaire (HAQ) (Hawley & Wolfe 1991), the degree of self-assessed disability in FMS has been found to be similar to that in other rheumatic diseases, e.g. RA and OA. Cathey and associates (1988) administered 5 standardised work tasks to 28 patients with FMS, 26 with RA and 11 normal healthy controls. FMS patients performed 58.6% and RA patients 62.1% of the work done by normal controls; work performance was strongly associated with pretest HAQ scores ($r = 0.705$).

In a six-centre study of work and disability status among 1604 patients with FMS in the USA (Wolfe et al 1997), the overall disability by HAQ was found to be similar to that found in RA in other studies. More than 16% reported receiving US social security disability, the highest (35.7%) in San Antonio and the lowest (6.3%) in Peoria, as compared with 2.2% of the US population. The regional differences in reported disability perhaps reflect the demographic and socioeconomic differences between the populations studied. HAQ scores, pain and unmarried status predicted disability by multivariate analysis. However, 64% reported being able to work all or most days.

Quality of life (QOL) is significantly impaired in FMS (Burckhardt et al 1993, Henriksson 1994, Martinez et al 1995). Burckhardt and colleagues (1993) measured QOL by Quality of Life Scale in FMS in comparison with other chronic diseases, such as RA, OA, permanent ostomies, chronic obstructive pulmonary disease, insulin-dependent diabetes, and healthy controls, and found that QOL scores were among the lowest in all domains among the patients with FMS (low score meaning low satisfaction with life).

Martinez and his associates (1995) measured function, impact of disease on life, pain, sleep difficulties and socioeconomic impact among 44 women with FMS and 41 with RA, and concluded that the FMS had a negative impact on life, similar to RA. Henriksson (1994) found similar negative impact of FMS in the daily life of patients, both at home and at work; 75% reported that FMS had adversely affected their job, and more than 70% stated that their disease had unfavourably affected their relationship with family members as well as those outside the family. FMS patients took longer to complete a task in daily life because of their symptoms and needed to take frequent rests during the day.

CENTRAL SENSITIVITY SYNDROMES

The concept of central sensitivity syndromes (CSS) has received increasing recognition in recent years (Yunus 1984, 1994, 2000a, Yunus et al 1989c). Beginning with the first description of an association of FMS with IBS, tension-type headaches and migraine as compared with matched normal controls (Yunus et al 1981), it became increasingly clear that many other similar conditions share several clinical characteristics as well as a common biophysiological glue that binds them. Besides FMS, IBS and headaches, other members of this group of diseases include chronic fatigue syndrome, myofascial pain syndrome, temporomandibular pain and dysfunction syndrome, restless legs syndrome, periodic limb movement disorder and primary dysmenorrhoea (Fig. 16.3). With further studies, the number of these similar conditions will undoubtedly grow in the future.

Recognising that the common biophysiological mechanism for these illnesses or diseases involves neuroendocrine dysfunctions. Yunus (1994) had earlier called this group of conditions 'dysfunctional spectrum syndrome'. However, more recently, it has become clear that these neuroendocrine factors are likely to embody central sensitisation as a common link, as discussed above under 'Biopathophysiological mechanisms of FMS'. Considering that the central nervous system may not be sensitised in response to a peripheral stimulus in all cases, and that the sensitisation may be inherently present in many patients, these conditions have now been collectively called 'central sensitivity syndromes' (Yunus 2000a, 2000b).

The evidence for central sensitivity leading to a hyperalgesic state in FMS has been presented above. However, as discussed by Yunus (2000b), similar evidence exists for other members of the CSS, e.g. MPS (Bendtsen et al 1996a), IBS (Mertz et al 1995), chronic tension-type headache (Bendtsen et al 1996b) and migraine (Nicolodi et al 1998).

In 1989, Hudson and Pope had suggested the nomenclature 'affective spectrum disorder' (ASD) for several members of the CSS family as well as several psychiatric conditions, e.g. depression (Hudson & Pope 1989, 1990). ASD is a mixture of medical and psychiatric disorders and the very term 'affective' implies depression. However, we have argued in this chapter and previously (Yunus 1994) that depression and FMS (and most likely other members of the CSS family) are biologically different conditions.

Apart from the fact that the members of the CSS family are statistically associated with each other, these conditions share many other clinical characteristics (Yunus 1994, 2000b), including pain, fatigue, poor sleep and paraesthesia in varying degrees. Additionally, the gender (mostly female) and age distribution (usually 30–60 years) are also similar. One of the striking similarities among the CSS members is the fact that none of them has hard objective findings (such as swelling of joints, objective muscle weakness or neurological deficit), and none has been convincingly

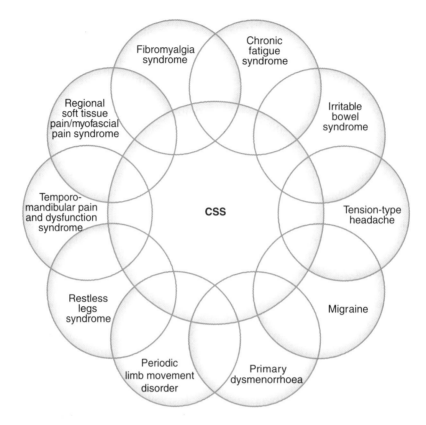

Figure 16.3   The members of the central sensitivity syndromes (CSS) share overlapping features and a common biophysiological mechanism of neuroendocrine function/central sensitivity. (Adapted from Yunus (1994), with permission.)

demonstrated to have structural pathology, e.g. inflammation, necrosis or degeneration. Thus, the usual laboratory tests are normal with unremarkable erythrocyte sedimentation rate or an absence of structural damage by radiography. However, as in FMS, a large number of neurobiochemical tests are abnormal in other members of the CSS (Yunus 2000b).

Although a subgroup of patients among the CSS diseases have a significant psychological or psychiatric problem, the frequencies of such problems are not remarkably different from a control group with another chronic illness or disease. Also, as mentioned above, FMS (and most likely other members of the CSS family) are biologically different from psychiatric diseases. Thus, CSS does not fit either into the traditional structural pathology paradigm or into the psychiatric paradigm. Hence Yunus (1998, 2000b)

has described the CSS diseases as belonging to the 'third paradigm' of central sensitivity–neurohormonal dysregulation. Although the psychiatric diseases are also based on neuroendocrine dysfunctions, the types of these dysfunctions are generally different from those found in CSS (Yunus 1994, 2000b).

CSS as a concept is useful for many reasons. CSS does not fit into the traditional structural pathology–psychiatry dichotomy, but to the 'third paradigm' as mentioned above. However, it should be recognised that none of these three paradigms are rigidly compartmentalised. Psychological factors, for example, can significantly influence the symptoms and the outcome of the so-called 'organic' diseases with structural pathology, such as rheumatoid arthritis, and psychological distress can also modulate symptoms in the CSS group of illnesses.

Recognition of CSS has significant implications for diagnosis, management and scientific investigations of these disorders. Research on these syndromes should focus on the neuroendocrine area as well as genetic contributions. Since the CSS members are related disorders, any clue to a pathophysiological mechanism or treatment of one of the members may apply to the other.

CSS is most likely the commonest group of illnesses for which a patient seeks help from a physician. An estimated 30–35 million persons in the USA probably has one or more of these distressing syndromes. These conditions cause significant disability and a huge financial burden on society. Therefore a better understanding of CSS by physicians and other health care providers is essential. Importantly, a greater research effort with much higher level of funding is of crucial importance.

SUMMARY

FMS is a clinically recognisable common condition that causes much pain and disability. It is not a disease of exclusion, but should be diagnosed by its own clinical characteristics of widespread musculoskeletal pain and many tender points. The major symptoms are pain, fatigue and poor sleep, as well as other associated symptoms, such as headaches, IBS and paraesthesia.

While the biopathophysiological mechanisms are incompletely understood, it is now clear that the major problem involves a neuroendocrine dysregulation, leading to an aberrant central pain mechanism with central sensitivity. Significant psychological distress in a subgroup of patients, as well as poor sleep, deconditioning, trauma and genetic factors, are important contributory factors for amplification of pain and other symptoms of FMS.

CSS is an important concept. The members of the CSS group, e.g. FMS, chronic fatigue syndrome, headaches, IBS and restless legs syndrome, are based on a central sensitivity–neuroendocrine dysregulation paradigm, which is different from psychiatric illnesses. Physicians should be familiar with FMS and other members of the CSS for a proper diagnosis and management of these conditions.

REFERENCES

Aaron L A, Bradley L A, Alarcon G S, Alexander R W, Triana-Alexander M, Martin M Y, Alberts K R 1996 Psychiatric diagnoses in patients with fibromyalgia are related to health care-seeking behavior rather than to illness. Arthritis and Rheumatism 39(3):436–445

Adler G K, Kinsley B T, Hurwitz S, Mossey C J, Goldenberg D L 1999 Reduced hypothalamic-pituitary and sympathoadrenal responses to hypoglycemia in women with fibromyalgia syndrome. American Journal of Medicine 106(5):534–543

Affleck G, Urrows S, Tennen H, Higgins P, Abeles M 1996 Sequential daily relations of sleep, pain intensity, and attention to pain among women with fibromyalgia. Pain 68(2–3):363–368

Ahles T A, Yunus M B, Riley S D, Bradley J M, Masi A T 1984 Psychological factors associated with primary fibromyalgia syndrome. Arthritis and Rheumatism 27(10):1101–1106

Ahles T A, Yunus M B, Masi A T 1987 Is chronic pain a variant of depressive disease? The case of primary fibromyalgia syndrome. Pain 29(1):105–111

Ahles T A, Khan S A, Yunus M B, Spiegel D A, Masi A T 1991 Psychiatric status of patients with primary fibromyalgia, patients with rheumatoid arthritis, and subjects without pain: a blind comparison of DSM-III

diagnoses. American Journal of Psychiatry 148(12):1721–1726

Alfici S, Sigal M, Landau M 1989 Primary fibromyalgia syndrome–a variant of depressive disorder? Psychotherapy and Psychosomatics 51(3):156–161

Amsterdam J D, Maislin G, Winokur A, Kling M, Gold P 1987 Pituitary and adrenocortical responses to the ovine corticotropin releasing hormone in depressed patients and healthy volunteers. Archives of General Psychiatry 44(9):775–781

Arroyo J F, Cohen M L 1993 Abnormal responses to electrocutaneous stimulation in fibromyalgia. Journal of Rheumatology 20(11):1925–1931

Bagge E, Bengtsson B A, Carlsson L, Carlsson J 1998 Low growth hormone secretion in patients with fibromyalgia – a preliminary report on 10 patients and 10 controls. Journal of Rheumatology 25(1):145–148

Banki C M, Bissette G, Arato M, O'Connor L, Nemeroff C B 1987 CSF corticotropin-releasing factor-like immunoreactivity in depression and schizophrenia. American Journal of Psychiatry 144(7): 873–877

Bendtsen L, Jensen R, Olesen J 1996a Qualitatively altered nociception in chronic myofascial pain. Pain 65(2–3):259–264

Bendtsen L, Jensen R, Olesen J 1996b Decreased pain detection and tolerance thresholds in chronic tension-type headache. Archives of Neurology 53(4):373–376

Bendtsen L, Norregaard J, Jensen R, Olesen J 1997 Evidence of qualitatively altered nociception in patients with fibromyalgia. Arthritis and Rheumatism 40(1):98–102

Bengtsson A, Henriksson K G, Jorfeldt L, Kagedal B, Lennmarken C, Lindstrom F 1986a Primary fibromyalgia. A clinical and laboratory study of 55 patients. Scandinavian Journal of Rheumatology 15(3):340–347

Bengtsson A, Henriksson K G, Larsson J 1986b Reduced high-energy phosphate levels in the painful muscles of patients with primary fibromyalgia. Arthritis and Rheumatism 29(7):817–821

Bennett R M 1996 Fibromyalgia and the disability dilemma. A new era in understanding a complex, multidimensional pain syndrome. Arthritis and Rheumatism 39(10):1627–1634

Bennett R M 1999 Emerging concepts in the neurobiology of chronic pain: evidence of abnormal sensory processing in fibromyalgia. Mayo Clinic Proceedings 74(4):385–398

Bennett R M, Clark S R, Campbell S M, Burckhardt C S 1992 Low levels of somatomedin C in patients with the fibromyalgia syndrome. A possible link between sleep and muscle pain. Arthritis and Rheumatism 35(10):1113–1116

Bennett R M, Cook D M, Clark S R, Burckhardt C S, Campbell S M 1997 Hypothalamic-pituitary-insulin-like growth factor-I axis dysfunction in patients with fibromyalgia. Journal of Rheumatology 24(7):1384–1389

Bennett R M, Clark S C, Walczyk J 1998 A randomized, double-blind, placebo-controlled study of growth hormone in the treatment of fibromyalgia. American Journal of Medicine 104(3):227–231

Besson J M 1999 The neurobiology of pain. Lancet 353(9164):1610–1615

Bonafede R P, Downey D C, Bennett R M 1995 An association of fibromyalgia with primary Sjogren's syndrome: a prospective study of 72 patients. Journal of Rheumatology 22(1):133–136

Bonnet M H, Arand D L 1997 Heart rate variability: sleep stage, time of night, and arousal influences. Electroencephalography and Clinical Neurophysiology 102(5):390–396

Bradley L A, Alberts K R, Alarcon G S et al 1996 Abnormal brain regional cerebral blood flow (rCBF) and cerebrospinal fluid (CSF) levels of substance P (SP) in patients and non-patients with fibromyalgia (FM). Arthritis and Rheumatism 39(suppl 19):S212

Branco J, Atalaia A, Paiva T 1994 Sleep cycles and alpha-delta sleep in fibromyalgia syndrome. Journal of Rheumatology 21(6):1113–1117

Branco J C, Taveres V, Abreu I, Correia M M, Machado-Caetano J A 1996 HLA studies in fibromyalgia. Journal of Musculoskeletal Pain 4(3):21–27

Bromm B, Treede R D 1991 Laser-evoked cerebral potentials in the assessment of cutaneous pain sensitivity in normal subjects and patients. Revue Neurologique (Paris) 147(10):625–643

Burckhardt C S, Clark S R, Bennett R M 1991 The fibromyalgia impact questionnaire: development and validation. Journal of Rheumatology 18(5):728–733

Burckhardt C S, Clark S R, Bennett R M 1993 Fibromyalgia and quality of life: a comparative analysis. Journal of Rheumatology 20(3):475–479

Burda C D, Cox F R, Osborne P 1986 Histocompatibility antigens in the fibrositis (fibromyalgia) syndrome. Clinical and Experimental Rheumatology 4(4):355–358

Buskila D, Neumann L 1997 Fibromyalgia syndrome (FM) and nonarticular tenderness in relatives of patients with FM. Journal of Rheumatology 24(5):941–944

Buskila D, Neumann L, Hazanov I, Carmi R 1996 Familial aggregation in the fibromyalgia syndrome. Seminars in Arthritis and Rheumatism 26(3):605–611

Campbell S M, Clark S, Tindall E A, Forehand M E, Bennett R M 1983 Clinical characteristics of fibrositis. I. A 'blinded' controlled study of symptoms and tender points. Arthritis and Rheumatism 26(7):817–824

Carette S, McCain G A, Bell D A, Fam A G 1986 Evaluation of amitriptyline in primary fibrositis. A double-blind, placebo-controlled study. Arthritis and Rheumatism 29(5):655–659

Carette S, Dessureault M, Belanger A 1992 Fibromyalgia and sex hormones. Journal of Rheumatology 19(5):831

Carette S, Oakson G, Guimont C, Steriade M 1995 Sleep electroencephalography and the clinical response to amitriptyline in patients with fibromyalgia. Arthritis and Rheumatism 38(9):1211–1217

Carmon A, Friedman Y, Coger R, Kenton B 1980 Single trial analysis of evoked potentials to noxious thermal stimulation in man. Pain 8(1):21–32

Cathey M A, Wolfe F, Kleinheksel S M 1988 Functional ability and work status in patients with fibromyalgia. Arthritis Care and Research 1:85–98

Clark S, Campbell S M, Forehand M E, Tindall E A, Bennett R M 1985 Clinical characteristics of fibrositis. II. A 'blinded,' controlled study using standard psychological tests. Arthritis and Rheumatism 28(2):132–137

Coderre T J, Katz J, Vaccarino A L, Melzack R 1993 Contribution of central neuroplasticity to pathological pain: review of clinical and experimental evidence. Pain 52(3):259–285

Cott A, Parkinson W, Bell M J, Adachi J, Bedard M, Cividino A, Bensen W 1992 Interrater reliability of the tender point criterion for fibromyalgia. Journal of Rheumatology 19(12):1955–1959

Crofford L J, Demitrack M A 1996 Evidence that abnormalities of central neurohormonal systems are key to understanding fibromyalgia and chronic fatigue syndrome. Rheumatic Disease Clinics of North America 22(2):267–284

Crofford L J, Pillemer S R, Kalogeras K T et al 1994 Hypothalamic-pituitary-adrenal axis perturbations in patients with fibromyalgia. Arthritis and Rheumatism 37(11):1583–1592

Dailey P A, Bishop G D, Russell I J, Fletcher E M 1990 Psychological stress and the fibrositis/fibromyalgia syndrome. Journal of Rheumatology 17(10):1380–1385

Devor M 1988 Central changes mediating neuropathic pain. Proceedings of the Vth World Congress on Pain. Elsevier Science Publishers BV, Amsterdam, pp 114–128

Donald F, Esdaile J M, Kimoff J R, Fitzcharles M A 1996 Musculoskeletal complaints and fibromyalgia in patients attending a respiratory sleep disorders clinic. Journal of Rheumatology 23(9):1612–1616

Donnerer J, Schuligoi R, Stein C 1992 Increased content and transport of substance P and calcitonin gene-related peptide in sensory nerves innervating inflamed tissue: evidence for a regulatory function of nerve growth factor in vivo. Neuroscience 49(3):693–698

Drewes A M, Andreasen A, Jennum P, Nielsen K D 1991 Zopiclone in the treatment of sleep abnormalities in fibromyalgia. Scandinavian Journal of Rheumatology 20(4):288–293

Drewes A M, Nielsen K D, Taagholt S J, Bjerregard K, Svendsen L, Gade J 1995a Sleep intensity in fibromyalgia: focus on the microstructure of the sleep process. British Journal of Rheumatology 34(7):629–635

Drewes A M, Gade J, Nielsen K D, Bjerregard K, Taagholt S J, Svendsen L 1995b Clustering of sleep electroencephalopathic patterns in patients with the fibromyalgia syndrome. British Journal of Rheumatology 34:1151–1156

Dubner R, Ruda M A 1992 Activity-dependent neuronal plasticity following tissue injury and inflammation. Trends in Neurosciences 15(3):96–103

Fassbender K, Samborsky W, Kellner M, Muller W, Lautenbacher S 1997 Tender points, depressive and functional symptoms: comparison between fibromyalgia and major depression. Clinical Rheumatology 16(1): 76–79

Ferraccioli G, Cavalieri F, Salaffi F, Fontana S, Scita F, Nolli M., Maestri D 1990 Neuroendocrinologic findings in primary fibromyalgia (soft tissue chronic pain syndrome) and in other chronic rheumatic conditions (rheumatoid arthritis, low back pain). Journal of Rheumatology 17(7):869–873

Ferraccioli G, Guerra P, Rizzi V, Baraldo M, Salaffi F, Furlanut M, Bartoli E 1994 Somatomedin C (insulin-like growth factor 1) levels decrease during acute changes of stress related hormones. Relevance for fibromyalgia. Journal of Rheumatology 21(7):1332–1334

Gibson S J, Littlejohn G O, Gorman M M, Helme R D, Granges G 1994 Altered heat pain thresholds and cerebral event-related potentials following painful CO_2 laser stimulation in subjects with fibromyalgia syndrome. Pain 58(2):185–193

Giovengo S L, Russell I J, Larson A A 1999 Increased concentrations of nerve growth factor in cerebrospinal fluid of patients with fibromyalgia. Journal of Rheumatology 26(7):1564–1569

Gold P W, Loriaux D L, Roy A 1986 Responses to corticotropin-releasing hormone in the hypercortisolism of depression and Cushing's disease. Pathophysiologic and diagnostic implications. New England Journal of Medicine 314(21):1329–1335

Goldenberg D L, Felson D T, Dinerman H 1986 A randomized, controlled trial of amitriptyline and naproxen in the treatment of patients with fibromyalgia. Arthritis and Rheumatism 29(11):1371–1377

Gormley G J, Lowy M T, Reder A T, Hospelhorn V D, Antel J P, Meltzer H Y 1985 Glucocorticoid receptors in depression: relationship to the dexamethasone suppression test. American Journal of Psychiatry 142(11):1278–1284

Granges G, Littlejohn G 1993 Pressure pain threshold in pain-free subjects, in patients with chronic regional pain syndromes, and in patients with fibromyalgia syndrome. Arthritis and Rheumatism 36(5):642–646

Griep E N, Boersma J W, de Kloet E R 1993 Altered reactivity of the hypothalamic-pituitary-adrenal axis in the primary fibromyalgia syndrome. Journal of Rheumatology 20(3):469–474

Griep E N, Boersma J W, de Kloet E R 1994 Pituitary release of growth hormone and prolactin in the primary fibromyalgia syndrome. Journal of Rheumatology 21(11):2125–2130

Griep E N, Boersma J W, Lentjes E G, Prins A P, van der Korst J K, de Kloet E R 1998 Function of the hypothalamic-pituitary-adrenal axis in patients with fibromyalgia and low back pain. Journal of Rheumatology 25(7):1374–1381

Harding S M 1998 Sleep in fibromyalgia patients: subjective and objective findings. American Journal of the Medical Sciences 315(6):367–376

Hawley D J, Wolfe F 1991 Pain, disability, and pain/disability relationships in seven rheumatic disorders: a study of 1,522 patients. Journal of Rheumatology 18(10):1552–1557

Hawley D J, Wolfe F 1993 Depression is not more common in rheumatoid arthritis: a 10-year longitudinal study of 6,153 patients with rheumatic disease. Journal of Rheumatology 20(12):2025–2031

Hawley D J, Wolfe F, Cathey M A 1988 Pain, functional disability, and psychological status: a 12-month study of severity in fibromyalgia. Journal of Rheumatology 15(10):1551–1556

Henriksson C M 1994 Longterm effects of fibromyalgia on everyday life. A study of 56 patients. Scandinavian Journal of Rheumatology 23(1):36–41

Holsboer F, Von Bardeleben U, Gerken A, Stalla G K, Muller O A 1984 Blunted corticotropin and normal cortisol response to human corticotropin-releasing factor in depression. New England Journal of Medicine 311(17):1127

Horne J A, Shackell B S 1991 Alpha-like EEG activity in non-REM sleep and the fibromyalgia (fibrositis) syndrome. Electroencephalography and Clinical Neurophysiology 79(4):271–276

Horven S, Stiles T C, Holst A, Moen T 1992 HLA antigens in primary fibromyalgia syndrome. Journal of Rheumatology 19(8):1269–1270

Houvenagel E, Forzy G, Leloire O et al 1990 Cerebrospinal fluid monoamines in primary fibromyalgia. Revue Du Rhumatisme Et Des Maladies Osteo-Articulaires 57(1):21–23

Hrycaj P, Stratz T, Muller W 1993 Platelet 3H-imipramine uptake receptor density and serum serotonin levels in patients with fibromyalgia/fibrositis syndrome. Journal of Rheumatology 20(11):1986–1988

Hudson J I, Pope H G 1989 Fibromyalgia and psychopathology: is fibromyalgia a form of 'affective spectrum disorder'? Journal of Rheumatology Supplement 19:15–22

Hudson J I, Pope H G 1990 Affective spectrum disorder: does antidepressant response identify a family of disorders with a common pathophysiology? American Journal of Psychiatry 147(5):552–564

Hudson J I, Hudson M S, Pliner L F, Goldenberg D L, Pope H G 1985 Fibromyalgia and major affective disorder: a controlled phenomenology and family history study. American Journal of Psychiatry 142(4):441–446

Hyyppa M T, Kronholm E 1995 Nocturnal motor activity in fibromyalgia patients with poor sleep quality. Journal of Psychosomatic Research 39(1):85–91

İnanıcı F, Yunus M B, Aldag J C 1999 Clinical features and psychologic factors in regional soft tissue pain: comparison with fibromyalgia syndrome. Journal of Musculoskeletal Pain 7(1–2):293–301

Jacobsen S, Main K, Danneskiold-Samsoe B, Skakkebaek N E 1995 A controlled study on serum insulin-like growth factor-I and urinary excretion of growth hormone in fibromyalgia. Journal of Rheumatology 22(6):1138–1140

Jennum P, Drewes A M, Andreasen A, Nielsen K D 1993 Sleep and other symptoms in primary fibromyalgia and in healthy controls. Journal of Rheumatology 20(10):1756–1759

Jubrias S A, Bennett R M, Klug G A 1994 Increased incidence of a resonance in the phosphodiester region of ^{31}P nuclear magnetic resonance spectra in the skeletal muscle of fibromyalgia patients. Arthritis and Rheumatism 37(60):801–807

Kang Y-K, Russell I J, Vipraio G A, Acworth I N 1998 Low urinary 5-hydroxyindole acetic acid in fibromyalgia syndrome: evidence in support of a serotonin-deficiency pathogenesis. Myalgia 1(1):14–21

Kirmayer L J, Robbins J M, Kapusta M A 1988 Somatization and depression in fibromyalgia syndrome. American Journal of Psychiatry 145(8):950–954

Korszun A, Sackett-Lundeen L, Papadopoulos E et al 1999 Melatonin levels in women with fibromyalgia and chronic fatigue syndrome. Journal of Rheumatology 26(12):2675–2680

Kosek E, Hansson P 1997 Modulatory influence on somatosensory perception from vibration and heterotopic noxious conditioning stimulation (HNCS) in fibromyalgia patients and healthy subjects. Pain 70(1):41–51

Kramis R C, Roberts W J, Gillette R G 1996 Non-nociceptive aspects of persistent musculoskeletal pain. Journal of Orthopaedic and Sports Physical Therapy 24(4):255–267

Kravitz H M, Katz R, Kot E, Helmke N, Fawcett J 1992 Biochemical clues to a fibromyalgia-depression link: imipramine binding in patients with fibromyalgia or depression and in healthy controls. Journal of Rheumatology 19(9):1428–1432

Lario B A, Teran J, Alonso J L, Alegre J, Arroyo I, Viejo J L 1992 Lack of association between fibromyalgia and sleep apnea syndrome. Annals of the Rheumatic Diseases 51(1):108–111

Lautenbacher S, Roscher S, Strian D, Fassbender K, Krumrey K, Krieg J C 1994 Pain perception in depression: relationships to symptomatology and naloxone-sensitive mechanisms. Psychosomatic Medicine 56(4):345–352

Leal-Cerro A, Povedano J, Astorga R et al 1999 The growth hormone (GH)-releasing hormone-GH-insulin-like growth factor-1 axis in patients with fibromyalgia syndrome. Journal of Clinical Endocrinology and Metabolism 84(9):3378–3381

Lentjes E G, Griep E N, Boersma J W, Romijn F P, de Kloet E R 1997 Glucocorticoid receptors, fibromyalgia and low back pain. Psychoneuroendocrinology 22(8):603–614

Lima D 1998 Anatomical basis for the dynamic processing of nociceptive input. European Journal of Pain 2(2):195–202

Lorenz J, Grasedyck K, Bromm B 1996 Middle and long latency somatosensory evoked potentials after painful laser stimulation in patients with fibromyalgia syndrome. Electroencephalography and Clinical Neurophysiology 100(2):165–168

Lundberg J M, Franco-Cereceda A, Lacroix J S, Pernow J 1990 Neuropeptide Y and sympathetic neurotransmission. Annals of the New York Academy of Sciences 611:166–174

McCain G A, Tilbe K S 1989 Diurnal hormone variation in fibromyalgia syndrome: a comparison with rheumatoid arthritis. Journal of Rheumatology Supplement 19:154–157

Maes M, Lin A, Bonaccorso S, Van Hunsel F et al 1998 Increased 24-hour urinary cortisol excretion in patients with post-traumatic stress disorder and patients with major depression, but not in patients with fibromyalgia. Acta Psychiatrica Scandinavica 98(4):328–335

Martinez J E, Ferraz M B, Sato E I, Atra E 1995. Fibromyalgia versus rheumatoid arthritis: a longitudinal comparison of the quality of life. Journal of Rheumatology 22(2): 270–274

Martinez-Lavin M, Hermosillo A G, Mendoza C et al 1997 Orthostatic sympathetic derangement in subjects with fibromyalgia. Journal of Rheumatology 24(4):714–718

Martinez-Lavin M, Hermosillo A G, Rosas M, Soto M E 1998 Circadian studies of autonomic nervous balance in patients with fibromyalgia: a heart rate variability analysis. Arthritis and Rheumatism 41(11):1966–1971

Mertz H, Naliboff B, Munakata J, Niazi N, Mayer E A 1995 Altered rectal perception is a biological marker of patients with irritable bowel syndrome. Gastroenterology 109(1):40–52

Middleton G D, McFarlin J E, Lipsky P E 1994 The prevalence and clinical impact of fibromyalgia in systemic lupus erythematosus. Arthritis and Rheumatism 37(8):1181–1188

Moldofsky H, Scarisbrick P, England R, Smythe H 1975 Musculoskeletal symptoms and non-REM sleep disturbance in patients with 'fibrositis syndrome' and healthy subjects. Psychosomatic Medicine 37(4):341–351

Moldofsky H, Lue F A, Smythe H A 1983 Alpha EEG sleep and morning symptoms in rheumatoid arthritis. Journal of Rheumatology 10(3):373–379

Moldofsky H, Lue F A, Mously C, Roth-Schechter B, Reynolds W J 1996 The effect of zolpidem in patients with fibromyalgia: a dose ranging, double blind, placebo controlled, modified crossover study. Journal of Rheumatology 23(3):529–533

Molony R R, MacPeek D M, Schiffman P L, Frank M, Neubauer J A, Schwartzberg M, Seibold J R 1986 Sleep, sleep apnea and the fibromyalgia syndrome. Journal of Rheumatology 13(4):797–800

Mountz J M, Bradley L A, Modell J G et al 1995 Fibromyalgia in women. Abnormalities of regional cerebral blood flow in the thalamus and the caudate nucleus are associated with low pain threshold levels. Arthritis and Rheumatism 38(7):926–938

Mukerji B, Mukerji V, Alpert M A, Selukar R 1995 The prevalence of rheumatologic disorders in patients with chest pain and angiographically normal coronary arteries. Angiology 46(5):425–430

Neeck G, Riedel W 1992 Thyroid function in patients with fibromyalgia syndrome. Journal of Rheumatology 19(7):1120–1122

Nemeroff C B, Widerlov E, Bissette G et al 1984 Elevated concentrations of CSF corticotropin-releasing factor-like immunoreactivity in depressed patients. Science 226(4680):1342–1344

Nicolodi M, Volpe A R, Sicuteri F 1998 Fibromyalgia and headache. Failure of serotonergic analgesia and N-methyl-D-aspartate-mediated neuronal plasticity: their common clues. Cephalalgia 18 (suppl 21):41–44

Offenbaecher M, Bondy B, de Jonge S, Glatzeder K, Kruger M, Schoeps P, Ackenheil M 1999 Possible association of fibromyalgia with a polymorphism in the serotonin transporter gene regulatory region. Arthritis and Rheumatism 42(11):2482–2488

Olsen N J, Park J H 1998 Skeletal muscle abnormalities in patients with fibromyalgia. American Journal of the Medical Sciences 315(6):351–358

Park J H, Kari S, King L E, Olsen N J 1998 Analysis of ^{31}P MR spectroscopy data using artificial neural networks for longitudinal evaluation of muscle diseases; dermatomyositis. NMR in Biomedicine 11(4–5):245–256

Pellegrino M J 1990 Atypical chest pain as an initial presentation of primary fibromyalgia. Archives of Physical Medicine and Rehabilitation 71(7):526–528

Pellegrino M J, Waylonis G W, Sommer A 1989 Familial occurrence of primary fibromyalgia. Archives of Physical Medicine and Rehabilitation 70(1):61–63

Perlis M L, Giles D E, Bootzin R R, Dikman Z V, Fleming G M, Drummond S P, Rose M W 1997 Alpha sleep and information processing, perception of sleep, pain, and arousability in fibromyalgia. International Journal of Neuroscience 89(3–4):265–280

Pillay A L, Sargent C A 1999 Relationship of age and education with anxiety, depression, and hopelessness in a South African community sample. Perceptual and Motor Skills 89(3):881–884

Pillemer S R, Bradley L A, Crofford L J, Moldofsky H, Chrousos G P 1997 The neuroscience and endocrinology of fibromyalgia. Arthritis and Rheumatism 40(11):1928–1939

Pincus T, Callahan L F 1995 What explains the association between socioeconomic status and health: primarily access to medical care or mind–body variables? Journal of Mind–Body Health 11(1):4–36

Press J, Phillip M, Neumann L, Barak R, Segev Y, Abu-Shakra M, Buskila D 1998 Normal melatonin levels in patients with fibromyalgia syndrome. Journal of Rheumatology 25(3):551–555

Price D D, Mao J, Frenk H, Mayer D J 1994 The N-methyl-D-aspartate receptor antagonist dextromethorphan selectively reduces temporal summation of second pain in man. Pain 59(2):165–174

Raadsheer F C 1994 Increased activity of hypothalamic corticotropin-releasing neurons in aging. Alzheimer disease and depression [dissertation]. University of Amsterdam.

Reilly P A, Littlejohn G O 1992 Peripheral arthralgic presentation of fibrositis/fibromyalgia syndrome. Journal of Rheumatology 19(2):281–283

Ren K 1994 Wind-up and the NMDA receptor: from animal studies to humans. Pain 59(2):157–158

Russell I J 1998 Advances in fibromyalgia: possible role for central neurochemicals. American Journal of the Medical Sciences 315(6):377–384

Russell I J, Michalek J E, Vipraio G A, Fletcher E M, Wall K 1989 Serum amino acids in fibrositis/fibromyalgia syndrome. Journal of Rheumatology Supplement 19:158–163

Russell I J, Vaeroy H, Javors M, Nyberg F 1992a Cerebrospinal fluid biogenic amine metabolites in fibromyalgia/fibrositis syndrome and rheumatoid arthritis. Arthritis and Rheumatism 35(5):550–556

Russell I J, Michalek J E, Vipraio G A, Fletcher E M, Javors M A, Bowden C A 1992b Platelet ^{3}H-imipramine uptake receptor density and serum serotonin levels in patients with fibromyalgia/fibrositis syndrome. Journal of Rheumatology 19(1):104–109

Russell I J, Orr M D, Littman B et al 1994 Elevated cerebrospinal fluid levels of substance P in patients with the fibromyalgia syndrome. Arthritis and Rheumatism 37(11):1593–1601

Schatzberg A F, Rothschild A J, Stahl J B et al 1983 The dexamethasone suppression test: identification of subtypes of depression. American Journal of Psychiatry 140(1):88–91

Simms R W 1998 Fibromyalgia is not a muscle disorder. American Journal of the Medical Sciences 315(6):346–350

Simms R W, Goldenberg D L 1988 Symptoms mimicking neurologic disorders in fibromyalgia syndrome. Journal of Rheumatology 15(8):1271–1273

Simms R W, Hrovat M 1995 Role of phosphodiesters (PDE) in muscles of patients with fibromyalgia syndrome. Arthritis and Rheumatism 38(9):S229

Simms R W, Roy S H, Hrovat M et al 1994 Lack of association between fibromyalgia syndrome and abnormalities in muscle energy metabolism. Arthritis and Rheumatism 37(6):794–800

Sorensen J, Bengtsson A, Backman E, Henriksson K G, Bengtsson M 1995 Pain analysis in patients with fibromyalgia. Effects of intravenous morphine, Lidocaine, and ketamine. Scandinavian Journal of Rheumatology 24(6):360–365

Sorensen J, Graven-Nielsen T, Henriksson K G, Bengtsson M, Arendt-Nielsen L 1998 Hyperexcitability in fibromyalgia. Journal of Rheumatology 25(1):152–155

Sprott H, Bradley L A, Oh S J et al 1998 Immunohistochemical and molecular studies of serotonin, substance P, galanin, pituitary adenylyl cyclase-activating polypeptide, and secretoneurin in fibromyalgic muscle tissue. Arthritis and Rheumatism 41(9):1689–1694

Thorner M O, Vance M L, Laws E R, Horvath E, Kovacs K 1998 The anterior pituitary. In: Wilson J D, Foster D W, Kronenberg H M, Larsen P R (eds) Williams textbook of endocrinology, 9th edn. WB Saunders, Philadelphia, pp 249–340

Torpy D J, Papanicolaou D A, Lotsikas A J, Wilder R L, Chrousos GP, Pillemer S 2000 Responses of the sympathetic nervous system and the hypothalamic-pituitary-adrenal axis to interleukin-6: a pilot study in fibromyalgia. Arthritis and Rheumatism 43(4):872–880.

Tunks E, McCain G A, Hart L E et al 1995 The reliability of examination for tenderness in patients with myofascial pain, chronic fibromyalgia and controls. Journal of Rheumatology 22(5):944–952

Turk D C, Okifuji A, Sinclair J D, Starz T W 1996 Pain, disability, and physical functioning in subgroups of patients with fibromyalgia. Journal of Rheumatology 23(7):1255–1262

Turk D C, Okifuji A, Sinclair J D, Starz T W 1998 Interdisciplinary treatment for fibromyalgia syndrome:

clinical and statistical significance. Arthritis Care Research 11(3):186–195

Uveges J M, Parker J C, Smarr K L et al 1990 Psychological symptoms in primary fibromyalgia syndrome: relationship to pain, life stress, and sleep disturbance. Arthritis and Rheumatism 33(8):1279–1283

Vaeroy H, Helle R, Forre O, Kass E, Terenius L 1988a Elevated CSF levels of substance P and high incidence of Raynaud phenomenon in patients with fibromyalgia: new features for diagnosis. Pain 32(1):21–26

Vaeroy H, Helle R, Forre O, Kass E, Terenius L 1988b Cerebrospinal fluid levels of β endorphin in patients with fibromyalgia (fibrositis syndrome). Journal of Rheumatology 15:1804–1806

Vaeroy H, Qiao Z G, Morkrid L, Forre O 1989 Altered sympathetic nervous system response in patients with fibromyalgia (fibrositis syndrome). Journal of Rheumatology 16(11):1460–1465

Vaeroy H, Nyberg F, Terenius L 1991 No evidence for endorphin deficiency in fibromyalgia following investigation of cerebrospinal fluid (CSF) dynorphin A and met-enkephalin-arg^6-phe^7. Pain 46(2):139–143

van Denderen J C, Boersma J W, Zeinstra P, Hollander A P, van Neerbos B R 1992 Physiological effects of exhaustive physical exercise in primary fibromyalgia syndrome (PFS): is PFS a disorder of neuroendocrine reactivity? Scandinavian Journal of Rheumatology 21(1):35–37

Watson R, Libmann K O, Jenson J 1985 Alpha-delta sleep: EEG characteristics, incidence, treatment, psychological correlates in personality. Sleep Research 14:226

Welin M, Bragee B, Nyberg F, Kristiansson M 1995 Elevated substance P levels are contrasted by a decrease in met-enkephalin-arg-phe levels in CSF from fibromyalgia patients. Journal of Musculoskeletal Pain 3(suppl 1):4

Whalley L J, Borthwick N, Copolov D, Dick H, Christie J E, Fink G 1986 Glucocorticoid receptors and depression. British Medical Journal (Clinical Research Edition) 292(6524):859–861

White K P, Speechley M, Harth M, Ostbye T 1999 The London Fibromyalgia Epidemiology Study: the prevalence of fibromyalgia syndrome in London, Ontario. Journal of Rheumatology 26(7):1570–1576

Wikner J, Hirsch U, Wetterberg L, Rojdmark S 1998 Fibromyalgia – a syndrome associated with decreased nocturnal melatonin secretion. Clinical Endocrinology (Oxford) 49(2):179–183

Wolfe F 1990 Fibromyalgia. Rheumatic Disease Clinics of North America 16(3):681–698

Wolfe F 1998 What use are fibromyalgia control points. Journal of Rheumatology 25(3):546–550

Wolfe F, Cathey M A, Kleinheksel S M 1984 Fibrositis (Fibromyalgia) in rheumatoid arthritis. Journal of Rheumatology 11(6):814–818

Wolfe F, Smythe H A, Yunus M B et al 1990 The American College of Rheumatology 1990 Criteria for the Classification of Fibromyalgia. Report of the Multicenter Criteria Committee. Arthritis and Rheumatism 33(2):160–172

Wolfe F, Ross K, Anderson J, Russell I J, Hebert L 1995a The prevalence and characteristics of fibromyalgia in the general population. Arthritis and Rheumatism 38(1): 19–28

Wolfe F, Ross K, Anderson J, Russell I J 1995b Aspects of fibromyalgia in the general population: sex, pain

threshold, and fibromyalgia symptoms. Journal of Rheumatology 22(1):151–156

Wolfe F, Anderson J, Harkness D et al 1997 Work and disability status of persons with fibromyalgia. Journal of Rheumatology 24(6):1171–1178

Woolf C J 1983 Evidence for a central component of post-injury pain hypersensitivity. Nature 306(5944):686–688

Woolf C J, Thompson S W 1991 The induction and maintenance of central sensitization is dependent on N-methyl-D-aspartic acid receptor activation; implications for the treatment of post-injury pain hypersensitivity states. Pain 44(3):293–299

Yunus M B 1984 Primary fibromyalgia syndrome: current concepts. Comprehensive Therapy 10(8):21–28

Yunus M B 1992 Towards a model of pathophysiology of fibromyalgia: aberrant central pain mechanisms with peripheral modulation. Journal of Rheumatology 19(6):846–850

Yunus M B 1994 Psychological aspects of fibromyalgia syndrome: a component of the dysfunctional spectrum syndrome. Baillière's Clinical Rheumatology 8(4):811–837

Yunus M B 1996 Fibromyalgia syndrome: is there any effective therapy? Consultant 36:1279–1285

Yunus M B 1998 Dysregulation spectrum syndrome: a unified new concept for many common maladies. Multidisciplinary Approaches to Fibromyalgia, FMS Resources Group, LTD. Anadem Publishing, Columbus, Ohio, pp 243–251

Yunus M B 2000a Fibromyalgia and related syndromes. Current Practice of Medicine On line serial [http://praxis.md/index.cfm?page=cpmref&article=CPM 02%2DRH393]

Yunus M B 2000b Central sensitivity syndromes: a unified concept for fibromyalgia and other similar maladies. Journal of Indian Rheumatism Association 8(1):27–33

Yunus M B 2000c Genetic aspects of fibromyalgia syndrome. Journal of Rheumatology and Medical Rehabilitation 11(2):143–145

Yunus M B, Masi A T 1993 Fibromyalgia, restless legs syndrome, periodic limb movement disorder, and psychogenic pain. In: McCarty D J, Koopman W J (eds) Arthritis and Allied Conditions: A Textbook of Rheumatology, 12th edn. Lea and Febiger, Philadelphia, pp 1383–1405

Yunus M B, Masi A T, Calabro J J, Miller K A, Feigenbaum S L 1981 Primary fibromyalgia (fibrositis): clinical study of 50 patients with matched normal controls. Seminars in Arthritis and Rheumatism 11(1):151–171

Yunus M B, Denko C W, Masi A T 1986 Serum beta-endorphin in primary fibromyalgia syndrome: a controlled study. Journal of Rheumatology 13(1): 183–186

Yunus M B, Kalyan-Raman U P, Masi A T, Aldag J C 1989a Electron microscopic studies of muscle biopsy in primary fibromyalgia syndrome: a controlled and blinded study. Journal of Rheumatology 16(1):97–101

Yunus M B, Berg B C, Masi A T 1989b Multiphase skeletal scintigraphy in primary fibromyalgia syndrome: a blinded study. Journal of Rheumatology 16(11): 1466–1468

Yunus M B, Masi A T, Aldag J C 1989c A controlled study of primary fibromyalgia syndrome: clinical features and association with other functional syndromes. Journal of Rheumatology Supplement 19:62–71

Yunus M B, Ahles T A, Aldag J C, Masi A T 1991 Relationship of clinical features with psychological status in primary fibromyalgia. Arthritis and Rheumatism 34(1):15–21

Yunus M B, Dailey J W, Aldag J C, Masi A T, Jobe P C 1992a Plasma and urinary catecholamines in primary fibromyalgia: a controlled study. Journal of Rheumatology 19(1):95–97

Yunus M B, Dailey J W, Aldag J C, Masi A T, Jobe P C 1992b Plasma tryptophan and other amino acids in primary fibromyalgia: a controlled study. Journal of Rheumatology 19(1):90–94

Yunus M B, Aldag J C, Dailey J W, Jobe P C 1995 Interrelationships of biochemical parameters in classification of fibromyalgia syndrome and healthy normal controls. Journal of Musculoskeletal Pain 3: 15–24

Yunus M B, Khan M A, Rawlings K K, Green J R, Olson J M, Shah S 1999 Genetic linkage analysis of multicase families with fibromyalgia syndrome. Journal of Rheumatology 26(2):408–412

Yunus M B, İnanıcı F, Aldag J C, Mangold R F 2000 Fibromyalgia in men: comparison of clinical features with women. Journal of Rheumatology 27(2):485–490

17

Management of fibromyalgia syndrome

Fatma İnanıcı
Muhammad B. Yunus

INTRODUCTION

The aetiology and biopathophysiological mechanisms of symptoms in fibromyalgia syndrome (FMS) are not completely understood. It is a complex and multifactorial disorder with considerable variations among patients. Many different factors interact to cause symptoms, with their relative importance varying from patient to patient. Furthermore, with regard to drug therapy, because the pain processing mechanisms are not the same for everyone with FMS it follows that not all patients respond to the same drugs (Sorensen et al 1997).

The management of fibromyalgia, which is both challenging and time-consuming, includes patient education and reassurance; elimination of aggravating factors; and the use of drugs and non-pharmacological interventions (Box 17.1).

PATIENT EDUCATION AND REASSURANCE

As with any chronic condition, education of the patient is essential in FMS (Burckhardt & Bjelle 1994). This includes discussing currently known biophysiological mechanisms, the non-inflammatory, non-malignant nature of the illness, and its aggravating factors. The patient should be reassured that although the disorder is a very painful one, it does not cause tissue damage,

---

Box 17.1 Important components of management of fibromyalgia syndrome

- Positive and empathetic attitude of the physician
- Firm diagnosis
- Patient education and reassurance
- Individualisation of management
- Addressing aggravating factors
- Non-pharmacological interventions
  1. Physical fitness training
  2. Physical therapy modalities, e.g. TENS, ultrasound, massage, manipulation
  3. EMG biofeedback
  4. Acupuncture/Electroacupuncture
  5. Cognitive behavioural therapy
  6. Use of other non-pharmacological approach, e.g. hypnotherapy
  7. Interdisciplinary group treatment
- Pharmacological management
- Tender point injections

Box 17.2 Factors that may aggravate the symptoms of FMS (adapted from Yunus 1996, p.1281, with permission)

1. Neurohormonal/muscular factors
   - Non-restorative sleep
   - Physical deconditioning
   - Poor posture
   - Muscle overload
   - Hypothyroidism
   - Medication side-effects
2. Psychological factors
   - Stress
   - Anxiety
   - Depression
   - Poor coping skills
3. Environmental factors
   - Hot or cold temperature
   - Chilling
   - Humidity
   - Excess air conditioning
   - Noise
4. Occupational factors
   - Repetitive trauma
   - Ergonomic factors
   - Prolonged sitting/standing/walking
   - Weight lifting/bending
   - Mental/physical stress
   - Poor sleep (shift workers)
5. Co-morbid conditions
   - Headache
   - Irritable bowel syndrome
   - Restless legs syndrome
   - Periodic limb movement disorder
   - Chronic fatigue syndrome
   - Arthritis
   - Hyperlaxity
   - Neuropathy
6. Family/social factors
   - Lack of social and family support
   - Excess family demands
   - Lack of hobbies and recreation

---

reduced life expectancy, deformity or crippling (Bennett 1997, Yunus 1996). Experience suggests that calling it a 'benign condition' is often resented by patients disabled by severe, unremitting pain.

Educational material in the form of an information sheet or booklet is frequently helpful.

Patients need to accept that although their pain is likely to remain chronic, the aim of the treatment is to make them more active (Rosen 1994) and to reduce the level of pain so as to improve the quality of their lives (Yunus 1996).

Burckhardt et al (1994) evaluated the effectiveness of education and physical training in decreasing FMS symptoms and concluded that they are useful, especially in increasing patients' self-reliance.

ADDRESSING AGGRAVATING FACTORS

Aggravating factors are not the same for everyone. It is therefore important to identify those present in each individual patient (Box 17.2).

Sleep disturbances

Most patients with FMS have various kinds of sleep difficulties. It is not clear whether disturbed sleep is a cause or a consequence of it, although experimental sleep deprivation in healthy controls causes FMS-like symptoms and increased tender points (TP) (Moldofsky & Scarisbrick 1976). Because poor sleep contributes to pain, fatigue and impaired physical and mental performance (Harding 1998), improving its quality is essential (Box 17.3).

Drugs that are helpful for this purpose include tricyclic antidepressants (Bennett et al 1988, Carette et al 1994, Goldenberg 1989, Branco et al 1996), alprazolam (Russell et al 1991), zolpidem

---

Box 17.3 Important elements for improving sleep quality

1. A complete history of patient's sleeping habits
   - Sleep/wake time cycle,
   - Caffeine intake, alcohol, smoking
   - Exercising habits
   - Sleep environment, noise
2. Addressing sleep difficulties/disorders
   - Non-restorative sleep (awakening feeling tired or unrefreshed)
   - Difficulty falling asleep
   - Frequent awakening during sleep
   - Early morning awakenings
   - Sleep apnoea
   - Restless legs syndrome
   - Periodic limb movements of sleep
3. Addressing psychological factors
   - Stress
   - Anxiety
   - Depression
4. Restoring sleep hygiene
   - A regular sleep/wake schedule
   - Adequate sleep time (i.e. at least 7 or 8 hours/night)
   - Daily exercise
   - Avoiding heavy meals before bedtime
   - Avoiding caffeine, smoking and alcohol within several hours of bedtime
   - Treating rhinitis, acid reflux
   - Eliminating environmental disturbances (e.g. noise, light)
   - Relaxation
5. Pain management
6. Avoiding pharmacological agents that may disrupt sleep (e.g. narcotics, cocaine, clonidine, beta blockers, sympathomimetic drugs)
7. Medications that facilitate sleep

(Moldofsky et al 1996) and zopiclone (Drewes et al 1991, Gronblad et al 1993).

Patients with sleep apnoea usually require treatment with continuous positive airway pressure or surgery (Bennett 1997).

Restless legs syndrome and periodic limb movements during sleep can be treated with L-dopa 100–200 mg/day or clonazepam 0.5–1.5 mg/day (Boghen et al 1986, Krueger 1990, Montplaisir et al 1986).

Physical deconditioning

Musculoskeletal pain and fatigue contribute to inactivity in FMS, and many patients have muscle deconditioning. Deconditioned muscles use excess energy for a given task and may therefore contribute to fatigue. Such muscles are also susceptible to microtrauma-induced damage, which then aggravates the pain (Bennett et al 1991, Bennett 1997). Thus, patients should be encouraged to exercise progressively and regularly. Stretching exercises provide short-term help. Aerobic exercises are the most beneficial. The types of exercise should be individualised according to the patient's choice and pain severity. The key is to start exercising at a low level for 5 to 10 minutes and to increase this gradually to 30 to 40 minutes daily (Yunus 1996). Aerobic exercises should be done three to four times a week at about 70% of maximum pulse rate (Clark 1994). Patients also benefit from brisk walking, swimming in a warm pool, and bicycling. Treadmill exercise is helpful, particularly in the winter months with a low outside temperature.

Psychological factors

Significant psychological distress (varying degrees of anxiety, depression, mental stress and poor coping skills) has been observed in about 30–40% of patients with FMS (Yunus 1994). Pain, irrespective of its cause, is significantly influenced by psychological factors and accentuated by stress, anxiety and depression. In many patients, the proper management of psychological factors helps, but does not completely alleviate the symptoms of FMS. It includes emotional support and psychotherapy and the use of antidepressant and anxiolytic drugs. Only a minority of patients with severe psychiatric problems need referral to a psychiatrist.

Occupational factors

Waylonis et al (1994) described various occupational activities that are associated with increased pain symptoms. Job or workplace modification is often beneficial in the management of FMS (Parziale 1999, Yunus 1996). Every attempt should be made to keep FMS patients employed, as this gives them less time to focus on their pain, and it also provides them with a sense of self-worth, which is particularly important with chronic illness (Yunus 1996).

Management of concomitant conditions

The presence of concurrent diseases, such as arthritis, hypothyroidism, neurological diseases, restless legs syndrome, bowel problems and migraine, often adds to the global distress of a patient and should be appropriately managed.

NON-PHARMACOLOGICAL INTERVENTIONS

There are a number of non-pharmacological interventions that have been found to be helpful in controlled studies (Table 17.1).

Physical fitness training

Exercise training leads to improved conditioning and resistance to microtrauma, enhancement in strength, endurance and flexibility, higher levels of general activity, and an increased sense of control. It also has an antidepressant and relaxing effect (Bennett et al 1991, McCain 1986, Sim & Adams 1999). Additionally exercise has pain modulating effects. Following aerobic exercise, increas-

es in levels of beta-endorphin-like products, prolactin and growth hormone were reported, with a resultant decreased pain sensitivity (Sim & Adams 1999). McCain (1989) proposed that exercise may normalise the hypothalamic-pituitary-adrenal axis (HPA) dysfunction that plays an important role in the development of pain, fatigue and sleep difficulties in FMS (see Ch. 16).

McCain et al (1988) compared the efficacy of a 20-week supervised cardiovascular fitness training with supervised simple flexibility and stretching exercises in a randomised controlled trial of 42 patients with FMS. At the end of the study, significant improvements in both patient and physician global assessments and TP thresholds were recorded in the cardiovascular fitness training group, but not in the simple flexibility group.

Low-intensity endurance training has been studied in a randomised trial (Mengshoel et al 1992). During a period of 20 weeks 18 patients with FMS participated in a 60-minute continuous, modified, low-impact aerobic dance programme. Training intensity was kept at a heart rate of 120–150 beats/minute. As a control group, 17 patients were asked not to change their physical activity level. At the end of the programme, the intensity of pain, fatigue or sleep had not changed in either group but the patients in the

Table 17.1 Randomised, controlled, blinded trials of non-pharmacological interventions in FMS

Intervention	Study	Control intervention	No. of points	Study duration (weeks)	Effective
Cardiovascular fitness training	McCain et al 1988	Simple flexibility and stretching exercises	42	20	Yes
Low intensity endurance training	Mengshoel et al 1992	No change in physical activity	35	20	No
Aerobic exercise	Wigers et al 1996	Usual treatment group	60	14	Yes
Aerobic, flexibility and strengthening exercises	Martin et al 1996	Relaxation training	60	6	Yes
Exercise and education	Gowans et al 1999	Waiting list controls	41	6	Yes
Hydrogalvanic bath	Gunther et al 1994	Progressive muscle relaxation	25	5	No
Balneotherapy	Yurtkuran & Celiktas 1996	Relaxation exercises	40	2	Yes
EMG biofeedback	Ferraccioli et al 1987	Sham	12	24	Yes
Electroacupuncture	Deluze et al 1992	Sham	70	3	Yes
Cognitive behavioural therapy	Vlaeyen et al 1996	Waiting list controls	131	6	No
Cognitive behavioural therapy	Nicassio et al 1997	Education	86	10	No
Hypnotherapy	Haanen et al 1991	Physical therapy	40	12	Yes
Interdisciplinary group treatment[a]	Keel et al 1998	Relaxation training	32	24	Yes

[a] Patients were allowed to continue their pharmacological treatment.

training group reported that exercise had increased their feelings of general wellbeing.

Clark (1994) argued that the pain experienced following exercise may be a result of too much eccentric work (contracting and lengthening a muscle) and/or working at too high an intensity. She advocates educating patients regarding this, and prescribing stretching followed by activities that minimise eccentric workload. In addition, she emphasises the importance of taking into account a patient's initial fitness level when determining a suitable exercise intensity.

Short- and long-term effects of aerobic exercise were studied in a controlled, blinded study by Wingers et al (1996). They compared the effects of aerobic exercise, stress management and 'usual treatment' in 60 patients. Patients were randomly placed in one of these three treatment groups for 14 weeks. At the end of this time, patients in both the aerobic exercise group and stress management group improved more than 'the usual' treatment group, but 4-year follow-up data showed no obvious group differences in symptom severity. The authors noted a considerable compliance problem with long-term aerobic exercise programmes.

Similarly, Martin et al (1996) reported the short-term benefit of an exercise programme which included aerobic, flexibility and strength training exercises in a randomised, controlled, blinded trial of 60 patients. Patients met 3 times a week for 6 weeks for 1 hour of supervised exercise or relaxation. Measures such as number of TPs, degree of tenderness and aerobic fitness level were improved in the exercise group.

A randomised controlled trial of exercise and education was performed by Gowans et al (1999). Forty-one fibromyalgia patients with severe disability, according to the physical impairment subscale of the Fibromyalgia Impact Questionnaire (FIQ) and 6-minute walk distance, participated in a 6-week exercise and education programme or served as waiting list controls. The physical function, sense of wellbeing and self-efficacy of patients in the exercise and education group improved significantly. This improvement was maintained up to 3 months. However, it was not possible to determine whether exercise or education or both contributed to it.

Physical therapy

Stretching and strengthening of muscles, massage, manipulation, mobilisation and the application of heat, ice, ultrasound, electrical stimulation, mechanical pressure, light energy and electromagnetic energy are widely used adjunctive forms of treatment (Rosen 1994). Some of them can be applied in the patient's own home environment and may be useful in achieving muscle relaxation, relieving pain and muscle spasm, and in activating endogenous opioids (Rosen 1994). However, no controlled studies with adequate sample size and study design have confirmed their efficacy in patients with FMS.

Transcutaneous electrical nerve stimulation (TENS)

TENS was applied to 40 patients with FMS and in an open study found to produce transient benefit in 70% of the patients (Kaada 1989).

Hydrogalvanic bath therapy (HBT)

HBT was compared with progressive muscle relaxation in a randomised controlled trial of 25 patients with FMS, and was not found to be effective (Gunther et al 1994).

Balneotherapy

The effect of balneotherapy (warm mineralised bath) and that of relaxation exercises were compared by Yurtkuran & Celiktas (1996) in a randomised controlled trial of 40 patients with FMS. In the balneotherapy group, pain and algometer scores were improved significantly at the end of 2 weeks treatment and 6 weeks follow-up. No significant changes were observed in the relaxation exercises group.

Manual medicine techniques

Chiropractors are the most frequently consulted complementary medicine practitioners by patients with FMS (Pioro-Boisset et al 1996).

However, there is only one study that reports the efficacy of chiropractic management in FMS (Blunt et al 1997). In this study, 21 patients received chiropractic management consisting of soft tissue massage, stretching, spinal manipulation and education, administered three to five times a week for 4 weeks in 21 patients. At the end of this time, the cervical and lumbar ranges of motion, straight leg raise and pain levels in the chiropractic group improved more than they did in a waiting list control group.

EMG-biofeedback

Ferraccioli et al (1987) conducted true EMG-biofeedback or false EMG-biofeedback in 20-minute sessions twice weekly for a total of 15 sessions in 12 patients. They suggested that there was a decrease of plasma ACTH and beta-endorphin levels during EMG-biofeedback training. However, the blindness of this study is uncertain. Sarnoch et al (1997) conducted an open study in 18 patients. In both trials an improvement in FMS symptoms was reported.

Acupuncture

Deluze et al (1992) evaluated the efficacy of electro-acupuncture in a double-blind controlled trial. Seventy patients were randomised to electro-acupuncture or a sham procedure. Pain intensity, pain threshold, number of analgesic tablets used, regional pain score, sleep quality and patients' and physicians' global assessment were improved in the electro-acupuncture group. Lewis (1993) pointed out the uncertainty of the acupuncture points and the sham procedure in this study. Recently, Sprott et al (1998) carried out an open study of 29 patients treated with acupuncture over 6 weeks. They reported a decreased pain level and number of TPs, and also an increase of serotonin and substance P levels in serum. Based on these results, the authors suggested a physiological mechanism of acupuncture for pain relief.

The National Institutes of Health consensus conference statement on acupuncture (1998) concluded that in some situations, including fibromyalgia, 'acupuncture may be useful as an adjunct treatment or an acceptable alternative or may be included in a comprehensive management program'.

Cognitive behavioural therapy

Cognitive behavioural therapy (CBT) includes relaxation training, reinforcement of healthy behaviour patterns, reducing pain behaviour, coping skills training, and the restructuring of maladaptive beliefs about a person's ability to control pain (Bradley 1989, Nielson et al 1992). Several studies have reported the efficacy of inpatient and outpatient programmes of CBT (Goldenberg et al 1994, Nielson et al 1992, Singh et al 1998, Vlaeyen et al 1996, White & Nielson 1995).

Nielson et al (1992) evaluated CBT in a preliminary study of 3 weeks' duration that included medical, psychological, social work, physiotherapy, occupational therapy and nursing interventions based on the cognitive behavioural model. They reported significant improvements in perceived pain severity, distress, and the ability to cope with pain liable to interfere with normal activities. A follow-up study (White & Nielson 1995) found that improvement persisted 30 months after the treatment. Singh et al (1998) found similar results in an 8-week CBT study. Such findings, however, must be regarded with some caution as these trials were not randomised, controlled trials.

The effectiveness of cognitive educational treatment was evaluated by Vlaeyen et al (1996) in a randomised controlled trial. One hundred and thirty-one patients with FMS were randomly assigned to three outpatient programmes: cognitive/educational programme (ECO), group education and group discussion programme (EDI) or waiting list control (WLC). The authors reported improvement in pain coping in both ECO and EDI groups, but there was no difference between these two groups on any outcome measures.

Nicassio et al (1997) recently carried out a similar trial. Eighty-six patients with FMS were included in a 10-week treatment and 6-month follow-up programme. The behavioural intervention focused on the development of diverse pain coping skills, while the education/control condition presented information on a range of health-related topics without emphasising skill acquisition. Similar improvements were found in both groups. Multiple regression analyses revealed that changes in helplessness and passive coping were associated with improvement in some of the clinical outcomes.

Buckelew et al (1998) compared biofeedback/relaxation treatment with exercise training. They randomised 119 patients to one of four groups: (1) biofeedback/relaxation training; (2) exercise training; (3) a combination treatment; or (4) an educational/attention control programme. Improvement in self-efficacy for physical function was best maintained by the combination group at the end of 2-year follow-up.

Overall, CBT seems helpful in FMS and should be utilised in difficult cases.

Hypnotherapy

There is increasing interest in the use of hypnotherapy for the management of chronic pain syndromes (NIH Technology Assessment Panel, 1996). But there has been only one study of its use in the management of FMS (Haanen et al 1991). Forty patients with FMS were randomised to receive either hypnotherapy or physical therapy for 12 weeks. Pain intensity, morning fatigue, sleep, patient global assessment and psychological scores were reported to improve significantly in the hypnotherapy group. At 24-week follow-up, beneficial effects were maintained.

Interdisciplinary group treatment

Masi (1994) has advocated a multimodal psychotherapeutic approach aimed at modifying the effects of life stresses in FMS. He described a combination of physical therapy, medication and psychological treatment that may improve patients' wellbeing and TP ratings.

Recently Bennett et al (1996) emphasised the usefulness of multidimensional group treatment in a 6-month programme in 104 patients with FMS. It included education, behaviour modification, fitness training, muscle awareness training, 'spray and stretch' procedures, and management of associated problems, such as depression, anxiety and irritable bowel syndrome. Total FIQ score, FIQ subscales, number of TPs, total myalgic score, quality of life index, 6-minute walking distance, depression and anxiety scores, fibromyalgia attitude index and coping skills questionnaire subscales improved by an average of at least 25%. Results were encouraging, but unfortunately the study was uncontrolled and unblinded.

In a randomised controlled study carried out by Keel et al (1998) 32 patients received either integrated group therapy or group relaxation training. The authors reported significant improvements in clinical parameters and pain intensity in those receiving integrated group therapy at 4 months follow-up.

Turk et al (1998) evaluated the effects of a 4-week outpatient integrated group programme of education, exercise therapy, functional re-education, and CBT in 67 patients with FMS. At the end of the programme, pain severity, anxiety, depression, affective distress, and fatigue were improved. The authors noted that pretreatment levels of psychological distress and improvement in pain severity were closely related. At 6-month follow-up, apart from fatigue, the improvements persisted. Randomised, blinded and controlled studies with appropriate sample size are necessary in this area.

PHARMACOLOGICAL MANAGEMENT

A substantial number of randomised, placebo-controlled trials have demonstrated that several pharmacological agents are beneficial in FMS (Table 17.2). In view of the biopathophysiology of FMS (see Ch. 16), centrally acting agents are most likely to be useful in its management. Buskila (1999) has emphasised the necessity of developing new drugs and the importance of long-term comparative trials of both their efficacy and toxicity.

Table 17.2   Controlled, blinded trials of pharmacological agents in fibromyalgia syndrome

Agent	Reference	Design	Trial duration	No. of pts	Dose	Control group	Effective
Antidepressants							
Amitriptyline	Carette et al 1986	Parallel	9 weeks	70	10–50 mg/day	Placebo	Yes
Amitriptyline	Goldenberg et al 1986	Parallel	6 weeks	62	25 mg/day	Placebo	Yes
Amitriptyline	Scudds et al 1989	Crossover	10 weeks	36	50 mg/day	Placebo	Yes
Amitriptyline	Jaeschke et al 1991	N-of-1	2 weeks	23	10 mg/day	Placebo	Yes
Cyclobenzaprine	Bennett et al 1988	Parallel	12 weeks	120	10–40 mg/day	Placebo	Yes
Cyclobenzaprine	Reynolds et al 1991	Crossover	8 weeks	12	30 mg/day	Placebo	Yes
Cyclobenzaprine	Fossaluzza & De Vita 1992	Parallel	10 days	32	10 mg/day	C+Ibuprofen	No
Cyclobenzaprine	Carette et al 1994	Parallel	6 months	208	10 mg/day	Placebo	Yes
Dosulepin (dothiepin)	Caruso et al 1987	Parallel	8 weeks	60	75 mg/day	Placebo	Yes
Clomipramine	Bibolotti et al 1986	Crossover	3 weeks	37	75 mg/day	Placebo	No
Fluoxetine	Wolfe et al 1994	Parallel	6 weeks	42	20 mg/day	Placebo	Yes
Fluoxetine	Goldenberg et al 1996	Crossover	4x6 weeks	19	20 mg/day	Placebo	Yes
Fluoxetine+amitriptyline	Goldenberg et al 1996	Crossover	4x6 weeks	19	20 mg/day F 10 mg/day AMI	Fluoxetine AMI	Yes Yes
Citalopram	Norregaard et al 1995	Parallel	8 weeks	22	20–40 mg/day	Placebo	No
Sertraline	Alberts et al 1998	Parallel	10 weeks	14	—[b]	Placebo	Yes
Trazodone	Branco et al 1996	Crossover	2 months	13	—[b]	Placebo	Yes
Moclobemide	Hannonen et al 1998	Parallel	12 weeks	130	450–600 mg/day	Placebo	No
Pirlindole	Ginsberg et al 1998	Parallel	4 weeks	100	75 mg b.i.d.	Placebo	Yes
SAMe	Tavoni et al 1987	Crossover	3 weeks	17	200 mg/day i.v.	Placebo	Yes
SAMe	Jacobsen et al 1991	Parallel	6 weeks	44	800 mg/day p.o.	Placebo	No
SAMe	Valkmann et al 1997	Crossover	10 days	34	600 mg/day i.v.	Placebo	No
SAMe	Tavoni et al 1998	Parallel	15 days	30	400 mg/day i.v.	Placebo	Yes
Benzodiazepines							
Alprazolam	Russell et al 1991	Parallel	6 weeks	78	0.5–3 mg/day	Placebo	No
Bromazepam	Quijada-Carrera et al 1996	Parallel	8 weeks	164	3 mg/day	Placebo	No
Temazepam	Hench et al 1989	Crossover	12 weeks	10	15–30 mg/day	Placebo	Yes
Hypnotics							
Zopiclone	Drewes et al 1991	Parallel	12 weeks	41	7.5 mg/day	Placebo	Yes[a]
Zopiclone	Gronbald et al 1993	Parallel	8 weeks	33	7.5 mg/day	Placebo	Yes[a]
Zolpidem	Moldofsky et al 1996	Crossover	16 days	19	5–10–15 mg/day	Placebo	Yes[a]
Anti-inflammatory agents							
Ibuprofen	Yunus et al 1989b	Parallel	3 weeks	46	600 mg q.i.d.	Placebo	No
Prednisone	Clark et al 1985	Crossover	28 days	20	15 mg/day	Placebo	No
Naproxen	Goldenberg et al 1986	Parallel	6 weeks	62	1000 mg/day	Placebo	No
Tenoxicam	Quijada-Carrera et al 1996	Parallel	8 weeks	164	20 mg/day	Placebo	No
Analgesics							
Tramadol	Biasi et al 1998	Crossover	Single dose	12	100 mg	Placebo	Yes
Tramadol	Russell et al 1998	Parallel	6 weeks	69	50–400 mg/day	Placebo	Yes
Others							
Chlormezanone	Pattrick et al 1993	Parallel	6 weeks	42	400 mg/day	Placebo	No
Malic acid	Russell et al 1995	Parallel	4 weeks	24	600 mg/day	Placebo	No
SER282	Kempenaers et al 1994	Parallel	8 weeks	36	20 mg × 3/week	Placebo	No
Growth hormone	Bennett et al 1998	Parallel	9 months	50	0.0125 mg/kg/day	Placebo	Yes
5-Hydroxytryptophan	Caruso et al 1990	Parallel	30 days	50	100 mg t.i.d.	Placebo	Yes
Ritanserin	Olin et al 1998	Parallel	16 weeks	51	10 mg/day	Placebo	No
Human interferon alpha	Russell et al 1999	Parallel	6 weeks	120	50 IU/day	Placebo	Yes
Salmon calcitonin	Bessette et al 1998	Crossover	1 month	11	100 IU/day	Placebo	No

AMI, amitriptyline; C, cyclobenzaprine; F, fluoxetine; SAMe, S-adenosylmethionine; i.v., intravenously; p.o., by mouth; b.i.d., twice a day; q.i.d., four times a day; t.i.d., three times a day.
[a] Effective as a hypnotic agent without improvement in pain or tender points. [b] Not known.

Antidepressant agents

As disturbed sleep and pain are prominent features in FMS (Moldofsky & Scarisbrick 1976) and the neurotransmitter serotonin modulates both of these, serotonergic antidepressant agents have been evaluated and found to be useful in the management of FMS. These drugs, by blocking the reuptake of serotonin, provide analgesia in chronic pain syndromes and most of them also increase the time spent in stage 4 sleep (Godfrey 1996).

Tricyclic antidepressants (TCAs)

Amitriptyline is the most widely prescribed pharmacological agent for the treatment of FMS (Leventhal 1999). Wolfe et al (1997a) reported a 7-year study at six rheumatology centres showing that 40% of the fibromyalgia patients at these centres used amitriptyline during the course of the investigation. Its beneficial effects on FMS symptoms have been demonstrated in randomised controlled trials (Carette et al 1986, 1994, 1995, Goldenberg et al 1986, Jaeschke et al 1991, Scudds et al 1989).

Carette et al (1986) performed a 9-week, double-blind placebo-controlled trial of 70 patients with FMS who received an escalated dose of amitriptyline from 10 mg/day to 50 mg/day or placebo. They reported that duration of morning stiffness, pain analogue scales, sleep quality, patient and physician overall assessment were improved in the amitriptyline group, but not in the placebo group. TP scores measured with a dolorimeter did not improve significantly in either of the groups.

Goldenberg et al (1986) randomised 62 patients to receive 25 mg of amitriptyline at night, 500 mg of naproxen twice daily, both amitriptyline and naproxen, or placebo, in a 6-week double-blind trial. They reported significant improvement in all outcome measures, including pain, sleep difficulties, morning fatigue, global assessment and TP score, in patients who received amitriptyline. Naproxen was ineffective, with little synergistic effect with amitriptyline. Scudds et al (1989) found similar results with amitriptyline in a randomised, double-blind, crossover trial of 36 patients with FMS.

Jaeschke et al (1991) conducted 23 N-of-1 randomised controlled trials of amitriptyline. They concluded that 25% of patients with FMS derived clinically significant benefit from amitriptyline and noted rapid improvement, generally within 1 week. They found that a low dose, i.e. 10 mg at bedtime, is effective in some patients and that it avoids the drug's anticholinergic side-effects.

The only study to examine the long-term effects of TCAs showed that the benefit of amitriptyline therapy obtained at 1 month was lost at 3 and 6 months because of the development of tolerance (Carette et al 1994).

Side-effects of TCAs, such as dry mouth, daytime sedation, weight gain, constipation, orthostatic hypotension, fluid retention, nightmares, paradoxical insomnia, occurred in up to 20% of patients (Wallace 1997). The recommended starting dose of amitriptyline is 10 mg, taken 1 to 3 hours before bedtime. If there are no side-effects, the dosage can be gradually increased to 50 to 75 mg/day. Since not all patients with FMS benefit from amitriptyline, it is reasonable to try the drug for 4 to 6 weeks. If there is no benefit, the drug can be gradually withdrawn and another tricyclic, such as nortriptyline or cyclobenzaprine, can be given (Creamer 1999). Since tolerance may occur after 2 to 3 months of continued treatment, a 2- to 4-week amitriptyline-free period is advised (Russell 1996). During this time, Russell (1996) suggests employing alprazolam. This drug is likely to be particularly useful in anxious patients.

Cyclobenzaprine, another TCA, has been marketed as a muscle relaxant because of its ability to reduce brainstem noradrenergic function and motor neuron efferent activity (Barnes et al 1980). In a 12-week, double-blind, randomised, controlled study of 120 patients with FMS, it was found to decrease the severity of pain significantly, and improve the quality of sleep from weeks 2 to 12 (Bennett et al 1988). Fatigue improved during weeks 2 to 4, but not weeks 8 to 12. Withdrawal rates were 52% in the placebo group and 16% in the cyclobenzaprine-treated group. Reynolds et al (1991) evaluated its effect in a 4-week, randomised, double-blind, crossover study of 12 patients. They reported improvement in evening fatigue and total sleep time, but there was no effect on pain, TPs, mood ratings and other sleep parameters. However, because the sample size and the duration of this study were inadequate a definite conclusion as to its value could not be reached.

Santandrea et al (1993) evaluated the efficacy and tolerability of two different regimens of cyclobenzaprine in a double-blind crossover study. Patients received either a single dose of 10 mg/day cyclobenzaprine at bedtime or 30 mg/day cyclobenzaprine in three equal doses daily for 15 days. After a 15-day washout period, the groups were crossed over to the other regimen. The authors noted that both regimens resulted in a significant improvement in the number of TPs, quality of sleep, anxiety, fatigue, irritable bowel syndrome and stiffness. The higher dose, however, did not have a better therapeutic effect but did have an increased incidence of side-effects.

In a 6-month, double-blind, randomised, comparative trial of amitriptyline, cyclobenzaprine and placebo in 208 patients with FMS, Carette et al (1994) found that 21%, 12% and 0% of the amitriptyline, cyclobenzaprine and placebo patients had significant clinical improvement after 1 month (amitriptyline versus placebo $P = 0.002$, cyclobenzaprine versus placebo $P = 0.02$, amitriptyline versus cyclobenzaprine P not significant). At 3 months and 6 months, however, the proportion of the responders was no different between the three groups. A normal Minnesota Multiphasic Personality Inventory profile at baseline was predictive of clinical improvement at 1-month evaluation.

Several trials have utilised other TCAs in FMS. In a double-blind placebo-controlled study of 60 patients, Caruso et al (1987) reported that 75 mg/day dothiepin at bedtime reduced TP score and pain. Clomipramine 75 mg/day and maprotiline 75 mg/day were compared with placebo in a triple-crossover, randomised study of 37 patients over a 3-week period (Bibolotti 1986). It was found that clomipramine, which preferentially decreases serotonin uptake, significantly reduced the number of TPs, and maprotiline, which has more effect on noradren-

aline (norepinephrine), improved psychological scores.

Wysenbeek et al (1985) treated 30 patients with imipramine for 3 months but obtained no beneficial therapeutic effect with it.

In summary, overall improvement with TCAs has in general occurred in one-third of the patients studied. Benefit from these agents is generally seen within the first 2 weeks. Serotonergic drugs, such as amitriptyline, dothiepin or clomipramine, may be more beneficial in relieving pain and improving sleep whereas drugs that affect noradrenaline (norepinephrine) reuptake, such as cyclobenzaprine and maprotiline, improve fatigue and psychological outcomes more effectively (Wilke 1995).

Selective serotonin reuptake inhibitors (SSRIs)

Fluoxetine, a selective serotonin reuptake inhibitor, has been studied in FMS. Most case reports, open label and controlled studies have shown that it improves sleep disturbances and depression, but has no positive effect on pain relief or TP score (Finestone & Ober 1990, Geller 1989, Wolfe et al 1994).

An exception to this was a 6-week, double-blind, randomised, crossover study of 19 patients carried out by Goldenberg et al (1996), who found that a combination of amitriptyline and fluoxetine was better than either drug used alone, although both drugs were individually beneficial. Major concerns about this study, however, are that it had a small sample size, short follow-up, and also high dropout rate, with nearly one-third of patients withdrawing due to adverse drug effects or worsening symptoms.

Citalopram, another SSRI, showed no symptom improvement in a randomised, double-blind, placebo-controlled study (Norregaard 1995).

Sertraline has been evaluated by Alberts et al (1998) in a double-blind placebo-controlled trial on 14 patients with FMS. The trial showed that patients treated with this drug have increased pain thresholds at both tender and control points. Furthermore, there was a significantly increased blood flow in both left and right frontal cortical regions, a finding that led the authors to suggest that the drug may act by enhancing activation of the pain inhibition network.

Other antidepressant agents

Although clinical experience led Wilke (1995) and Yunus (1996) to believe that 50 to 100 mg trazodone, a heterocyclic antidepressant, taken at bedtime is beneficial, there is only one controlled study with this agent (Branco et al 1996). The clinical and polysomnographic effects of trazodone were evaluated in a double-blind, crossover, placebo-controlled, 2-month study of 12 patients with FMS. Branco et al (1996) concluded that trazodone normalises REM latency and the alpha-delta pattern, but is not superior to placebo in improving the psychological profile, symptoms and functional parameters.

Venlafaxine, another heterocyclic antidepressant, which inhibits both serotonin and noradrenaline (norepinephrine) reuptake, significantly improved pain, fatigue, sleep quality, morning stiffness, depression, anxiety, and patient global assessment in a small, open label, clinical trial (Dwight et al 1998).

Moclobemide, an inhibitor of monoamine oxidase A (MAO-A) (which inhibits the deamination of serotonin, noradrenaline and dopamine), has not been shown in a randomised, double-blind, placebo-controlled study to be helpful in alleviating fibromyalgia symptoms (Hannonen et al, 1998).

Conversely, another MAO-A inhibitor, pirlindole, was found to be superior to a placebo with respect to pain, TP score, and global evaluation by the patients and a medical assessor in a 4-week double-blind study of 100 cases of FMS (Ginsberg et al 1998). However, MAO-A inhibitors should be used with caution in the treatment of this disorder, and should never be prescribed in combination with other serotonergic and noradrenergic drugs.

S-adenosylmethionine (SAMe), an anti-inflammatory drug with analgesic and antidepressant effects, has had its efficacy and tolerability in FMS evaluated (Jacobsen et al 1991, Tavoni et al 1987, 1998, Valkmann et al 1997).

Tavoni et al (1987), in a 3-week, double-blind, placebo-controlled crossover trial of 17 patients with FMS, found that the number of TPs and painful anatomic sites decreased after intramuscular administration of SAMe, but not after placebo treatment. In addition, depression scores improved after SAMe administration.

The efficacy of 800 mg orally administered SAMe daily versus placebo for 6 weeks was investigated in 44 patients with FMS in a double-blind trial carried out by Jacobsen et al (1991). They suggested that SAMe has some beneficial effects on fibromyalgia and could be an important option in the treatment of this condition.

Tavoni et al (1998) used 400 mg/day intravenous SAMe for 15 days in 30 fibromyalgia patients with connective tissue disease (Sjögren's syndrome in 8, systemic lupus erythematosus in 7, rheumatoid arthritis in 4, systemic sclerosis in 3, mixed connective tissue disease in 3, mixed cryoglobulinaemia in 2, and Raynaud's disease in 2 patients) in a randomised double-blind trial. They reported a significant decrease in pain. In contrast to this, Valkmann et al (1997) administered intravenous SAMe 600 mg/day or placebo for 10 days in 34 patients with fibromyalgia in a crossover trial and reported no beneficial effect of SAMe. Overall, SAMe seems to be useful in FMS.

Anxiolytic drugs

Benzodiazepines

Several clinical trials have assessed the efficacy of benzodiazepines in FMS. Russell et al (1991) randomised 78 patients with FMS to receive ibuprofen and/or alprazolam in a double-blind placebo-controlled trial. They reported that clinical improvement in patient rating of disease severity and in the severity of tenderness upon palpation was most apparent, but not significant, in patients who were receiving ibuprofen plus alprazolam. The study was followed by an open label extension for 52 patients, who all received a combination of ibuprofen and alprazolam for 8 weeks. At the end of 8 weeks, small but statistically significant levels of improvement were seen in several outcomes. The authors concluded that treatment with a combination of alprazolam and ibuprofen is beneficial for some patients with FMS. Another benzodiazepine, bromazepam, was evaluated in 164 patients with FMS by Quijada-Carrera et al (1996). They reported that bromazepam and tenoxicam in combination was more effective than tenoxicam alone, although no statistically significant difference was seen between combination treatment and placebo. Hench et al (1989) compared the efficacy of amitriptyline, temazepam and placebo in a double-blind crossover study of 10 patients and noted a significant improvement in patient and physician global assessment, sleep disturbance and morning stiffness in patients treated with temazepam. Finally, lorazepam was found to have a beneficial effect on pain scores of patients with refractory fibromyalgia evaluated with a retrospective chart analysis (Holman 1998).

Benzodiazepines are not recommended for the long-term treatment of FMS because of the potential dependence and withdrawal seizures associated with them (Leventhal 1999).

Hypnotics

Zopiclone was evaluated in two double-blind placebo-controlled studies of 41 and 33 patients, respectively, which reported similar results (Drewes et al 1991, Gronbald et al 1993). Both studies found zopiclone to be helpful in improvement of subjective sleep complaints, but not pain. Similarly zolpidem, another hypnotic agent, was also reported to be beneficial for sleep and daytime energy, but it was not effective in pain relief (Moldofsky et al 1996). Thus, hypnotic agents appear to help sleep, but not pain, in FMS.

Tranquillisers

The major tranquilliser chlorpromazine, 100 mg, was compared with L-tryptophan, 5 g, both given at bedtime in a double-blind controlled trial of 15 patients (Moldofsky et al 1976). Both drugs significantly increased time spent in stage 4 sleep but only chlorpromazine improved TP

and subjective pain scores. The number of patients studied was thus small. Chlorpromazine is not recommended in FMS because of its potentially serious neurological side-effects.

Anti-inflammatory agents

Despite the fact that there is no evidence of tissue inflammation in FMS (Simms 1998, Yunus et al 1989a), anti-inflammatory agents are used by 91% of patients (Wolfe et al 1997a). In clinical trials, therapeutic doses of naproxen (Goldenberg et al 1986) and ibuprofen (Yunus et al 1989b) were not significantly better than placebo. The combinations of naproxen and amitriptyline (Goldenberg et al 1986), ibuprofen and alprazolam (Russell et al 1991), and tenoxicam and bromazepam (Quijada-Carrera et al 1996) resulted in slightly more improvement in some of the outcome measures than either drug used alone, which suggests these combinations may confer slight synergistic analgesic benefit. These differences were not statistically significant. In general, most FMS patients do not get considerable benefit from non-steroidal anti-inflammatory drugs, but such agents can take the edge off the pain enough to be therapeutically worthwhile (Simms 1994). However, risk factors for gastrointestinal, renal or hepatic side-effects should be carefully considered before prescribing a non-steroidal anti-inflammatory drug.

Prednisone was found to be ineffective in a 2-week, double-blind, placebo-controlled, crossover trial involving 20 patients with FMS (Clark et al 1985). This is consistent with the fact that FMS is not an inflammatory condition and that hypocortisolaemia in FMS is of central origin (see Ch. 16).

Analgesics

Although there is no controlled trial available regarding its efficacy, paracetamol (acetaminophen) is used frequently for pain control in FMS. Wolfe et al (1997a) reported that paracetamol (acetaminophen) was used by 59% of 538 patients with FMS in a 7-year study at six rheumatology centres, whereas 75.5% was reported recently in another study of 286 patients with FMS (Wolfe et al 2000). In the latter study, 27% of the FMS patients reported paracetamol (acetaminophen) not to be effective at all, 46% slightly effective, 25% moderately effective and 2% very effective. The patients compared the effectiveness of paracetamol (acetaminophen) and non-steroidal anti-inflammatory drugs (NSAIDs); 66% reported that paracetamol (acetaminophen) was less effective than NSAIDs, 26% that it was about the same and 8% that it was more effective (Wolfe et al 2000).

The prescription of narcotic analgesics for patients with fibromyalgia should be generally avoided (Buskila 1999). However, tramadol, a centrally acting analgesic, with both mu-opioid receptor binding and noradrenaline (norepinephrine) and serotonin reuptake inhibition that contribute to its antinociceptive effect, may be useful for the treatment of pain in FMS. Russell (1997, 1998) conducted an open label trial of 50–400 mg/day tramadol in 100 patients with fibromyalgia. At the end of 21 days, 69 patients who tolerated tramadol and had adequate pain relief were randomised to receive either tramadol or placebo for 42 days. The time before withdrawal due to inadequate pain relief was significantly longer and the withdrawal rate was significantly lower in the tramadol group than in the placebo group. Statistically significant improvements in patient reported pain scores and pain relief ratings were also demonstrated. Bennett et al (1998a) examined the efficacy and safety of tramadol in a 6-week, double-blind, placebo-controlled trial. They reported similar results to Russell et al (1997). Biasi et al (1998), employing a single 100 mg intravenous dose of tramadol in a double-blind, placebo-controlled, crossover study of 12 patients, found that the tramadol group had greater pain relief than the placebo group, but the number of TPs did not change. Overall, tramadol seems to be a useful drug in FMS. Results of a larger study on this drug are awaited.

Clinical experience shows that a small dose of codeine, e.g. 15–30 mg three times a day, is well tolerated, even on a long-term basis, but it should only be used occasionally (Yunus 1996).

Other pharmacological agents

Carisoprodol is a muscle relaxant and an analgesic agent. Soma Compound, a combination of carisoprodol (1200 mg/day), paracetamol (acetaminophen) and caffeine was shown to be more effective than placebo in an 8-week double-blind trial of 58 patients (Vaeroy et al 1989).

Chlormezanone is an effective muscle relaxant that probably acts via reduction of the gamma efferent discharge to motor fibres of muscle spindles. It also has some benzodiazepine-like effects on sleep physiology, but does not cause reduction in stage 4 sleep. Pattrick et al (1993) found it to be ineffective in the treatment of FMS.

A combination of malic acid and magnesium (200 mg malic acid plus 50 mg magnesium per tablet), both of which are involved in the generation of adenosine triphosphate, was evaluated in the treatment of FMS, on the presumed basis of deficient high energy phosphate in muscles in FMS (Russell et al 1995). Symptoms were not alleviated during a 4-week, double-blind, placebo-controlled trial at a dose of three tablets twice daily. A subsequent open label, dose escalation trial showed improvement in fibromyalgia symptoms. Thus, the efficacy of either malic acid or magnesium in FMS is doubtful.

The efficacy of an antidiencephalon immune serum, SER282, was evaluated in 36 patients with fibromyalgia (Kempenaers et al 1994). Treatment consisted of either SER282 (20 mg/ml) or amitriptyline (50 mg/day) or placebo over an 8-week treatment course. A moderate effect on pain and a tendency to promote stage 4 sleep were reported with SER282.

Bennett et al (1998b) studied the efficacy of human growth hormone in fibromyalgia patients who had low insulin growth factor-1 (IGF-1) levels. Fifty women were included in a double-blind placebo-controlled trial of 9 months. An initial dose of 0.0125 mg/kg/day was given for the first month, which was adjusted at monthly intervals to maintain an IGF-1 level of about 250 ng/ml. There was an improvement in FIQ scores and number of TPs after 9 months of therapy. Pain alone was not evaluated as an outcome measure.

On the basis of serotonin deficiency in patients with fibromyalgia (see Ch. 16), the serotonin precursor 5-hydroxytryptophan was evaluated in the treatment of FMS in a double-blind placebo-controlled trial for 30 days (Caruso et al 1990), and in a 90-day open study (Puttini & Caruso 1992). The drug was shown to be effective in improving fibromyalgia symptoms.

The blockade of the serotonin receptor subtype 5-HT3 with tropisetron (Samborski et al 1996, Faerber et al 1999) and ondansetron (Hrycaj et al 1996) and subtype 5-HT2 with ritanserin (Olin et al 1998) has been studied in the treatment of fibromyalgia. Limited beneficial effects of these 5-HT receptor blockers were reported. Further studies are needed.

In an open label study of 11 patients with fibromyalgia, gamma hydroxybutyrate was given at a dose of 2.25 g at bedtime and again 4 hours later for 1 month (Scharf et al 1998). Patients reported significant decreases in pain and fatigue and improvement in overall well-being, but objective sleep measurements were not significantly improved in this small group.

Low dose sublingual human interferon-alpha was found to be beneficial in a 6-week, double-blind placebo-controlled study of 112 patients with FMS (Russell et al 1999). The authors reported that there was no change in the TP index at the end of the 6-week trial, but morning stiffness and physical function improved significantly.

There are several studies that evaluate the possible role of melatonin, a pineal hormone, in FMS, since it involves synchronising circadian systems, and has sleep-promoting properties. Contradictory results have been reported for melatonin levels in patients with FMS, i.e. higher than controls (Korszun et al 1999), lower than controls (Wikner et al 1998) or similar to controls (Press et al 1998). Citera et al (2000) evaluated the possible effect of melatonin treatment on disturbed sleep, fatigue and pain in a 4-week open study of 21 patients with FMS. Improvements in TP counts, severity of pain and sleep disturbances, and patient and physician global assessments, were reported with 3 mg melatonin at bedtime. The authors suggested that melatonin could be an alternative and safe treatment for patients with FMS. Further controlled studies with large numbers will be needed to evaluate the efficacy of this nutritional supplement.

In a randomised, double-blind, crossover trial, salmon calcitonin was administered subcutaneously at a daily dose of 100 IU for 1 month with no beneficial effect (Bessette et al 1998).

Combining stellate ganglion blockade followed by regional sympathetic blockade was examined in a 28-patient, comparative, blinded trial (Bengtsson & Bengtsson 1988). Bupivacaine stellate ganglion blockade was found to be more effective than guanetidine blockade in reducing the number of TPs as evaluated 24 hours after the injection. But no long-term studies of regional sympathetic blockade are available.

Janzen & Scudds (1997) examined the efficacy of sphenopalatine blocks with lignocaine (lidocaine) in the treatment of pain in 42 patients with FMS and 19 with myofascial pain. They reported that 4% lignocaine (lidocaine) was no better than placebo. Intravenous lignocaine (lidocaine) was studied in a 6-day open label trial of 10 patients with FMS (Bennett & Tai 1995). Pain relief and improvement in mood scores was reported at 7 and at 30 days follow-up.

TENDER POINT INJECTIONS

Another therapeutic approach in the treatment of FMS is the administration of serial local injections in the TPs. It is a very valuable adjunctive therapy. In an open study of 41 patients with FMS, a mixture of 1% lignocaine (lidocaine) 1/2 cc and triamcinolone diacetate 1/4 cc (10 mg) was injected in TPs (Reddy et al in press, Yunus et al 1998). Average duration of pain relief per injected site was 13 weeks. Injection of TPs is particularly useful if the patient can localize one to four areas that are most bothersome. After the injections patients should apply local ice for several hours and rest the injected areas for 24 to 48 hours to minimise postinjection flare. Figuerola et al (1998) found the increase in met-enkephalin levels similar after the injection of TPs by lignocaine (lidocaine), saline or dry needling. They suggested that some of the benefits of TP injection might be attributed to the mechanistic effects of needling, rather than the pharmacological agent.

Baldry (2000) has found that superficial dry needling alone is useful in patients with FMS. In order to avoid temporary exacerbation of pain, he inserts the needle to a depth of about 2–3 mm into the subcutaneous tissues overlying an intramuscular TP and leaves it in situ for about 5–10 seconds. Multiple TPs may be treated this way. Frequent treatments are necessary, since initially the benefit lasts only for a few days. Repeated treatment, however, results in worthwhile relief of pain for as long as 6–8 weeks with improvement in a patient's functions without side-effects. It is suggested that dry needling alone causes stimulation of alpha-delta nerve fibres in the skin and subcutaneous tissues, which in turn, activate pain-inhibiting mechanisms in the spinal cord (Baldry 1995).

PROGNOSIS

The prognosis in FMS is one of chronic pain and disability. Hawley et al (1988) evaluated pain, functional disability and psychological status by monthly questionnaires for 12 months and found that these parameters remained stable from month to month among the patients as a group, but there was considerable individual variations among the patients.

In a six-centre study in the USA, Wolfe and his associates (1997b) assessed outcome of symptoms and function among 538 patients with FMS in a longitudinal study over a period of 7 years. Overall, all the parameters evaluated, including pain, fatigue, sleep difficulties, psychological status, global severity and functional disability, remained unchanged over time. In the same study, a follow-up of 85 patients from the Wichita centre over a mean period of 11.5 years was also reported and the outcome was found to be similar. Ledingham et al (1993) from the United Kingdom also reported that FMS symptoms overall remained unchanged after a mean follow-up period of 4 years.

Factors that may affect prognosis positively includes patients' level of education, younger age, and increased time spent doing exercise.

Factors associated with poor prognosis are the initial degree of global severity and pain, depressed mood and a large number of pain sites (Felson & Goldenberg 1986, Granges et al 1994, Henriksson 1994).

Although follow-up studies show that symptoms in fibromyalgia patients as a group do not change significantly overall, there is a lot of variation between individual patients. Many patients have their symptoms improved with appropriate treatment over a relatively short period of time, during which they also experience better function.

SUMMARY

Since biopathophysiological mechanisms of FMS are incompletely understood, management of this condition remains unsatisfactory. Multiple factors interact to produce symptoms, and these factors vary among patients. Therefore individualisation of management is important.

A firm diagnosis, patient education and reassurance are important initial components of FMS management. The physician should adopt a positive and empathetic attitude. Management should be individualised according to a patient's symptoms and the severity of FMS. For successful management, possible aggravating factors should be identified so that they may be eliminated or modified.

Management of FMS includes a variety of non-pharmacological and pharmacological interventions. Aerobic exercise, EMG biofeedback, acupuncture, cognitive behavioural therapy and integrated group therapy have been shown to be beneficial by randomised controlled trials in FMS. Although physical therapies, such as heat, massage, ultrasound and TENS are widely used, and some patients report benefit, their effectiveness is not proven by controlled studies.

Among pharmacological agents, studies have focused mainly on serotonergic drugs. Several of these drugs have been shown to be effective in double-blind controlled trials. Amitriptyline at a dose of 10–50 mg at bedtime is beneficial and frequently prescribed in FMS. A combination of amitriptyline and fluoxetine has been reported to be more efficacious than either agent alone. The dose of both drugs should be kept low if used in combination. Cyclobenzaprine and trazodone are the other agents that are used frequently. Benzodiazepines are helpful in anxious patients. Hypnotics may be helpful for sleep disturbance, but they do not help pain. Tramadol appears to be a useful drug. Low dose codeine may be used during a flare up and in severe cases. Tender point injection is a very valuable adjunctive therapy.

The optimal management of FMS should include appropriate medical treatment of pain and sleep disturbances in combination with non-pharmacological interventions, especially aerobic exercises, cognitive behavioural therapy and interdisciplinary group treatment. The management plan outlined in this chapter is helpful in most patients.

REFERENCES

Alberts K R, Bradley L A, Alarcon G S 1998 Sertraline hydrochloride (Zoloft) alters pain threshold, sensory discrimination ability, and functional brain activity in patients with fibromyalgia (FM): a randomized controlled trial (RCT) (abstract). Arthritis and Rheumatism 41(Suppl):S259

Baldry P 1995 Superficial dry needling at myofascial trigger point sites. Journal of Musculoskeletal Pain 3(3):117–126

Baldry P 2000 Superficial dry needling. In: Chaltow L (ed) Fibromyalgia syndrome: a practitioner's guide to treatment. Churchill Livingstone, Edinburgh, ch 7.

Barnes C D, Fung S J, Gintautus J 1980 Brainstem noradrenergic system depression by cyclobenzaprine. Neuropharmacology 19:221–224

Bengtsson A, Bengtsson M, 1988 Regional sympathetic blockade in primary fibromyalgia. Pain 33(2):161–167

Bennett M I, Tai Y M 1995 Intravenous lignocaine in the management of primary fibromyalgia syndrome. International Journal of Clinical Pharmacology Research 15(3):115–119

Bennett R M 1997 The fibromyalgia syndrome. In: Kelley W N (ed) Textbook of Rheumatology. WB Saunders Company, Philadelphia, ch 34, pp 517–518

Bennett R M, Gatter R A, Campbell S M, Andrews R P, Clark S R, Scarola J A 1988 A comparison of cyclobenzaprine and placebo in the management of fibrositis. A double-blind controlled study. Arthritis and Rheumatism 31(12):1535–1542

Bennett R M, Campbell S M, Burckhardt C S et al 1991 A multidisciplinary approach to fibromyalgia management. Journal of Musculoskeletal Medicine 8(11):21–32

Bennett R M, Burckhardt C S, Clark S R, et al 1996 Group treatment of fibromyalgia: a 6 month outpatient program. Journal of Rheumatology 23:521–528

Bennett R M, TPS-FM Study Group 1998a A blinded, placebo-controlled evaluation of tramadol in the management of fibromyalgia pain. Journal of Musculoskeletal Pain 6(Suppl 2):146

Bennett R M, Clark S C, Walczyk J 1998b A randomized, double-blind, placebo-controlled study of growth hormone in the treatment of fibromyalgia. American Journal of Medicine 104(3):227–231

Bessette L, Carette S, Fossel A H, Lew R A 1998 A placebo controlled crossover trial of subcutaneous salmon calcitonin in the treatment of patients with fibromyalgia. Scandinavian Journal of Rheumatology 27(2):112–116

Biasi G, Manca S, Manganelli S, Marcolongo R 1998 Tramadol in the fibromyalgia syndrome: a controlled clinical trial versus placebo. International Journal of Clinical Pharmacology Research 18(1):13–19

Bibolotti E, Borghi C, Paculli E et al 1986 The management of fibrositis: a double blind comparison of maprotiline, chlorimipramine and placebo. Clinical Trials Journal 23:269–280

Blunt K L, Rajwani M H, Guerriero R C 1997 The effectiveness of chiropractic management of fibromyalgia patients: a pilot study. Journal of Manipulative and Physiological Therapeutics 20(6):389–399

Boghen D, Lamothe L, Elie R, Godbout R, Montplaisir J 1986 The treatment of the restless legs syndrome with clonazepam: a prospective controlled study. Canadian Journal of Neurological Sciences 13(3):245–247

Bradley L A 1989 Cognitive-behavioral therapy for primary fibromyalgia. Journal of Rheumatology 19(Suppl):131–136

Branco J C, Martini A, Palva T 1996 Treatment of sleep abnormalities and clinical complaints in fibromyalgia with trazodone (abstract). Arthritis and Rheumatism 39(Suppl):59

Buckelew S P, Conway R, Parker J et al 1998 Biofeedback/relaxation training and exercise interventions for fibromyalgia: a prospective trial. Arthritis Care and Research 11(3):196–209

Burckhardt C S, Bjelle A 1994 Education programs for fibromyalgia patients: description and evaluation. Baillière's Clinical Rheumatology 8(4):935–955

Burckhardt C S, Mannerkorpi K, Hedenberg L, Bjelle A 1994 A randomized, controlled clinical trial of education and physical training for women with fibromyalgia. Journal of Rheumatology 21(4):714–720

Buskila D 1999 Drug therapy. Baillière's Best Practice and Research on Clinical Rheumatology 13(3):479–485

Carette S, McCain G A, Bell D A, Fam A G 1986 Evaluation of amitriptyline in primary fibrositis. A double blind, placebo-controlled study. Arthritis and Rheumatism 29(5):655–659

Carette S, Bell M J, Reynolds W J, et al 1994 Comparison of amitriptyline, cyclobenzaprine, and placebo in the treatment of fibromyalgia. Arthritis and Rheumatism 37(1):32–40

Carette S, Oakson G, Guimont C, Steriade M 1995 Sleep electroencephalography and the clinical response to amitriptyline in patients with fibromyalgia. Arthritis and Rheumatism 38(9):1211–1217

Caruso I, Sarzi Puttini P C, Boccassini L et al 1987 Double-blind study of dothiepin versus placebo in the treatment of primary fibromyalgia syndrome. Journal of International Medical Research 15(3):154–159

Caruso I, Sarzi Puttini P, Cazzola M, Azzolini V 1990 Double-blind study of 5-hydroxytryptophan versus placebo in the treatment of primary fibromyalgia syndrome. Journal of International Medical Research 18(3):201–209

Citera G, Arias M A, Maldonado-Cocco J A, et al 2000 The effect of melatonin in patients with fibromyalgia: a pilot study. Clinical Rheumatology 19(1):9–13

Clark S, Tindall E, Bennett R M 1985 A double blind crossover trial of prednisone versus placebo in the treatment of fibrositis. Journal of Rheumatology 12(5):980–983

Clark S R 1994 Prescribing exercise for fibromyalgia patients. Arthritis Care and Research 7(4):221–225

Creamer P 1999 Effective management of fibromyalgia. Journal of Musculoskeletal Medicine 16:622–637

DeLuze C, Bosia L, Zirbs A, Chantraine A, Vischer T L 1992 Electroacupuncture in fibromyalgia: results of a controlled trial. British Medical Journal 305(6864):1249–1252

Drewes A M, Andreasen A, Jennum P, Nielsen K D 1991 Zopiclone in the treatment of sleep abnormalities in fibromyalgia. Scandinavian Journal of Rheumatology 20(4):288–293

Dwight M M, Arnold L M, O'Brien H, Metzger R, Morris-Park E, Keck P E Jr 1998 An open clinical trial of venlafaxine treatment of fibromyalgia. Psychosomatics 39(1):14–17

Faerber L, Stratz T, Michael S et al 1999 Efficacy and safety of a 5-HT3 receptor antagonist (Tropisetron) in primary fibromyalgia (abstract). Arthritis and Rheumatism 42(Suppl 9):S395

Felson D T, Goldenberg D L 1986 The natural history of fibromyalgia. Arthritis and Rheumatism 29:1522–1526

Ferraccioli G, Ghirelli L, Scita F et al 1987 EMG-biofeedback training in fibromyalgia syndrome. Journal of Rheumatology 14(4):820–825

Figuerola M L, Loe W, Sormani M, Barontini M 1998 Met-enkephalin increase in patients with fibromyalgia under local treatment. Functional Neurology 13(4):291–295

Finestone D H, Ober S K 1990 Fluoxetine and fibromyalgia. Journal of the American Medical Association 264(22):2869–2870 (letter)

Fossaluzza V, De Vita S 1992 Combined therapy with cyclobenzaprine and ibuprofen in primary fibromyalgia syndrome. International Journal of Clinical Pharmacology Research 12(2):99–102

Geller S A 1989 Treatment of fibrositis with fluoxetine hydrochloride (Prozac). American Journal of Medicine 87(5):594–595

Ginsberg F, Joos E, Geczy J, Bruhwyler J, Vandekerckhove K, Famaey J P 1998 A pilot randomized placebo controlled study of pirlindole in the treatment of primary fibromyalgia. Journal of Musculoskeletal Pain 6(2):5–17

Godfrey R G 1996 A guide to the understanding and use of tricyclic antidepressants in the overall management of fibromyalgia and other chronic pain syndromes. Archives of Internal Medicine 156(10):1047–1052

Goldenberg D L 1989 A review of the role of tricyclic medications in the treatment of fibromyalgia syndrome. Journal of Rheumatology 19(Suppl):137–139.

Goldenberg D L, Felson D T, Dinerman H 1986 A randomized, controlled trial of amitriptyline and naproxen in the treatment of patients with fibromyalgia. Arthritis and Rheumatism 29(11):1371–1377

Goldenberg D L, Kaplan K H, Nadeau M G, Brodeur C, Smith S, Schmid C H 1994 A controlled study of stress-reduction, cognitive behavioral treatment program in fibromyalgia. Journal of Musculoskeletal Pain 2:53–66

Goldenberg D, Mayskiy M, Mossey C, Ruthazer R, Schmid C 1996 A randomized, double-blind crossover trial of fluoxetine and amitriptyline in the treatment of fibromyalgia. Arthritis and Rheumatism 39(11):1852–1859

Gowans S E, deHueck A, Voss S, Richardson M 1999 A randomized, controlled trial of exercise and education for individuals with fibromyalgia. Arthritis Care and Research 12(2):120–128

Granges G, Zilko P, Littlejohn G O 1994 Fibromyalgia syndrome: assessment of severity of the condition two years after diagnosis. Journal of Rheumatology 21:523–529

Gronblad M, Nykanen J, Konttinen Y, Jarvinen E, Helve T 1993 Effect of zopiclone on sleep quality, morning stiffness, widespread tenderness and pain and general discomfort in primary fibromyalgia patients. A double-blind randomized trial. Clinical Rheumatology 12(2):186–191

Gunther V, Mur E, Kinigadner U, Miller C, 1994 Fibromyalgia – the effect of relaxation and hydrogalvanic bath therapy on the subjective pain experience. Clinical Rheumatology 13(4):573–578

Haanen H C, Hoenderdos H T, van Romunde L K et al 1991 Controlled trial of hypnotherapy in the treatment of refractory fibromyalgia. Journal of Rheumatology 18(1):72–75

Hannonen P, Malminiemi K, Yli-Kerttula U, Isomeri R, Roponen P 1998 A randomized, double-blind, placebo-controlled study of moclobemide and amitriptyline in the treatment of fibromyalgia in females without psychiatric disorder. British Journal of Rheumatology 37(12):1279–1286

Harding S M 1998 Sleep in fibromyalgia patients: subjective and objective findings. American Journal of Medical Sciences 315(6):367–376

Hawley D J, Wolfe F, Cathey M A 1988 Pain, functional disability, and psychological status: a 12-month study of severity in fibromyalgia. Journal of Rheumatology 15(10):1551–1556

Hench P K, Cohen R, Mitler M M 1989 Fibromyalgia: effects of amitriptyline, temazepam and placebo on pain and sleep. Arthritis and Rheumatism 32(Suppl):S47

Henriksson C M 1994 Long-term effects of fibromyalgia on everyday life: a study of 56 patients. Scandinavian Journal of Rheumatology 23:36–41

Holman A J 1998 Effect of lorazepam on pain score of refractory fibromyalgia. Arthritis and Rheumatism 41 (Suppl):S259

Hrycaj P, Stratz T, Mennet P, Muller V 1996 Pathogenic aspects of responsiveness to ondansetron (5-hydroxytryptamine type 3 receptor antagonist) in patients with primary fibromyalgia syndrome – a preliminary study. Journal of Rheumatology 23:1418–1423

Jacobsen S, Danneskiold-Samsoe B, Andersen RB 1991 Oral S-adenosylmethionine in primary fibromyalgia. Double-blind clinical evaluation. Scandinavian Journal of Rheumatology 20(4):294–302

Jaeschke R, Adachi J, Guyatt G, Keller J, Wong B 1991 Clinical usefulness of amitriptyline in fibromyalgia: the results of 23 N-of-1 randomized controlled trials. Journal of Rheumatology 18(3):447–451

Janzen V D, Scudds R 1997 Sphenopalatine blocks in the treatment of pain in fibromyalgia and myofascial pain syndrome. Laryngoscope 107(10):1420–1422

Kaada B 1989 Treatment of fibromyalgia by low-frequency transcutaneous nerve stimulation. Tidsskrift For Den Norske Laegeforening 109:2992–2995

Keel P J, Bodoky C, Gerhard U, Muller W 1998 Comparison of integrated group therapy and group relaxation training for fibromyalgia. Clinical Journal of Pain 14:232–238

Kempenaers C, Simenon G, Vander Elst M et al 1994 Effect of an antidiencephalon immune serum on pain and sleep in primary fibromyalgia. Neuropsychobiology 30(2–3):66–72

Korszun A, Sackett-Lundeen L, Papadopoulos E et al 1999 Melatonin levels in women with fibromyalgia and chronic fatigue syndrome. Journal of Rheumatology 26(12):2675–2680

Krueger B R 1990 Restless legs syndrome and periodic limb movements of sleep. Mayo Clinic Proceedings 65:999–1006

Ledingham J, Doherty S, Doherty M 1993 Primary fibromyalgia syndrome – an outcome study. British Journal of Rheumatology 32:139–142

Leventhal L J 1999 Management of fibromyalgia. Annals of Internal Medicine 7131(11):850–858

Lewis P J 1993 Electroacupuncture in fibromyalgia (letter, comment). British Medical Journal 306(6874):393

McCain G A 1986 Role of physical fitness training in the fibrositis/fibromyalgia syndrome. American Journal of Medicine 2981(3A):73–77

McCain G A 1989 Nonmedicinal treatments in primary fibromyalgia. Rheumatic Disease Clinics of North America 15(1):73–90

McCain G A, Bell D A, Mai F M, Halliday P D 1988 A controlled study of the effects of a supervised cardiovascular fitness training program on the manifestations of primary fibromyalgia. Arthritis and Rheumatism 31(9):1135–1141

Martin L, Nutting A, MacIntosh B R, Edworthy S M, Butterwick D, Cook J 1996 An exercise program in the treatment of fibromyalgia. Journal of Rheumatology 23(6):1050–1053

Masi A T 1994 An intuitive person-centered perspective on fibromyalgia syndrome and its management. Baillière's Clinical Rheumatology 8(4):957–993

Mengshoel A M, Komnaes H B, Forre O 1992 The effects of 20 weeks of physical fitness training in female patients with fibromyalgia. Clinical and Experimental Rheumatology 10(4):345–349

Moldofsky H, Scarisbrick P 1976 Induction of neurasthenic musculoskeletal pain syndrome by selective sleep deprivation. Psychosomatic Medicine 37:341–351

Moldofsky H, Benz B, Luc F et al 1976 Comparison of chlorpromazine and L-tryptophane on sleep, musculoskeletal pain, and mood in fibrositis syndrome. Sleep Research 5:76

Moldofsky H, Lue F A, Mously C, Roth-Schechter B, Reynolds W J 1996 The effect of zolpidem in patients with fibromyalgia: a dose ranging, double blind, placebo controlled, modified crossover study. Journal of Rheumatology 23(3):529–533

Montplaisir J, Godbout R, Poirier G, Bedard M A 1986 Restless legs syndrome and periodic limb movements in sleep: physiopathology and treatment with L-dopa. Clinical Neuropharmacology 9:456–463

NIH Consensus Conference 1998 Acupuncture. Journal of the American Medical Association 280:1518–1524

NIH Technology Assessment Panel on integration of behavioral and relaxation approaches into the treatment of chronic pain and insomnia. 1996 Integration of behavioral and relaxation approaches into the treatment of chronic pain and insomnia. Journal of the American Medical Association 276:313–318

Nicassio P M, Schuman C, Kim J, Cordova A, Weisman M H 1997 Psychosocial factors associated with complementary treatment use in fibromyalgia. Journal of Rheumatology 24(10):2008–2013

Nielson W R, Walker C, McCain G A 1992 Cognitive behavioral treatment of fibromyalgia syndrome: preliminary findings. Journal of Rheumatology 19(1):98–103

Norregaard J, Volkmann H, Danneskiold-Samsoe B 1995 A randomized controlled trial of citalopram in the treatment of fibromyalgia. Pain 61(3):445–449

Olin R, Klein R, Berg P A 1998 A randomized double-blind 16-week study of ritanserin in fibromyalgia syndrome: clinical outcome and analysis of autoantibodies to serotonin, gangliosides and phospholipids. Clinical Rheumatology 17(2):89–94

Parziale J R 1999 The clinical management of fibromyalgia. Medicine and Health, Rhode Island 82(9):325–328

Pattrick M, Swannell A, Doherty M 1993 Chlormezanone in primary fibromyalgia syndrome: a double blind placebo controlled study. British Journal of Rheumatology 32(1):55–58

Pioro-Boisset M, Esdaile J M, Fitzcharles M A 1996 Alternative medicine use in fibromyalgia syndrome Arthritis Care and Research 9(1):13–17

Press J, Phillip M, Neumann L, et al 1998 Normal melatonin levels in patients with fibromyalgia syndrome. Journal of Rheumatology 25(3):551–555

Puttini P S, Caruso I 1992 Primary fibromyalgia syndrome and 5-hydroxy-L-tryptophan: a 90-day open study. Journal of International Medical Research 20(2):182–189

Quijada-Carrera J, Valenzuela-Castano A, Povedano-Gomez J, et al 1996 Comparison of tenoxicam and bromazepan in the treatment of fibromyalgia: a randomized, double-blind, placebo-controlled trial. Pain 65(2–3):221–225

Reddy S S, Yunus M B, İnanıcı F, Aldag J C Tender point injections are beneficial in fibromyalgia syndrome: a descriptive, open study. Journal of Musculoskeletal Pain (in press)

Reynolds W J, Moldofsky H, Saskin P, Lue F A 1991 The effects of cyclobenzaprine on sleep physiology and symptoms in patients with fibromyalgia. Journal of Rheumatology 18(3):452–454

Rosen N B 1994 Physical medicine and rehabilitation approaches to the management of myofascial pain and fibromyalgia syndromes. Baillière's Clinical Rheumatology 8(4):881–916

Russell I J 1996 Fibromyalgia syndrome: approaches to management. Bulletin on Rheumatic Diseases 45(3):1–4

Russell I J 1998 Efficacy of Ultram (tramadol HCL) treatment of fibromyalgia syndrome: secondary outcome report. TPS-FM Study Group(abstract). Journal of Musculoskeletal Pain 6(Suppl 2):147

Russell I J, Fletcher E M, Michalek J E, McBroom P C, Hester G G 1991 Treatment of primary fibrositis/fibromyalgia syndrome with ibuprofen and alprazolam. A double-blind, placebo-controlled study. Arthritis and Rheumatism 34(5):552–560

Russell I J, Michalek J E, Flechas J D, Abraham G E 1995 Treatment of fibromyalgia syndrome with Super Malic: a randomized, double blind, placebo controlled, crossover pilot study. Journal of Rheumatology 22(5):953–958

Russell I J, Kamin M, Sager D, et al 1997 Efficacy of Ultram (tramadol HCL) treatment of fibromyalgia syndrome: preliminary analysis of a multi-center, randomized, placebo controlled study (abstract). Arthritis and Rheumatism 40(Suppl 9):S117

Russell I J, Michalek J E, Kang Y K, Richards A B 1999 Reduction of morning stiffness and improvement in physical function in fibromyalgia syndrome patients treated sublingually with low doses of human interferon-alpha. Journal of Interferon Cytokine Research 19(8):961–968

Samborski W, Stratz T, Lacki J K, Klama K, Mennet P, Muller W 1996 The 5-HT3 blockers in the treatment of the primary fibromyalgia syndrome: a 10–day open study with Tropisetron at a low dose. Materia Medica Polona 28(1):17–19

Santandrea S, Montrone F, Sarzi-Puttini P, Boccassini L, Caruso I 1993 A double-blind crossover study of two cyclobenzaprine regimens in primary fibromyalgia syndrome. Journal of International Medical Research 21(2):74–80

Sarnoch H, Adler F, Scholz O B 1997 Relevance of muscular sensitivity, muscular activity, and cognitive variables for pain reduction associated with EMG biofeedback in fibromyalgia. Perceptual Motor Skills 84(3 Pt 1):1043–1050

Scharf M B, Hauck M, Stover R, McDannold M, Berkowitz D 1998 Effect of gamma-hydroxybutyrate on pain, fatigue, and the alpha sleep anomaly in patients with fibromyalgia. Preliminary report. Journal of Rheumatology 25(10):1986–1990

Scudds R A, McCain G A, Rollman G B, Harth M 1989 Improvements in pain responsiveness in patients with fibrositis after successful treatment with amitriptyline. Journal of Rheumatology 19(Suppl):98–103

Singh B B, Berman B M, Hadhazy V A, Creamer P 1998 A pilot study of cognitive behavioral therapy in fibromyalgia.Alternative Therapies in Health and Medicine 4(2):67–70

Sim J, Adams N 1999 Physical and other non-pharmacological interventions for fibromyalgia. Baillière's Clinical Rheumatology 13(3):507–523

Simms R W 1994 Controlled trials of therapy in fibromyalgia syndrome. Baillière's Clinical Rheumatology 8(4):917–934

Simms R W 1998 Fibromyalgia is not a muscle disorder. American Journal of Sciences 315:346–350

Sorensen J, Bengtsson A, Ahlner J, Henriksson K G, Ekselius L, Bengtsson M 1997 Fibromyalgia – are there different mechanisms in the processing of pain? A double blind crossover comparison of analgesic drugs. Journal of Rheumatology 24(8):1615–1621

Sprott H, Franke S, Kluge H, Hein G 1998 Pain treatment of fibromyalgia by acupuncture (letter). Rheumatology International 18(1):35–36

Tavoni A, Vitali C, Bombardieri S, Pasero G 1987 Evaluation of S-adenosylmethionine in primary fibromyalgia. A double-blind crossover study. American Journal of Medicine 83(5A):107–110

Tavoni A, Jeracitano G, Cirigliano G 1998 Evaluation of S-adenosylmethionine in secondary fibromyalgia: a double-blind study (letter). Clinical and Experimental Rheumatology 16(1):106–107

Turk D C, Okifuji A, Sinclair J D, Starz T W 1998 Interdisciplinary treatment for fibromyalgia syndrome: clinical and statistical significance. Arthritis Care Research 11:186–195

Vaeroy H, Abrahamsen A, Forre O, Kass E 1989 Treatment of fibromyalgia (fibrositis syndrome): a parallel double blind trial with carisoprodol, paracetamol and caffeine (Somadril comp) versus placebo. Clinical Rheumatology 8(2):245–250

Valkmann H, Norregaard J, Jacobsen S, Danneskiold-Samsoe B, Knoke G, Nehrdich D 1997 Double blind, placebo controlled crossover study of intravenous S-adenosyl-L-methionine in patients with fibromyalgia. Scandinavian Journal of Rheumatology 26:206–211

Vlaeyen J W, Teeken-Gruben N J, Goossens M E, et al 1996 Cognitive-educational treatment of fibromyalgia: a randomized clinical trial. I. Clinical effects. Journal of Rheumatology 23(7):1237–1245

Wallace D J 1997 The fibromyalgia syndrome. Annals of Medicine 29:9–21

Waylonis G W, Ronan P G, Gordon C 1994 A profile of fibromyalgia in occupational environments. American Journal of Physical Medicine and Rehabilitation 73:112–115

White K P, Nielson W R 1995 Cognitive behavioral treatment of fibromyalgia syndrome: a follow-up assessment. Journal of Rheumatology 22(4):717–721

Wigers S H, Stiles T C, Vogel P A 1996 Effects of aerobic exercise versus stress management treatment in fibromyalgia. A 4.5 year prospective study. Scandinavian Journal of Rheumatology 25(2):77–86

Wikner J, Hirsch U, Wetterberg L, Rojdmark S 1998 Fibromyalgia – a syndrome associated with decreased nocturnal melatonin secretion. Clinical Endocrinology 49(2):161–162

Wilke W S 1995 Treatment of 'resistant' fibromyalgia. Rheumatic Disease Clinics of North America 21(1):247–260

Wolfe F, Cathey M A, Hawley D J 1994 A double-blind placebo controlled trial of fluoxetine in fibromyalgia. Scandinavian Journal of Rheumatology 23(5):255–259

Wolfe F, Anderson J, Harkness D et al 1997a A prospective, longitudinal, multicenter study of service utilization and costs in fibromyalgia. Arthritis and Rheumatism 40(9):1560–1570

Wolfe F, Anderson J, Harkness D, et al 1997b Health status and disease severity in fibromyalgia: results of a six-center longitudinal study. Arthritis and Rheumatism 40(9):1571–1579

Wolfe F, Zhao S, Lane N 2000 Preference for nonsteroidal antiinflammatory drugs over acetaminophen by rheumatic disease patients. Arthritis and Rheumatism 43(2):378–385

Wysenbeek A J, Mor F, Lurie Y, Weinberger A 1985 Imipramine for the treatment of fibrositis: a therapeutic trial. Annals of Rheumatic Diseases 44(11):752–753

Yunus M B 1992 Towards a model of pathophysiology of fibromyalgia: aberrant central pain mechanisms with peripheral modulation. Journal of Rheumatology 19(6):846–850

Yunus M B 1994 Psychological aspects of fibromyalgia syndrome – a component of the dysfunctional spectrum syndrome. Baillière's Clinical Rheumatology 8(4): 811–837

Yunus M B 1996 Fibromyalgia syndrome: is there any effective therapy? Consultant 36:1279–1285

Yunus M B, Kalyan-Raman U P, Masi A T, Aldag J C 1989a Electron microscopic studies of muscle biopsy in primary fibromyalgia syndrome; a controlled and blinded study. Journal of Rheumatology 16:97–101

Yunus M B, Masi A T, Aldag J C 1989b Short term effects of ibuprofen in primary fibromyalgia syndrome: a double blind, placebo controlled trial. Journal of Rheumatology 16(4):527–532

Yunus M B, Reddy S S, İnanıcı F, Aldag J C 1998 Tender point injections are beneficial in fibromyalgia (abstract). Journal of Rheumatology 25(Suppl 52):M58

Yurtkuran M, Celiktas M 1996 A randomized, controlled therapy of balneotherapy in the treatment of patients with primary fibromyalgia syndrome. Physikalische Medizin Rehabilitationsmedizin Kurortmedizin 6:109–112

Index

Soleus muscle, 286–287
  pedal exercise, 287
  periostalgia syndrome, 287, 289
Soma Compound, 391
Somatisation disorder, 49
Somatostatin, 32
Soreness, post-treatment, 105, 110, 133
  hamstring muscles, 272
Spatial disorientation, whiplash injury, 139–140
Sphenopalatine blocks, FMS treatment, 392
Spinal accessory nerve, 133
Spinal cord
  dorsal horn *see* Dorsal horn, spinal cord
  laminae, **22**, 27–28
  self-perpetuating circuits between MTrPs and, 70–72
Spinoreticular tract *see* Paleo-spino-diencephalic pathway
Spinothalamic tract, 28
Splenius cervicis, 124, **137**
Spondylolisthesis, degenerative, 255, 257
Spondylosis
  cervical, 145–147
  lumbar, 254–255
Spontaneous electrical activity (SEA), MTrP sites, 61, **62**
Stalked cells *see* Enkephalinergic inhibitory interneurons
Steindler, Arthur, 12
Sternalis, 304–305
Sternoclavicular joint arthropathy, 309–310
Sternocleidomastoid, 128–129
  TrP sites and pain referral, 129
    chest wall pain, 304
    TrP-induced headache, 203
    whiplash injury, 140
Steroids
  epidural, 144, 252
  plantar fasciitis, 299–300
  rotator cuff tendinitis, 166
  see also Corticosteroids
Stiffness, fibromyalgia, 352
Stimulation-produced analgesia, 37–38
Stockman, Ralph, 4, 6, 67
Straight leg raising test
  hamstring TrP-evoked restriction, 272
  intervertebral disc prolapse, 250, 253
Strauss H, 5
Stress
  FMS, 367
  RSI, 195
  and TrP activity, 47
Stress fracture
  calcaneum, 299
  tibia, 287
Stroke
  central post-stroke pain, 86
  post-stroke MTrP pain, 64, 86
Strong responders, 114, 133

'Stuck patella', 268
Subacromial bursa, triamcinolone injection, 166
Subacromial decompression, 167
Subchondral bone pain, 275
Subclavius, 307–**308**
Subcutaneous tissue thickening, 74
Subnucleus interpolaris, 28
Subnucleus oralis, 28
Subnucleus caudalis, 28, 204, 206, 207, 211, 213
Subnucleus reticularis dorsalis, 211
Subscapularis, 162, 163
Substance P, 24, 32, 69, 205, 207, 357
  in CSF, FMS, 360
Substantia gelatinosa (lamina II), 27, 31–32
  opiate receptors, 33
Sudeck's atrophy, 96
Sudomotor changes, CRPS type I, 98, 99
Suggestions Relating to the Study of Somatic Pain, Lewis, 7
Sumatriptan, 205, 208
Superficial dry needling, 36, 37–39, 103, 111–112
  electrically generated current, 113, 114
  indications
    cervical MTrP pain syndrome, 133
    chest wall pain, 326
    FMS tender points, 393
    lateral pterygoid muscle, 219
    lumbar disc herniation pain, 252
    migraine prophylaxis, 211
    periarticular tender points, knee joint, 276
    quadratus lumborum muscle, 236
    shoulder pain, 164
    whiplash injury, 144
  optimum stimulus, determination, 114–115
  responders, strong, average and weak, 114, 133
Supinator, 178–180
Supraspinatus, 152–154
Sydenham, Thomas, 3, 4
Sympathetic activity, nocturnal in FMS, 360, 361
Sympathetic changes, MTrP activity associated, 68–69
Sympathetic efferent activity, 71, 72
Sympathetic overdrive syndrome (SOS) *see* Complex regional pain syndrome (CRPS type I)
Sympathetic-sensory coupling, 83
Syndrome of the sagging shoulder, 122
Synovial pain, knee joint, 275
Systemic lupus erythematosus (SLE) and FMS, 353, 354, 357

T

Tabes dorsalis, 85
  sensory tests, 18–19

Tactile allodynia, 84
Taut bands, MTrP-related, 65–66
  palpation, 74, 76
Temazepam, **386**, 390
Temperament and response to pain, 46
Temporal summation, 357, 358
Temporalis, 214–215
  TrP sites and pain referral, 203, 214, **216**
Temporo-facial pain, 214–221
  differential diagnosis, 220–221
  lateral pterygoid muscle, 217–219
  masseter muscle, 215–217
  medial pterygoid muscle, 219–220
  temporalis muscle, 203, 214–215, **216**
Temporomandibular joint pain
  extra-articular, 222–223
  intra-articular, 221–222
Tender points (TPs), 5–6, 9, 75
  abdominal wall pain, 331
  FMS, 353, **354**
    injections, 392–393
  migraine, 205–206
  osteoarthritis, knee joint, 274, 275, 276
Tennis elbow *see* Lateral epicondylitis
Tenosynovitis of wrist, 191, 196–197
Tenoxicam, **386**, 390
Tension-type headaches, 28, 47, 212–214
  continuum with migraine, 212–213
  myofascial-supraspinal-vascular model, 206, 213
  pathogenesis, 212
  prophylaxis, 213–214
  relationship to temporomandibular MTrP pain syndrome, 223
Tensor fasciae latae, 232, 264–265
Teres major, 162, **163**
Teres minor, 156
Terminological confusion, 3–7
Testosterone levels, FMS, 364
Thalamic syndrome, 85–86
Thalamus, 33
Thermal pain threshold, FMS, 359
Thermographic studies, 68–69
Thigh, MTrP pain syndrome
  anterior, lateral and medial aspect, 264–269
    hip adductors, 265–266
    quadriceps femoris group, 266–269
  differential diagnosis, 273, 274–278
  posterior muscles, 269–274, **270**
    biceps femoris, 271–274
    popliteus, 273
    semitendinosus and semimembranosus, 270, **271**
  see also Iliopsoas muscle; Piriformis muscle
Thoracic outlet syndrome, 135–136
Thoracolumbar paravertebral muscles, 230–233
  anatomical relationships, 230